Psychosocial Occupational Therapy

Proactive Approaches

Edited by
Rita P. Fleming Cottrell, MA, OTR

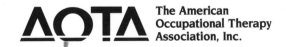

The American Occupational Therapy Association, Inc.

Disclaimers

"This publication is designed to provide accurate and authoritative information in regard to the subject matter covered. It is sold or distributed with the understanding that the publisher is not engaged in rendering legal, accounting, or other professional service. If legal advice or other expert assistance is required, the services of a competent professional person should be sought."

— From the Declaration of Principles jointly adopted by the American Bar Association and a Committee of Publishers and Associations.

It is the objective of the American Occupational Therapy Association to be a forum for free expression and interchange of ideas. The opinions and positions expressed by the contributors to this work are their own and not necessarily those of either the editors or the American Occupational Therapy Association.

Anne Rosenstein, AOTA Director of Publications

Edited by Laura Farr Collins
Designed by Anthony Rubino, Jr.

Printed in the United States of America.

ISBN 0-910317-96-8

Table of Contents

Section III: The Practice of Occupational Therapy Along the Mental Health Continuum of Care

Section IV: Humanistic Approaches in Mental Health: The Patient Perspective

Section V: Family Interaction and Social Supports: Promoting Adaptive Behaviors

Section VI: Program Evaluation: The Assurance of Quality in Clinical Practice

Section VII: Neuroscientific and Research Considerations for Occupational Therapists

Section VIII: Psychosocial Considerations for the Nonpsychiatric Client: Expanding Occupational Therapy's Role

Section IX: Professional Career Development: The Attainment and Maintenance of Excellence

Appendix A: Supplemental Reference Lists

Appendix B: Supplemental Resource Lists

Index

Preface

This text is a natural and direct extension of my professional experience as an occupational therapy (OT) educator and clinician specializing in mental health. My career in psychosocial occupational therapy has been and continues to be a rewarding and enriching experience. It has enhanced my professional development and facilitated my personal growth. I have never regretted my decision to become an occupational therapist, and I am continually excited by the wealth of opportunities my occupational therapy career in mental health has afforded me.

However, my professional entry into psychosocial occupational therapy took a rather long, roundabout route through my personal life. When I was a young child my older brother, Kevin, was diagnosed with Friedreich's Ataxia, a progressive neuromuscular disorder. Since we were only 2 years apart in age, his lifelong journey through the disease process became my journey also.

Initially, my childhood naiveté prompted me to decide to become a physician who would cure my brother and all others with devastating illnesses. However with age comes realism, and as I grew I began to recognize that cures were infrequent, especially for such rare diseases as my brother's. While I realized that extensive research would hopefully one day find a cure (or at least an effective treatment) my brother needed something done during his lifetime to help him manage his progressive illness. Therefore, as an adolescent I began to explore the profession of physical therapy (PT). Throughout high school I formalized my decision to become a physical therapist and subsequently entered New York University as a "pre-PT" student. At this point, Kevin's disease had progressed significantly, and he could not participate in many activities of daily living. He was an avid reader and a music aficionado, but still many hours were filled with boredom and depression.

In my search to find ways to improve the quality of Kevin's life, I discovered the field of occupational therapy. It was a perfect match. Occupational therapy's holistic approach, which maximized abilities, minimized disabilities, and provided adaptive strategies and compensation methods to enable the individual to live a productive, satisfying life, was just what Kevin and I had been searching for.[1] I quickly changed my major to occupational therapy and became a "sponge" to absorb all the information and skills we had been seeking for so many years (without even knowing what we had been looking for). While we clearly regretted the previously "wasted" years, we now seized the opportunities my occupational therapy education was affording us. Kevin entered New York University during my senior year. We adapted his dorm, and he began a successful academic career—typing his papers from memory with one finger while maintaining a B average! He obtained his bachelor's and master's degrees within five years, developed friendships, attended concerts, dined in restaurants, and traveled to England and a multitude of American states. A definite quality of life had replaced the boredom and depression of our "pre-OT" years.

With Kevin empowered to live his own life, I began my clinical affiliations with the determination that I would become an occupational therapist specializing in pediatric physical disabilities. My goal was to prevent children and their families from traveling our convoluted route to obtain a quality of life. However, as I completed my affiliations in physical rehabilitation, mental health, and pediatrics, I began to recognize the need to separate one's personal and professional lives.

Working in physical disabilities and/or pediatrics was just too close to home for me at that point in my life, so when I received my occupational therapy certification I began to work in mental health. Initially, I viewed this specialty choice as a temporary decision. However, as

---

[1] Kevin had the unfortunate "luck" to be born prior to the development of childhood intervention programs and the expansion of occupational therapy into community, home-care, and school settings; therefore, his contact with therapists was virtually non-existent. Hopefully, in this day and age it would not take a lifetime for a family to obtain proper interventions for themselves and their loved ones.

the years progressed, my appreciation for the qualitative difference occupational therapy makes in the lives of those with mental illness deepened, and I realized I had found my professional niche. Over the years I worked in acute care, community day treatment, and transitional living programs. I found each setting effective and rewarding. On a personal level, my increased awareness and improved skills in psychosocial issues and interventions greatly aided Kevin and me as we continued to deal with the challenges of his progressive disease.

My search to increase my knowledge of and competence in psychosocial occupational therapy led me to pursue continuing education avidly, accumulate professional literature, and eventually obtain my post-professional master's degree. Throughout this learning process my recognition of the depth and breadth of excellence in occupational therapy practice in mental health was greatly expanded. The love of this dynamic field resulted in my becoming a clinical educator and then an academic educator, specializing in psychosocial occupational therapy.

I began my academic career recognizing that many students might have a negative view of psychosocial occupational therapy practice, as societal stigma remain strong against the mentally ill, and many professionals unfortunately denigrate the value of occupational therapy practice in mental health. Therefore, I set out to counter these potential biases by culling the "best of the best" in professional literature to share with my students. I wanted to expose them to the wealth of opportunities and depth of professional excellence practiced by many psychosocial occupational therapists. My goal was not to persuade all students to specialize in mental health; rather, my aim was to ensure that students developed a balanced view and appreciation of the relevance and efficacy of psychosocial occupational therapy. My emphasis was (and continues to be) that mental health is generic and vital to all persons, regardless of age or diagnosis; therefore, its study and application are relevant to all areas of clinical practice.

Fortunately, many of my students have integrated this message and reflect positive views of psychosocial occupational therapy. They have frequently commented on the excellence of the articles utilized in class and have asked for copies to share with their clinical fieldwork supervisors. The favorable response of students, clinicians, and colleagues to this literature has led me to the development of this text.

In completing this publication, I have carefully selected timely and relevant articles on occupational therapy practice in mental health to assist the occupational therapy educator, student, and clinician in their study of this dynamic field. This anthology is well-researched and compiles numerous scholarly articles from quality, juried professional publications. The articles are organized into topical sections with thought-provoking introductions challenging readers to analyze their perceptions and to integrate personal issues with their current knowledge and developing clinical skills.

While articles were judiciously selected to reflect accurately the depth and breadth of psychosocial occupational therapy, there are realistic parameters to the text. Extensive reviews of occupational therapy frames of reference, models of practice, and evaluation methods are not provided, as there are a number of excellent publications already available that provide in-depth information on these critical professional topics. Readers are urged to utilize the reference lists at the end of each chapter and the appendixes at the end of the text to study these topics and other relevant issues further. Readers are encouraged to employ these references and resources on an ongoing basis throughout their professional careers.

Readers should also note that because all the chapters in this text are reprinted from other sources, they vary in style (Please see the "Note to Readers" on page *iv*, and refer to the appendixes for more current information.)

I would also encourage readers to join the American Occupational Therapy Association's (AOTA's) Special Interest Sections and to subscribe to *Hospital and Community Psychiatry* and *Occupational Therapy in Mental Health*, as these resources are invaluable in increasing knowledge of current occupational therapy practice in today's health care system. Many of the chapters in this text are compiled from these superb resources and clearly reflect a proactive stance towards psychosocial occupational therapy in mental health.

While some individuals may maintain negative perspectives on occupational therapy practice in mental health, it is my hope that the quality of the chapters in this text will foster an increased awareness and appreciation of the relevance, variety, and richness of skilled, dynamic psychosocial occupational therapy practice. Current trends within the health care system demand the utilization of holistic and functional approaches in the evaluation of and intervention for persons with disabilities. Employing the proactive philosophies and practices described in this text will enable the reader to meet professional challenges positively and to develop a rich occupational therapy career, regardless of specialty choice. This positive outcome will serve to greatly enhance the quality of life for clients and their families. Based upon my life experiences and values, this is the primary goal and the true art of occupational therapy.

Acknowledgments

I would like to thank my clients and students, who have challenged and enriched my clinical and academic work; my husband, Michael, who has lovingly supported my professional career development; my son, Christopher Michael, who has shared his boundless imagination and creativity to give my life endless joy; and my mother, Rita E. Fleming, who patiently and diligently typed this manuscript. This was truly a family effort.

Dedication

This book is dedicated to the memory of my brother, Kevin Michael Fleming, whose life underscored the vital need for a holistic therapeutic approach, regardless of clinical diagnosis, and the inherent value of meaningful, purposeful occupation in one's daily life. May his legacy live on and be celebrated in my teachings and in the reader's joyful pursuit of a fulfilling occupational therapy career.

Note to Readers

Due to the need to comply with copyright laws, all of the chapters in this text were reprinted as originally published— while editorial efforts were made to ensure grammatical accuracy and gender-neutral language, readers will note some inconsistencies in several chapters. These chapters contain relevant content, but their formats do not always adhere to the American Occupational Therapy Association's (AOTA's) publication guidelines. Areas of concern include various styles of referencing and usage, non-gender-neutral language, and potentially dated (or nonexistent) author credentials. Readers are advised to review all chapters critically—recognizing the strengths of each while acknowledging their limitations according to current professional standards.

Section I

Historical and Current Issues in Mental Health Practice

Introduction

Occupational therapy has been significantly influenced by sociopolitical issues throughout its professional history. The founders of occupational therapy were very concerned with the contemporary issues of their time, and these societal forces largely shaped occupational therapy's heritage (Peloquin, 1991). Over the ensuing years the development of occupational therapy continued to be responsive to changes in sociopolitical thought, values, and policies (Kielhofner & Burke, 1977). Contemporary occupational therapists are now confronted with new challenges in today's changing health care system. Advances in neuroscience and technology, increased demands for cost containment and quality assurance, decreased length of inpatient treatment stays, and increased emphasis on community integration are all current trends that are challenging the entire health care system. It is vital that occupational therapists are informed about these issues, as societal trends and public policy directly influence our practice (Baum, 1991; Palmer, 1988; Peloquin, 1991).

Many health care professionals (i.e., psychiatrists, nurses, and social workers) are now advocating and implementing functional approaches to treatment in response to the sociopolitical trends identified above (Ascher-Svanum & Krause, 1991; Fine, 1980; Lamb, 1976; Liberman, 1988). While some therapists may view this movement as a threat to our profession, others will view it as an opportunity as great as the one that led to the initial founding of the profession of occupational therapy (which was also led by doctors, nurses, and social workers) (Peloquin, 1991). Occupational therapists who are skilled in the evaluation and intervention of functional performance and who are knowledgeable about sociopolitical issues can seize this opportunity to become

leaders in today's mental health care system. Our holistic approach to improving a client's functional performance and enhancing quality of life is highly congruent with the current demand for cost-effective, high quality, consumer-oriented treatment emphasizing independent living skills.

The chapters in this section emphasize the unique ability of occupational therapists to respond constructively and in a proactive way to the current sociopolitical trends and professional challenges influencing the mental health care system. Ellek begins this section with an historical review of mental health public policy. She discusses the economic, social, and political factors that influenced major mental health care policy initiatives. Institutionalization, deinstitutionalization, community-based care, and community support programs are the four major policies defined and discussed. Ellek provides a thoughtful analysis of the values, benefits, and limits of each of these historic public policy initiatives.

Current health care policy is the focus of chapter 2. Gibson reviews five major trends that have significantly influenced the recent delivery of mental health services. The impact of these trends on occupational therapy practice is realistically analyzed. Practical, constructive recommendations for responding to these changes in a proactive manner are presented by the author.

A positive view of the potential for occupational therapists to respond effectively to the changing health care system is also presented in chapter 3. Fidler argues that the current, shorter lengths of inpatient treatment stays require occupational therapists to expand their professional view beyond the hospital walls and into the community. She poses a series of questions that challenge therapists to assess their values, opinions, and practices in response to the demands of the changing health care system. Suggestions for ensuring continuity of care, multidisciplinary team collaboration, and role clarification are provided to assist readers in effectively meeting "the challenge of change."

Issues related to short-term, acute hospitalization and the changing health care system are further explored in chapter 4, by Jackson, who also emphasizes viewing short-term treatment as an initial step in the rehabilitation continuum. In his analysis of the implications of current trends for occupational therapy practice, Jackson proposes a number of realistic modifications to occupational therapy treatment approaches that maintain a solid theoretical base and a clear professional role for the occupational therapist. He argues that the current evolution of occupational therapy practice in mental health will enhance and expand occupational therapy's role across the entire mental health continuum of care.

The expansion of mental health care into the community and the emphasis on functional living skills treatment for persons with mental illness have greatly increased the need for occupational therapists to provide community-based services. However, according to Dasler, there is a significant shortage of occupational therapists working in community mental health. In chapter 5 Dasler analyzes reasons for this shortage of community-based occupational therapists and describes an effective strategy used by an occupational therapy network to increase the employment of occupational therapists in community mental health. This successful, well-organized, resourceful approach can be easily transferred to other states and situations in which a shortage of occupational therapists is an area of concern. Dasler advises occupational therapists to look beyond traditional occupational therapy job offerings, as our professional education and training enable us to be successfully employed in a diversity of professional roles within the community.

The need for occupational therapists to adapt their traditional role functioning is also explored in this section's final chapter. However, in their presentation, Hemphill and Werner focus on the changing role of occupational therapy within the state hospital system. The impact of the community mental health movement and deinstitutionalization on state hospitals is explored by the authors. Changes in patient population characteristics, geographic isolation, structural deficits, funding limitations, and staff shortages present unique challenges for the provision of quality care within the state hospital. Hemphill and Werner discuss these problems and provide a practical analysis of the reasons to support continuation of state hospitals as specialized treatment, research, and training facilities. The role of occupational therapists in the current and future state hospital system

is clearly described. The authors advocate that occupational therapy programs change their focus from the provision of diversionary activities to the implementation of comprehensive, holistic evaluation and intervention in independent living skills. They emphasize a collaborative, interdisciplinary treatment approach and provide practical suggestions for the development of a viable role for occupational therapy within the "new" state hospital.

The development of proactive roles for occupational therapists working in the current mental health care system is a theme that is explored further in this text. In-depth presentations on program development, implementation, and evaluation across the entire mental health continuum of care are provided in subsequent chapters. Readers are encouraged to analyze their own views about the challenges of the current health care system and their effect on the role of occupational therapy. It is hoped that readers will adopt the proactive stance of this section's authors and seize the opportunities that the current health care system is affording the profession of occupational therapy. Our professional emphasis on the holistic development of functional living skills qualifies us to become leaders in the provision of quality mental health services now and well into the 21st century (Fine, 1980; Peloquin, 1991).

Questions to Consider

1. How have public policy initiatives influenced the nature and scope of mental health service delivery? What are the implications of the different sociopolitical value systems identified by Ellek on patient care and occupational therapy practice?
2. What are current trends and issues affecting the mental health care system? How do these trends and issues impact the role of occupational therapy in acute care settings? In community mental health? In long-term institutions?
3. How can occupational therapists effectively adapt to these health care trends and professional role changes in a manner that is consistent with occupational therapy frames of reference/models of practice? What professional knowledge and skills can occupational therapists uniquely offer to define proactive roles for themselves in the changing mental health care system?
4. What are the implications of current issues and trends in mental health practice for occupational therapy evaluation and intervention? How can occupational therapy evaluation procedures and

intervention methods be realistically adapted within the context of these changes and in a manner congruent with occupational therapy's philosophical base?

5. How will occupational therapy be viewed in the 21st century? What steps can occupational therapists take to ensure that our profession attains and maintains a leadership role in the provision of quality care across the mental health continuum?

References

Ascher-Svanum, H., & Krause, A. A. (1991). *Psychoeducational groups for patients with schizophrenia*. Rockville, MD: Aspen Publishers.

Baum, C. (1991). Professional issues in a changing environment. In C. Christiansen & C. Baum (Eds.), *Occupational therapy: Overcoming human performance deficits* (pp. 805-817). Thorofare, NJ: Slack.

Fine, S. B. (1980). Psychiatric treatment and rehabilitation: What's in a name? *Journal of the National Association of Private Psychiatric Hospitals, 11*(5), 8-13.

Kielhofner, G., & Burke, J. P. (1977). Occupational therapy after 60 years: An account of changing identity and knowledge. *American Journal of Occupational Therapy, 31*, 675-689.

Lamb, R. (1976). An educational model for teaching living skills to long-term patients. *Hospital and Community Psychiatry, 27*, 875-877.

Liberman, R. (Ed.). (1988). *Psychiatric rehabilitation of chronic mental patients*. Washington, DC: American Psychiatric Press.

Palmer, F. (1988). The present context of service delivery. In S. C. Robertson (Ed.), *Mental health focus: Skills for assessment and treatment* (pp. 1-28—1-36). Rockville, MD: American Occupational Therapy Association.

Peloquin, S. M. (1991). Looking back: Occupational therapy service: Individual and collective understandings of the founders, part 2. *American Journal of Occupational Therapy, 45*, 733-743.

Chapter 1

The Evolution of Fairness in Mental Health Policy

Donalda Ellek, PhD, OTR/L

Anyone who is involved in health policy, whether as a patient, a health professional, a payer, or an administrator, has at some time experienced feelings about the fairness of a policy. Policies stir intense controversy about who is getting what benefits from a policy, and why. The purpose of this article is to examine fairness in mental health policy as it has evolved over several decades. Because the mental health system has been heavily dependent on public funds and public policy, especially for those persons with the most chronic and severe mental illness, this discussion will be limited to public policy in mental health.

States differ in the quality of mental health care and the amount of money earmarked for mental health, but the intent of mental health policy from one state to another is strikingly similar. Thus, the fairness of mental health policy can be discussed as a national issue. Those policies that have been applied in every state throughout the United States are broadly described as institutionalization, deinstitutionalization and community-based care, and the community support program.

Many groups of people have a role in the development of policy as well as a personal stake in its outcome. Professionals in the mental health field have traditionally been advocates for patients' interests but also have spoken for the economic and political interests of their various professions. The government must advocate for the interests of society as a whole, consider the effect of policies on persons with mental illness as a particular group within society, and be responsive to particular lobbies. In recent years, persons with mental illness and their families have formed organizations and begun to advocate for their interests in mental health policy. Rarely do all interested parties benefit equally from a policy; often, benefits are realized by one group over another, and some groups may suffer a loss.

The fairness of the allocation of benefits can be viewed from the perspective of theories of social justice, which present reasons for or explanations of how the benefits and losses that occur in a society should be allocated and, most importantly, why they should be allocated in a particular way. As might be expected, the *why* reflects a value system of what is important in society (Veatch, 1981). These value systems are very different from one another, and I think they are the crux of controversy about health policy.

An analysis of major mental health policy initiatives (i.e., institutionalization, deinstitutionalization and community-based care, and the community support program) shows that mental health policy does not share one common underlying theory of justice. Rather, policy development has been an evolutionary process in which the particular interests of persons with mental illness have been addressed differently at various stages.

Institutionalization

Prior to the 20th century, there was widespread belief that mental illness was due to possession by the devil or to immorality. In either case, it was viewed as an uncontrollable phenomenon to which the individual's own weakness contributed. People were fearful that the person with mental illness would cause physical harm to others or in some way negatively influence their morality. This fear was perhaps the most basic reason why persons with mental illness were extruded from society and locked in poorhouses and jails against their will. In essence, institutionalization was viewed as a method of protecting society from the physical harm and moral wrongdoing of persons with mental illness (Mechanic, 1969).

Around the mid-1800s, social reformers began advocating that persons with mental illness be treated more humanely, pointing out that the state could provide care more efficiently in large institutions than communities were providing it in poorhouses and jails. Thus, by 1900, state governments had assumed responsibility for persons with mental illness (Gruenberg & Archer, 1979).

Institutionalization of persons with mental illness provided several benefits: (a) society was protected from the physical harm it was feared persons with mental illness would inflict; (b) treatment offered the potential of a cure along with the potential future economic benefits of a healthy and productive member of society; and (c) economies of scale could be realized through the provision of care in large institutions where it could be handled en masse with personnel working to their fullest capacity.

The fairness of institutionalizing persons with mental illness can be best explained by a utilitarian concept of justice. Utilitarian theory evaluates social actions strictly in terms of their impact on general human welfare (Veatch, 1981). If society is happier or has increased "utility," the policy is fair. Certainly, the general society seemed to benefit from institutionalization—From its perspective, it was being protected from the dangerousness of persons with mental illness.

However, utilitarianism also generally places a great value on individual liberty; thus, institutionalization seems to conflict with utilitarianism. While society was protecting its safety, it was depriving persons with mental illness of liberty. But the utilitarian doctrine accounts for this. John Stuart Mill, a utilitarian philosopher, wrote:

> The sole end for which mankind are warranted, individually or collectively, in interfering with the liberty of action of any of their number is self-protection.
>
> That the only purpose for which power can be rightfully exercised over any member of a civilized community, against his will is to prevent harm to others. (Mill, 1956, pp. 72-73).

Thus, if members of society believed they were in danger from persons with mental illness, they were just in depriving those persons of their liberty.

The harm principle is a widely accepted principle to limit liberty, but its extensive applicability to persons with mental illness is doubtful. In some cases, it is true that persons diagnosed as mentally ill are dangerous and present a serious threat of physical harm to others. It does not follow, though, that every mentally ill person poses a threat to others. Studies have shown either that mentally ill people, as a group, are no more dangerous than others or that, if they are, the differences are so small that they allow little success in predicting dangerousness.

This harm principle, then, has limited applicability to persons with mental illness, at least in the present day. It might be asked if it was fair to apply the harm principle in previous times, when society believed that persons with mental illness were dangerous. Because society had to decide based on the information available at that time, it was fair to apply the harm principle. It did not conflict with the principle of liberty as explained under utilitarianism.

In later years, the perceived dangerousness of persons with mental illness diminished somewhat, but institutionalization remained with the argument that persons with mental illness could not care for themselves and often were not rational enough to determine their own best interests. This protection of persons with mental illness fits within fairness under the utilitarian concept because mentally ill persons are not able to look after themselves. In assigning a high value to individual liberty, the utilitarians also define instances in which paternalistic intervention is appropriate, in order to bring the greatest good to the greatest number.

Another factor that figured into the welfare of society is the economic cost of providing care for persons with mental illness. These costs were paid by society through taxes. However, society attached great value to having the objectionable behavior of persons with mental illness removed from society's view. In this respect, while institutionalization generated cost, it also generated benefits equal to the value of the nonpecuniary cost no longer imposed on society by the behavior of persons with mental illness. Thus, institutionalization was just, according to utilitarian doctrine, because it protected society, provided certain economic gains over the nonsystem of care in communities, and benefited society overall.

Deinstitutionalization and Community-Based Care

During the 1950s, several factors coincided, beginning a policy of deinstitutionalizing seriously mentally ill (then called chronically mentally ill) patients, discharging them to live in the community and receive care on an outpatient basis. An important factor that spurred this policy change was the burgeoning population of mentally ill people and the increasing economic strain on the states to maintain psychiatric patients in state hospitals (Rose, 1979). Also, the development of psychotropic medications was advancing, making it possible to better control the overt symptomatology of mental illness. This made it more possible for patients to live in the community. Another important factor was that the federal government became aware of a national problem presented by psychiatric illness when 1.75 million Americans were rejected for service during World War 11 (Greene, 1984). This prompted Congress to pass the National Mental Health Act of 1946 (Public Law 79-487). This act established the National Institute of Mental Health (NIMH), which served as a major advocate of mental health care on a national level (U.S. Department of Health and Human Services, 1980).

For several years, there was controversy over government's role in mental health care and whether federal funds should be directed toward preventive, acute, or chronic care. In 1961, President Kennedy appointed a committee to study the federal role in mental health care. The committee came up with the community mental health plan, which led to the Community Mental Health Centers Act of 1963 (Public Law 88-164). Through this act, the federal government provided funding to establish community mental health centers (Bachrach, 1983).

Public Law 88-164 was enacted with a wide base of support and seemed to have the potential to give something to everyone. It was expected to increase the accessibility and availability of mental health services to the public; expand the professional area of psychiatrists and other mental health professionals into primary prevention; and decrease the costs associated with state hospital care (Rose, 1979). It also was expected to benefit persons with serious mental illness by reintegrating them into the community where they could, with the aid of medication, live more independently and participate meaningfully in community life. The community mental health centers and the state hospitals were expected to function together to provide a broad array of services (Bachrach, 1983).

In a short time, many problems began to surface. Because of the funding structure of Public Law 88-164, community mental health centers could be federally funded and operate independently of state hospitals and state mental health authorities. Because no economic link existed between them, no communication link developed (Clarke, 1979). Patients were discharged from state hospitals, but their linkage to a community mental health center was tenuous. Even when seriously mentally ill patients were linked to a community mental health center, few services were designed to meet their needs.

In addition to the lack of community-based services for seriously mentally ill patients, legal issues further tested the treatment of these persons. Legal cases were increasingly concluding that serious deprivation of liberty (i.e., hospitalization) could only be justified if adequate treatment was given. This principle was known as the "right to treatment." The economic implication was that more effective demand (by the courts) for better quality care, with no shifts in available supply, raised the costs of care to the states. Along with the right to treatment, another ruling essentially said that a person should be deprived of liberty only to the extent absolutely necessary. Thus, patients hospitalized either voluntarily or involuntarily could demand to be treated in the least restrictive environment. All of these legal rulings created an effective demand for community-based care.

As a result of these political and legal developments, it became increasingly apparent that the state hospitals had not developed after-care services and that community mental health centers were focused on prevention and acute care. This meant that chronic patients being discharged into the community were not receiving necessary services.

In reviewing the long, complicated history of the deinstitutionalization and community-based care policy initiative, one is faced with the question of who benefited from the policies and whether their benefit was fair. The state governments seemed to have benefited economically overall. Several studies suggest that, after considering all costs (i.e., cost shifting between levels of government, the cost of supporting community inpatient services and state hospital back-up care), the cost of deinstitutionalization was less than that of inpatient care provided through the hospital alone (Buck, 1984; Nash & Argyle, 1984; Rose, 1979). Additionally, the census in state hospitals decreased.

The general public also seemed to benefit in that more psychiatric services were available for persons who needed psychiatric care but were not necessarily severely or chronically mentally ill. Also, mental health professionals grew in number and kind and had opportunities to expand their roles and professional skills.

People with serious mental illness, however, were in a questionable position. Although they gained their liberty, it became clear that many of them were mentally disabled to the extent that they could not provide for their own basic human needs. After-care services were sparse and often did not address their special needs. As a result, some patients had frequent rehospitalizations, some lived in unhealthy or unsafe conditions, and others were in the dubious circumstance of depending entirely on their family members. Persons with serious mental illness essentially traded security for liberty.

The fairness of the deinstitutionalization and community-based care policy initiative can best be explained from the perspective of the Pareto doctrine (Pareto, 1935), which considers an action, or policy, to be fair if no one is worse off. Another important element of the Pareto doctrine is that each person is the sole determiner of his or her own welfare. However, this concept is based on the premise that all rational people seek to maximize their welfare.

Persons with mental illness clearly did not express any particular interests to spur the policy initiative, and it is debatable whether they would be considered rational enough to do so. However, advocates for these persons served as spokespersons, advocating liberty as the goal. Liberty was achieved. On balance, persons with serious mental illness received the benefit of liberty, but gave up some security. The fact that they benefited the least of all interested parties is insignificant under the Pareto doctrine.

Community Support Program

The NIMH developed the community support program in 1977 as a policy initiative aimed specifically at improving the quality of life for the chronically and severely mentally ill people who were deinstitutionalized and living in the community. The community support program provided funding for states to set up a community support system, which was intended to address the comprehensive needs of persons with serious mental illness and drew on elements from the medical rehabilitation and social support models of care (Stroul, 1984). The 10 essential components of a community support system were as follows:

1. Identification of the target population
2. Assistance in applying for entitlements
3. Crisis stabilization in the least restrictive environment
4. Psychosocial rehabilitation services
5. Supportive services of indefinite duration
6. Medical and mental health care
7. Backup support to families, friends, and community members
8. Involvement of concerned community members
9. Protection of clients' rights
10. Case management (Turner & Ten Hoor, 1978).

The community support system model was flexible in that implementation was not prescribed; every state was expected to implement it according to their own particular needs, circumstances, and resources (Stroul, 1984).

Legal rulings, coupled with public moral outrage, seemed to have prompted the community support program initiative. As mentally ill people lived in the community, the public could see the deplorable living conditions of many of them. The public media also began to expose the plight of persons with mental illness. The low level of benefits received by persons with serious mental illness, in comparison to the much greater benefits received by others, was obviously unjust, and public opinion was that the deinstitutionalization and community-based care policy was unsatisfactory.

Another factor might be at least equally important in explaining how interest in the community support program initiative was generated. The legal rulings regarding civil commitment, the right to treatment in the least restrictive setting, and the right to refuse treatment all stood as rights to be asserted by persons with serious mental illness. These rulings provided a legal mandate to the public sector to develop services that respect patients' rights.

The Omnibus Reconciliation Act of 1981 (Public Law 97-35) combined formerly categorical grant programs and established block grants to states (Nash & Argyle, 1984). This resulted in a reduction of the federal contribution to mental health care by approximately 25% (Buck, 1984). However, state mental health departments did not abandon their commitment to provide service to persons with serious mental illness as a priority population (Jerrell & Larsen, 1985).

The disappointment with the community mental health center concept and its failure to provide service to persons with serious mental illness, as contrasted with the community support program and its particular attention to persons with serious mental illness, raises an interesting issue. Community mental health centers were equally available and accessible to all categories of mentally ill people. That is, any mentally ill person who went to a community mental health center and requested service could theoretically receive service (assuming he or she lived in the catchment area and was able to use the services that were offered). In this sense, there was equal access and availability. What really seemed to hinder the provision of services to persons with serious mental illness was a lack of consideration for their special needs. For example, these persons often were not capable of following the intake procedures of the community mental health center, such as making and keeping an appointment. They also spent a great deal of effort attending to their basic needs, which could preclude their ability to participate in traditional therapeutic regimens. In this sense, access and availability were equal but not equitable, because persons with serious mental illness did not have the same capacity as the general population to seek services in a community mental health center.

The Rawlsian concept of justice (also referred to as the egalitarian concept of social justice) accounts for inequities of opportunity (Rawls, 1971). The Rawlsian concept of justice is that those persons with the greatest need should benefit the most, and the allocation of benefits should be available in consideration of equal opportunity, or ability, to seek potential benefits. Those persons not able to seek benefits should be given additional help. Thus, a policy such as the community support program, which gives special consideration to persons with serious mental illness, would be fair under the Rawlsian concept of social justice.

In contrast to the Rawlsian theory of justice, the Pareto theory, which could explain deinstitutionalization and community-based care, does not consider the individual's initial level of welfare or his or her ability to use established procedures.

Conclusion

The mental health policy initiatives have been formed by interdependent economic, social, and political factors. Social factors that have affected mental health policy have sometimes been specific to mental health, such as perceptions and public attitudes toward mental illness and definitions of mental illness. However, these social factors usually operate in tandem with broader social factors. The decade of Public Law 88-164 (late 1960s and early 1970s) illustrates this point because it was marked by public disappointment in and distrust of government and a movement toward social change across many aspects of society. During that time, systems changed to promote public welfare. The Social Security Amendments of 1965 (Public Law 89-97) were enacted, and court decisions affirmed the rights of persons with mental illness. The mental health system, by advancing the rights of persons with mental illness, participated in the activism to promote social change.

Once social change is in the air, the political process responds. Special interest groups want to be sure that their best interests are considered during a time of change; often, public interest takes a secondary position to the narrower interests of politicians and others in the policy-making arena as they pursue economic benefits and personal power. Thus, the political process shapes an idea for change to suit the diverse needs of the most powerful segments of society. In this way, social factors can lose some of their strength in creating change.

Economic factors also enter into the mental health care policy-making process as either constraints or opportunities. The crisis in state hospital care that led to deinstitutionalization was presented as an economic problem created by a rising census and overcrowding. The economy of scale of large institutions was outstripped. The solution to this economic problem was either to allocate more funds to state mental hospitals, and thus increase the supply of services, or to decrease the use of services (i.e., decrease demand), and so decrease the cost of mental health care to the states. The choice was made to decrease the use of state mental hospital services.

Social justice reflects the values of society at a given point in time. These values are most directly expressed as public opinion and social movements for change. The political process responds to these values but tempers them and determines the specifications of policy.

The fairness of mental health policy has evolved with these social, political, and economic factors. It evolved from the institutionalization policy of the mid-1800s, when society's idea of fairness was providing the greatest good to the greatest number of people, through the deinstitutionalization and community-based care era of the 1960s and 1970s, when society thought everyone could benefit to some degree and fairness meant that no one should lose, to the 1980s, when society began dealing with perceived limitations in resources and designated special populations to receive greater benefits. This latter policy perspective aims to address issues of equity in addition to issues of equality.

Whether or not a policy is fair is still a matter of values at a particular point in time, in the context of social, political, and economic factors. One particular social justice theory cannot always be fair under all circumstances. However, social justice theories are useful in explaining the most common perspectives on fairness. Society has appeared to formulate mental health policy within social justice theories of one kind or another as society's values and circumstances have evolved.

References

Bachrach, L. (1983). An overview of deinstitutionalization. *New Directions for Mental Health Services, 17*, 5-14.

Buck, J. (1984). Block grants and federal promotion of community mental health services, 1946-65. *Community Mental Health Journal, 20*(3), 236-247.

Clarke, G. (1979). In defense of deinstitutionalization. *Milbank Memorial Fund Quarterly/Health and Society, 57*(4), 461-479.

Community Mental Health Centers Act of 1963 (Public Law 88-164).

Greene, B. (1984). Evolving mental health policy. *Journal of Health Administration Education, 2*(2), 193-220.

Gruenberg, E., & Archer, J. (1979). Abandonment of responsibility for the seriously mentally ill. *Milbank Memorial Fund Quarterly/ Health and Society, 57*(4), 485-505.

Jerrell, J., & Larsen, J. (1985). Policy and organizational changes in state mental health systems. *Administration in Mental Health 12*(3), 184-191.

Mechanic, D. (1969). *Mental health and social policy.* Englewood Cliffs, NJ: Prentice Hall.

Mill, J. S. (1956). *On liberty.* New York: Liberal Arts Press.

Nash, M., & Argyle, N. (1984). Services for the mentally ill: A reversal in federal policy. *Administration in Mental Health, 11*(4), 263-276.

National Mental Health Act of 1946 (Public Law 79-487).

Omnibus Reconciliation Act of 1981 (Public Law 97-35). 42 U.S.C., §1396.

Pareto, V. (1935). *The mind and society: A treatise on general sociology.* New York: Dover.

Rawls, J. A. (1971). *A theory of justice.* Cambridge, MA: Harvard University Press.

Rose, S. (1979). Deciphering deinstitutionalization: Complexities in policy and program analysis. *Milbank Memorial Fund Quarterly/ Health and Society, 57*(4), 429-459.

Social Security Amendments of 1965 (Public Law 89-97).

Stroul, B. (1984). *Toward community support systems for the mentally disabled.* Rockville, MD: National Institute of Mental Health.

Turner, J., & Ten Hoor, W. (1978). The NIMH community support program: Pilot approach to a needed social reform. *Schizophrenia Bulletin, 4*(3), 319-344.

U.S. Department of Health and Human Services. (1980). *Toward a national plan for the chronically mentally ill.* Washington, DC: U.S. Government Printing Office.

Veatch, R. M. (1981). *A theory of medical ethics.* New York: Basic.

Chapter 2

The Challenge of Adaptation: Shaping Service Delivery to Meet Changing Needs

Diane Gibson, MS, OTR/L

Profound changes in medical economics and in the preferred practices regarding the health care delivery system have pressed practitioners, including occupational therapists, to plan proactively for their impact (1). The steps that occupational therapists and other health care providers can take to react effectively to current trends are the focus of this column.

National Trends

Five major trends have had a significant impact on the scope and complexion of mental health services. Decreased length of stay has occurred concomitantly with increased severity of illness in acute care settings. Although short-term care may be the optimal treatment for patients with lower levels of pathology (2,3), it may be all that is available to seriously ill patients who may need more. Chronic schizophrenic patients, however, benefit from short-term hospitalization followed by "successful community adjustment" (4). Discharge planning is increasingly critical to the quality of care.

The range of available treatment settings is also changing service structure. Quarterway and halfway houses, residential treatment facilities, and supervised apartments provide longer-term services after the diagnostic, medication, and evaluation services provided in short-term settings.

Knowledge about the etiology of mental illness has expanded exponentially in the past ten years. The emphasis on diagnosis and medication has increased significantly. Programs designed to change behavior through didactic education, gradation of activity, and experiential learning are more common.

Consumerism and public awareness also have increased. Interest in public education and consumerism has been further developed and consolidated in America by a growing opinion that one can and should assume responsibility for one's health.

Finally, personnel shortages are particularly grave in the field of mental health. Long-vacant occupational therapy positions have been filled by people with different professional backgrounds. Changing roles are expected to increase negotiations about the functions of various disciplines in many institutions.

Responding to Changes

Allied health professionals must respond to changes in the provision of mental health treatment in a manner that is cost-effective, preserves high-quality care, and maintains the viability of their roles. For example, occupational therapists make key contributions to functional assessment and functional improvement, the cornerstones of treatment for patients with biopsychosocial dysfunction. Occupational therapists have responded by adapting program designs and incorporating variations in approaches to patient interventions. The recommendations that follow incorporate specific changes in process and structural components of psychiatric intervention. Although they focus on occupational therapy, all allied mental health disciplines could consider such strategies.

Short-Term Acute Care Programs

Occupational therapists play an important role in helping patients adapt to change. They assess what rehabilitation can accomplish in acute care within short treatment time frames, such as one to three weeks. The services offered in acute care settings where the length of stay is more than one month are less viable in the growing number of facilities with shorter lengths of stay. For example, activities that require a longer period of time to finish, such as building a table or making a set of ceramic dishes, may be valuable for longer term rehabilitation. However, short-term treatment objectives may be better addressed by activities that require a lesser investment of time and are relevant to acute care needs; some examples are psychoeducational modules such as stress management, assertiveness training, and discharge planning. It is important to retain purposeful activities as a method for the patient to meet selected goals, whether they are short term or long term.

Psychiatric occupational therapists have an opportunity to highlight functional evaluation in acute settings (5,6). Using functional evaluations to predict community adjustment and to select appropriate housing and vocational discharge plans may be their most important role. By focusing on the patients' discrete levels of functioning in emotional, interpersonal, cognitive, and motor areas, the occupational therapist can assist the interdisciplinary team in identifying the performance areas that facilitate patients' successful postdischarge adjustment in work, play, and self-care. Insurance carriers and managed care utilization review officers in particular are interested in measures that predict expected length of stay, especially when the predictions indicate treatment plans that are less expensive than hospitalization.

Treatment Formats and Settings

Another area in which occupational therapists have adapted service delivery to change is the format of activity programs and the structure of treatment settings. The typical format for treatment groups includes two one-hour segments each week, not on weekends, which minimizes the number of sessions acute inpatients can attend during a two-week stay. Structuring more frequent presentations of core activities, such as training in daily living skills, and interpersonal, physical, and vocational activities, may better meet the needs of acute psychiatric inpatients.

Philosophy of Treatment

Occupational therapy's approach to intervention is amenable to changes caused by the trends in health care. In addition to assisting with proper discharge placement through predictive functional assessment, the occupational therapist of the 1990s may find a psychoeducational structure useful. For example, leveled instructional modules in independent living skills—such as stress and time management, mental health and illness education, interpersonal and assertiveness skills, and self-care skills—will be more common approaches to treatment. When vocational, recreation, or expressive therapies are not otherwise available to patients, the occupational therapist may also offer vocational planning, leisure education, and expressive activities. Regular physical exercise and recreational opportunities are also needed to complete the holistic rehabilitation program.

Staffing Patterns

How programs are staffed greatly affects the effectiveness and quality of service delivery. The ratio of direct-contact hours to indirect-contact hours requires regular examination and revision. Careful organization of personnel is essential for occupational therapists to provide patients with sufficient contact time during short hospitalizations and to meet the stringent utilization review demands of third-party payers. Staff with experience in evaluation and placement are essential.

Documentation

The time required for documentation has a direct influence on the number of available contact hours, and therefore organization influences the quality of treatment. Rodriguez (7) has stated that "because medical records as well as defined therapeutic outcomes will become vehicles of quality assessment, more emphasis will be placed on detailed, organized, objective, and relevant clinical information that can be assessed against standards of care." Although a reasonable amount of indirect service delivery is important, the number of hours spent documenting progress will drop significantly when therapists move from narrative assessment and progress notes to checklist formats or documentation by exception criteria. Furthermore, indirect hours can be significantly reduced by consolidating forms or eliminating unnecessary documentation.

Indirect Service Delivery

Critical examination of the numerous demands on allied health personnel to support direct patient contact with indirect service delivery is essential. Occupational therapists have a professional responsibility to add timesaving measures and delete unnecessary, redundant, and poorly focused activities. For example, some clinical and administrative meetings can be dropped in an effort to pick up more direct hours. The increased emphasis on direct care may cause a decrease in the proportion of time spent on indirect care in many occupational therapy programs. The most important principles are to balance time spent on direct and indirect service delivery and to maintain consistent communication among staff.

Responding to Consumerism and Public Awareness

An emerging but undeveloped role for occupational therapists rests in more fully addressing patients' needs and rights. Occupational therapy stresses growth in mastery, competence, and assertive communication—skills that enable patients to play a determining rather than a passive role in changing the hospital environment or treatment program. As occupational therapists respond to the consumer-patient, they may play a liaison role between the patients and the hospital administration.

Occupational therapists also have a strong position in broadening public awareness of mental health services. Speaking on radio or television or to community groups represents an exciting dimension of occupational therapy, one that gives public visibility to the field and to mental health issues. Occupational therapists are trained in psychopathology, stress management, assertive communication, human development, and the use of purposeful activity as a healing agent. All of these skills can be easily adapted to public information regarding disease prevention and health promotion (8).

Dealing with Staff Shortages

The shortage of occupational therapy personnel is a critical and frustrating national problem. Between 1977 and 1986 the proportion of registered occupational therapists in mental health positions decreased by 11.3 percent (9). Hospital administrators have attempted to solve the problem by abolishing occupational therapy positions, by filling the positions with other providers, or by using occupational therapists working under contract to assess patients and supervise paraprofessional staff.

Although these interim measures are often used, there is no quick solution to the shortage. Filling occupational therapy positions with personnel of different backgrounds changes the complexion of treatment, and not enough research has been conducted to determine the optimal pattern of services to decrease dysfunction in patients and maximize their functional independence.

Occupational therapy educational programs actively examine entry-level coursework in mental health with an eye to strengthening the didactic and fieldwork curricula. With the decrease of occupational therapy positions in mental health there are fewer proper fieldwork sites for on-the-job training, a critical component of the total educational process in the profession.

Lower salaries in psychiatry than in other areas of medicine compound the staffing problem. These conditions will remain until long-term efforts upgrade the academic training, prestige, and salaries across the board in psychiatry. In the meantime, the roles in mental health of occupational therapists and other allied health professionals are becoming more consultative and are focusing increasingly on program design, functional evaluation, quality assurance, and supervision of a multidisciplinary staff.

Conclusions

The completion of service delivery in psychiatry, particularly the roles and functions of allied health professionals, is evolving in response to economic, political, legal, and social changes. Understanding that change is inevitable, knowing that services shift to meet changing consumer needs, and effectively designing and developing suitable programs that address social changes are skills that have enabled occupational therapists to become change agents. Occupational therapists are able and willing to cooperate in a dedicated effort to improve the functional abilities of those with psychiatric illnesses. Engaging in a collaborative effort to refine mental health services to meet consumer needs while respecting system constraints is a joint effort. Efficient use of experienced personnel to develop the optimal solution to the effects of shrinking resources, staff shortages, and the demands of more educated consumers will result in the best the system has to offer.

References

1. Sharfstein SS, Muszynski S, Myers E: Health Insurance and Psychiatric Care: Update and Appraisal. Washington, DC, American Psychiatric Press, 1984.

2. Herz M, Endicott J, Spitzer R: Brief hospitalization: a two-year follow-up. American Journal of Psychiatry 134:502-507, 1977.

3. Glick I: Short-term intensive psychiatric hospital treatment: which treatment for whom? Journal of the National Association of Private Psychiatric Hospitals 9:8-11, 1977.

4. Kaplan K: Introduction to short-term treatment in occupational therapy. Occupational therapy in Mental Health 4:29-45, 1984.

5. Allen CK: Occupational Therapy for Psychiatric Diseases: Measurement and Management of Cognitive Disabilities. Boston: Little, Brown, 1985.

6. Williams SL, Bloomer JS: Bay Area Functional Performance Evaluation. Palo Alto, Calif, Consulting Psychologists Press, 1987.

7. Rodriguez A: The effects of contemporary economic conditions on availability and quality of mental health services, in Handbook of Quality Assurance in Mental Health. Edited by Stricken G, Rodriguez A. New York, Plenum, 1988

8. Jaffe E: Nationally speaking: the role of occupational therapy in disease prevention and health promotion. American Journal of Occupational Therapy 40:749-752, 1986.

9. Membership Data Survey. Rockville, Md, American Occupational Therapy Association, 1977, 1982, 1986.

Chapter 3

The Challenge of Change to Occupational Therapy Practice

Gail S. Fidler, OTR, FAOTA

I t has been evident for some time that the health care system is in the process of significant change. Increasing medical and social problems, accelerating development of complex technology, reductions in federal funding, spiraling health care costs and public demand for increased accountability have all contributed to the reordering of priorities and alterations in the system. These are evident in the cost containment efforts of governments and insurance companies and in the shift of responsibility for monitoring care from professionals to third party payers. The resulting change from the provision of long term hospital care to short term care, efforts to develop alternatives to hospitalization such as case management and mobile care units, [and] the establishment of productivity standards all significantly impact the practice of occupational therapy. There are drastic changes in the context of our practice. Such change challenges us to examine the validity of occupational therapy, demonstrate its effectiveness and reexamine our professional values, ethics and motivations.

What is the nature of this challenge? The challenge is in the rethinking, in confronting what it is we do and why we do it. It is in sitting out and in clarifying the core focus of occupational therapy, how this then defines the nature and parameters of hospital practice and how we conceptualize and plan for post hospital services. The challenge is in reassessing professional standards, values, expectations, roles, functions, and priorities.

When the length of a hospital stay is open ended, one can rely on time for sorting out essentials, time for the process itself to evolve a direction and focus. When time is limited, the early clarity of purpose becomes critical and there are necessary shifts in priorities. It is not so much the length of time as it is how that time is used that makes the difference.

This challenge then of scrutiny, reassessment and analysis should address at least four major questions:

1. What adaptations will need to be made in how the delivery system is viewed?
2. What adaptations will need to be made in the content of the treatment/remedial process? In other words, what should our in-hospital practice look like?
3. What alterations will need to be made in our patterns of communication? And finally,
4. What adaptations will need to occur in our values, attitudes and expectations?

With a shortened hospital stay, in-patient treatment can no longer be viewed as a self contained system, responsible for providing the full spectrum of treatment. Reliance on community based services becomes essential. A continuity of treatment and rehabilitation requires a range of intact community based services well beyond the traditional out-patient psychotherapy. Out-patient clinics, partial care programs, day treatment centers, the family, all become significant agents and must be viewed as sharing with the hospital and the patient responsibility for treatment outcomes. It becomes a partnership! Thus, the meaning of discharge is altered. Rather than signaling an end to a comprehensive treatment regimen, it marks the beginning of a next level in the continuity of care and treatment.

Development of a collaborative working relationship between occupational therapists, other hospital staff and the staff of community agencies becomes crucial. Furthermore, experience has demonstrated that at this time, much of such relationship building is still up to the occupational therapist. Traditional attitudes and role expectations change slowly and change initiatives such as these require a persistence, a sensitivity, and practice, practice.

The challenge then is to come to understand and define the role of occupational therapy within these changed perspectives so that remediation plans with the patient extend beyond the here and now of the hospital setting. [It is necessary to ensure] that information sharing and recommendations for the focus of post hospital remediation programs are clearly provided and that these are supported by dialogue with the relevant external persons or agency. And finally, [it is imperative] that such functions are conceptualized as an inherent role responsibility of an occupational therapy staff.

One of the challenges to the broader system is to come to understand the system as a system and to provide services to patients accordingly. Although the "delivery system" is a frequently used term, what often exists in reality is not a system but rather a number of services in competition with one another for the diminishing dollar. Organizationally and functionally there is, traditionally, a clear line separating hospital services and community services. Funding practices furthermore reinforce such separation in both public and private enterprises. For example, it was disturbing to learn recently that the New Jersey Governor's Advisory Council was charged with making recommendations for a plan for mental health services. Not for a mental health system, but for services! The separations, the fragmentation is at risk of continuing. In such models, a shortened hospital stay can indeed pose problems for the patient and hospital staff. Many of our values, attitudes and territoriality get in the way of evolving a truly comprehensive system with interdependent parts. The question then is how do we describe our role within this context? As you critique your system's operations, what adaptations will need to be made?

What plans and initiatives will need to be generated in order to facilitate such change? In terms of the functions of occupational therapy? In relation to the roles of colleagues, and the role of the patient? Internalizing the belief that patient care extends beyond the hospital, that it is not necessarily a short term of care but a shorter time in the hospital will, like all attitudinal change, take work and time.

The second question to be examined is, *What adaptations will need to be made in the content of our remedial process?* Addressing this question requires, first of all, taking a second, very critical look at the principal focus of how we define the core concern of our discipline.

Short term care brings the reality of time and priorities clearly to the fore. It is indeed the time of "when push comes to shove"! The questions are: what stays, what goes? what needs to be done now? what later? To use time efficiently and effectively, in the best interest of the patient, requires a clarity of focus and well organized, incremental steps for getting there.

A reexamination of one's frame of reference, one's treatment model or paradigm and how it is being operationalized should be undertaken periodically. When faced with a shortened timeframe, such scrutiny is essential. To sustain the quality of care while accommodating to a shortened hospital stay, requires a truly critical assessment and consensus about fundamentals. It is only from such a base that adaptations can be made. To do otherwise places quality at risk. There is no viable short cut for such a process. Without this step there is great risk that time pressures will force structural and/or technologic changes without the support of conceptual substance. Such a dichotomy dooms most initiatives to failure! At the very least it erodes quality. What must now be asked is: What is your fundamental core focus and how does this determine decisions? What gets relinquished and what are established as top priorities?

For example, my perspective is that as occupational therapists, as specialists in the rehabilitation process our fundamental focus is performance. Thus the content of intervention relates directly to the patient's ability to perform those roles and tasks of daily living which are relevant to their age, to their social-cultural norms and interests, and to the social-cultural norms and expectations of the social structure in which they live: their family and the community. The explicit purpose of such a focus is to enable the patient to evolve a lifestyle, a way of living that is more satisfying than not to self and to the significant others with whom he or she lives.

How do you articulate your frame of reference? Your core focus? What consensus have you established?

If my thesis is tenable, then it follows that all assessments and rehabilitation plans will address four very basic questions:

1. What is it that the patient must be able to do? What performance skills are essential for this patient at this time and at what level?
2. What can the patient do? What are the strengths, abilities, and interests of the patient, what are the resources of the external environment?
3. What can the patient not do? What internal/external factors interfere?
4. What interventions, what remedial activity must be taken and in what order of priority so that the patient will be able to move toward fulfilling relevant lifestyle performance expectations?

Are such questions relevant to your formulations? What factors determine the parameters of your assessments, of your plans of intervention? What questions are the organizers for your assessment and planning?

The process of clarifying what the content of interventions should be and thus what adaptations will be needed, involves taking a look at several additional factors. If indeed occupational therapy is in the business of making it possible for the individual to evolve a lifestyle more satisfying than not to the person and to his or her society, then it becomes necessary to come to closure with regard to identifying and categorizing what is considered to be the major roles and tasks of daily living. What are the components of a lifestyle? How should these be categorized so that relevant functional skills can be defined and measured? Without a model that sets such criteria, assessment and treatment initiatives with patients risk hanging in limbo, without context, without meaning or relevance to the patient or to others, credibility is at high risk and time becomes poorly used.

A second issue related to what criteria should be used to determine what are relevant functions and a relevant lifestyle for a given patient. What are the interdependent variables among the resources, the expectations, the potential of the community, of the family and of the patient which help to define relevance? With whom does one collaborate in addressing such questions? Without such a formula, it is unlikely that a truly individualized rehabilitation plan will be designed, especially under the pressures of time.

Assessment is critical and should not be short changed. Designing a rehabilitation plan that extends into the community requires some very solid and complex information. Obviously, in a short hospital stay more information must be gathered in a shorter period of time. Knowing what to look for (and) how to obtain and use the information reduces time. The use of a comprehensive (and comprehensive must be emphasized), functional skills assessment instrument is an extremely valuable organizing, data collection procedure. When there are limits on time, the use of such an instrument is essential. It must, however, accommodate to age and cultural variations and have a clear relevance to the definition of one's focus and frame of reference. A functional skills assessment instrument facilitates consensual planning, concertizes goals and progress, measures and documents outcomes and provides an M.I.S. base for quality assurance and program evaluation.

One needs to be regularly reminded that treatment and assessment are interrelated. There is no treatment without assessment and no information gathering without therapeutic gain. Our action oriented groups and activities are rich laboratories for simultaneous remediation and assessment. This reality maximizes the effective use of time to the benefit of the patient.

The patient's participation in the design of his/her rehabilitation plan takes on added significance in a short term setting. Shared planning and reaching consensus more frequently than not generate a sense of ownership on the part of the patient. Such investment pays dividends during hospitalization and is more likely to make a difference in the incentive to follow through after hospitalization. Furthermore, the shared planning, the negotiating, compromise and consensus regarding plans and priorities is an important learning opportunity. It is an exercise in volition, an experience in assessing one's alternatives, making decisions and planning for follow through. It is learning about being one's own agent and having some influence over one's life, an essential ingredient in a satisfying lifestyle.

Content adaptations will require a new look at community resources. Not only in terms of their role in post hospital programs but their significance as part of in-hospital programming. The use of community resources while the patient is still hospitalized provides an important bridge to the community. What educational, vocational, recreational resources, what peer support groups exist in the patient's community? What can they provide and what can be done to foster their involvement? This kind of bridging is so important to the young borderline and substance abuse patient. For the schizophrenic patient it compensates for problems with generalizing function and provides some essential mapping.

A hospital environment with fluid boundaries between itself and community resources is an environment that maximizes the potential of the patient to cope with the community and can reduce the need for continued stay. An experience early in my career in a small psychoanalytic hospital with remarkable collaborative relationships with and use of community resources, was a lesson I will always remember. I have since viewed the self contained or total hospital with self contained programs and services, with at least a jaundiced eye.

Scrutiny of the content of occupational therapy practice should also address our intervention strategies and methodologies. These are related to both the expeditious use of time and to the critical variable within time of role clarification. Although the temptation to embark on a discourse regarding the importance and meaning of activities is great, it is acknowledged that this is not the purpose of this paper. Suffice it to say that the use of purposeful activity (or occupation if you prefer) is without question our intervention of choice. It is purposeful action, the process of doing as remediation, which is the essence of our expertise, in contrast to the expertise and technologies of verbal expression and dialogue. Implicit in this thesis is the tenet that feelings, perceptions and behaviors are shaped and changed as the result of action experiences. Psychomotor activity is a fundamental learning process. In these respects we are different from other traditionally recognized health professionals.

A second and related point of differentiation is our primary attention to the strengths, capacities, intact skills and interests of the patient. Ours is an overriding concern for the discovery of such assets and their use in the process of successful doing. Our principal focus is maximizing the healthy aspects of the patient in contrast to a focal concern about pathology or disease. We are different and our difference brings a critical dimension to conceptualizing and implementing the curative process.

Time and again there is evidence of the ongoing risk of our getting lost, of losing our unique identity in the practice setting. The risk increases in environments where strong leadership and role modeling comes from outside of our profession. Upward mobility is the hallmark of a mobile society such as our western culture. The incentive to assume, to emulate the characteristics and behaviors of those who occupy a more privileged status, is a universal phenomenon. The health care system is no exception. The psychologist strives to emulate the physician; the occupational therapist tries to emulate the psychologist and so on. The occupational therapist's white uniform as a newcomer to the hospital system was no small effort to be seen as more like the influential registered nurse than like ourselves. Today, several rungs up the ladder, we take on testing behaviors and the clinical white coat! Abandonment of the ubiquitous uniforms in psychiatric hospitals seems to have had more to do with the politics of social class and power than patients' needs.

To be more like others rather than different is a strong social pull. However, when we lose our purposeful activity focus, we resign our responsibility and fail the patient. It is differences in perspectives, methodologies and expertise that best and most expeditiously serve the patient. That is the value of the interdisciplinary team, it provides a wide angle lens and a diversity of focus and methods!

For many years I have understood a functional difference in the meaning of treatment and the meaning of rehabilitation. In practice, treatment most characteristically references those interventions, those processes which are directed toward the reduction or elimination of pathology. Rehabilitation by contrast most generally connotes relearning, redevelopment, as Webster states, "to restore to suitability." The focus is on function. The coin has two sides, each different, distinguishable, but integrated to form the whole. So it is with treatment and rehabilitation each different and distinguishable, each interrelated and essential to form the whole.

Ongoing role clarification is critical, particularly when hospital stay is brief. It relates to time, efficiency and the comprehensive quality of care. Knowing who does what well, having different expertise available makes it possible to expeditiously use special expertise, as well as to share some roles and functions without threat to the integrity of care to the patient.

No one needs to be convinced that communication is vital to the life of any organization, any endeavor, any group or dyad. Over time institutions develop their own unique patterns of communication. These generally relate to the mission of the institution and in particular to its organizational and operational philosophy. Communication patterns reflect an institution's values, locus of power and influence and thus how it goes about achieving its mission. Who talks to whom about what is the mirror of operations and philosophy of care. Thus, for example, the typical long term psychoanalytic hospital has its unique patterns of communication which reflect, support and reinforce its psychoanalytic values, standards, ethics and beliefs. Within this context, communication around patient care and treatment decisions generally tend to be exploratory, speculative, thoughtful and without the pressure of time. It is understood that there is always time to work things through, and this process (the working through) is viewed many times as more significant than the coming to closure.

When hospital stays are shortened, when there are the inevitable alterations in the delivery system, when priorities are necessarily reshuffled, many of the traditional patterns of communication no longer support the goals of the institution. Some, because of changed circumstances, become counterproductive.

Clearly any change calls for a reexamination of patterns of communication. In light of the adaptations which you identify as needing to occur in your delivery system, and in the content and focus of your interventions, what should your communication network look like? Among yourselves, with patients, with other staff, and with the community? What should be the content of each of such dialogues? How do you facilitate and/or bring about the needed change and adaptations?

Values clarification is perhaps such an overused phrase that hearing it no longer elicits a sense of challenge. Nevertheless, it seems evident that most of the issues which have been raised here for consideration involve values, beliefs, ethics and sets of expectations. Our values set the stage for our decisions and for our performance. Getting clear on one's own values and beliefs is a first and necessary step in addressing response and adaptations to the complex and challenging issues of short term hospitalization. A critical reassessment of your values and beliefs is fundamental to coming to grips with the challenge.

Finally, meeting the challenge means confronting the threat of change. We have learned to explain the resistance to change as response to the threat to one's power, influence and control to the bureaucratic investment in the status quo, to job security, and the like. The constructs are so generalized and have become such cliches that frequently they are of only limited help to us in understanding why in the face of pending change we feel as we do and thus what might be done to reduce our anxiety and free us to act. Over the years, I have come to understand how resistance to change is caused not so much by the fear of change itself but rather, by the threat of change. It is the uncertainty, the numerous, open-ended possibilities, the ambiguities that are frightening and that threaten to unlock the "ghosts" in our closet. With many unknown possibilities, with untested waters, our ability to predict is threatened. Familiar cause and effect formulas no longer seem so reliable. Our ghosts of questionable competence, adequacy and validity of our

practice begin to stir. The old fears of being able to cope and to manage begin to reemerge and urge us to reaffirm that indeed a bird in the hand is preferable to two in a bush. In her impressive book *The Change Masters*, R. K. Kantor suggests that the threat of change implies loss of control when it is assumed that one does not have the resources to make the transition possible. Furthermore, she goes on to say that "the threat of change arouses anxiety when it is still a threat, not an actuality." Certainly, my experience has shown that when we confront the threat by planning, our resources and capabilities are disclosed and reaffirmed. In the process of scrutinizing the challenge, in planning for change we assume control over events and the "too many possibilities" become known and manageable. The threat of change then becomes the challenge of opportunity.

I have raised more questions than suggested solutions. First, because I have always believed that understanding the question is the essence of resolution. Additionally, and more important perhaps, my purpose has been to provoke analytic dialogue among you knowing that through this process you are capable of making those decisions which will maximize the potential inherent in each of you, inherent in the patient and in the system.

Chapter 4

Short-Term Psychiatric Treatment: How Will Occupational Therapy Adapt?

Gary A. Jackson, MS, OTR

Inpatient psychiatric treatment has been undergoing significant change stimulated by a multitude of forces within and outside of the psychiatric establishment. A new accountability to the consumer and to the sources of funding increasingly demand proof of the efficacy and cost-effectiveness of treatment. The abhorrence of "warehousing" the mentally ill has been mobilized in the spirit of deinstitutionalization, and laws protecting individual rights have narrowed the criteria both for admission as well as for the continuation of involuntary hospitalization. Third-party payers have become a major influence in the provision of psychiatric treatment. To control costs, insurance carriers have reduced the maximum number of hospital days covered and have been increasingly restrictive in determining what services will be reimbursable.

Medicare, the largest single payer for inpatient services, has recently introduced a prospective pricing system where fixed payments will be made for each diagnosis-related group (DRG). This will undoubtedly have far-reaching implications for the availability of many services. Faced with limitations of time and funding, can hospitals "afford" to provide any rehabilitative services beyond crisis intervention? Choices must be made about what can and cannot be provided that will enable the patient to return to the community without imminent risk of harm to himself or others. Consequently, most rehabilitative services which address the chronic and extensive impact of many psychiatric disorders must take place elsewhere.

Occupational therapists face serious questions concerning the scope and purpose of their services in short-term inpatient treatment. What role is to be played by professionals who have previously been concerned in large part with relatively long-term rehabilitative services? With the rising number of psychiatric beds being established in acute care general hospitals, more occupational therapists are likely to align themselves with the medical model which predominates in these settings. Emphasis on symptom reduction and other short range, problem-oriented interventions may overshadow the more holistic philosophy of occupational therapy. Does this orientation risk what Phillip Shannon described as "derailment" from the essence of occupational therapy (Shannon, 1977)? This appears entirely possible if we modify our approach primarily as an accommodation to the medical model. Shannon further warned that derailment could lead to a loss of legitimacy of the profession and ultimately, absorption of services by other health care professionals. There are few interventions that are the sole domain of a single profession in mental health care. It is not uncommon to find different disciplines providing similar services within the same hospital. It is even more advantageous in short-term treatment to have these multiple options so as to provide a service rapidly and efficiently. It is a mistake to look upon modalities as territory that defines professional identity. This can occur all too easily if at the same time occupational therapists abandon their traditional rehabilitative orientation because it appears impractical in short-term treatment. As a result, occupational therapists would not be members of a legitimate profession. Rather, they would more accurately be considered as health care technicians with an assortment of isolated skills. Occupational therapy services must change in order to be relevant and effective in these settings. Needed change is possible without losing sight of underlying theories of practice. Development or reestablishment of functional independence in major life activities through purposeful activity is a task that unquestionably requires time beyond that of a brief hospital stay. Occupational therapists must therefore begin with direct hands-on service but extend treatment beyond hospitalization with long-range plans that more fully utilize community resources. Occupational therapists are particularly well-suited to assess and select appropriate activities to further treatment goals regardless of whether these are hospital based or whether they originate in the community. This concept marks a shift in the methods used to deliver services but does not alter essential working assumptions. To the contrary, the use of resources in the community may do more to promote normalization of life-style than would be possible by the heavy reliance on hospital-based activity programs prevalent in long-term treatment facilities.

Concurrent with the significant impact that reduced treatment time has upon the practice of occupational therapy, other pressures are rapidly becoming major issues. Accountability will have important implications for practice. Funding with be jeopardized in the near future unless the need for services and the efficacy of these services are demonstrated convincingly to hospital administrators and third-party payers. For too long, occupational therapists have not been held accountable in clarifying treatment principles. Therapists have been allowed to freely explore a wide variety of treatment approaches so long as no harm has resulted. This form of "benign neglect" has resulted in occupational therapy practices nearly as varied as the number of settings but has provided little incentive for practitioners to develop the necessary skills to objectively evaluate their own services. In addition, many therapists practice in "pockets of isolation" (Gillette, 1978). The small psychiatric units in general hospitals often employ a single occupational therapist. This condition precludes the benefit of day-to-day collaboration with professional peers and increases the likelihood that such diversity will occur. The potential for role blurring is great, and touchstones for professional identity must be sought outside of the workplace. At this time, there is not a representative body of literature specific to short-term treatment to guide the therapist. Consequently, the therapist must adapt theory and practice that often originated out of traditional long-term treatment and may or may not be appropriate to this different setting. How to determine what is appropriate and effective treatment has been an elusive issue for occupational therapists as well as for other psychiatric professionals. The problem cannot be resolved by a single practitioner, yet this is the situation that most occupational therapists face when working in isolation. The lack of a specialized knowledge base which is supported by research also does not further the occupational therapist's role as a full-fledged professional among peers and ultimately limits one's effectiveness in treatment. The question is whether or not occupational therapists will develop the skills necessary for effective adaptation, skills central to a true profession.

A blueprint for professionalism was outlined in a special session for the Representative Assembly of the American Occupational Therapy Association in 1978 (AOTA Monograph, 1979). This was not the first, nor will it be the last examination of the prerequisites of a full-fledged profession. Yet, progress towards this goal has been slow. With the demise of "benign neglect," that which will be expected of occupational therapists practicing in mental health pertains directly to professionalism. The development of a specific knowledge base and specialized training in short-term psychosocial treatment, more extensive research, and greater accountability in the clinic cannot continue at a slow pace without serious repercussions. Psychiatric health care is rapidly changing and with it, occupational therapists must upgrade their professional skills or face increased erosion of their relevance within this system. Complacency or efforts to maintain the status quo mark the inevitable decline of an organism or of a philosophy. Is this less true of an art or a science? It is incumbent upon the profession to make these determinations objectively, and in so doing, occupational therapists will also gain the respect and trust of their constituency as well as that of the professional community. The risk is that we recognize our shortcomings, but the potential rewards far outweigh the mediocrity assured by inaction.

An urgent professional need, and perhaps one that may be addressed most readily, concerns reaching the isolated therapist with current state of the art evaluation and treatment methods specific to short-term psychiatric settings. What evaluation methods obtain necessary information rapidly and with a minimum of the redundancy common to multidisciplinary treatment team approaches? Modifications to traditional treatment approaches used in long-term institutions must be made. What is reasonable to accomplish in such a short time frame? Habit formation and the development of major skills are unlikely to occur, but learning effective alternatives to a specific and immediate problem may be possible. Brief in-hospital efforts to improve self-esteem may be insignificant for patients who have experienced years of failure. The value of "doing" is reflected in our philosophy, but time constraints often favor the immediacy of verbal interventions as the expedient approach of choice. To what extent is this consistent with our philosophy? What are the varieties of symptom reduction interventions available from occupational therapists, and in what context are these also consistent with our philosophy? Craft-based task groups may be ineffective in facilitating basic task skills given the time frame, but craft groups may have greater use as initial and ongoing assessments of a patient's readiness to return to major life activities, such as work or school. As previously noted, discharge planning is an extension of treatment into the community where much of the "doing" must take place. The occupational therapist's role in this process should be strong. These are but a few issues pertinent to the increasing number of clinicians providing short-term treatment. A means of compiling and disseminating this information to practicing clinicians must be established. The American Occupational Therapy Association's TOTEMS project to strengthen services in the school system did just that. Their planned development of a similar project in the area of mental health holds great potential for addressing these urgent needs.

A long-range issue for therapists specializing in mental health concerns the profession's role in the changing configuration of health care delivery systems. The un-

precedented shift away from institution-based psychiatric treatment and the reductions of inpatient insurance coverage open the door to those who can provide viable service alternatives. Similarly, the limitations of acute care, which preclude a significant portion of traditional occupational therapy services in these facilities, lead to a greater emphasis on referral to community programs. Many researchers believe that community-based models of service, in which facilitation of basic work habits and independent living skills play a central role, may have significant impact on recovery from mental illnesses (Anthony et al., 1978; Beard et al., 1978). The parallels between these programs and the philosophy of occupational therapy are strong and suggest that occupational therapists would be well-suited to work directly within such programs. However, the growth and development of our profession has historically followed its funding. Unless and until outpatient services are reimbursable by third-party payers or other funding mechanisms are developed, this expansion is unlikely to occur to any substantial extent. The strength of our national association and the collective grassroots support embodied in our local organizations must play a key role in securing these funding changes.

Ongoing and comprehensive efforts to upgrade the profession must also be undertaken as a long-range goal. All too commonly, noteworthy accomplishments of individual therapists are developed in relative isolation and remain unnoticed by the professional community. The evolution of occupational therapy services must rest more heavily upon the collective and cumulative efforts of the profession. In this regard, the appearance of the *Mental Health Special Interest Section Newsletter*, and journals, such as *Occupational Therapy in Mental Health* and *The Occupational Therapy Journal of Research*, have expanded the national forum. Not only must evaluation and treatment interventions be given greater exposure, but they must also be validated by research. To do this, graduates of at least the Master's degree level with significant training in research methodology are needed in greater numbers. Even with training in this area, there must be opportunities to carry out research in the field. The premium placed on direct services, particularly in short-term units, discourages the allotment of limited staff time for such endeavors. Increasingly common fee-for-service reimbursement is also a negative factor when the cost of staff time for research cannot be recovered. Larger departments may be more able to "write off" a small portion of staff time for research. Joint ventures between teaching hospitals and universities may be another avenue in this regard. Alternative funding for research, such as grants, must be aggressively sought. The complexities of such a task would suggest that these efforts are best initiated (as some have been) by the national and state professional associations and by the academic community. The subsequent benefits of these activities would strengthen clinical practice and also provide educators with a more unified body of current knowledge from which to teach.

This article has reviewed some of the major changes in mental health care which have significantly reduced the practical application of traditional occupational therapy modalities. Emphasis on symptom reduction, although consistent with short-term care, risks dilution of the profession's essential strength unless brief inpatient treatment is seen as part of a longer continuum of rehabilitation. Active participation in the discharge planning process and greater involvement with community-based resources are effective means for occupational therapists to extend the rehabilitative impact of treatment. Increasing demands for accountability further emphasize the need for research and the upgrading of clinician's skills in the field—formidable tasks requiring support and coordination at the national level. Although many of the newer pressures and limitations in the field of mental health care will continue to be problematic, the evolution of occupational therapy practice may ultimately lead to a stronger, more effective role in a health care continuum that extends beyond traditional hospital treatment.

References

American Occupational Therapy Association. *Occupational Therapy: 2001 AD* (Monograph), Rockville, MD: American Occupational Therapy Association, 1979.

Anthony, W. A., Cohen, M. R., & Vitalo, R. The Measurement of Rehabilitation Outcome. *Schizophrenia Bulletin.* 1978, *4*, 365-380.

Beard, J. H., Malmaud, T. J., & Rossman, E. Psychiatric Rehabilitation and Rehospitalization Rates: The Findings of Two Research Studies. *Schizophrenia Bulletin*, 1978, *4*, 622.

Friedson, E. *Professional Dominance.* NY: Atherton Press, Inc., 1970.

Gillette, N. Practice, Education, and Research. *Occupational Therapy: 2001 AD* (Monograph), 18-25, Rockville, MD: American Occupational Therapy Association, 1979.

National Institute of Mental Health. Mental Health Series Reports and Statistical Notes. *Division of Biometry and Epidemiology*, 1981.

Shannon, P. D. The Derailment of Occupational Therapy. *American Journal of Occupational Therapy*, 1977, *31*(4), 229-234.

Spiro, H. R. Reforming the State Hospital in a Unified Care System. *Hospital and Community Psychiatry*,1982, *33*, 722 -728.

Vollmer, H. M. & Mills, D. L. (Eds.) *Professionalization.* Englewood Cliffs, NJ: Prentice Hall, 1966.

Chapter 5

Deinstitutionalizing the Occupational Therapist

Patricia J. Dasler, MA, OTR

For the past twenty years efforts have continued to move patients and services in rehabilitation into the community. With such relocation of disabled persons who need help in returning to normal daily roles, the need for occupational therapy services seems obvious. Yet, in many communities there are relatively few occupational therapists working outside of traditional centers. This situation suggests the question: If occupational therapists are not the ones assisting patients in learning daily living skills, socialization and adaptation to homes and jobs, who is? In a 1978 descriptive study of community mental health centers the National Institute of Mental Health found that social workers and nurses were the staff most frequently employed. In their study of core professionals in mental health, occupational therapists were not even mentioned. [1]

In another study that surveyed how patients were being trained in activities of daily living in day treatment centers it was shown that such training was done by social workers, nurses, psychologists and teachers. [2] Further, more than half of the centers providing daily living skills training did not even have an occupational therapist on their staff. Occupational therapy has a long established philosophy and practice of training disabled persons in independent living skills. [3] The education process for the occupational therapy profession includes acquiring understandings of the pathology of disabling conditions, the cognitive, motoric, perceptual and psycho-social components of successful independent functioning, and an awareness of how both environment and individual can be adapted to enable the disabled person to function as independently as possible in his daily life. Yet, the occupational therapist, the professional best prepared to do this widely called-for teaching of daily living skills in the community is scarcely there. The purpose of this paper is to examine why so few occupational therapists work in community settings. In addition, one strategy that was successfully used to increase employment of occupational therapists in one community will be described.

Movement of the Disabled Population

Reflecting a change in treatment policy, many large state residential social and health care institutions have reduced the numbers of their beds drastically. Some have even been closed. These include schools for the blind and deaf and hospitals for the mentally ill and mentally retarded. The change occurs not because these patients have been "cured" or even fully rehabilitated. Rather they were discharged to their communities in an effort to "normalize" their lives. Unfortunately it cannot be assumed that these disabled persons possess the skills they need to function independently outside of institutions. In fact it is true that many of these patients find it difficult simply to maintain their current levels of functioning if they do not have the structure and support of an institution and programs such as occupational therapy.

Many references speak about mentally ill persons living in communities who still need training in the activities of daily living, socialization and leisure skills.[4-6] It is known that for patients who do not generalize well, hospitals are not an ideal or appropriate setting in which to be taught these personal skills. Persons should be taught daily life skills in the environments in which they will actually be needed and used. Test and Stein called this "in vivo" training.[7] Further, in current mental health treatment hospitalization is being used only to stabilize patients, largely with medication. Such approaches thus become interventive measures and not rehabilitation efforts. Under emerging treatment philosophies rehabilitation is thought to be best conducted in the community where patients live and need to function.

The Non-Movement of Occupational Therapists

From the above one can see that disabled persons moved from hospitals to the community are still in need of services occupational therapists regularly give. However, now it seems that to provide such services it is the occupational therapists who must be "deinstitutionalized". Like their patients, occupational therapists must break away from the security offered by institutional practice. For patients, the price of institutional security is loss of freedom. For our profession, the price is dilution of the ability to move patients toward meaningful activity by continuing to use the artificial environments of residential facilities for training. Like their

patients, occupational therapists need to adapt their skills to fit the new "outside" environment of the community. It is only in the community that the daily problems of living with a disability will become as clear to the therapist as it is for patients.

The reasons behind the small numbers of occupational therapists working in the community are many and complex. It is not fair to blame the health care delivery system for this situation. The profession must accept some responsibility for not deinstitutionalizing itself. If therapists continue to insist on the more secure and more lucrative jobs in traditional and well established "clinics" in institutions, they may find they have sealed the fate of the profession by not being available where the population is that most needs them. Others in the community will fill the gap left by the occupational therapists' absence.

Discrepancies in levels of educational preparation between occupational therapists and other health workers and the large salary differences also pose major problems for therapists wishing to break into the community mental health field. The largest competition comes from the social work field, where most have Master's degrees. Jobs in mental health not requiring a Master's degree are generally on the level of a mental health assistant and may currently pay less than any occupational therapy personnel would expect to make. In some cases occupational therapists working in the community, even having Master's degrees, find themselves making less than their counterparts in hospitals. Because of the salary levels of available jobs in mental health, often new graduates eager to find employment are the only ones attracted. This trend further complicates the situation as these inexperienced therapists may not function optimally as occupational therapists because of the role blurring that tends to occur in community mental health settings. Without confidence built through experience young therapists often abandon traditional activity-centered treatment for maximizing independent functioning in patients in favor of the seemingly more accepted model of "talk" therapy. The potential for activity-based daily living programming does exist and can be developed even though the occupational therapist in a community health facility is in most instances required to function as a generalist and is often also responsible for case management, a clinical skill readily identified with the social worker.

Because of this generalist role pattern job titles tend to obscure professional identity and training. The job descriptions of such titles as program specialist, mental health specialist, skills trainer and case manager show a distinct fit with occupational therapy function. However, if occupational therapists' job searches focus solely on positions listed as "occupational therapist" they are not apt to find employment in a community mental health facility.

Another factor confounding the deinstitutionalization of the occupational therapist is the small pool of therapists interested in mental health positions. Fewer therapists countrywide are choosing to work in the mental health field. In the state of Oregon, for example, the number of occupational therapists registered in the Oregon Mental Health Special Interest Section has not grown in over two years. So while administrators of some agencies may not see the need for occupational therapy staff, it is still not uncommon to hear administrators in other agencies complain that they gave up looking for occupational therapy staff because none applied after extensive advertising efforts. While the limited labor pool and how to resolve it are not the focus of this paper they are issues needing attention in many parts of the country if more mental health occupational therapy services are to be made available.

Strategy for Change

Moving occupational therapists to jobs in mental health in the community presents many problems. These will be solved only by the combined efforts of many dedicated individuals using strategies that match the complexities of the problems. A single therapist would find solutions difficult if not impossible. A plan for such change was developed and successfully used in Portland, Oregon to increase the number of occupational therapists in the community. That was the goal identified. The plan consisted of five interrelated components made operational by a vital network of persons serving various roles. Each component of the plan will be discussed with examples of the Oregon experience shared for illustration. The components needed to implement this plan are as follows:

1. A network of people to coordinate strategy efforts
2. Advocates of the plan from within the occupational therapy profession
3. Advocates other than occupational therapists
4. A labor pool of qualified therapist applicants
5. Interested health agency administrators who understand occupational therapy services
6. Regulatory support for the positions

Building a Network

A network of professionals interested in participating in planning and implementing a strategy must be assembled as the first step. The functions appear to be: to serve as information sources, to gather the human resources

for the other components of the strategy, and to maintain frequent contact to assure that the plan's efforts are coordinated. Employees in state facilities are prime resources for change information since they often are first to know about shifts in funding and target populations in health care programs. Besides information sources other people are needed to gather and coordinate the advocates (#s 2 and 3 above) and the labor pool (#4 above), core essentials of the plan. Frequent informal telephone contacts and several actual meetings of network persons help to create the organized system needed to move the strategy ahead as planned. For example, it does little good if occupational therapy applicants (labor pool) approach administrators before such persons have been contacted and prepared for interviewing occupational therapists.

The network in Oregon was formed after occupational therapists from one state hospital alerted members of the Mental Health Special Interest Section that the State was reducing the number of beds at the hospital and diverting operating money for services in the community. Thereby jobs were to be created, several of which carried the title of skills trainer. The proposed duties of these trainers seemed to be a description of an occupational therapist's function yet no occupational therapists were being sought or hired in those positions. Armed with this information a group of interested individuals got together, made a plan and gathered resources targeted on placing occupational therapists in those jobs. The network used the telephone to stay in touch and to share information and report progress.

Assembling Advocates from Within the Profession

Occupational therapists themselves must join in the effort to move jobs to the community. In this case therapists who have some experience in community health centers can prove very valuable. These advocates can either brief people who go to speak with mental health administrators or can contact the administrators themselves to state the concerns and solicit interest in hiring occupational therapists. Another use of these advocates is as consultant/references in case administrators have questions about the role of occupational therapy services in their facilities. Advocates might later be asked by administrators to serve in the agencies as ongoing consultants, to provide assistance in continued planning, to provide in-service education sessions, or to orient and supervise newly hired staff. Continued consultation by an experienced occupational therapist is particularly helpful in an agency when a newly hired therapist happens to be inexperienced.

Getting Advocates from the Community

Advocates from outside of occupational therapy are co-workers such as psychiatrists, social workers and administrators, or consumers who value occupational therapy services. As advocates such persons serve as references and vocal supporters of the use and effectiveness of occupational therapy services. Agency administrators often welcome the possibility of contact with reputable community persons to assist in decision-making about staffing and programming. It is particularly good if such advocates are persons whose names are recognized locally. Further, having a printed list of community advocates to give to administrators during discussions with them is a most useful strategy. Cultivating non-occupational therapy advocates is an important part of a plan like this. They lend credibility and establish the value of occupational therapy services in a way that no therapist could.

Establishing a Pool of Applicants

A ready pool of qualified occupational therapy personnel is vital to the success of the plan. Once agency administrators become responsive to hiring therapists it is necessary to have persons ready to apply for the jobs. If a list of possible candidates for jobs is not available a pool must be assembled before any other public relations efforts are made. Actually getting a pool of applicants together can be more difficult than creating the jobs to be filled. The network must be active in this phase to put out the word that jobs may be opening up and to identify suitable applicants. Directors of educational programs often are helpful since they seek to place graduates. Or the network persons can advertise their role and the job potentials in state or national newsletters seeking candidate resumes which can be shared with likely agencies as a beginning step. This idea can prove to be very effective in targeting occupational therapists for positions as often notices of mental health positions produce a plethora of local applicants from other disciplines before occupational therapists are even aware of the openings.

It is important to consider the levels and experience of those in the labor pool so that public relations efforts can be aimed at creating jobs that are possible to fill. In Oregon there are fewer registered therapists than might be expected because there is no professional level educational program to produce local graduates. However, a class of occupational therapy assistants had just graduated from the local community college so it was concluded that this class would be the immediate labor pool. Accordingly, in this plan efforts at creating jobs were centered around those which COTAs could fill.

Making Health Agency Contacts

Discussions with mental health agency administrators to develop specific occupational therapy awareness should be undertaken as soon as networking is solid and there are possible applicants available. These discussions are best done by therapists not seeking employment themselves even though they may be willing to serve as consultants. Here is where the occupational therapy advocates are particularly effective, for the goal of these contacts is to make sure that administrators understand the scope of services offered by occupational therapists as well as the educational backgrounds and appropriate functions of the OTR and COTA.

It is helpful in this process to review with the administrator the needs of mental health patients and how these needs are addressed by occupational therapy personnel. A good example to use is the lack in many patients of independent living skills such as cooking and money management, and the difficulties such patients have in learning and then transferring skills learned to actual living situations unless they learn by doing, a function of occupational therapy.

Other issues of concern to administrators are reimbursement for services, salaries, and job descriptions for therapists according to program and services given. Both community and occupational therapy advocates are helpful in discussing these issues and should be prepared for them.

Understanding and Using Regulations

Regulations impact most health care programs today. Those directly related to community mental health services and personnel must be understood and applied as the plan develops. Networkers should be certain what positions are required in mental health settings and which personnel are to fill them. If licensing of occupational therapists is in effect they should determine if occupational therapy functions in mental health settings are being done by non-OT personnel. This is one way to identify jobs for occupational therapists though it is generally better to gain jobs by persuasion than by coercion. Other regulations regarding supervision, reimbursement and scope of treatment may also exist or need amending in order to open positions for therapists.

In Oregon through discussion with personnel in Mental Health and on the Licensing Board, occupational therapy roles were clarified and distinguished from personnel currently serving as trainers. It is now hoped that a letter will be issued by the Department of Mental Health recommending that occupational therapists be hired for these positions in the future.

Results of the Strategy for Change

Within nine months of the first meeting of the network group, four occupational therapists were hired in community agencies. Three COTAs have become full-time employees at three different agencies. One COTA was hired as a skills trainer to work directly with patients placed in a semi-independent apartment program. Two were hired to provide socialization activities in their centers. One OTR has reached full-time employment in private practice, consulting with the COTAs at two of the agencies. The agencies hiring these personnel had never had occupational therapy staff before. Four new positions now exist.

While the original network and its activities seem to have been discontinued, the four hired therapists have formed their own network or support group and meet once a month to share information about their jobs and developments in their agencies. With the OTR leading, specific in-service sessions have been conducted to focus on issues that have arisen in their exchanges or in individual consultation with the OTR.

Summary

This paper has discussed the problems created by the deinstitutionalization from state health facilities of large numbers of disabled persons who need but are not receiving occupational therapy services in the community. It has been demonstrated that these persons continue to need the support and training previously offered to them by occupational therapists. Many things contribute to the lack of therapists in community agencies to provide such services. Among them are the apparent reticence of occupational therapists to fit into the current mental health care structure and the salary discrepancies, unclear role functions and competition for jobs with less trained personnel.

A strategy was presented for moving occupational therapists to community positions. It resulted after a one year effort in four therapists being hired in community mental health practice. While mental health practice was highlighted, the problem of moving occupational therapists to the community is not just a problem in mental health, but exists in all areas of OT practice. Occupational therapists need to band together to plan strategies such as the one described to assure the delivery of needed services to the increasing populations of disabled persons living in the community. The state association special interest sections seem to provide a ready vehicle for the operation of such strategies to deinstitutionalize the occupational therapist. As more community health services are developed occupational therapy will survive only if the profession plans for and makes definite moves to serve in those areas.

References

1. National Institute of Mental Health: *Series B, No. 16, CMHC Staffing: Who Minds the Store?* DHEW Publications No. (ADM) 78-686, Superintendent of Documents, U.S. Government Printing Office, Washington, D.C. 1978.

2. Dasler, P: A descriptive study: the practice of training activities of daily living in psychiatric day-treatment centers.Unpublished Master's thesis, University of Southern California, Los Angeles, California, 1981.

3. American Occupational Therapy Association: *Occupational Therapy 2001 AD.* Rockville, MD: American Occupational Therapy Association, 1979.

4. Lamb R: Treating long term schizophrenic patients in the community. In *Progress in Community Mental Health*, (Vol. III), L Bellak and H Barton, Editors. New York: Brunner/Mazel, 1975.

5. Marx A, Test M and Stein L: Extrohospital management of severe mental illness. *Arch Gen Psychiatry*, 29: 505-511, 1973.

6. Turner J: Comprehensive community support systems and adults with seriously disabling mental health problems. *Psychosocial Rehabilitation Journal*, 1:39-47, 1977.

7. Test M, Stein L: Practical guidelines for the community treatment of the markedly impaired patients. *Community Ment Health J*, 12: 72-82, 1976.

Chapter 6

Deinstitutionalization: A Role for Occupational Therapy in the State Hospital

Barbara J. Hemphill, MS, OTR, FAOTA
Pamela Carr Werner, BS, OTR

This chapter was previously published in *Occupational Therapy in Mental Health*, 10(2), 85-99. Copyright © 1990, Haworth Press. Reprinted by permission.

State institutions, which for the past century have been built and maintained as major care sites for the chronically mentally ill (Morrissey, Goldman, 1984; Pepper, Ryglewicz, 1985), no longer serve that purpose in many localities. For the past two decades, debate has raged over the issue of deinstitutionalization of mentally disabled patients. The combination of humanitarian zeal and the desire to contain costs has resulted in the release or diversion of hundreds of thousands of patients from state mental hospitals into community centers (Craig & Laska, 1983).

Tuason, Rair-Riedesel and Hoffmann (1982) defined deinstitutionalization as:

> . . . the movement of individuals who have difficulty functioning independently and who need continuing care of various kinds from more to less restrictive settings. In the mental health sector, the term describes the transfer of patients from public mental hospitals to community settings. The intent is that community living confers a better quality of life on these formerly hospitalized individuals while participating in the necessary outpatient, day care, or other rehabilitation programs. (page 697)

The deinstitutionalization movement grew haphazardly, without careful long-range social planning. Its development and progress reflected social values, funding priorities and ethical factors in contemporary American society (Markson, 1985) that left state hospitals struggling with overwhelming burdens.

The remaining inpatients included the seriously mentally ill and nondischargeable elderly. Although the young adult inpatients show a profile of difficult behavior and challenging demands that mandate institutionalization (Pepper & Ryglewicz, 1985), debate continues as to whether state mental hospitals should be closed. Because their mission is unclear, they are markedly understaffed, have inadequate programming and financial resources, and lack rehabilitative programs. For example, the number of occupational therapists is grossly inadequate. Many of the programs occupy only a small part of the patient's day and do not teach skills relevant to life in the community (Okin, 1983).

This paper examines the current status of deinstitutionalization and its effect on the delivery of mental health services in state hospitals. It examines the future of state hospitals and the role of occupational therapists in this setting.

Deinstitutionalization

Downsizing in state institutional population resulted from five major forces (Pepper & Ryglewicz, 1985, page 231):

1. The open-hospital concept, which led to community-based treatment.
2. The development of powerful psychotropic medications that made it possible to rapidly control the most flagrant symptoms of mental illness.
3. The application of civil rights laws as applied to persons considered mentally ill.
4. The rapid acceleration to an unmanageable level of the inpatient-care cost.
5. The availability of federal funds—Social Security Disability payments and Medicaid—to provide community care for the mentally ill.

In 1963, deinstitutionalization became the federal government's formal policy on mental illness (Gronfein, 1985). The goals were to reduce the inpatient populations of state and county mental hospitals and to provide community-based programs for the care and treatment of the chronically mentally ill (President's Commission on Mental Health, 1978).

Community mental health centers, first proposed in 1963, were fully funded by 1965. They were designed specifically to increase discharges and decrease admissions to state hospitals. Part of their mission was to reduce state hospital populations by 50% in ten years (Gronfein, 1985). It was hoped that community-based treatment programs would replace state institutions, the traditional places of care for the mentally ill for more than 150 years (Winslow, 1982).

The success of community mental health centers has been debated in recent years. Originally, the centers were permitted and even encouraged to ignore the chronically and seriously mentally ill people coming out of the state hospitals, to focus primarily on prevention. By the mid 1970s, the error was realized; it was evident that many homeless and unemployed were former state hospital patients. The centers were unprepared for, underfunded, and slow to address these populations.

In November 1977, the General Accounting Office issued the final report on state mental hospital deinstitutionalization. The report contained little new information on the consequences of the rapid phase out of state mental hospitals. It criticized federal support of the phase out policy and called for immediate action to deal with the needs of the thousands of chronic patients who were released to local communities without adequate provision for their care (Morrissey & Goldman, 1984). There is increasing recent evidence that numbers of the mentally ill are in jails (Lamb, 1984), single rooms of seedy hotels, half-way houses, and single-room-occupancy residential hotels. Forty percent of nursing home residents are mentally ill. Most of these facilities provide inadequate treatment or living quarters. Many mentally ill rely on soup kitchens for food, emergency shelters for lodging, and subway tunnels to escape from the cold. At least 25% of the homeless are mentally ill (Garlnick, 1985; Okin, 1985; Morrissey & Goldman, 1984); however, studies show that severely ill people can live in the community if given adequate services (Braun, Kochansky, Shapiro, 1981; Polak & Kirby, 1976; Kinard, 1981).

The passage of the Mental Health Systems Act of 1980 provided federal funding for state and local agencies to establish community support systems and other community-based mental health services. Although the act represented major reform in the care of chronically mentally ill persons, the ability of these community programs to maintain patients outside state hospitals is not necessarily conclusive evidence of their clinical superiority. Even though some patients seem to experience an increased sense of well-being, it does not prove that their quality of life while living in the community is better than it would be if they were living in state hospitals (Garlnick, 1985).

The tragedy of large numbers of homeless mentally ill in American cities has stimulated renewed debate as to whether deinstitutionalization has failed and should be abandoned as social policy. Several authors suggest revitalizing the state hospital system (Craig & Laska, 1983; Garlnick, 1985).

The Changing Role of the State Mental Institution

Many observations of the current status of state hospitals provide reasons for not having state hospitals as part of the delivery of mental-health care (Pepper & Ryglewicz, 1985). There are, however, reasons for maintaining state hospitals. The changing role of state hospitals is studied from five perspectives—population, quality of care, isolation, funding, and integration.

Population

The population increasingly is dominated by the more difficult and volatile young adult patient group, by "revolving-door" patients, and by the serious nondischargeable mentally ill. Gudeman and Shore (1984) identified five groups of the nondischargeable patients: (1) elderly patients suffering from a combination of dementia, psychosis, and medical illness, making them dangerous to themselves or others; (2) mentally retarded persons with psychiatric illness and assaultive and aggressive behavior—a group not tolerated by community settings; (3) patients with a serious loss of impulse control due to brain damage from head injuries or degenerative diseases; (4) patients with schizophrenia who are unremittingly assaultive and suicidal; and (5) chronically schizophrenic patients who are not acutely dangerous to themselves or others, but exhibit behavior that makes them vulnerable to exploitation.

Over the past five years, young adult admissions to state centers have increased, as have their lengths of stay. Weinstein and Morris (1984) report that patients admitted to state hospitals are admitted sicker, more hostile, and more difficult to treat. Patients age 18 to 44 constitute nearly half of the patients hospitalized for periods of three months to five years. More than 20% of the young adult males admitted now stay three months or longer, a marked increase since 1977. The trend is similar for women, although less pronounced. Former state hospital patients comprise more than 70% of the admissions age 21 to 44. The diagnoses of young patients has changed. Schizophrenia has decreased, while the major affective disorders and other psychoses have increased.

The young adult population is difficult to treat and resists entering the mental health system, as these people are highly mobile and prefer autonomy. Substance abuse is prevalent among them, and the suicide-attempt rate is high. The young adults become alienated from society and are fearful, suspicious, and disorganized (Bachrach, 1982; Lamb, 1984; and Pepper & Ryglewicz, 1985). Populations needing services, therefore, are the young adults between the ages of 18 to 44 who have never been institutionalized and former patients who, as a result of deinstitutionalization, are homeless and chronically mentally ill.

Quality of Care

Current standards of quality of care and legal and medical accountability consume valuable staff time and have made substantial additions in staff necessary in many states. Okin (1985) states that the majority of state facilities are old, barren, and inadequately staffed, and offer only limited programs for patients. The quality of care is not inferior, it simply is the wrong kind of care, in the wrong treatment setting. A survey of all state mental hospitals found that 65% were not in compliance with regulations because they were inadequately staffed or had insufficient nursing coverage to ensure patient safety (Okin, 1983). These deficiencies led to the closing of some state hospitals.

Isolation

It is difficult to provide quality care in a large institution with physically outmoded and deteriorating facilities. In some cases, the administrative structures and clinical methodologies are also outmoded because the institutions have failed to adopt contemporary models of care that are based on up-to-date scientific knowledge (Pepper & Ryglewicz, 1985). Instead of being homelike, these institutions are sterile and faceless. Instead of providing private rooms for patients, they have large wards for 8-20 patients. Instead of giving patients the opportunity to learn to be self-sufficient, thereby increasing their level of functioning, they centralize support services, which is efficient, but permits patients to be passive and dependent (Okin, 1983).

In addition, the geographic remoteness of state hospitals creates barriers to family involvement in treatment. Continuity of care between the state hospital and community programs is either inconsistent or absent and depends on the personal relationships among facilities (Okin, 1985). The facilities and the geographic isolation must change if state hospitals are to improve.

Funding

State hospitals do not enjoy the advantages of a capitation system or a fee-for-service reimbursement system. Unlike health maintenance organizations, they cannot control their use, and their revenues do not increase in proportion to their patient census. Their line-item budget structure makes it impossible to transfer resources from one function to another without permission from another part of the state governmental unit. Line-item budget inflexibility discourages innovation and reduces the ability to change the environment or patient mix (Okin, 1983, 1985).

Inflationary costs place a heavy burden on the state institutional system. As state hospitals consume the major share of state mental health budgets, funds are not available to undertake large-scale modernization of either facilities or programs (Okin, 1982). Funding for the state hospitals cannot be substantially increased because community service programs legitimately require increased state support. This situation is worsened by the present reduction of mental health and other human services funding at the federal level (Pepper & Ryglewicz, 1985).

Integration

In many states and localities the state hospital system is not fully integrated with community services and, therefore, is unable to maintain continuity of care or to plan long-term treatment. Consequently, patients who are chronically mentally ill may be actively treated only for acute problems, spending most of their time in the community as voluntary outpatients (or nonpatients) before again passing through the institution's revolving door (Pepper & Ryglewicz, 1985). Ecklund (1978), Miller (1981) and Bachrach (1986) advocate that state hospitals be accepted as an integral and necessary component of a comprehensive mental health system and that they serve as centers for research, professional training, and continuing education.

A Policy for Continuation of the State Hospital

While a national commitment to deinstitutionalization continues and funds are passed from the national to the state and then to the local level, no clear policy about the role of the state hospital in the delivery of mental health services seems to exist. There are as many valid reasons for closing state hospitals as there are against; however, the need for state hospitals for certain types of patients is recognized.

Despite this ambivalence, there is some support for continuing state hospitals. Keeping patients out of the hospital and in the community does not always prevent chronicity and disability. Even though 80% of first admissions are treated as outpatients in community-based programs, many of these patients progress toward a chronically disabled state, and that number seems to be increasing (Winslow, 1982). Moving patients from state hospitals to the community shifted some of the financial responsibility to the federal government. Unfortunately, many patients were moved to nursing homes and penal institutions. Neither of these settings is less costly to the states or to society, and it has not been proven that more humane care is provided.

Between 1981 and 1983, nearly 500,000 disability beneficiaries, a disproportionate number of whom were mentally ill, were removed from the social security and social disability rolls. This action was designed to save federal resources and shift the cost to the states (Andrulis & Mazada, 1983). It also contributed to increases in the population of homeless mentally ill and created a new demand for admission to state mental hospitals (Goldman & Taube, 1985). Perhaps these individuals need to be evaluated and provided with a safe environment in which to learn skills that will enable them to survive in the community. Okin (1982) stressed a need for state hospitals to care for patients who are simply too disturbed to be treated in the existing community system.

The Diagnosis Related Groups that determine payment rates to hospitals under Medicare could increase the transfer of clients to state mental hospitals. The incentives of this payment system to hospitals are shorter stays, less treatment, multiple admissions, and transfers to other facilities. The implementation of a prospective payment system for psychiatric hospitals is now under study. Use of such a system could reverse the trend toward deinstitutionalization (Goldman & Taube, 1985). This does not imply reinstitutionalization, but rather that deinstitutionalization will stabilize. Greater importance would be placed on functional impairment as it relates to treatment and discharge planning. Length of stay would be determined by functional capacity instead of diagnosis. Prospective payment therefore, would be based on Axis V of the DSM III-R. Axis V determines functional status. Mezzich and Coffman (1985) showed that adaptive functioning is considered an important factor in determining length of hospital stay.

The role of the state institution is changing because the community has failed to provide treatment for new nonschizophrenic young adult populations, to provide services for violent and aggressive patients, or to deal with homeless, and former state hospital mental patients. The literature cited cases of state hospital patients who remained in the state hospitals, but needed discharge planning, treatment, or maintenance of functioning. The primary role of the state hospital would be to treat patients who are too sick to function in the community, to help patients maintain the highest possible level of function, and to offer training programs in community survival skills. These are some of the reasons to support the continuation of the state hospital.

There are indications that the state hospital will survive (Bachrach, 1986), but continue to shrink in size. Perhaps a smaller population will facilitate better care with custodial institutions becoming active treatment settings. A balance between size and population will be achieved in the financing of care. Acute care hospitals will continue to resist treating difficult patient populations.

Essentially, the survival of state hospitals depends on their receiving adequate funding, being integrated into the total mental health service policy, and having a specially trained staff that is able to deliver quality care. If the state hospital is to deliver quality mental health services, the role of the occupational therapist must change.

Role of the Occupational Therapist

The literature clearly pointed out that the treatment focus and services provided by state hospitals needed examination and upgrading. The use of rehabilitative treatment models has proved effective and beneficial to the population most frequently served by psychiatric hospitals (Liberman, Mueser, Wallace, Jacobs, Eckman

& Massel, 1986). The goal of these models is to enhance the level of functioning, encourage adaptation, and provide the least restrictive living environment possible. Occupational therapists can play an important service delivery role in these areas. In state institutions, medication alone cannot provide the teaching and training tools needed to help a patient develop the coping skills required to survive in the community (Liberman & Foy, 1983).

Occupational therapists' educational background and skills make them ideally suited to help patients build the rehabilitative skills necessary to function outside the state hospital. To meet the rehabilitative goals that are needed by this population, the role of occupational therapists in state-run psychiatric hospitals must change.

Currently, occupational therapists in most state hospitals are used as activity providers. In this role, the therapists often provide recreational, diversional, and leisure-time activities. Although woodworking, volleyball, papier-mâché, socials, and ceramics can be very beneficial to patients, depending on the goal, for many receiving only these types of treatment adds to the unreality of institutional life, and deprives them of the opportunity to develop community survival skills.

To be effective, the occupational therapist should focus on providing the rehabilitative service needs that are common to a population in this setting. [He or she] should provide comprehensive, holistic treatment programming in independent living skills training; for example nutritional meal planning, comparative shopping, medication knowledge, money management, and the knowledge of community resources.

Skill building and rehabilitative training should be available to all hospital residents. One approach to delivering these services is through providing programming, whereby patients are referred for training. The patients are assigned to various skill-building classes in a central location. Programs to increase the patients' functional level and provide environmental adaptations, as necessary, must be emphasized. Survival skill training programs for psychiatric patients could lead to reduced hospital recidivism rates and more cost-effective treatment.

Occupational therapists should collaborate with other health care professionals to provide functional assessments and evaluations, particularly during the admission and discharge treatment planning process. A comprehensive functional assessment should be completed on all individuals at the time of hospitalization and prior to discharge. This approach would replace the diagnostic assessment often seen in state hospitals. The functional assessment determines the patient's level of functioning, including strengths and limitations, that will impact treatment. The functional assessment also identifies a patient's independent living skill deficits and

guides the therapist in prioritizing the patient's most urgent treatment needs. Functional assessment findings are directly pertinent to planning and implementing the treatment process (Hargrove & Spaulding, 1988). Hargrove and Spaulding (1988) further report that specific cognitive, attention, psychophysiological, social, and vocational measures may be taken to identify deficits that can become the focus of treatment interventions. The occupational therapist can provide functional assessments for all patients, promoting a holistic and interdisciplinary team approach in addressing rehabilitative programming needs. A functional assessment prior to a patient's discharge assists the treatment team to determine the most appropriate placement for the patient to better ensure the likelihood of community adjustment. It also helps the team identify specific independent living skills that need improvement and provides community mental health agencies with an additional treatment focus for aftercare planning. This specifically relates to Axis V of the DSM III-R.

Because adaptive functioning is an important criterion for discharge into the community, occupational therapists need to work closely with other mental health personnel to identify strengths and impairments in activities of daily living (Fine, 1986). Working closely together, hospital and community mental health personnel provide a continuum of comprehensive services for patients being discharged from state institutions.

The occupational therapist among other qualified professionals, should provide comprehensive vocational services for patients. The literature demonstrates the importance of vocational programs in state hospitals. The absence of work contributes to psychiatric problems (Perfetti & Bingham, 1983; Landau, Neal, Meisner & Prudic, 1980). A correlation exists between job loss and an increase in diagnosed cases of mental illness and use of mental health services (Barling & Handal, 1980; Frank, 1981). The vocational literature stresses the importance of employment in relation to the state hospital population. The opportunity to work decreases psychopathological symptoms and leads to a more normalized lifestyle (Jacobs, Kardashian, Kreinbring, Ponder & Simpson, 1984). In addition, a significant relationship exists between unemployment and psychiatric readmission rates (Franklin, Kittredge & Thrasher, 1975). Rubin and Roessler (1978) report that employment is a major factor in reducing recidivism rates among psychiatric patients. This directly demonstrates that vocational programs are cost-effective in reducing further hospitalizations for individuals with mental illness.

The vocational programs should go beyond interview and job placement. To determine the specific vocational level at which the patient is functioning, a functional

---

analysis should be completed before placing a patient in a vocational environment. The occupational therapist is an appropriate staff member to develop, coordinate, and implement patient vocational programs within the state hospital. Job training for realistic careers that promote skills transferable to community-based employment must be offered to all patients who might benefit from a therapeutic work assignment. Employment skill classes to train patients in job seeking areas, such as completing applications, interviewing, finding job leads, and writing resumes must be provided to assist patients in attaining employment in the community once discharged.

Student occupational therapy internship programs should be a part of all state hospitals' commitment to increase, update, and deliver innovative programs to hospitalized patients. Relationships between hospitals and universities must be strengthened to provide patients and therapists with innovative ideas and programs offered by occupational therapy curricula. The hospitals must become research and training facilities to increase the literature available to professionals working with the chronic mentally ill. If this position were adopted by state institutions, they could provide leadership in the field of mental health. Occupational therapists can provide technical assistance to facilitate this leadership role in state hospitals.

Many occupational therapists in psychiatric hospitals are only able to address the psychological and emotional needs of patients. Physical rehabilitative programs for traumatic brain injuries, cardiovascular accidents, diabetes, amputees, joint dysfunctions, and vision impairments are rarely implemented by occupational therapists in state hospitals. The geriatric population frequently exhibits physically disabling conditions in addition to their psychiatric illness. Occupational therapists could offer this population services, such as positioning techniques, splinting, independence training in grooming and hygiene tasks, feeding and swallowing programs, transfer techniques and, range of motion exercises. Most state hospitals subcontract these services to other professionals who are limited in the programming they are able to provide given their time constraints and caseloads. By using occupational therapists holistically, the patients would receive both the physical and psychological programs necessary for rehabilitation.

Conclusion and Summary

The purpose of this article was to examine the future of state hospitals. The literature indicated that deinstitutionalization has not been completely successful. The goals were to reduce the population of state hospitals and to develop community-based programs. It appears that these two goals were achieved; however, the result is a patient population that continues to be neglected and produces the strongest argument for the continued existence of state hospitals. Deinstitutionalization has not dealt successfully with the chronically mentally ill, the new mentally ill young adult, or the nondischargeable population. These authors take the position that the state hospital must continue to function.

Clearly, treatment methods must change if the state hospital is to survive. The therapist's role also must change from a caretaker to an evaluator, functional capacity assessor, trainer, and community supporter. We suggest that occupational therapists provide leadership and consultation services to change the environment to a place where independence is fostered. Arts and crafts no longer are the state-of-the-art treatment. Treatment should reflect an holistic approach that includes programming in activities of daily living, vocational rehabilitation, and experiences that are relevant to community living.

References

Andrulis, B. & Mazada, N. J. (1983). American mental health policy: Changing directions in the 80s. *Hospital and Community Psychiatry, 34*, 601.

Bachrach, L. (1982). Young adult chronic patients: An analytical review of the literature. *Hospital and Community Psychiatry, 33*, 189.

Bachrach, L. (1986). The future of the state mental hospital. *Hospital and Community Psychiatry, 37*, 467.

Barling, P. & Handal, P. (1980). Incidence of utilization of public mental health facilities as a function of short term economic decline. *American Journal of Community Psychology, 8*, 31-39.

Craig, T. & Laska, E. (1983). Deinstitutionalization and the survival of the state hospital. *Hospital and Community Psychiatry, 34*, 616.

Ecklund, L. (1978). The role of a regional treatment center in a model mental health delivery system. *Hospital and Community Psychiatry, 29*, 379.

Fine, S. (1986). Trends in mental health. In S. Robertson (Ed.), *Scope: Strategies, Concepts, and Opportunities for Program Development and Evaluation* (p. 19). Rockville, MD: The American Occupational Therapy Association, Inc.

Frank, J. (1981). Economic change and mental health in an uncontaminated setting. *American Journal of Community Psychology, 9*, 395-410.

Franklin, J., Kittredge, L., & Thrasher, D. (1975). A survey of factors related to mental hospital admissions. *Hospital and Community Psychiatry, 26*, 749-751.

Goldman, H., Adams, N., & Taube, C. (1983). *Hospital and Community Psychiatry, 34*, 129.

Goldman, H., Taube, C., Regier, D., & Witkin, M. (1983). The multiple functions of the state mental hospital. *American Journal of Psychiatry, 140*, 296.

Garlnick, A. (1985). Build a better state hospital: Deinstitutionalization has failed. *Hospital and Community Psychiatry, 36*, 738.

Gronfein, W. (1985). Incentives and intentions in mental health policy: A comparison of the medicaid and community mental health programs. *Journal of Health and Social Behavior, 26*, 192.

Gudeman, J. & Shore, M. (1984). Beyond deinstitutionalization: A new class of facilities for the mentally ill. *New England Journal of Medicine , 311*, 832.

Hargrove, D. & Spaulding, W. (1988) Training Psychologists to Work with the Chronic Mentally Ill. *Community Mental Health Journal, 24*, 283.

Jacobs, H., Kardashian, S., Kreinbring, R., Ponder, R. & Simpson, A., (1984). A skills oriented model for facilitating employment among psychiatrically disabled persons. *Rehabilitation Counseling Bulletin, 28*, 87-96.

Lamb, H. (1984). Deinstitutionalization and the homeless mentally ill. *Hospital and Community Psychiatry, 35*, 899.

Landau, S., Neal, D., Meisner, M. & Prudic, J. (1980). Depressive symptomology among laid off workers. *Journal of Psychiatric Treatment and Evaluation, 2*, 5-12.

Liberman, R. & Foy, D. (1983). Psychiatric rehabilitation for chronic mental patients. *Psychiatric Annals, 13*, 539.

Liberman, R., Mueser, T., Wallace, C., Jacobs, H., Eckman, T. & Massel, K. (1986). Training skills in the psychiatrically disabled: Learning and competence. *Schizophrenia Bulletin,12*, 631.

Markson, E. (1985). After deinstitutionalization, what? *Journal of Geriatric Psychiatry,18*, 37.

Miller, R. (1981). Beyond the old state hospital: New opportunities ahead, *Hospital and Community Psychiatry, 32*, 29.

Morrissey, J. & Goldman, H. (1984). Cycles of reform in the care of the chronically mentally ill. *Hospital and Community Psychiatry, 35*, 785.

Okin, R. (1982). State hospitals in the 1980s. *Hospital and Community Psychiatry, 33*, 717.

Okin, R. (1983). The future of state hospitals: Should there be one? *American Journal of Psychiatry,140*, 577.

Okin, R. (1985). Expand the community care system: Deinstitutionalization can work. *Hospital and Community Psychiatry, 36*, 742.

Pepper, B. & Ryglewicz, H. (1985). The role of the state hospital: A new mandate for a new era. *Psychiatric Quarterly, 57*, 230.

Perfetti, L. & Bringham, W. (1983). Unemployment and self-esteem in mental refinery workers. *Vocational Guidance Quarterly, 31*, 195-202.

Report to the President from The President's Commission on Mental Health (1978). (Volume 1). Washington, DC: U.S. Government Printing Office.

Rubin, S. & Roessler, R. (1978). Guidelines for successful vocational rehabilitation of the psychiatrically disabled. *Rehabilitation Literature, 38*, pp. 70-74.

Tuason, V., Rair-Riedesel, P. & Hoffmann, N. (1982, November). Effects of deinstitutionalization on acute care psychiatric facilities. *Minnesota Medicine*, 697.

Weistein, A. & Morris, C. (1984). Young chronic patients and changes in the state hospital population. *Hospital and Community Psychiatry, 35*, 595.

Winslow, W. (1982). Changing trends in cmhcs: Keys to survival in the eighties. *Hospital and Community Psychiatry, 33*, 273.

Section II

Strategies for Program Development and Team Collaboration

Introduction

To respond proactively to the issues and trends identified in the preceding section, the occupational therapist must have a solid foundation in program development and team collaboration skills. The knowledge and competence that occupational therapists utilize to provide direct patient care (i.e., evaluation, clinical reasoning, treatment implementation, and reevaluation) can be naturally extended to the development of occupational therapy treatment programs (Ostrow, 1985; Scammahorn, 1985). Competent program planning and development is essential for ensuring that occupational therapy is available to a diversity of patient populations across the entire health care continuum (Ostrow, 1985; Schwartz, 1988).

Effective program planning in today's complex and changing health care system requires occupational therapists to collaborate with other professionals to ensure comprehensiveness and excellence in their provision of professional services (Gilfoyle, 1987). Adequate knowledge and understanding of the roles and functions of other professionals are essential to the development of a close collaborative relationship which will result in the most comprehensive program plan and the best possible treatment outcome for the client (Bonder, 1990; Bonder, 1991; Schwartz, 1988).

The therapist who collaborates with other professionals to plan and implement programs must have a solid foundation in occupational therapy philosophy, theories, frames of reference, and models of practice (Barris, Kielhofner, & Watts, 1983; Fidler, 1991). Ambiguity about occupational therapy's role within an interdisciplinary health care system limits our ability to make a unique and focused contribution to the health care of persons with disabilities (Barris, Kielhofner, & Watts,

1983). Therefore, readers are urged to study and work actively on establishing a strong professional identity based on sound occupational therapy theory and frames of reference. (References for a number of excellent sources on occupational therapy theory, practice models, and frames of reference are provided at the end of this text). The formation of a solid professional identity will enable the occupational therapist to develop treatment programs and collaborative professional relationships that reflect professional excellence and are responsive to the complexities of the current health care system (Bonder, 1991; Fidler, 1991; Gilfoyle, 1987; Schwartz, 1988).

The chapters in this section support the development of excellence in program planning and team collaboration skills based upon a strong foundation in occupational therapy theory. In chapter 7, Grossman and Bortone present a four-step model for program development. Each step is systematically and comprehensively described. The provision of practical suggestions and methodologies for clinical application of this program development model makes the process understandable and manageable.

The clinical application of program development principles based on sound occupational therapy theoretical concepts is expanded upon in chapter 8. Robinson and Avallone review the current challenges affecting occupational therapy practice on acute, inpatient psychiatric units. To meet these challenges effectively, the authors developed a program that clearly defined occupational therapy's role on their unit and provided relevant evaluation and goal-oriented intervention for the inpatient, psychiatric client. Their emphasis on an activities health approach and multidisciplinary collaboration is relevant to a diversity of occupational therapy treatment settings. The provision of clear practical descriptions of each step in the program development process can assist readers in the clinical application of program development principles.

One of the most frequent outcomes of occupational therapy program development is the formation and implementation of occupational therapy treatment groups. In chapter 9, Haiman reviews current health care issues that influence the use of groups in occupational therapy practice. According to Haiman, effective, relevant groups are selected and designed based on a needs assessment and utilize clinical reasoning skills throughout their development and implementation (in contrast to a "cookbook" approach). Based on these principles, Haiman presents a group protocol selection system that readers will find applicable to any clinical setting and patient population that utilizes groups for evaluation and intervention.

The interdisciplinary team approach to patient care is another aspect of the current health care system that is utilized in a diversity of treatment settings. In chapter 10, Reed argues that occupational therapists "armed with a knowledge" of the dynamics and functions of an interdisciplinary team can make significant contributions as either team members or team leaders, which will result in improved patient care and enhanced professional satisfaction. Reed discusses six key issues that are critical to the effectiveness of an interdisciplinary team. These relevant issues are vital for the occupational therapist to consider prior to joining a team as either its leader or as a member of its staff. Addressing these issues proactively will maximize the team's effectiveness and ensure its continued viability.

One of the major issues confronting an interdisciplinary treatment team is the need for an organized, collaborative, client-focused approach to treatment planning. In chapter 11, Lang and Mattson discuss one setting's approach to developing an effective, comprehensive, multidisciplinary treatment plan to replace discipline-specific treatment plans, which had resulted in fragmentation of treatment. The year-long process to develop and implement this treatment plan is clearly and realistically described. Concrete behavioral examples, supplemented by well-designed figures, provide a clear outline of relevant patient problems and goals for the disciplines of occupational therapy and vocational rehabilitation. Implementation of this multidisciplinary treatment plan resulted in numerous benefits for patients and staff, including increased appreciation for the efficacy of activities therapies, more relevant goal formation, and improved collaboration between patients and staff.

The ability of occupational therapists to develop and implement program changes, and to assume leadership roles within their clinical settings, is often dependent upon their communication skills. In this section's last chapter, Robertson and Schwartz define strategic communication and explore this vital link between occupational therapy and the practice setting. Environmental, organizational, and professional factors influencing communication and clinical decision making are explored. Strategies for developing effective communication skills are described. A practice-oriented framework for utilizing strategic communication within a clinical setting is presented. The efficacy of applying strategic communication principles to clinical practice is highlighted by two relevant examples.

The ability of occupational therapists to utilize their unique professional knowledge, along with their effective communication and clinical reasoning skills, to plan treatment programs and assume leadership roles in today's health care system is strongly supported in this section. These issues are further emphasized and expanded upon in section III, which discusses the practice of occupational therapy along the mental health continuum of care.

Questions to Consider

1. How can occupational therapists apply their knowledge and skills in patient care to the development of treatment programs? What are important differences between patient treatment planning and population-focused program planning?

2. What are current issues and trends that influence program planning? What are the essential steps to developing an effective occupational therapy program?

3. How does an occupational therapist's frame of reference influence program planning? Which frames of reference are compatible with the treatment program needs of today's health care system? Which frames of reference(s) would you utilize in developing an occupational therapy program for an acute, inpatient unit? An outpatient, day treatment program? A long-term residential facility?

4. What are current issues and important factors for occupational therapists to consider when designing group interventions? How can the clinical decision making process facilitate the development and selection of relevant group protocols? What clinical reasoning skills are vital to utilize in the implementation and evaluation of therapeutic groups?

5. What are key issues for the occupational therapist to consider prior to joining a treatment team? How can an occupational therapist proac-

tively respond to these issues to enhance a team's functioning, improve patient care, and develop a clear and satisfying professional role?

6. How can occupational therapists increase team collaboration in treatment planning and program implementation? What are the benefits and limits of a multidisciplinary treatment plan as compared to individual discipline-specific treatment plans?

7. What are the issues and factors that influence effective communication within today's health care system? What principles and methods can an occupational therapist utilize to develop strategic communication skills? How can these strategies be applied in a clinical setting to enhance the role of occupational therapy?

References

Barris, R., Kielhofner, G., & Watts, J. H. (1983). *Psychosocial occupational therapy: Practice in a pluralistic arena.* Laurel, MD: RAMSCO.

Bonder, B. (1990). Disease and dysfunction: The value of Axis V. *Hospital and Community Psychiatry, 41*, 959-960, 964.

Bonder, B. R. (Ed.). (1991). *Psychopathology and function.* Thorofare, NJ: Slack.

Fidler, G. (1991). The challenge of change. *Occupational Therapy in Mental Health, 11*(1), 1-11.

Gilfoyle, E. M. (1987). Nationally speaking—creative partnerships: The profession's plan. [Presidential address]. *American Journal of Occupational Therapy, 41*, 779-781.

Ostrow, P. (1985). Strategic planning. In J. Bair & M. Gray (Eds.), *The occupational therapy manager* (pp. 29-48). Rockville, MD: American Occupational Therapy Association.

Scammahorn, G. (1985). Program planning. In J. Bair and M. Gray (Eds.), *The occupational therapy manager* (pp. 49-64). Rockville, MD: American Occupational Therapy Association.

Schwartz, S. C. (1988). Service management strategies for occupational therapy. In S. C. Robertson (Ed.), *Mental health focus: Skills for assessment and treatment* (pp. 1-37—1-43). Rockville, MD: American Occupational Therapy Association.

Chapter 7

Program Development

Judy Grossman, MS, OTR, FAOTA
Jody Bortone, MA, OTR

This chapter was previously published in S. C. Robertson (Ed.), *Mental health scope: Strategies, concepts, and opportunities for program development and evaluation* (pp. 91-99). Rockville, MD: The American Occupational Therapy Association, Inc. (AOTA). Copyright © 1986, AOTA.

To provide mental health services in occupational therapy, the program manager must develop competencies on several levels, grouped under the broad "micro" and "macro" levels of planning. The micro level represents clinical management issues for a patient. The macro level represents programmatic issues for a population. The micro and macro levels actually parallel each other in the sequencing of problem identification, planning, implementation, and outcome. Both patient treatment and population-focused planning require good clinical judgment and analytical skills for assessment and intervention. They differ, however, in some important respects that will be discussed in this chapter.

Micro—Patient	Macro—Population
Screening and evaluation	Needs assessment
	Program planning
Treatment planning	Program implementation
Treatment intervention	Program evaluation and
Reevaluation	quality assurance

The changing nature of mental health services delivery, the needs of chronic mentally ill patients, and the acute staffing shortage are all driving forces behind the need for increased competencies in program development. Good planning skills will have an effect on patient care and career mobility in occupational therapy.

The most critical step in program development is the shift to population-based planning. The objective in developing an occupational therapy program is to design the most effective program for the most people.

There are four basic steps in program development:
1. Needs assessment
2. Program planning
3. Program implementation
4. Program evaluation

Step 1—Needs Assessment: This step involves data gathering and problem identification, including a description of the population to be served and an assessment of the treatment needs and the resources available to meet these needs.

Step 2—Program Planning: This step integrates the treatment needs and resources with theoretical frame(s) of reference. It also establishes goals and objectives for problem-focused planning.

Step 3—Program Implementation: This step focuses on documentation, communication, and coordination with other providers. It also requires the appropriate selection of assessments and interventions for each patient/client.

Step 4—Program Evaluation: This step involves systematic review and analysis of the program based on the established goals and objectives.

Program development is a progressive and cyclical process in which the therapist continually monitors and adjusts the program to meet the needs of the target population. This process is depicted graphically in Figure 1.

Needs Assessment

Needs assessment is very important, yet is often the most overlooked step in program development. Collecting appropriate information about the target population is necessary in order to design an effective program. This

step deserves adequate time and attention.

Needs assessment takes place on several levels from the patient/client level (micro) to the community at large level (macro), as shown in Figure 2.

For example, the occupational therapist will first want information on an identified patient/client. The therapist who is implementing a treatment program will put the most effort into assessing the individual patient/client and the target clinical population of which the patient is a member (for example, a young adult chronic patient in a transitional unit). The therapist will then want to obtain information about the target population in the community in order to locate resources or develop programs for continuity of care (for example, day treatment programs for deinstitutionalized chronically mentally ill patients/clients). Finally, the therapist will want information about the community to which the patient/client will return (the expected environment) and the functional skill requirements that the community will demand. To develop a program in which any patient/client will participate, information must be gathered on all these levels using micro and macro perspectives.

Needs assessment requires a systematic approach to data gathering. The steps in this systematic approach include (a) describing the community, (b) describing the target population, (c) identifying needs, and (d) identifying resources.

Describing the Community

This first step in gathering data for needs assessment is important for planning relevant programs and developing realistic discharge plans. A sensitive therapist should understand the patient's/client's natural environment and the daily routines of community residents. This step involves both quantitative and qualitative data gathering. The following information will be helpful to the therapist during this stage:

1. *Sociodemographic Data on Community Residents*

   These data may include information on age, sex,

Figure 1. Program Development

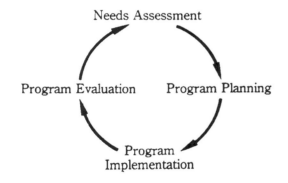

Figure 2. Levels of Needs Assessment

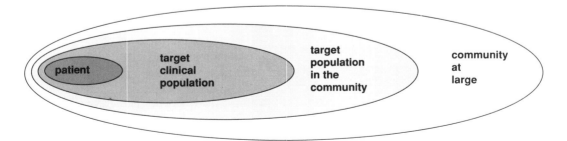

family structure, religious and ethnic background, education, income, occupational level, and employment.

2. *Community Description*

A community description provides information on the physical, social, cultural, and economic factors that are relevant for mental health planning. The physical description of the community should include the boundaries of the geographic area or catchment area, physical landmarks, and the location of essential services. This information relates to the utilization and accessibility of essential services and community resources. The social and cultural description provides information about attitudes, beliefs, expectations, proscribed roles, and standards of behavior. It is critical to appreciate the value system of community residents and the patterns of work and leisure-time activities. An economic description provides information on the power structure in the community, support for essential services, and the economic livelihood of residents.

3. *Community Trends and Populations at Risk*

It is often helpful to have information on community trends, such as the stability or transitional nature of different neighborhoods. While conducting the needs assessment, it is possible to identify populations at risk in the community that may need additional services and resource development. At-risk populations can be defined according to developmental status (e.g., geriatric, adolescent), life crises (e.g., divorce, hospitalization of family member), or chronic strains (e.g., multiproblem families). The identified population for occupational therapy programming may or may not be recognized as one of the high-risk groups.

Describing the Target Population

The second step in gathering information for needs assessment is to define the target population, that is, those people for whom an occupational therapy program is to be designed.

Demographic data must also be gathered on the target population, and it is often helpful to compare these data to the community data. The targeted population may constitute a distinct subgroup in the community or be representative of a particular culture or socioeconomic strata in the community. To conduct population-focused planning, it is helpful to categorize the target population in a way that will emphasize the similarities of the targeted group, such as the diagnosis or prognosis of the illness or disorder or perhaps the level of function. Other useful information that may be collected from medical records is the average length of stay, number of hospitalizations, and level of premorbid functioning.

To develop programs for the target population, it is important to be familiar with the clinical description of the disability. It is necessary to review the theoretical and research literature to understand each disorder and to be alert to significant manifestations, associated signs and symptoms, prognosis, and functional abilities and disabilities.

Identifying Needs

The third step in gathering information for needs assessment is to identify the specific needs of the target population. In many cases, specific treatment needs appear obvious, but a more systematic approach is warranted.

There are different levels of needs. First are the *felt* needs of the patients/clients. While these are not always realistic, they provide the basis for collaboration between the therapist and patient. Within this context, felt needs can be modified or shaped. Occupational therapy personnel should always ask patients about what they need to work on or what they want to get out of the program.

Second are the *perceived* needs reported by others. Occupational therapy personnel may wish to interview or survey department staff, treatment providers in both the present system and the expected environment, or significant others such as family members or teachers. It is important to consider patient/client needs from the perspective of other people.

Third are the *real* needs that describe the true functional abilities and disabilities of the population, as measured by objective evaluation instruments. Therapists must systematically use a battery of evaluation instruments to determine if the patient/client population has a deficiency. For example, 60% of the people may be deficient in work skills, whereas only 20% may not be independent in activities of daily living. It is important to understand the actual and full range of abilities and disabilities of the target population. This information is usually gathered for individual patients/clients and must be synthesized in aggregate form for use in planning occupational therapy programs.

Once needs are assessed, it is helpful to determine any discrepancy between felt and real needs. This process is important to communicate goals and objectives to all people concerned, including the consumer, providers of service, and family members.

The purpose of the needs assessment is to identify *unmet* needs and to categorize them in priority order for planning. To establish priorities, it is necessary to assess how the needs match the expectations of the general population. For example, the feasibility of vocational training in a given job market or the value placed on certain social activities will influence the emphasis placed on meeting certain population needs.

Identifying Resources

The last step in gathering information for needs assessment is to evaluate the resources available for implementing the program. Resources can be categorized as both formal and informal sources of support. *Formal*, or institutional, resources include administrative support: staff, supplies and equipment, space, time, and money. Staff support includes occupational therapy staff, as well as other professional staff.

In evaluating institutional resources, it is important to know what programs exist and whether they are meeting real needs. Some services are offered on an inpatient basis, and others are available after discharge. Analysis of the services provided by the institution should encompass not only those delivered by occupational therapy personnel but also those delivered by other team members.

Some questions to consider in assessing resources are whether services are available, accessible, and effective. The full range of services currently available should be analyzed to determine what real needs have not yet been met. Any gaps in services should become apparent, and these will enter into the formulation of goals and objectives for the occupational therapy program.

It may also be appropriate to identify formal resources in the community such as educational, recreational, health, and social services. Occupational therapy personnel should become familiar with community programs: the referral process, expectations of the agency, and, most important, the ways the program is addressing real needs.

It is also essential to identify *informal* resources to support the program itself or the population it serves. These resources may be either institutional or community-based. They may be advocates of occupational therapy in the hospital, or support personnel who will help implement the occupational therapy program. Social supports such as family, friends, religious and cultural figures, and self-help groups may be identified in the community. The various contributions of informal care givers should also enter into the program planning done by occupational therapy personnel.

Needs Assessment Methods

There are many ways to assess needs. A good place to start is the sociodemographic and descriptive information that is readily available in communities. This information may be found in documents and reports from the U.S. Census Bureau, state and local government, health departments, health planning agencies, community planning boards, mental health associations, research departments of community mental health centers, and universities. These sources can be located through the town hall, local library, and telephone directory. Specific program information may be obtained by contacting facilities directly or the state mental health agency.

Objective information on the community should be supplemented with subjective information. The occupational therapist's personal experience and conversations with community residents, community care givers, social service agencies, and school personnel, for example, may provide a perspective that complements or reinforces the objective assessment.

Objective methods include the use of surveys, key informants, community forums, rates under treatment, and social indicators.

The *survey method* is a reliable and comprehensive way to collect a great deal of information. The survey can involve interview or self-report, and it may be directed to any group, such as the target population, the providers of service, or community residents. For this method, it is important to select a representative sample and to develop a relatively reliable survey.

The *key informant approach* is a method of surveying key people who are in a position to perceive patterns of needs, rather than sampling the entire population. It is simple, less expensive, and less time-consuming than the survey method. There may, however, be bias in the sampling or in the interviewing technique.

The *community forum* is a method that achieves broad representation through panels or public meetings. This approach is most applicable to problems that affect the entire community or significant subgroups. A potential disadvantage of this method is that these groups may not be representative of the community at large and that their opinions may represent a bias.

The *rates under treatment* approach is really a measure of service utilization gathered through records and reports. Caution should be exercised in relying on this approach, since statistics reflect those in treatment and not necessarily those in need.

Social indicators are actually indirect measures of need. Social indicators are social and environmental factors that correlate with mental health problems and are therefore used to predict problems or derive inferences about a population. This type of analysis can be conducted through statistics available through such sources as the U.S. Census Bureau.

Program Planning

After needs have been assessed, the second step in population-based program development is program planning. Program planning uses the information obtained in the needs assessment about the needs of the population and the present resources available to address those needs. To plan a program, one must integrate this information with appropriate frames of reference to establish the program's goals and objectives.

A comprehensive plan for any program will also include the establishment of standards for the program's outcome, a timetable, methods of integrating the program with the existing system, the definition of roles, and the establishment of a referral system that details how people enter and leave the program.

The program planning step is a systematic integration of factual information with theoretical frames of reference in order to define a comprehensive program plan designed to address the needs of the target population in a prescribed sequence. The steps for developing a program plan follow:

1. Defining a focus
2. Adopting frame(s) of reference
3. Establishing goals and objectives
4. Establishing methods to integrate the program into the existing system
5. Developing referral systems

Defining a Focus

The ability to define a focus for a program depends on an analysis of the needs assessment results. The needs assessment will yield a massive amount of information that the program planner must categorize and establish priorities for, so that a focus for the program can be determined.

The *content* focus of a program can be determined by first categorizing the needs (felt and real) identified according to the various occupational performance areas and component skill functions, and then identifying those areas and skills that are deficient for a specific percentage of the target population. Since the intent of program development is to address the unmet needs of the target population, only those skill areas that are deficient for the majority of the target population will be given priority in content focus.

By comparing the functional skill deficit areas with the skill demands of the expected environment, the therapist can identify occupational performance areas and component skill functions that are crucial for the program to address. This list of priorities may then be further refined by evaluating available resources and patterns of use. If the therapist identifies needs that are already being addressed by other resources, it will not be necessary to duplicate those services. Close coordination of services is, however, essential. Occupational therapy should focus the program on needs deficits and skills deficits that are not adequately addressed and that could not be addressed by other resources.

The *level* of difficulty of the occupational performance and component skills addressed in the program must be incorporated into its design. The level of any program is not static, but includes a range of levels so that a larger percentage of the target population can be served. The program can thereby include a coherent sequence by which people can progress through the program with increasing challenge.

The range of levels should begin at the current lowest level of functioning of the clear majority of the target population. The lower, or minimal, functional level of a program is the set of minimal expected behaviors and skills that people must have to enter the program. This level of the program is determined by assessing the real needs of the target population, using assessment and evaluation instruments.

The upper, or maximal, functional level of the program is the set of maximum or most difficult skills and behaviors that can be offered by the program. Again, this level of the program is obtained by assessing felt and perceived needs and is determined by the level of functional skills demanded by the expected environment. The program's content addresses only the needs or functional skills of the target population that are considered deficient in relation to the skill functions at the level demanded by the expected environment.

Adopting Frames of Reference

Frame(s) of reference give the therapist the *criteria* by which findings of the needs assessment can be categorized into content areas and levels. In the context of the program planning stage, however, the therapist must now evaluate and choose the frames of reference that are most likely to be successful in addressing and resolving the needs that constitute the program's focus.

Reevaluating and selecting alternative frames of reference can be systematically completed by paying attention to three basic considerations. First, therapists must consider their own experiences and familiarity and comfort with the various occupational therapy frames of reference. Second, therapists must be familiar with relevant clinical and research literature that will offer guidelines about those frames of reference found helpful in addressing specific functional needs of specific populations. Finally, it is essential that the therapist have a thorough understanding of the frames of reference that are used and emphasized in the institution or treatment system.

It is important for the occupational therapist to be familiar with a variety of frames of reference. For example, therapists who develop a program based only on a frame of reference with which they are familiar may indeed develop a perfectly balanced program according to that frame of reference. But this program may not specifically address the needs of the target population, or it may include treatment approaches that have been found to be ineffective with the target population. It may also be a program that, by its very design, constantly conflicts with the rest of the treatment system.

A review of the clinical and research literature may validate the therapist's choice of a particular frame of reference and/or may pinpoint new frames of reference that the therapist should understand and incorporate into the program design.

The occupational therapist must consider the frames of reference used and considered primary by the institutional system. It is important to select a frame of reference for the occupational therapy program that is compatible with those of the institutional system. Each profession has its own frames of reference. Compatible definitions of a functional or dysfunctional state may differ among professions, and treatment goals and methodologies differ. Major conflicts in the system's and a program's frame of reference may place the program and its therapists in a difficult position.

Establishing Goals and Objectives

Establishing goals and objectives is the next step in developing a program plan. The goals and objectives of the treatment program are specifically related to the focus of the program The goals should be problem-oriented and should be described in behavioral terms, specifying the level of performance expected at the outcome. Goals should paint a clear picture of what patients/clients will be able to do once they complete the program.

When establishing treatment goals for patients/clients in the program, it is also important to establish standards for the program as a whole. In this way, quality assurance becomes an integral part of the overall program plan. Standards should project the acceptable percentage of the target population that is served by the program, the percentage of patients/clients who enter and complete the program, and the percentage of patients/clients who actually reach the goals. Such standards need to be set during the program planning stage. By establishing standards ahead of time, the therapist will have guidelines for documenting information in order to evaluate the efficacy and efficiency of the program over an extended period. Goals and standards are crucial to any program evaluation and must therefore be established in the planning phase.

Establishing Methods to Integrate the Program

The next step in program planning describes exactly how the program will be integrated into the existing treatment system. It involves the establishment of time-tables and the definition of therapists' roles and areas of collaboration with other professionals. The identification of potential obstacles to the implementation of the program and of key resources that could be helpful in implementation is also essential.

The first part of this integration process is the establishment of a realistic timetable. This timetable should show when the program will be implemented and in what sequence. In establishing this timetable, it is desirable to involve professional groups within the system who are key to the success or failure of the program.

Definition of the roles of various disciplines is the second part of this integration process. Roles should be defined in accordance with professional competencies and affiliations. The success or failure of a program depends on appropriate staff assignments.

Definition of roles may well include areas of collaboration with other professionals when appropriate. Consultation among professionals and co-leadership of program components should be considered carefully and should be formally established only when suited to the program's focus. For example, one component of a program for alcohol abusers might be to help them develop more appropriate parenting skills with their children. An occupational therapist and a social worker might collaborate on this process. The social worker provides expertise in family therapy and the occupational therapist provides expertise in interpersonal skill development through purposeful activities with their children.

The final consideration in integrating a program is identifying potential obstacles to implementation. Conflicts over professional turf and competition for patients'/clients' time could interfere with the implementation of the best-planned program. Once obstacles have been identified, program developers should then find ways to deal with these obstacles *before* the program is implemented. Once again, collaboration with other professional groups is beneficial.

Developing Referral Systems

The final step in designing a new program is the development of patient/client referral systems. Mechanisms must be designed that establish how people enter a program, how they move through the program, and how they will be discharged from the program. Referral systems require the integration of the micro and macro levels of planning. A referral system must account for the needs of each person and must offer a mechanism by which each patient/client is able to have a complete program suited to his or her own needs and goals.

Referral systems include four basic components: evaluation protocols, criteria for entry into the program, criteria for entering and leaving each level of the program, and exit or discharge criteria.

Evaluation protocols include all evaluation instruments and procedures that will be completed for each patient/client. The purpose of having a standardized protocol is twofold: (1) to standardize the kinds of information obtained, and (2) to determine the appropriate treatment program for each person.

Criteria for entry into the program may include some procedural prerequisites as well as minimum expected behaviors and functional skill levels. Criteria for entering and leaving each level of the program will also be necessary so that both the patient/client and therapist know when advancement through the program is appropriate.

Finally, exit or discharge criteria are necessary to determine when the maximum gain has been achieved. Exit criteria are defined by the goals of the program. Usually, when a person has achieved the goals described for the program, he or she has met the exit criteria.

Program Implementation

Program implementation is the third step in developing a program. It includes not only the actual implementation of the program plan but also the documentation, communication, and coordination.

Implementation of the program plan involves starting the program and its components according to the timetable and sequence described in the planning stage.

An important part of program implementation is documentation of what is going on in the program and how the program is being used. Documentation leads to program evaluation. To document the program, the therapist will have to gather statistics to assess the efficacy and efficiency of the program and to evaluate whether the program goals and standards have been achieved. Specific guidelines on what and how to document are fully discussed in the literature on quality assurance. Items that may be documented include the following:

1. The total number of patients/clients evaluated
2. The percentage of the target population referred into the program
3. The percentage of patients/clients referred into the program who remained until discharge (vs. those who dropped out before discharge)
4. Use of the therapists' time: hours in direct patient/client care, hours in indirect patient care, and so forth
5. Administrative and supervisory time
6. The percentage of the target population served by the program

To maintain a program, communication and coordination are required within the occupational therapy department and among other parts of the institutional system. Those who develop and implement the program must continually monitor and identify obstacles as they occur, communicate about them internally, and coordinate problem-solving efforts.

Program Evaluation

The aim of program evaluation is to measure the effects of a program against the goals it is designed to accomplish. The objective is to improve programming. Program evaluation guides the decision-making process by providing data that will help determine if programs should be continued, discontinued, or changed. The purpose of program evaluation is to answer program-related questions, such as what the best intervention is, who benefits from the program, what the optimum program duration is, and what the best format is for the program.

The initial stage of program evaluation begins with the development of clear, specific, and measurable goals and objectives. In stating goals, it is critical to be specific rather than general and to state goals in terms of behavioral change. Determination of the measures for the goals and objectives of the program occurs early in the development process and must be directly aligned with the program itself.

Program goals are actually measures of outcome, such as improved functional capacity, improved role functioning, or improved coping or social skills. The most common outcome measures in mental health are recidivism and employment figures, but these are gross indications of function. Other measures of outcome cited in the literature include the degree of independent living, level of symptomatology, social behavior, skill gain, patient/client satisfaction with services, and cost-effectiveness. A good program evaluation study typically includes multiple outcome measures.

Several specific steps for conducting program evaluation are described below:

1. Description of program goals and objectives. Differentiation between short- and long-term goals should be the first step in deciding on meaningful outcome criteria.
2. Description of program inputs that include, for example, the type of program or intervention, staff, population served, location, and length of treatment.
3. Design of the evaluation study. All forms of research design are appropriate depending on the nature of the study, such as descriptive, quasi-experimental, case study, or time-series design.
4. Selection of methods of collecting information,

such as the interview, the questionnaire, the observation, tests, and the record review. The method selected will depend on the nature of the study and the characteristics of the sample.

5. Analysis and reporting of the results and limitations of the study. The results may be used to support the efficacy of occupational therapy intervention.

Conclusion

The four basic steps of program development, as described in this chapter, constitute a working model for occupational therapy personnel employed in institutional or community-based settings. Program development is an ongoing process, each step of which contributes to overall program effectiveness. Inherent in this process is a clear and well-defined view of the role of occupational therapy in the selected setting. It also requires appropriate collaboration with other service providers to create well-designed and specifically targeted programs. This model of program development can be used by all occupational therapy personnel to improve existing programs and/or to create new programs.

Strauss, J. S., & Carpenter, W. T. (1977). Prediction of outcome in schizophrenia. *Archives of General Psychiatry, 34,*159-163.

Struening, E. L., & Guttentag, M. (Eds.). (1975). *Handbook of evaluation research* (Vol. 2). New York: Sage Publications. Ch. 1.

Weiss, C. H. (1983). Evaluation research in the political context. In E. Struening & M. Brewer (Eds.) *Handbook of evaluation research* (pp. 31-43). New York: Sage Publications.

Weiss, C. (1972). *Evaluation research: Methods of assessing program effectiveness.* Englewood Cliffs, NJ: Prentice Hall.

Williamson, J. W., Ostrow, P. C., & Braswell, H. R. (1981). *Health accounting for quality assurance: A manual for assessing and improving outcomes of care.* Rockville, MD: American Occupational Therapy Association.

Resources

Anthony, W. A., Cohen, M. R., & Vitalo, R. (1978). The measurement of rehabilitation outcome. *Schizophrenia Bulletin, 4,* 365-383.

Bachrach, L. (1984). Principles of planning for chronic psychiatric patients: A synthesis. In J. Talbott (Ed.), *The chronic mental patient: Five years later.* New York: Grune and Stratton.

Braun, P., Kochansky, G., Shapiro, R. (1981). Overview: Deinstitutionalization of psychiatric patients: A clinical review of outcome studies. *American Journal of Psychiatry, 138,* 736-749.

Cubie, S. H., Kaplan, K. L., & Kielhofner, G. (1985). Program development. In G. Kielhofner (Ed.), *A model of human occupation* (pp. 156-176). Baltimore, MD: Williams and Wilkins.

Frey, W. R. (1985). Planning is a continuous process. *Occupational Therapy Forum, 1*(23), 20-21.

Kamis. (1981). Sound of target compassion: Assessing the needs of and planning services for deinstitutionalized clients. In *Planning for Deinstitutionalization: A Review of Principles, Methods, and Applications.* Human Services Memograph No. 28, 23-33.

Morrissey, J. P., & Goldman, H. H. (1984). Cycles of reform in the care of the chronically mentally ill. *Hospital and Community Psychiatry, 35,* 785- 792.

Suchman, E. A. (1968). *Evaluative research: Principles and practice in public service and social action programs.* New York: Russell Sage Foundation.

Chapter 8

An Activities Health Approach to Program Development

Anne Mazur Robinson, MA, OTR
Joan Avallone, MS, OTR

The activities that we do every day provide a foundation for our lives. Psychiatric illness often interferes with a person's ability to perform the activities that are part of everyday living. When one considers the kinds of symptoms that psychiatric patients exhibit (e.g., disturbances in thinking, judgment, reality testing, and communication; social withdrawal, anhedonia, and dysphoria), problems in daily functioning are not surprising. Functional difficulties are most severe when symptoms are exacerbated to the extent that hospitalization is required.

It is a widely accepted assumption in the mental health field that psychiatric illness has an impact on day-to-day functioning. It has been observed that in the course of patient assessments professionals from virtually all of the disciplines involved in the treatment of psychiatric inpatients comment on the degree to which these patients are able to carry out daily activities. Reasons for hospitalization are often described in terms of the person's inability to function adequately in the community, and improvement in psychiatric status is often first noted in improved hygiene and grooming, improved orientation to unit routines, a greater ability to keep one's hospital room orderly, and more appropriate social interactions.

The gradual shortening of lengths of stay for psychiatric inpatients has raised important questions about the role of occupational therapy in acute, short-term hospital settings. Occupational therapists, who are concerned with the improvement of daily functioning, are often frustrated by the lack of time available for treating long-standing functional problems (Jackson, 1984; Short, 1984). Given the realities of briefer stays in inpatient settings, how can the role of the occupational therapist best be defined? What kind of program would meet the overall occupational therapy objectives for patients at the acute stage of psychiatric care?

In this article, we will address these questions by briefly reviewing the changing patterns of service provision affecting inpatient psychiatry and by discussing the implications for the practice of occupational therapy in short-term hospital settings. We will then describe a model for occupational therapy practice in short-term, acute inpatient psychiatry that is in its early stages of development at the 100-bed inpatient service of the Department of Psychiatry at St. Vincent's Hospital and Medical Center of New York. Included is a step-by-step approach to program development that can be applied to a variety of inpatient psychiatric settings.

Changing Patterns of Inpatient Hospitalization

Since the deinstitutionalization of chronic psychiatric patients began in the 1970s, there has been a movement toward shortening lengths of stay in most psychiatric facilities. With lengths of stay hovering at 30 days and under, diagnostic assessment, control of acute symptoms, and early discharge planning have logically assumed the greatest priority. The implementation of a prospective payment system in inpatient psychiatry (Scherl, English, & Sharfstein, 1988) will probably shorten hospitalizations even further. The results of a survey of New Jersey psychiatrists who have worked with a diagnosis-related groups system indicate that the primary impact on practice has been the increased pressure to discharge and refer. The psychiatrists noted that the inpatient milieu treatment model is being replaced by a model focused on crisis intervention, management of symptoms, and discharge of patients who are often at lower levels of functioning than previously (Sargent, Scherl, & Muszynski, 1988). Even in states where prospective payment systems have not yet been instituted, the priorities of short-term inpatient settings are quite similar.

Reasons for reductions in length of stay go beyond economics. Outcome research has suggested that patients resume adult roles in the community more quickly following short-term hospitalizations, perhaps because the person's identity is maintained (Talbott & Glick, 1988). Length-of-stay studies have demonstrated no advantage for chronic schizophrenic patients treated for 30 to 90 days as compared with treatment periods of under 30 days (Talbott & Glick, 1988). However, it is noted in the literature that although the evidence suggests that there are advantages to briefer hospitalizations, follow-up outpatient treatment in day programs is seen as an important factor in the promotion of successful outcomes with this chronic psychiatric population (Talbott & Glick, 1988). This finding underscores the importance of careful assessment of the kinds of outpatient services the chronic psychiatric patient needs, in order to effectively address more long-term functional problems.

Dilemmas Inherent in Inpatient Occupational Therapy Practice

The acute exacerbation of chronic psychiatric illness often results in the deterioration of the patient's ability to adequately fulfill roles assumed in everyday living. Because the physical environment, sociocultural surroundings, and pattern of activities of an inpatient psychiatric unit bear little resemblance to everyday living, and because the very nature of each activity changes when separated from its natural context, hospitalized patients lose contact with the familiar activities associated with life roles, which compounds the role dysfunction that is often triggered by the exacerbation of symptoms. Addressing issues of daily functioning in an inpatient setting therefore presents a fundamental challenge to the occupational therapist.

Guiding Principles and Overall Objectives

The approach to inpatient occupational therapy programming presented in this article incorporates the concept of *activities health*, which is based on the premise that health in an activities sense (or function) is possible even in the presence of a chronic illness. Activities health has been defined as a state of being in which a person is able to perform the activities of everyday living in ways that are comfortable, satisfying, and socioculturally acceptable (Cynkin & Robinson, 1990). The distinction between an activities health approach and more traditional approaches may be difficult to discern at the start. The primary difference lies in the degree of emphasis on diagnosis and symptoms. In a more traditional approach, the amelioration of symptoms is often a major focus of intervention. In an activities health approach, symptoms are of concern only insofar as they interfere with the patient's ability to achieve activities health. For a particular patient, for example, a traditional approach might be to identify symptom-specific needs such as increased concentration, socialization, and self-esteem. In an activities health approach the therapist would assess the patient's ability to perform activities needed for the particular roles to be assumed in particular environments after discharge in ways that are comfortable, satisfying, and socioculturally acceptable. Thus, an activities health approach emphasizes the importance of understanding both the typical patterns of activities as they occur in the patient's everyday life and the inextricable connections that exist between the activities and the natural contexts in which they take place (i.e., time, place, and sociocultural surroundings).

Given the hospitalized person's need to remain in

contact with familiar activities associated with life roles and the limitations that are present when addressing activities-related problems out of context, the objectives of occupational therapy in acute, short-term inpatient treatment are as follows:

1. Provide the patient with a normalizing, structured routine, integrating meaningful activities from the various aspects of daily living (i.e., self-care, chores, work, leisure, sleep).
2. Provide opportunities for the patient to participate in daily simulations of activities associated with his or her roles outside of the hospital, to maintain partial contact with the roles to be resumed after discharge.
3. Monitor the degree to which treatment interventions (e.g., medication, behavioral management) are affecting the patient's ability to manage everyday activities in the milieu. The treatment team can use this information as one of many indicators of the patient's recovery from an acute episode.
4. Obtain information about the patient's roles and daily routine outside the hospital. This includes the identification (with the patient) of those aspects of his or her activities life that are in need of change.
5. Make recommendations to the treatment team regarding the kinds of services the patient will need upon discharge to improve everyday functioning, and convey assessment findings and long-term occupational therapy goals to the agency to which the patient is referred.

The inpatient occupational therapy program is viewed as a point of entry into a long-term progression toward a more desirable state of activities health—a progression that is likely to extend well beyond the inpatient stay if the goal is to be fully achieved. The patient's ability to manage activities in a hospital situation does not necessarily indicate an ability to do similar activities within the context of everyday living. Recognizing this fact helps the inpatient therapist provide more accurate functional assessments, because it brings a clearer understanding of what can and cannot be inferred from observations of patients on an inpatient unit. Once what can and cannot be accomplished in a hospital setting is understood, it becomes incumbent upon the therapist to consider and make provision for the steps that need to be taken after discharge to help the patient integrate gains made in treatment into everyday life outside the hospital. Thus, functional assessment and participation in discharge planning are integral parts of the inpatient occupational therapist's role.

The Programming Process

The following is a step-by-step approach to inpatient program development for an acute setting, to be followed once the objectives of occupational therapy at this level of care have been established.

Step 1: Assessing the Population and Setting

The patient population can be systematically assessed from two general perspectives: (a) characteristic lifestyles and (b) level of functioning (i.e., the degree to which the patient's psychiatric disturbance is affecting his or her performance of everyday activities).

First, the commonalities and variations of lifestyle within the group are examined to determine what aspects are characteristic of the population as a whole. Such information can be gathered from a variety of sources, including historical information from current and previous hospital records, verbal reports from other team members, and informal or formal interviews with the patient. All of this information is used together to determine the demographics of the population, the range of roles that the patients in any given setting are likely to assume outside the hospital, the specific activities required for these roles, and the prevailing norms and expectations of the sociocultural groups to which the patients belong. The Activities Health Assessment (Cynkin & Robinson, 1990) can be adopted to provide a means of eliciting information about commonalities and variations in the patients' activities lives.

The group's clinical status must also be assessed, including range of diagnoses, severity of symptoms, and level of functional abilities. Assessments administered by other team members (e.g., psychological reports, mental status examinations, nursing and social work assessments) can be used in conjunction with occupational therapy assessments designed to measure cognitive skills (Allen, 1988), social interaction skills (Mosey, 1986), and other specific components of activities performance.

Step 2: Assessing the Clinical Setting

In addition to analysis of the patient population, the characteristics of the clinical setting are examined, so that the programs that are planned can realistically be implemented given the existing unit structure and interdisciplinary goals. The therapist specifically investigates unit routines, the potential for modifying components of the routines (e.g., mealtimes, wake-up times, and procedures), and opportunities and limitations regarding the use of a variety of hospital and community environments.

Once all of this information has been gathered, efforts can be directed toward planning a program in collaboration with other disciplines that is meaningful to the patients, socioculturally relevant, realistic in view of the patients' levels of functioning, and feasible in view of the resources and limitations of the clinical setting.

Step 3: Determining the Overall Structure

In the context of everyday living, activities occur not as isolated events but in rhythms and patterns that are typical of each person. Therefore, to provide patients with an "orderly rhythm in the atmosphere . . . [to help them] become attuned to the larger rhythms of night and day" (Meyer, 1922/1977, p. 641), it is critical for milieu activities to be sequenced and timed in ways that are representative of out-of-hospital living. Similarly, it is important that opportunities be available for patients to participate in activities both alone and with others— again, in keeping with general patterns of everyday activities.

The unit schedule is best conceptualized as a 24-hour, 7-days-a-week sequence of activities. Consequently, it takes into account the patient's activities around the clock, even beyond the limits of the occupational therapist's workday. Collaboration with the nursing staff in designing the unit program is therefore an essential ingredient in this programming approach. The activities program in the milieu can be seen as a simulation of a group (or sociocultural) activities pattern, in which activities are arranged in rhythms and patterns that are typical of their at-home schedules. This provides opportunities to interweave activities in socioculturally relevant sequences. Such an activities pattern can be used to restore a sense of balance, structure, and variety in the patients' daily routines, while also providing opportunities for the assessment of each person's performance of activities. Because virtually all patients carry out activities that fall into the general categories of self-care, chores, work (or its analogue), leisure, and sleep, the program can be designed so that patients are expected to carry out familiar, relevant activities from each of these areas of everyday living, timed and sequenced whenever possible in keeping with life outside of the hospital. Examples will be described later in this paper.

Obviously, it is impossible to create a program that is representative of the specific activities pattern for each patient. Therefore, in addition to structuring communal activities that are relevant to the population as a whole, the occupational therapy program must also include means of examining the activities life of each person, including the exploration of the degree to which and ways in which each patient's psychiatric symptoms interfere with the performance of routine activities outside of the hospital. The rapid turnover of patients that is characteristic of short-term settings requires that the methods selected be efficient ones. Examples are discussed under Step 4.

Thus, the two major program components described above—providing opportunities for involvement in normalizing activities in the milieu and gathering lifestyle information from each patient—can be used together to achieve the overall occupational therapy objectives discussed earlier. Ultimately, it is the occupational therapist's job to systematically put all of this information together to make predictions about each patient's readiness to return to the demands of everyday living and to identify the kinds of supports and services that will be needed for successful functioning in the community.

Step 4: Determining Program Specifics

Once the program's overall structure has been established, appropriate activities can be selected and integrated into the schedule. Selected portions of the occupational therapy program at St. Vincent's Hospital are described as an example. These program developments are not in their final form; they represent the beginning of efforts to program activities in ways that specifically address the overall occupational therapy objectives identified. The descriptions are included for purposes of illustration and are not intended to be a blueprint for successful inpatient programming. As indicated earlier, it is important to arrive at a program design that is specific to the population of patients in each unique clinical setting.

Functional assessment. To assess each patient's degree of activities health, the occupational therapist gathers information from a variety of sources. Information presented on admission helps the occupational therapist begin to formulate a picture of the person's activities pattern, both at his or her optimal level of functioning and immediately prior to admission. As information is collected from the patient and significant others by various team members after admission, it can also be used to identify the roles that the patient has assumed by choice or necessity and the factors influencing success in carrying out these roles (Barris, Kielhofner, & Watts, 1983; Miller, 1988). From this information, the occupational therapist can then identify the performance components required for each of the activities needed for successful daily living (Mosey, 1986).

The patient is a necessary source of information for the assessment of activities health. The Activities Health Assessment provides a graphic pattern of the patient's activities life, which is used to explore the person's own perception of his or her lifestyle. The assessment begins with the graphic reconstruction of the patient's weekly activities schedule when at baseline and before admission. Once the pattern has been obtained, the patient is asked to categorize each activity (i.e., work, leisure alone, leisure with others, sleep, chores, self-care) and color-code it. This graphic pattern is used as the point of reference for an interview about the patient's activities life, which culminates in the patient's rating of his or her degree of overall satisfaction, overall comfort, and sense of sociocultural fit. Thus, the Activities Health Assessment is used to (a) identify those activities that are part of everyday living, (b) explore the patient's perception of specific activities, and (c) determine his or her degree of activities health.[1]

The milieu program. Each patient is given a schedule at the time of admission, including all prescheduled appointments, groups, and meetings he or she is expected to attend. Staff members from other disciplines are asked to refer to the patient's schedule when discussing appointment times, thereby reinforcing the importance of the schedule. The schedules are used as a point of departure for a Time Management Group, where the patients address difficulties in organizing time in concrete, specific terms, rather than in an abstract, hypothetical way. The ability to use a daily schedule, which is actually a representation of the various appointment books on which so many people passionately rely, is one important predictor of the patient's ability to return to work or participate in a day program following discharge.

Patients' ability to care for themselves and for their environment is monitored by observing them as they carry out their sequence of self-care activities and as they perform chores to maintain order in the environment. Such observations have traditionally been part of the nursing staff's assessment. To complement the nursing assessment, occupational therapy cooking groups are used to provide opportunities for patients to participate in yet another set of activities associated with a universal activity—eating. Information obtained during cooking groups is used to assess a patient's ability to assume partial or complete responsibility for the preparation of meals after discharge. Whenever feasible, cooking groups are held at mealtime, so that they retain as much reality as possible. Cooking, like many other activities, is both preceded and followed by a sequence of other related activities, so these related activities are also incorporated to the extent possible. Meal planning, budgeting, shopping for supplies, setting the table, eating, clearing the table, and washing the dishes are some of the antecedent and consequent activities inextricably tied to the activity of meal preparation.

Depending on each patient's living situation in the community, he or she may assume anywhere from no responsibility to total responsibility for preparing meals at home. Patients who live with their families may not prepare the whole meal, but may be responsible for a related task like setting the table or cleaning up. On the other hand, a patient who lives in a group residence may not be involved in any of the meal preparation activities, but may simply be served food and be expected to eat meals with other residents. The therapist focuses on each patient's ability to engage in the activity in the way that will be required of him or her in the community.

Some of these related activities are rather easily simulated; others, like shopping, present logistical problems. More realistic activities will be substituted during the outpatient stage of treatment.

The use of leisure time is frequently an area in which dysfunction is evident. To address this aspect of everyday living, both group and individual activities are used. Supplies for individual pursuits are made available (e.g., books, needlecrafts, stationery, games) so that the ability to plan leisure activities and follow through on such plans can be assessed. Leisure-planning groups conducted by the recreational therapist are used both for the planning of leisure time while the patient is in the hospital and for formulating long-term leisure plans that the patient can pursue after discharge. To obtain accurate leisure assessment information, it is critical that the materials supplied be relevant to the patients' lives outside the hospital. The tile trivits and ashtrays that unfortunately have proliferated in psychiatric settings are, therefore, to be avoided.

Physical exercise, which is widely viewed as a valuable activity for psychological and physical well-being, is also integral to the program. For some, exercise is perceived as self-care; for others it is considered leisure; still others classify it as a chore. Regardless of individual perceptions, exercise experiences are structured and conducted in much the same format as the classes that are popular in the community, although they are markedly less physically demanding. An adapted exercise program (Avallone, 1986) can either provide an introduction to an activity that may be of benefit upon discharge or can help reacquaint a patient with an activity that is, or has been, a part of everyday living for him or her.

Finally, the expressed interest of some patients in returning to a previous job or seeking new employment upon discharge must be reality-tested. Assessment of vocational readiness is particularly difficult in an inpatient setting, because it is impossible to replicate in a supportive institutional setting the kinds of pressures and environments that are characteristic of the workplace. Therefore, the patient's work history is used as the primary means of predicting whether or not the person will be able to work once acute symptoms are relieved.

---

[1] Some will note that the Activities Health Assessment bears a resemblance to the Barth Time Construction (Barth, 1978), in that they both use an activities configuration as a point of departure. An analysis of both instruments, however, reveals differences in purpose, design, and kind of information elicited.

For those patients who express the desire to work immediately after discharge, group activities (such as unit bake sales and patient-run thrift shops) can be used to supplement the examination of the patient's work history. These vocationally oriented groups are also valuable for patients for whom work is a long-term goal; they serve as preliminary work simulations for such patients and are used to monitor the patient's work-related and interpersonal skills, activities, habits, and attitudes.

Summary

This approach to occupational therapy in short-term psychiatric inpatient settings has been developed in response to questions that we and other occupational therapists have grappled with regarding our role in acute settings. Many persons, both inside and outside the field of occupational therapy, have an ample knowledge base yet have difficulty articulating the contribution that can be made at this level of care.

This approach is not revolutionary; clearly, some occupational therapists have already been assuming some of these roles and functions in their practice, and some occupational therapists have included therapeutic activities similar to those we have described. What is unique about this approach, however, is its emphasis on incorporating into treatment programs an understanding of activities as phenomena in and of themselves, paying attention to when, why, where, and how they occur in the course of everyday life. Also distinctive is the lack of emphasis on psychiatric diagnosis and symptoms per se; they are of concern only as they relate to the person's capacity to achieve activities health. This kind of perspective on activities helps the therapist to design simulations of everyday activities that are representative of the contents in which they naturally occur and focus individual functional assessments on the activities required to fulfill roles assumed outside the hospital. Efforts are directed toward structuring the inpatient milieu to (a) have as normalizing a routine as possible, (b) promote engagement in everyday activities, and (c) provide a means of assessing the person's ability to resume everyday life roles following discharge.

By maintaining an awareness of the inextricable connections between activities and the contexts in which they occur, the therapist can also be clear about the conclusions that can and cannot be drawn about the patient's functioning in the hospital. Functional assessment in an inpatient setting provides a valuable starting point, but it cannot be seen as a definitive predictor of functioning after discharge. Because the ultimate goal is to produce changes in patients' activities patterns, it is critical that discharge plans for those patients in need of further occupational therapy services include means for assessment of actual functioning in their everyday environments and means for helping patients carry over into the community gains made in the hospital.

Thus, if occupational therapy services in acute inpatient psychiatric care are understood as the initial steps of what is often a long-term progression toward greater activities health, both the therapist and the patient can direct their efforts toward attaining objectives that are meaningful and attainable within a brief stay. The role of the inpatient occupational therapist is a vital one, because the therapeutic process sets the stage for the postdischarge phases of treatment that ultimately can help the patient achieve a better quality of everyday living, even in the presence of chronic psychiatric illness.

Acknowledgments

We credit Simme Cynkin, MS, OTR, FAOTA, for many of the ideas that underlie this approach, and we thank her and Linda Silber, MA, OTR, for their valuable feedback during the writing of this article.

References

Allen, C. K. (1988). Occupational therapy: Functional assessment of the severity of mental disorders. *Hospital and Community Psychiatry, 39*(2), 140-142.

Avallone, J. (1986). *Any body can.* Los Angeles: Framework Books.

Barris, R., Kielhofner, G., & Watts, J. (1983). *Psychosocial occupational therapy practice in a pluralistic arena.* Laurel, MD: RAMSCO.

Barth, T. (1978). *Barth time construction.* New York: Health Related Consulting Services.

Cynkin, S., & Robinson, A. M. (1990). *Occupational therapy and activities health: Toward health through activities.* Boston: Little, Brown.

Jackson, G. (1984). Short-term psychiatric treatment: How will occupational therapy adapt? *Occupational Therapy in Mental Health, 4*, 11-17.

Meyer, A. (1977). The philosophy of occupational therapy. *American Journal of Occupational Therapy, 31*, 639-642. (Reprinted from the Archives of Occupational Therapy, 1922, *1*, 7-10).

Miller, B. R. J. (1988). Gary Kielhofner. In B. R. J. Miller, K. Sieg, F. Ludwig, S. Shortridge, & J. van Deusen (Eds.), *Six perspectives on theory for the practice of occupational therapy* (pp. 169-204). Rockville, MD: Aspen.

Mosey, A. C. (1986). *Psychosocial components of occupational therapy.* New York: Raven.

Sargent, S. C., Scherl, D. J., & Muszynski, J. D. (1988). The New Jersey experience with diagnosis-related groups. In D. Scherl, J. T. English, & S. Sharfstein (Eds.), *Prospective payment and psychiatric care.* Washington, DC: American Psychiatric Association.

Scherl, D., English, J. T., & Sharfstein, S. (Eds.). (1988). *Prospective payment and psychiatric care*. Washington, DC: American Psychiatric Association.

Short, J. (1984). Changing role expectations of psychiatric occupational therapists. *Occupational Therapy in Mental Health, 4,* 19-27.

Talbott, J. A., & Glick, I. D. (1988). The inpatient care of the chronic mentally ill. In J. R. Lion, W. N. Adler, & W. L. Webb, Jr. (Eds.), *Modern hospital psychiatry* (pp. 352-370). New York: Norton.

Chapter 9

Selecting Group Protocols: Recipe or Reasoning?

Susan Haiman, MPS, OTR/L

The health care delivery systems of the 1990s promise to be more demanding of evidence that occupational therapists provide essential services in psychosocial settings. Mandates to demonstrate predictable outcomes, relevance and efficiency require more research around theory and clearer definitions of practice. We can no longer justify reimbursement for occupational therapy by relying on the conventional wisdom. Instead, we must substantiate the efficacy of the various groups and programs we select as tools for intervention. We must take time from routinized methods of program planning to look anew at the use of occupational therapy's philosophy, domain of concern and theoretical bases for making sound clinical judgements. Refining our use of clinical decision-making and clinical reasoning enables us to determine: which groups best integrate our frames of reference/practice models; which groups are indicated for specific patients; when in the course of illness the groups are appropriate interventions; and in what settings groups should occur, e.g., acute or long term settings.

Using this opportunity to move slowly through the steps in the process of group protocol design or selection allows us to set the parameters within which occupational therapists can use reasoning, not recipes, to enhance practice. Of course, there are critical ingredients common to all groups, but let us take the time to blend them from scratch, rather than taking the shortcut of using a mix!

The first step is to look at group activities as interventions evolving from particular historical and environmental contexts. Next we will look at how to use the process of clinical decision-making, thus producing protocols that truly reflect our critical thinking around the techniques we believe to be effective (Parham, 1987; Pelland, 1987; Mattingly, 1988; Neuhaus, 1988). Finally, a case example will highlight some of the issues addressed in the more theoretical aspects of this paper.

Establishing the Context

It is not the purpose of this editorial to review the history of the role of groups in the era of moral treatment during the nineteenth century, or during the evolution of occupational therapy practice. Suffice it to say, that although patients were engaged frequently in tasks within group settings, it was not until the 1950s that theories of group dynamics and group process emerged, fostering the concept of groups as agents of change in addition to the traditional view of groups as vehicles for social interaction. During the 1950s group activity was used for skill building to enhance functioning. From [the] 1950s to [the] 1970s the focus was on intrapsychic or ego skill building, while in the 1980s the focus is on performance in occupational roles and activities of daily living (Howe & Schwartzberg, 1986; Mosey, 1979; Fidler, 1984).

As we move toward the 1990s, and look prospectively at group activity as a viable intervention, we must consider the environmental context in which our current practice occurs and the environmental context in which future practice will occur. None of us could be strangers to the crisis in health care, as it has had impact on every mental health care delivery system (Fine, 1987; Bonder, 1987). The reality is that resources are diminishing, while costs rise; consumer demands for quality care intensify in the face of increased pressure to shorten lengths of stay. These factors have forced practitioners in acute care settings to consider "re-evaluation of the objectives and methods for short lengths of stay…and rehabilitation interventions to provide basic foundation for posthospital adjustment" (Fine, 1987, p. 9). Similarly, occupational therapists in longer term inpatient and community settings must reassess their program goals and objectives in order to assume the task of working with patients who may be increasingly acutely ill, less stabilized on medications, and more chronically impaired than those in past years.

In addition to the impact of increased accountability and decreased resources, what are other environmental factors to bear in mind when designing group interventions? Some critical ingredients to consider include the facility's location and the relationship between the facility and the socio-economic level of the community. For example, the skills required to be a functional member of the community in New York City are not the same as those required in rural North Dakota. For example, negotiating crowded subways to get to work in New York City is quite different than relearning how to drive a tractor. Thus, group protocols dealing with independent living skills will have to be designed quite differently for those two geographical locations. In addition, knowing what resources are available to patients in the community is essential, in order that the objectives of groups designed to integrate patients into the "outside world" are relevant to the realities encountered. One must be careful about encouraging patients' participation in community center social activities, when their lack of social skills will only result in failure at being integrated into a group.

Consideration of the population's demographics served by the facility is important. For example, ages, ethnicity, educational levels, pre-morbid functioning diagnoses and prognoses of the patients must be considered when designing a group which is relevant to its context. Other important considerations are the average length of treatment and other intervention services available to the patients at the facility or in the outside community (Grossman, Bortone, 1986). Occupational therapy interventions should be appropriate, necessary, and unique, when balanced against the efforts of other members of the multidisciplinary team; they should meet patient needs, and needs identified by functional assessment, rather than meeting perceived needs of the staff (Grossman, Bortone, 1986). One example is of the psychiatrist who wouldn't allow the wife of a blue collar worker to go home until she could identify and explain her feelings, despite the fact that she could again cook for her family (Gibson, 1989).

Other questions to consider when designing group interventions are financial and legal constraints or mandates. Therapists should be aware of how facilities are funded and how occupational therapy services are reimbursed, i.e., per diem, as part of a set bed rate, or fee-for-services. Differences in reimbursement methods can influence how services are managed and whether or not groups are a cost-effective method of delivering care. For instance, fee-for-service departments might not support co-leadership of groups, while departments whose services are part of the per diem rate might be less concerned about the increased cost of co-leadership of group activities. Whether or not the department is able and encouraged to generate income is certainly a factor to weigh in designing programs or groups. Caseload size, session length, frequency of visits and reimbursement rates also contribute to feasibility of implementing certain activities.

Finally, as therapists, we must ask ourselves what are

the "legal" constraints on our group or programs. Every setting, whether public or private, large or small, acute or custodial, institutional or community based, must answer to the regulations imposed by federal, state and local governments, the courts and patients' rights organizations. Consider, for a moment, the impact of Medicare and the impact on reimbursement of Diagnostic Related Groups (DRGs). Other regulating bodies, such as Joint Commission on Accreditation of Health Organizations (JCAHO), licensure boards and peer review agencies also have the power to influence, and, at times control our practice. Even the American Occupational Therapy Association, representing our own professional standards, ethics and practice with uniform terminology, certification and registration procedures has policies we all incorporate into our daily role functioning in the field.

Narrowing the focus to occupational therapy services/departments, we can determine whether or not they will, or can, support particular group interventions. Is the department organized around a particular frame of reference? What level of staff experience is required to lead a new group? What special skills or training is required? Does the department have support from the facility's administration to engage in quality of life and rehabilitation efforts or is the setting strictly bio-medical (Cynkin, 1979)?

When the issues and questions raised above have been addressed, we are free to engage in the "ethics, science and art" (Rogers, 1983, p. 601) of clinical decision-making and clinical reasoning. By employing clinical decision-making and clinical reasoning we prevent occupational therapy from becoming "cookie cutter therapy," we individualize the treatment of our patients and we specifically address the functional problems they face (Parham, 1987).

Clinical Decision-Making and Clinical Reasoning

Clinical decision-making and clinical reasoning about development and/or selection of group protocols is a dynamic interactive systems process which for academic purposes will be divided into two phases. The descriptions of these phases are adapted from the work of Rogers (1983), Pelland (1987), Barris (1987) and Mattingly (1988), all of whom have written extensively on the subject. (See Figure 1.)

Clinical Decision-Making

Clinical decision-making, a four step process, represents the first phase, the one that occurs while sitting in the office, with the luxury of time to reflect on the results of the environmental analyses and assessments which pre-

cede group design. Step one in this phase is to *identify a frame of reference or practice model* which sets the framework for all of the planning to follow. A critical aspect of identifying a frame of reference/practice model is that it be consistent, or at least consonant with that of the department and of the institution. Imagine selecting a Cognitive Disabilities frame of reference (Allen, 1988) in a setting where psychoanalytic approaches are endorsed! That would be like submitting wok recipes to a French cookbook.

It is the frame of reference which delineates the continua of function and dysfunction, and defines the postulates for change (Denton, 1987; Robertson, 1988), thereby moving us to step two, that of *clarifying what specific*

Figure 1. Group Protocol Selection System

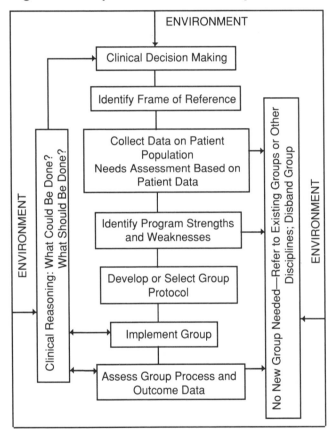

Adapted with permission from Pelland (*American Journal of Occupational Therapy, 41*[6], p. 353).

data we need about our population, and how to analyze activities for the best fit between patient and group design. For example, if a patient is given the Allen Cognitive Level Test, and achieves level 4 or below (Allen, 1988), it would be inconsistent with the Cognitive Disabilities frame of reference to place the patient in a group activity requiring the ability to think abstractly

(Denton, 1987; Pelland, 1987).

Step three in the decision-making process is *program assessment* of existing groups and individual intervention possibilities. This assessment is intended to identify strengths and weaknesses in departmental services as well as strengths and weaknesses in the services provided by other disciplines throughout the facility. Once again, the frame of reference/practice model helps identify ways in which occupational therapists can either offer unique services, or refer patients to other disciplines who share concerns, rather than duplicating services (Denton, 1987). In this instance the choice is not to develop a new group at all.

The fourth step in decision-making about groups is *selection or design of an appropriate protocol*. Required at this juncture is a return to the art and science of activity analysis, along with knowledge about group process and the critical elements of a group plan. As defined by Howe and Schwartzberg (1986, p. 141), these elements are structure and content. The structure includes: group name; time and length of meeting; place; whether group is open or closed; goals and outcome criteria for goal attainment stated in behavioral terms; criteria for patient selection; leadership roles and functions; nature of the group contract; and methods and procedures. Content refers to the medium used in the groups.

Group structure and content must be considered vis à vis the frame of reference as we develop the rationale for the activities we choose and establish goals and objectives for our group (Kaplan, 1988). The importance of clarity around these issues lies in the reality that occupational therapists must begin to produce observable, measurable evidence that demonstrates the link between our theory and practice; replicates and validates our interventions; and substantiates the strength of our clinical decision-making and clinical reasoning skills. Setting observable, measurable outcome criteria makes the task of quality assessment and/or research easier to manage. For example, specificity in group structure can be compared to the need for specificity in learning to cook! I remember asking my great-grandmother how to make chicken soup. Her response was, "First you take a chicken!" While some of us cook by intuition, others rely on recipes to insure our success each time we cook. So, too, there are those of us who run groups according to protocols, defining clear goals and objectives, and with a significant amount of preparation, while others make decisions about group design only moments before the arrival of the patients.

Clinical Reasoning

The transition from clinical decision-making to clin-

ical reasoning occurs at the moment we take the step to *implement* the group and *begin to evaluate it*, both as the group process emerges and as outcome data is generated. Mattingly (1988) has written about clinical reasoning in occupational therapy as a patient-centered approach which relies on the patient's perception and interpretation of his illness. In the clinical decision-making process theory is linked to group process skills, activity analysis, and generalized patient needs. In the clinical reasoning process, the focus is on applying theories in a very specific context, with specific patients, who bring their own symbolic and concrete meanings to the activities we offer in occupational therapy group. How many of us have had to do a fast reshuffling of group plans when the patients proclaim, "We hate that activity, it's boring!"

The essence of clinical reasoning is its dependence on patients' active participation in their choice of goals and definition of the methods for achieving them. "Efficacious treatment in occupational therapy relies on mobilizing patient commitment to the treatment process" (Mattingly, 1988, p. 1:86). When starting a group, clarifying "what therapeutic intervention would most effectively propel the patient in a positive direction" (Mattingly, 1988, p. 1:87) is as important as awareness about the context in which treatment occurs. Working with the patient requires us, as occupational therapists, to be conscious of therapeutic use of self, and to utilize the capacity to think on our feet or "reflect in action," when with the group (Shon, 1983; Mattingly, 1988).

On-going *assessment* of the group interaction and *evaluation of outcome data* is the step following implementation. This phase is also directly linked to both the clinical decision-making and clinical reasoning process. While the group is in progress, the therapist must continually use effective leadership skills to interact with patients and to respond to the ever changing nature of the individuals (Mosey, 1979; Kaplan, 1988); the nature of the environment and the nature of the activity. Neuhaus (1988) refers to this as constantly generating hypotheses and revising them to find the best fit between patients and activities.

The question of the efficacy of the group, as demonstrated by outcome data, is the last phase in the decision-making-reasoning cycle. Results at this point might suggest these possible options: continue the group as established; acknowledge the need to return to the decision-making phase; or end the group. Whichever choice is made depends on the consequences of each preceding phases.

To better demonstrate principles described above, let us look at a case example. Bear in mind that real life rarely fits perfectly into diagrams. Thus, the stages depicted in Figure 1 are somewhat obscured by demands of a brief narrative. Furthermore this case represents clinicians' thought processes. The content related to *actual* content of clinical decision-making and clinical reasoning will vary from occupational therapist to occupational therapist and depends upon the chosen frame of reference/practice model.

✳   ✳   ✳

Clinic A is a private, voluntary, non-profit, acute care psychiatric hospital. It is part of a university medical center located in the urban northeast. Of the one hundred four beds, a maximum of sixteen are available to adolescents in scatter-bed fashion, spread among three twenty-four bed general psychiatry units. Census ranges from zero to sixteen, depending on fluctuations in admissions.

The Department of Rehabilitation Services consists of occupational therapists, music, dance and recreation therapists and teachers. Services offered to adolescents are part of the per diem rate and are conceptualized from a bio-psycho-social frame of reference/ practice model.

Adolescents, ranging in age from thirteen to eighteen, are admitted for a full range of psychiatric and behavioral disorders, including major depression, acute psychotic disorders and conduct disorders. After a period of evaluation and observation on their units, patients are referred to a centralized adolescent rehabilitation program including school, occupational therapy, recreational therapy and dance therapy. In this way, patients from three units were gathered into peer groups which better replicate life outside the institution.

Clinic A is a tertiary care facility in which patients often come from great distances and from a variety of living situations including residential treatment centers and other social agencies. Third party payers, both public and private, bear the cost of hospitalization. Adolescents are from a wide spectrum of socio-economic backgrounds, from homeless to extremely wealthy; and attend public or exclusive private and parochial schools.

Patients perform at all levels of scholastic achievement, task, and interpersonal functioning as demonstrated through the Barth Time Construction evaluation. Wide variation exists on Axis IV and V diagnosis. At the time of this case example, most patients demonstrated the capacity to engage in peer group interaction despite the wide range of DSM-IIIR Axis I diagnoses and variability on Axis II diagnoses.

Patients were able to use multiple task group activities to practice social skills and gain mastery over new functional skills within the context of a setting that enhanced their capacity to cope with and adapt to the normative developmental tasks and roles of adolescence. Almost uniformly, patients spoke of and behaviorally demonstrated their difficulties with transition to

increased autonomy/independence. Often the concept of separation from home was the focus of individual psychotherapy and family therapy. This led to the development of intense attachments to co-patients and hospital staff, as hospitalization represented a crisis time in the transitional periods between early, middle and late adolescence.

As a result, there was a long history of patients staying in touch with co-patients after discharge, and of some even returning to the hospital cafeteria to meet for coffee and to touch base with the inpatient friends they left behind. Patients' return visits demonstrated the need to establish some mechanism for easing the transition from hospital to home, family and school. Even those who were discharged to residential treatment settings or long term hospitalization seemed to need an arena to deal with concerns about separation from the hospital. Discharge to the community for inpatients often meant return to school, friends and family, with some constellation of therapy at other agencies, but with no transitional intervention around re-integration into peer groups. That gaps were created by discharge from centralized adolescent programs seemed obvious.

One solution to this service gap was to establish a transitional group, designed around the old concept of "rap groups" for high school students. The bio-psycho-social frame of reference provided the theoretical foundation for the group, as it is consistent with departmental and institutional frames of reference, and pays particular attention to environmental issues. The "Rap Group" was to meet once weekly for one and a half hours (from 4:00 to 5:30 p.m.) in the department kitchen.

Led by an occupational therapist, this open-ended group is available to inpatients nearing discharge and outpatients who return to the clinic for approximately ten sessions. The rationale for the group is to provide a therapeutic forum in which issues around the difficult transition to life outside the hospital can be addressed, and thereby making it easier to separate from the inpatient experience at this hospital. This structured environment is intended to replace the informal "coffee klatches" in the hospital cafeteria.

Goals of the group include patients demonstrating the ability to loosen inpatient ties while tightening ties to post hospital dispositions, especially to follow-up therapy. Evidence for this ability is decreasing interest in attending the "Rap Group" and the patients' increasing ability to describe evidence of integration into other treatments and appropriate school community or peer groups.

Roles and functions of the group leader are to: assess and monitor interpersonal skills, aid in the development of increasingly adaptive capacities to separate successfully from the hospital, encourage independence rather than dependence, and monitor patients' ability to utilize disposition resources. In the face of failure to integrate post-discharge plans, the occupational therapist intervenes to facilitate integration or seeks consultation regarding whether or not plans could or should be altered.

Group methods include spending one half hour in preparation of snacks, drinks, coffee, etc. and informal "hellos," after which everyone is expected to settle into the more formal group discussion for approximately forty-five minutes. Especially important to formalize is saying "hello" to new members and "goodbye" to departing members. Psycho-education methods such as continually re-educating patients to group goals is an important aspect of this process. The final fifteen minutes of the group are used for cleanup, planning for snacks the next week, informal goodbyes and individual intervention, when necessary.

Establishment of the transitional "Rap Group" emerged from the process of sound clinical reasoning and clinical decision-making. It also emerged from an environmental analysis which both identified the absence of services to aid in the transition out of the hospital and enabled occupational therapy to formally become part of the services offered through the Child/Adolescent Outpatient Clinic. The addition of services by occupational therapists to this clinic increases the capacity of the Clinic to generate essential revenue through fee-for-service billing. Thus the group provides a good marketing strategy as well as a sound clinical service.

∗   ∗   ∗

With these thoughts in mind, I invite you to consider whether a "cookbook" approach to group protocol selection is the recipe we, as professionals, want to follow. Or, is it time to build scientific inquiry into our practice, by establishing group protocols which represent the use of critical thinking in occupational therapy (Barris, Keilhofner & Watts, 1983)? It is time to be reflective practitioners, designing and implementing treatment groups in collaboration with our patients, and with constant awareness of the fluid nature of the treatment environment. It is our professional obligation to continually re-assess and re-vamp our practice, both from the "safety" of our offices, as in clinical decisionmaking, and from the moment to moment context of groups in progress, through the clinical reasoning process (Parham, 1987; Robertson, 1988; Shon, 1983; Rogers, 1983).

References

Allen, C. (1988). Cognitive disabilities. In S. C. Robertson (Ed.). *Mental health focus: Skills for assessment and treatment.* Rockville, MD: The American Occupational Therapy Association, 3-18—3-34.

Barris R. (1987). Clinical reasoning in psychosocial occupational therapy: The evaluation process. *The Occupational Therapy Journal of Research*, 3, 148-162.

Barris, R., Keilhofner, G., & Watts, J. H. (1983). *Psychosocial occupational therapy/Practice in a pluralistic arena.* Maryland: RAMSCO.

Bonder, B. (1987). Occupational therapy in mental health: Crisis or opportunity? *American Journal of Occupational Therapy*, 41(7), 495-499.

Cynkin, S. (1979). *Occupational Therapy: Toward health through activities.* Boston: Little, Brown.

Denton, P. L. (1987). *Psychiatric occupational therapy: A workbook of practical skills.* Boston: Little, Brown.

Fine, S. B. (1987). Looking ahead: Opportunities for occupational therapy in the next decade. *Occupational Therapy in Mental Health*, 7(4), 3-11.

Gibson, D. (1989). *Personal Communication.*

Grossman, J., & Bortone, J. (1986). Program development. In S. C. Robertson (Ed.). *Mental health scope: Strategies, concepts and opportunities for program development and evaluation.* Rockville, MD: The American Occupational Therapy Association, 91-100.

Howe M. C., & Schwartzberg, S. L. (1986). *A functional approach to group work in occupational therapy.* Philadelphia: Lippincott.

Kaplan, K. L. (1988). *Directive Group Therapy: Innovative mental health treatment.* New Jersey: Slack.

Mattingly, C. (1988). Perspectives on clinical reasoning for occupational therapy. In S. C. Robertson (Ed.). *Mental health FOCUS: Skills for assessment and treatment.* Rockville, MD: The American Occupational Therapy Association, 1-81—1-88.

Mosey, A. C. (1979). *Activities Therapy.* New York: Raven Press.

Neuhaus, B. (1988). Ethical considerations in clinical reasoning: The impact of technology and cost containment. *American Journal of Occupational Therapy*, 42(5), 288-294.

Parham, D. (1987). Toward professionalism: The reflective therapist. *American Journal of Occupational Therapy*, 41(9), 555-561.

Pelland, M.J. (1987). A conceptual model for instruction and supervision of treatment planning. *American Journal of Occupational Therapy*, 41(6), 351-359.

Robertson, S. C. (1988). Reasoning in practice. In S. C. Robertson (Ed.). *Mental health FOCUS: Skills for assessment and treatment.* Rockville, MD: The American Occupational Therapy Association, 1-48—1-50.

Rogers, J. C. (1983). Eleanor Clarke Slagle Lectureship-1983: Clinical reasoning, the ethics, science and art. *American Journal of Occupational Therapy*, 37(9), 601-616.

Shon, D. A. (1983). *The reflective practitioner: How professionals think in action.* New York: Basic Books.

Chapter 10

Occupational Therapists in the Interdisciplinary Team Setting

Sherry M. Reed, OTR, MBA

The interdisciplinary team approach to patient management in the delivery of healthcare has resulted from a proliferation of specialities, the ensuing fragmentation of delivery, and increased confusion on the part of the patient and his family. It is likely that the movement towards specialization will continue and the team approach will be used to even a greater extent than it is used today in order to ensure coordinated and quality care. As promising a concept as the team approach is, however, it can be a difficult reality to implement and sustain. At its worst, the team effort can be a frustrating experience for all team members, detract from quality patient care, and ultimately fail. At its best, an effective health care team can do much to meet the various needs of today's patient and family as well as provide a stimulating working environment for its professionals.

A healthcare team's success or failure is largely determined by its administrative leadership. It is becoming less common for physicians to provide administrative as well as medical leadership, as each role is demanding, time consuming and different in focus. Today, professionals of any discipline who have the appropriate program development and personnel management skills are encouraged to apply for the position of administrative leader of the team.

As occupational therapists gain the management skills required to direct programs, they can be considered as serious candidates for leadership roles in interdisciplinary teams. They can meet this challenge knowing that their clinical skills of observation, problem identification, problem solving, and goal setting will be valuable assets in this new role.

As the administrative director of the team, occupational therapists can also exercise their clinical ability of thinking holistically. They can see the importance of dealing with healthcare megatrend issues such as healthcare costs, patient accessibility, competition with other facilities, patients as consumers, and government regulation to name but a few. By not ignoring the environment in which their program operates, they can make far reaching decisions whose effects will filter down to each patient and family member served by their program.

As staff members, occupational therapists fill a unique niche in the interdisciplinary setting. They, more than any other professional, have clinical skills in common with a number of the other team members, e.g. cognition with speech therapists, transfer training and muscle strengthening with physical therapists, recreational activities with recreation therapists, and activity of daily living with nursing. In the right environment, the occupational therapist will be enriched by this close working relationship with fellow teammates. However, in an ill-managed setting, the occupational therapist may become frustrated and discouraged by recurring role ambiguities, rivalries, and conflicts.

If occupational therapists want their team to succeed and thrive, they must have a working knowledge of how teams function. This paper discusses six key issues that the occupational therapist should be aware of before joining a team either as its leader or as a member of its staff. These issues are:
1. Program Philosophy;
2. Client Focus;
3. Role Clarification;
4. Collaboration and Information Sharing;
5. Policies and Procedures;
6. Supportive Staff.

Program Philosophy

The first task of the team leader and the program planning committee is to draft four important statements that will guide the program as it expands and matures. These are: (1) the program's mission statement, (2) admitting criteria, (3) continued stay criteria, and (4) discharge criteria.

These statements describe the purpose of the program and which patients will best be served by its efforts. They will also act as guidelines to keep the program on target as time passes. Once these statements have been drafted, they must be communicated to referring physicians, on-board and prospective staff, and the patients and their families who are being screened for admittance to the program. This will reduce the risk of disappointing patients and staff members whose expectations are not being met.

The mission statement is a short written statement that describes the scope of the service and the target population to be served. This statement gives the team identity and projects a certain image of it to the public. The admitting, continued stay, and discharge criteria ensure that the appropriate type of patients are served by the team for as long as they are improving but not longer.

The framework that the criteria provides will help screen out inappropriate referrals to the program. A common fault of health care teams is admitting or keeping patients that could be better served elsewhere. When this happens, the patient and his family are usually disappointed with the care and the staff becomes disillusioned as their best efforts do not seem to help the patient reach the unrealistic goals that have been set.

All the marketing and public relations efforts that relate to the program should reflect the program's philosophy. This will portray a strong and accurate image of the program to the public.

Without a carefully thought-out philosophy, a program runs the danger of disintegrating into ambiguity, meeting neither the patients' needs nor the professional staff's and public's expectations.

Client Focus

The team effort grew out of a need to provide better care to the client, and for this reason, the focus of all team effort must be continually directed towards the client. The team leader must remind the staff that the program is structured around the patients' needs and not the staff's convenience.

With the exception of nursing, many healthcare professionals expect to work a typical 40 hour Monday through Friday week. Oftentimes, this results in therapy scheduling conflicts, patients exhausted from trying to keep to an impossible schedule, and nurses pushed to find time to carry out their nursing tasks.

Client centered programs allow all seven days of the week to be used productively toward reaching the prescribed goals. Weekends and evenings do not have to be structured the same as weekdays in either intensity or content, but neither should they be times of inactivity and boredom. One solution is to devote weekends and evenings to the patient's educational or recreational needs. These activities may be done in a group setting. This provides the patient with the peer support and socialization which should be present in any good healthcare program, as well as requiring less people to staff.

When the focus of the program strays from the client to someone or somewhere else, the image and reputation of the service will suffer. This lack of client focus will be interpreted as a lack of commitment on the part of the team to put forth their best efforts. The physicians, consumers, regulatory agencies, and general public will eventually respond by withdrawing their support.

Role Clarification

In today's healthcare team, there are many gray areas among the staff members' fields of expertise and potential for misinterpretation and conflict. Oftentimes, well-meaning members will see a need in the patient's program and rush to plug a hole at the expense of their primary responsibilities. It is during the planning process that roles should be clarified, written and communicated to all concerned. Discussion should center on how to support and complement each others' efforts. If this structure is provided, the tone of the team will be one of smooth and coordinated effort. Team members will not feel a need to justify their existence or compete for recognition, and staff complaints of feeling unappreciated, misunderstood or overwhelmed can be minimized. The roles that the patient and family play as members of the team should also be formalized during the planning process. The primary decision to be made is if the patient will be an active or passive team member. As a passive member, the patient simply receives the benefits of the efforts that are directed towards him. As an active member, he actually takes part in the decision-making process and exercises a degree of control over the direction of his program. In most dynamic healthcare settings today, the patient plays an active role.

Usually the struggle for power and control that typifies many teams is a result of the staff's fear that their professional contribution will be eroded or engulfed by someone else. It is tragic when professionals spend their valuable time competing for power and control of the team in order to protect their professional integrity.

Collaboration and Information Sharing

If the team is to function effectively, the staff must work together by sharing information and collaborating regarding treatment on an ongoing basis. The make-up of the team must be one where members work together to identify patient care problems and possible solutions.

The key to effective problem solving is full problem identification. Both formal, as well as informal communication channels, must be utilized to ensure that information is transmitted within the healthcare team. Knowledgeable team members can make greater contributions and, thus, can be most effectively utilized. Therefore, a communication strategy should be mapped out that facilitates formal, informal, and spontaneous information sharing within the team.

Formal communications are usually accomplished through staff meetings and staff notes in the patient's chart. Staff should work together to see that the team meeting and charting methods are functional and effi-

cient. Each discipline can support the information sharing process by arriving at meetings on time armed with useful and relevant information. Likewise, staff should realize that charting is a necessary communication tool and that others are depending on their concise and timely information.

One method of facilitating informal communication among staff is space planning which places specific disciplines adjacent to one another. It is very effective, for example, to place the occupational and physical therapy clinics close together so that the therapists can observe one another at work and share valuable treatment information.

If staff offices must be shared, colleagues should be placed together who usually do not communicate enough due to lack of opportunity, such as the discharge planner and the nurse. This method of space allocation will foster team building and cement working relationships by allowing frequent and ongoing information sharing.

Armed with more complete information, team members can contribute fully to identifying patient care problems and solutions. The team leader should require that members agree on which problems take priority and that they work together towards solutions. If, for example, the team decides that an aphasiac patient's incontinence is hindering the patient's total rehabilitation effort, then everyone should contribute to the solution of this problem. For example, the speech therapist may design a method of communication between patient and staff that would signal staff when the patient needed to toilet. This signal would be used by all team members working with the patient. The physician and pharmacist could review the medications available for bladder control, the occupational therapist could concentrate on toilet transfers, and the physical therapist could work on trunk strengthening to increase the patients sitting balance on the commode. The counselor could help the patient deal with his feelings about being incontinent. In other words, an effective team approach would view incontinence as more than a nursing problem!

A team that is weak in collaboration and information sharing will not be able to effectively coordinate their efforts. Occasionally, management will attempt to knit a poorly functioning team together by hiring or appointing one person to act as coordinator. Typically, gaining a coordinator is not a solution to a problem, but a symptom of a situation where properly designed communication and collaboration systems are not in place.

Policies and Procedures

Effective policies and procedures will provide the team members with the structure they need to work together as a cohesive group. Examples of program-wide systems that may need developing are: (1) a procedure for coordinating the patient's program, (2) a procedure for scheduling patient treatments and conferences, (3) a procedure for orienting the patients and families to the program, and (4) a procedure for transporting patients between activities.

One of the hallmarks of an effective leader is the ability to recognize what policies and procedures need to be developed before problems occur. He must then have the analytical skills necessary to design systems that will meet most of the staff's needs most of the time. He must also possess the personnel management skills to get the systems accepted and successfully implemented. To function effectively in this capacity, the leader must have the appropriate level of authority and responsibility for setting policy and designing and monitoring the procedures that will govern all.

Without excellent working systems in place, the team effort risks failure as the patient continually arrives late to therapies, nurses are unable to join the team conferences because there is no one on the floor to relieve them, the patient was mistakenly scheduled for two activities at the same time, etc.

Orchestrating the efforts of a multidisciplinary team is a complex and challenging task. Even teams whose members try hard to make everything work need a leader who has an overview and the vision to draft effective policies and procedures.

As the program grows and changes, operational procedures must be continually updated to meet existing needs.

Supportive Staff

The success of the team effort hinges on the individual team member's ability to work effectively with others in a give-and-take environment. In a well-functioning team, each individual is valued for his specialized contribution but is not allowed to skew the team effort in his favor. An effective team is made up of members who understand, respect, and support the role of their colleagues.

The best time to focus on attracting suitable people for the team is during the recruitment process. During the interview, the program philosophy should be candidly discussed with the applicant. If the applicant is a team player, he will join the staff with enthusiasm; if he is not, he will look elsewhere for a position that provides more autonomy.

If an existing team has a member who is not a team player, immediate action should be taken. Even one uncooperative member can disrupt the effectiveness of the team effort and seriously affect staff morale. It is tempting to avoid an unpleasant confrontation, by ei-

ther working around that member or by giving in to his inappropriate demands. This temptation should be resisted, and if necessary, the individual should be replaced with someone who will wholeheartedly support the team process.

Conclusion

An increasing number of occupational therapists are opting to join interdisciplinary teams as staff members and team leaders. Armed with a knowledge of how effective teams work, these occupational therapists can affect change that will result in better care for their patients and increased professional satisfaction for themselves.

Chapter 11

The Multidisciplinary Treatment Plan: A Format for Enhancing Activity Therapy Department Involvement

Elissa Lang, CRC, MEd
Marlin Mattson, MD

A t a minimum, medical records must now specify the problems to be addressed, the treatment plan, and the expected outcomes or goals (1). Each discipline involved in inpatient treatment has traditionally developed its own treatment plan, which leads to a fragmentation of the patient's treatment and produces a variety of unrelated goals for the patient—goals that are "often confusing, sometimes contradictory, and many times conflicting" (2). A primary focus of the multidisciplinary treatment plan is to increase the collaboration between the individual disciplines in carrying out the plan (2,3).

In the traditional written treatment plan, nonmedical disciplines may abdicate to the physician the role they should play in helping to define problems to be dealt with during the patient's hospital stay. Physicians, on the other hand, may feel that their role in the written formal treatment plan is planning and carrying out the evaluation of problems that are clearly medical. This view is especially reflected in the discharge summary, which typically summarizes the physician's involvement with straightforward medical problems but pays relatively little attention to the other major problems that were managed in part or totally by the nursing, psychology, social service, or activity therapy staff. The physician's role should include ensuring that the plan is an integrated view of a patient's life problems, the many treatments administered for those problems, and the results.

Resistance to the documentation of a specific and meaningful treatment plan has grown as requirements for accountability have increased (4). Many medical staff members prefer verbal communication or object to the separation of the treatment plan from the progress notes in the medical record (5), as is done in the problem-oriented record or its adaptations. Others feel that writing things down may lead to criticism when patients fail to reach a defined goal.

Our review of medical records suggests that clinical staff are good at recording relevant data; less effective at documenting their assessment of that data; and least effective at documenting their priorities in treatment, the end points toward which they will work, and the evidence that suggests progress toward that end point. While one hears the words "treatment plan" more and more, the documented treatment plan often does not reflect what the actual plan has been. It is notable that when most of those outside the hospital who are interested in knowing what is going on with the patient (such as third-party payers and the Joint Commission on Accreditation of Hospitals) are turning to the documented treatment plan, the unit underplays the importance of this coordinated plan.

This paper describes an approach for integrating the activity therapy disciplines into the development of the comprehensive multidisciplinary treatment plan. We believe this approach can improve communication within and between disciplines, define activity treatment parameters, and educate other disciplines about activity therapy. Finally, for those who are writing more and enjoying it less, it can ease the burden of excessive documentation of treatment.

This approach was developed in the therapeutic activities department of the Westchester Division of New York Hospital—Cornell Medical Center, a 320-bed private psychiatric teaching hospital. The department is composed of 48 staff members from the six major activity disciplines of occupational, recreational, art, dance, and music therapies and vocational rehabilitation counseling. Each day the department provides treatment for an average of 270 inpatients of all ages and with all degrees of illness and 50 patients in the adult and children's day hospitals. These disciplines use different modalities and treatment interventions but hold in common the belief that the patient is "more than his or her illness" and can harness the abilities to overcome or compensate for the handicap of mental illness through accurate assessment of functional strengths and guided "purposeful doing" (6-10).

The use of a structured approach in determining, defining, describing, and delivering activity treatment for psychiatric patients is not new (6-8, 10). At the Westchester Division the various departments, including the therapeutic activities department, have used adaptations of the problem-oriented record for several years. However, in the therapeutic activities department oral and written communication about the treatment plan had been difficult. Most staff considered this responsibility the least attractive part of their work.

Evidence of communication problems about the treatment plan was seen in a 1978-79 patient care evaluation study that determined the percentage of patients actually using therapeutic activities services. This information was not evident from chart records. The study indicated that only 50 percent of the patients used the services at any given time, and that documentation of even these services was unsatisfactory. A subsequent survey of the department's treatment plans and documentation procedures showed that when activity staff did document treatment, they spent an inordinate amount of time recording information that few people read or understood, sometimes to the exclusion of actual service delivery. Staff solved the problem quite easily by simply not documenting on a regular basis.

Senior administrative staff were understandably concerned that the chart records in no way reflected the multitude of therapeutic activities services being delivered. Because records are considered to reflect the adequacy of patient care (5), the concern about inadequate treatment plan documentation reached even greater magnitude and lent impetus to developing a new format for therapeutic activities treatment plans.

Developing the treatment plan format involved asking the leaders of the six therapeutic activities disciplines to describe the scope of their disciplines' services. From these discipline overviews evolved the definitions used in constructing the treatment plan format and the structure of the plan itself. The steps were carried out in meetings held within the department over a 12-month period. The plan was then implemented through documentation seminars for therapeutic activities staff. The total development and implementation of the treatment plan format took place in three phases.

Phase 1: Defining the Format

Reporting human behavior requires that it be observable and measurable. Defining a problem to be treated requires a description of behavior, a description of the environmental or internal emotional matrix in which it is embedded, and someone's judgment that the behavior is a problem (1). Using this promise as an outline, meetings were held with discipline chiefs to decide on the initial direction of the treatment planning format. It was decided that the format should specify the following items:

- Problem areas that should be treated by members of the therapeutic activities disciplines and the goals that are commonly anticipated
- Treatment methods used to address problems and achieve goals
- Behaviors that signal improvement
- Which activity discipline is best qualified to treat a problem

The following definitions were then developed to be used in the treatment plan format:

The *problem* is a brief, concise description of the observable functional deficit or behavior being addressed. The problem can be stated in general terms (for example, history of poor interaction skills) or as a specific manifestation of a deficit area (for example, inability to communicate verbally, or fear of speaking to strangers).

The *goal* is a description of the optimal functional behavior that is anticipated as a result of the patient's participation in the therapeutic activities treatment of the stated problem. The goal should be observable and measurable so that progress toward the goal, or lack of progress, is evident to both patient and therapist. In many cases the goals addressed through therapeutic activities treatment should also reflect skills that the patient can be taught (10).

The *approach* or methodology is the general and specific progressive treatment steps patient and therapist take to reach the stated goal. The approach includes formal evaluation of the patient's skills and behaviors as the primary initial activities treatment step.

The *objective* or subgoal—also called a signal or anchor—is the general or specific skill or behavior designated by therapist and patient to signal graded progress toward the stated goal. For example, one subgoal might be talking to someone once during each one-hour socialization group every day for a week; the next subgoal might be talking to someone twice during the group every day for a week, and so on. The objectives should be specified in terms of observable graded behaviors indicating that the patient is progressing toward the goal.

The *discipline* is the specific therapeutic activity specialty most qualified to address the stated problem.

Phase 2: Developing the Format

In order to complete a sample plan, each discipline leader worked through the following sequence of questions:

Initial Steps

Step 1: What are the major service components of the department as a whole? Define your discipline and, in general, what special treatment services your discipline or program offers.

Step 2: What do you define as the major divisions of treatment within your particular discipline?

Problem and Goal

Step 3: What specific functional deficit areas are members of your discipline most qualified to treat in each of these treatment areas?

Method

Step 4: What specific evaluations, treatments, or groups do you offer in each major area, and which problems do they address?

Objective or Subgoal

Step 5: For each problem area, what are the general behaviors or skills that signal progress toward a goal or goal attainment? What specific behaviors or skill acquisitions will signify goal attainment for an individual patient?

Step 5 was the most time-consuming aspect of developing the treatment plan format. It was difficult to define, in developmental progression, observable and measurable behaviors that could act as anchor points, or signals, of functional progress. The process was facilitated by reviewing from start to finish the treatment of a "typical" patient exhibiting one or more of the originally defined functional problems. Discipline members were asked to describe step by step what they specifically looked for in assessing functional progress toward attaining goals.

In both steps 4 and 5, certain factors were so obvious that they were often left out of the treatment plan format. For example, the disciplines often minimized or overlooked the evaluation of a patient's behaviors and capabilities in preparing a treatment program because evaluation procedures were considered to be a "standard" part of treatment.

Another overlooked factor was the first general behavior, common to all activities, that signals a step toward functional reconstitution—regular attendance at a prescribed individual or group treatment activity. When attendance is set as the first objective, or signal, the next step may be a minimal level of participation in the activity.

Beginning with general observable signals made it much easier to define the specifics of the objectives. For example, if the general signal of progress is regular attendance, along with adherence to minimal levels of acceptable behavior, the first specific signal, or anchor, might include attending one-hour sessions three times a week, remaining seated for 20-minute intervals with five-minute breaks, and showing some interest in and concentration on the tasks of the session. The next signal might be attending sessions five times a week and showing interest and concentration for 25 minutes. Subsequent signals might be extensions of task concentration in five-minute intervals until a patient is able to sustain concentration for an entire treatment session.

Beyond such general signals or anchor points, the signals selected by therapist and patient to indicate the attainment of individual functional goals depend on the nature of the patient's original dysfunction, his or her abilities, the patient's particular manifestations of the problem, and the goals ultimately selected.

Once the discipline leaders worked through the five steps, each discipline leader developed a draft treatment plan. This phase included identifying program services, recording services using the defined format, and indicating how progress toward stated goals was observed, measured, and reported. Figures 1, 2, and 3 illustrate the results of the procedure. Figures 1 and 2 cover steps 1 through 3 for the disciplines of occupational therapy and vocational rehabilitation, and Figure 3 depicts steps 4 and 5 for vocational rehabilitation.

Phase 3: Implementing the Format

The new treatment plan was implemented beginning in 1982, through ongoing weekly one-hour documentation seminars for therapeutic activities staff. At first training was focused on newly hired staff who had not yet developed a "treatment plan style;" however, to our surprise other therapeutic activities staff began to ask to participate as well.

The documentation seminar stresses the importance and the function of cogently written treatment plans and progress notes that follow the defined format. Staff attend the seminar an average of three months; all new staff are required to complete the documentation training within their six-month probationary period to obtain permanent staff status.

Currently a trainer's manual and a staff workbook are being prepared. A study of staff's capabilities in documentation before and after participation in the seminars is underway, as is an audit to determine whether the training has affected the quality and quantity of documentation.

Using the Format: A Case Example

A case example and a sample treatment plan will illustrate how a therapeutic activities treatment plan is structured.

Margo was an 18-year-old, single, overweight young

Figure 1. Outline of Problems and Goals for the Discipline of Occupational Therapy

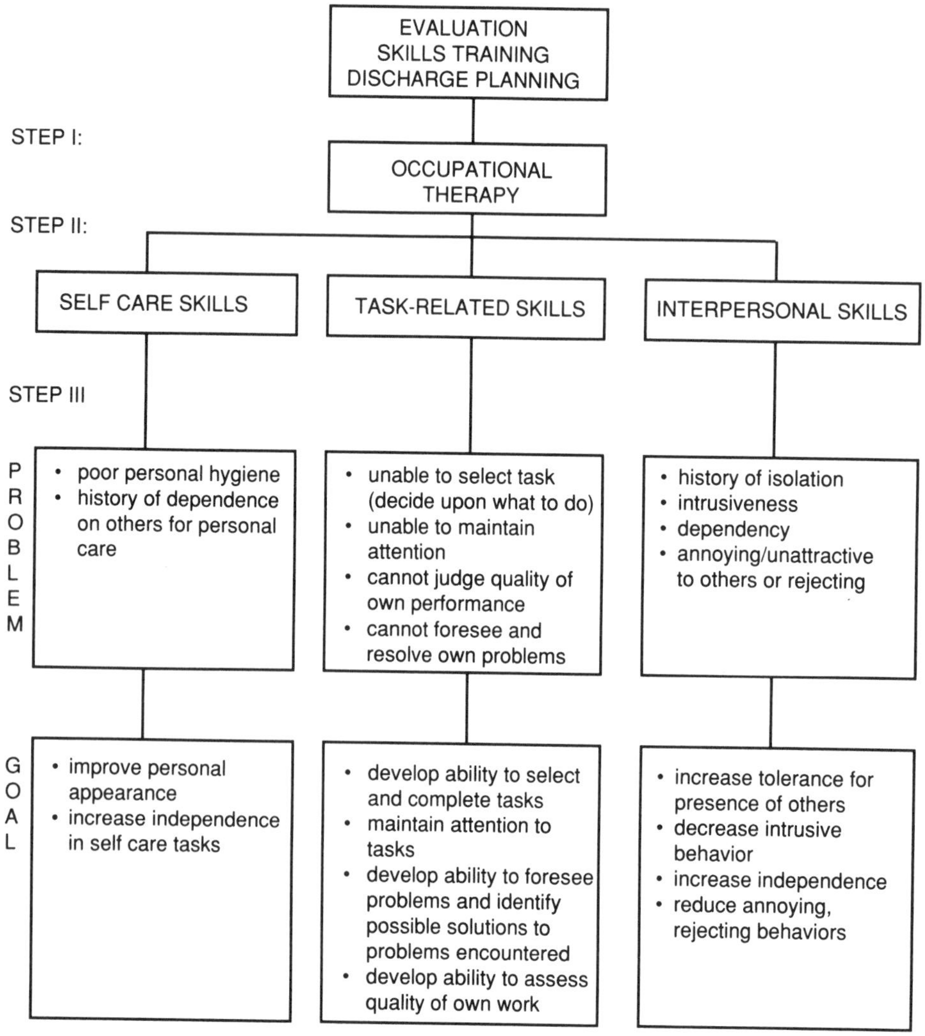

woman. She and her parents reported that she had experienced interpersonal and academic difficulties over the previous five years. With the help of private tutors, she had maintained a satisfactory grade-level performance and had graduated from high school. She completed one semester in a local community college but failed two of four courses. Her fear of returning to college after the semester break immobilized her; she became socially isolated and withdrawn and showed poor personal hygiene, decreased concentration, and erratic behavior, causing her parents to seek inpatient treatment for her. She had been in outpatient psychotherapy several times in the past, and she had received several courses of various psychotropic medications.

A three-month hospitalization for Margo was anticipated. Based on an evaluation of her capabilities by the therapeutic activities department and her stated goals, the following treatment plan was developed.

Weeks One Through Three

Problem: Poor task-related skills
Goal: Improve task-related skills
Approach: Occupational therapy: individual evaluation and skill development program
Objectives:
a) Attends evaluation sessions
b) Completes evaluation tasks
c) Reviews evaluation results with occupational therapist
d) Collaborates with occupational therapist to select two treatment goals
e) Selects one of two tasks to reach selected treatment goals
f) Describes how selected task will enable her to reach identified goal

Figure 2. Outline of Problems and Goals for the Discipline of Vocational Rehabilitation

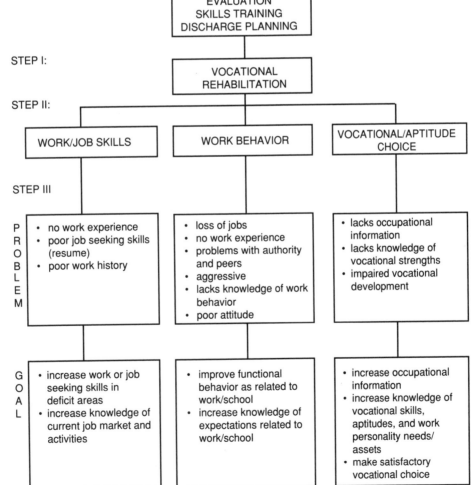

g) Attends one hour-long occupational therapy session daily. Arrives on time, and demonstrates attentiveness to tasks for entire session.
h) Arranges familiar needed materials and equipment without assistance
i) Follows written and verbal instructions, asking for clarification when needed
j) Notices and corrects mistakes with increasing independence
k) Identifies and describes possible solutions to problems encountered, selecting best solution
l) Assesses quality of own productions with fair degree of accuracy
m) Identifies and discusses skills acquired and their relationship to other life activities

Weeks One Through 12

Problem: Overweight

Goal: Reduce weight; improve nutrition; increase activity level
Approach: Recreation therapy: physical fitness activities. Occupational therapy: nutrition education
Objectives:
a) Attends physical fitness group once a day
b) Increases time in physical fitness group to full hour session each day
c) Discusses nutrition with therapist. Begins diet
d) Shows ability to retain information on diet and physical activity
e) Maintains diet and physical activity level
f) Shows increased physical activity level and growth
g) Loses two pounds each week
h) Maintains diet and activity on own initiative

Weeks Four Through Seven

Problem: Poor task-related and interpersonal skills

Figure 3. Outline of Methods and Objectives for the Discipline of Vocational Rehabilitation

STEP 3 PROBLEM:	STEP 3 GOAL:	STEP 4 APPROACH:	STEP 5 OBJECTIVES:
Poor work/job skills 1. poor work history. 2. unrealistic vocational goals. 3. history poor work relations.	Increase work/job skills 1. select appropriate vocation. 2. increase effective work behavior skills. 3. locate a job.	1. Individual Voc. Rehab. Counseling.	1 a. attends regularly. b. cooperates in reviewing work and school history. c. shows motivation to participate in vocational treatment planning.
		2. Vocational Test Battery.	2 a. attends testing sessions as scheduled. b. completes assigned voc. test battery. c. discusses test results with Counselor. d. shows understanding of own interests, aptitudes, and work personality traits by discussing with Counselor. e. selects tentative vocational goals.
		3. Vocational Exploration and Career Development Skills Group.	3 a. follows through on use of vocational reference materials to explore skill areas. b. shows ability to use materials. c. shows ability to integrate vocational information alone or with Counselor. d. adjusts vocational goals if necessary. e. seeks out vocational counselor for discussion of findings. f. selects vocational goal.
		4. Job Skills Group.	4 a. attends regularly. b. shows interests in learning or revising job skills. c. demonstrates ability to learn or revitalize job skills by completing assigned tasks (e.g., resume, school application). d. can discuss assets/deficits. e. transfers learning to own vocational goals.

Goal: Improve task-related and interpersonal skills

Approach: Occupational therapy: skill development program in task-oriented group

Objectives:

a) Clarifies task-related and interpersonal skill assets and deficits with occupational therapist

b) Selects two personal goals in collaboration with occupational therapist

c) Discusses how small task-oriented group will enable her to reach identified personal goals

d) Attends hour-and-a-half occupational therapy group sessions three times a week. Arrives on time and demonstrates attentiveness to group for full session

e) Participates appropriately in group goal-setting and task selection: remains in group; does not annoy other group members with intrusive, child-like behaviors; communicates suggestions and personal needs in constructive manner

f) Shows initiative in assuming responsibility for designated portion of group task, assembling necessary materials and equipment

Weeks Six Through Ten

Problem: Unclear vocational goals

Goal: Increase patient's knowledge of personal abilities

Approach: Vocational rehabilitation: individual and group counseling, vocational test battery; career exploration group

Objectives:

a) Meets regularly with vocational rehabilitation counselor as scheduled

b) Completes vocational aptitude, interest, and personality inventories within prescribed time

c) Discusses results with counselor

d) Demonstrates ability to use vocational exploration resources, such as career handbooks

e) Retains new vocational information and applies it to decision about returning to college

f) Makes decision about college reentry

Weeks Six Through 12

Problem: Fear of returning to college

Goal: Assist college reentry

Approach: Vocational rehabilitation: individual vocational counseling

Objectives:

a) Meets with vocational rehabilitation counselor as scheduled to discuss college reentry

b) Role-plays college reentry interview with therapist

c) Makes necessary phone calls and interviews to arrange appointments for readmission

d) Follows through with appointments and dis-cusses results with counselor

e) Identifies potential stress areas and recounts remedies independently

Discussion

Throughout the process of developing the treatment plan format, the task of dissecting and defining the behavioral treatment signals was exceedingly tedious. However, for most therapeutic activities staff the realization of the number of complex observation and treatment steps involved, and the formalization of those steps, was heartening.

In addition, presenting clear, observable behavioral expectations to patients, either verbally or by written treatment contract, proved to be a valuable treatment technique. Patients' participation in their own restoration increases when goals are clear and success signals are observable. The hospital environment often seems overwhelming to patients, and some clearly defined, action-oriented steps leading to observable personal goals can be a vital impetus for functional recovery.

With the new format, recording treatment methods and progress has become more focused, more meaningful, and certainly less time consuming. Treatment plans accurately reflect individual problems in functioning and individual successes in dealing with those problems. Thus the plans have more meaning for all team members, by allowing them to observe, understand, and reinforce the significance of progress in dealing with functional problems. By providing a structure that expects and encourages active patient participation and clear communication among patients and staff, the treatment plan format increases the therapeutic activities staff's sense of accountability for their part of patient care as well as providing maximum opportunity for genuine interdisciplinary planning and communication.

When the format was first introduced, therapeutic activities staff had difficulty recognizing how their work fit into the overall problem-oriented structure used by the hospital. Implementing the therapeutic activities treatment plan requires not only familiarity with the objectives defined but also the ability to communicate information about therapeutic activities to other treatment team members. In traditional treatment settings, information about patients' functioning is undervalued; information about psychodynamics clearly carries more weight. The treatment plan format can provide the basis for a common understanding and communication of parallel information among treatment team members. This understanding is a key factor in fostering activity therapy staff involvement in the treatment planning process.

Since activity therapists often characterize themselves as "doers," it is not surprising that communication of problems, treatment goals, and treatment methods between them and other treatment team members is often unclear, and descriptive literature about activity therapies is scarce. In addition, the "functional language" spoken by activity therapists may often be quite different from the clinical language spoken by other hospital-based mental health professionals. The patient described by an activity therapist as "exhibiting poor skills in activities of daily living, maladaptive work behavior, and disturbances in gross motor and leisure function" may be described by the physician as "depressed, withdrawn, agitated, and with blunted affect." The use of the activity treatment plan format increases understanding between the parallel languages of medicine and activities, a vital link in the development of a fully integrated individual treatment plan.

The scope, nature, and effectiveness of activity therapy may be the best-kept secret in psychiatry (Fine SB, personal communication, 1981). Most psychiatric hospitals employ activity therapists because of the vague belief that activities are important, but many hospital staff members are not sure exactly why they are important. The mystery that often surrounds the specific contributions of the activity therapies is reflected by the tendency to either exclude these so-called ancillary or support disciplines from active involvement in treatment planning, implementation, and clinical case conferences or to routinely include them without a genuine understanding of their value or function.

Refinement in the structure and function of the multidisciplinary treatment team requires greater involvement, integration, and skill on the part of all professional disciplines. Because activity therapists are now called on more frequently to participate in treatment planning, they face the challenge of role transition from a staff who are seen as "keeping patients busy" to treatment team members who must define and communicate the treatment goals and practices of the activity therapy disciplines. This transition carries with it greater responsibility and accountability for treatment delivered within the parameters of the activity disciplines and increased recognition by other hospital staff.

Recent legal decisions about quality of care (2) and the system-wide concern about accreditation and accountability make clear, sensible, integrated treatment a priority in mental health care. Perhaps more to the point is the impact that integrated treatment planning, through such mechanisms as the therapeutic activities treatment plan, has on patient care: by providing a clearly defined format, it decreases ambiguity in the patient record, focuses more attention on the patient, helps staff understand patients and their needs, increases patient participation in treatment, and helps prevent fragmented care.

References

1. Grant RL: The capacity of the psychiatric record to meet changing needs, in Psychiatric Records in Mental Health Care. Edited by Siegel C, Fischer SK. New York, Brunner/Mazel, 1981

2. National Institute of Mental Health: Individualized Treatment Planning for Psychiatric Patients. DHEW Publication ADM 77-399. Washington, DC, US Government Printing Office, 1977

3. Psychiatry in team work. Roche Report: Frontiers of Psychiatry 12:1,3-4, March 15, 1982

4. Task Force on the Problem-Oriented System: The Problem-Oriented System in Psychiatry. Washington, DC, American Psychiatric Association, 1977, pp 1-4

5. Siegel E, Fischer SK: Concluding remarks, in Psychiatric Records in Mental Health Care. Edited by Siegel E, Fischer SK. New York, Brunner/Mazel, 1981

6. Fine SB: Psychiatric treatment and rehabilitation: what's in a name? Journal: National Association of Private Psychiatric Hospitals 11(5):8-13, 1980

7. Anthony W: A rehabilitation model for rehabilitating the psychiatrically disabled. Rehabilitation Counseling Bulletin 24:6-21, 1980

8. Quinn P, Richman A: The contribution of a structured group rehabilitation approach. Rehabilitation Counseling Bulletin 24:118-129, 1980

9. Stone M: The evolution of activity therapies in transition from long-term psychoanalytic to a community health approach. Journal: National Association of Private Psychiatric Hospitals 7:(1)30-35, 1975

10. Anthony W: The Principles of Psychiatric Rehabilitation. Baltimore, University Park Press, 1980

Chapter 12

Strategic Communication for Occupational Therapy Practitioners in Mental Health

Susan C. Robertson, MS, OTR/L, FAOTA
Susan C. Schwartz, MPA, OTR

This chapter was previously published in S. C. Robertson (Ed.), *Mental health focus: Skills for assessment and treatment* (pp. 162-168). Rockville, MD: The American Occupational Therapy Association, Inc. (AOTA). Copyright © 1988, AOTA.

Communication is a highly complex human activity. It can be verbal, written, or nonverbal. Having effective communication skills in all three areas is essential for occupational therapy practitioners. It is not enough, however. Occupational therapy practitioners today must also have effective *strategic* communication skills to strengthen their position in the marketplace and to develop additional resources for optimal patient/client care.

This chapter explores the essence of strategic communication and its use in occupational therapy practice. The focus here is on verbal communication patterns and content. It is assumed that the reader is practiced in nonverbal communication and its therapeutic and nontherapeutic uses. For this reason, nonverbal communication is not dealt with separately but is integrated into the discussion of verbal communication.

Strategic Communication

Strategic communication takes place in an organizational setting and effectively mobilizes resources, accurately conveys departmental accomplishments and contributions, and positions the department to achieve internal and organizational goals. It is a complex but learnable skill that requires an understanding of the dynamics of the environment, organization, and profession.

Strategic communication is a means of linking program needs and goals to the patient/client, the organizational context, and the greater environment. Whereas effective communication is essential for relating assessment results to the patient/client, family, and treatment team, strategic communication is necessary for integrating occupational therapy services with other services provided in the setting. It strengthens team contributions in the organizational environment. Without strategic communication, patient care and client services may be compromised or be less than optimal. Strategic communication requires skill in organizational decision making that affects individuals and large and small groups in the system.

Factors that Influence Communication

Both external and internal factors influence the effectiveness of communication. Some external factors are found in the environment, others in the organization, and still others in the profession. Communication is also influenced by the experiences and skills of individual practitioners.

Psychosocial, political, legal, economic, and cultural issues from the external environment have an impact on the content of communication and the way in which it is delivered. By analyzing these forces, practitioners can specify both the content and style of their communications. Strategic communication can shape these external factors and, thereby, influence service delivery.

There is also a parallel set of psychosocial, political, legal, economic, and cultural influences in all organizational settings. By understanding the internal environment of these settings, a practitioner can effectively contribute to the informal communication of the team network and the more formal written and oral presentations needed by the organization. By defining the corporate culture (i.e., the values, norms, and habits of administrators and service providers), a practitioner can enhance the clarity, specificity, and relevance of all occupational therapy communication. Understanding other elements of the system helps define the receptiveness of the receiver of communication.

The occupational therapy profession itself influences communication among occupational therapy personnel. There are guidelines for the use of terminology in the profession, standards of behavior, and recommended formats for documentation. The defined domain of responsibility in the field also dictates how occupational therapy practitioners communicate with colleagues and others outside the profession.

Looking at the art of communication from another vantage point, the form, style, and type of communication are also influenced by the unique experiences and attributes of the individual who is sending information and the knowledge of the person who receives the information. Individual communication patterns can be assets or liabilities to effective communication. Each practitioner must adjust his or her personal style in order to be responsive to the demands of the individual patient/client, organization, or environment.

An Environmental Scan

The practice of occupational therapy must be well integrated within the organization and environment to be a viable and desirable component of the service delivery network. There are many elements in an environmental scan; only some of them are presented below. You will want to explore others that are unique to your particular setting.

On the national level, federal laws and regulations affect the delivery of mental health services nationwide. These include Medicare legislation, regulations for Medicare prospective payment, and the Community Mental Health Centers Act. Other national groups affect the practice of occupational therapy, including professional associations, such as the National Association of Private Psychiatric Hospitals, and accrediting organizations, such as the Joint Commission on the Accreditation of Healthcare Organizations. Both of these types of groups can have broad effects on service design and accountability.

Similar organizations exist on the state level and will be designated differently by each state. Each practitioner will want to examine the structure of service delivery within the state and identify groups that directly and indirectly affect the design of occupational therapy services and communication about them. There may be an office for statewide health planning, a department of health services, state and county commissions for health facilities, or an association of county mental health directors. There also may be medical associations, social service departments, and psychiatric societies on both the state and local levels.

An environmental scan consists of two activities: identifying external factors that influence the practice of occupational therapy in a particular setting and state, and analyzing the roles, functions, and procedures of the external factors as they relate to the goals and structure of the occupational therapy service. Because the set of external influences is very complex and always changing, it is important to scan the environment regularly. Once you have conducted one scan, it is relatively easy to update it on an ongoing basis. All practitioners should know which factors affect the delivery of occupational therapy services in general and in their own setting. Only by understanding the larger context can occupational therapy services be designed to maximize the use of resources.

An Organizational Analysis

A similar analysis is also conducted at the organizational level, where numerous economic, political, social, and cultural influences are assessed within the practice setting. This internal analysis is conducted for the inpatient unit or outpatient center, for example, and for the occupational therapy department and the institution as a whole.

The challenge facing every practitioner is to determine which unique set of factors affects the way occupational therapy services are designed in a given setting. One of the most critical factors in evaluating an organization is to determine how economic decisions are made and enforced. Finances often govern service delivery mechanisms, and, thus, it is critical to know how budgets are developed and approved and to understand what sources of income are available to the institution. Practitioners should also know how occupational therapy services bring revenue into the organization and how the occupational therapy department allocates expenses. With this understanding of the flow of authority and accountability, a practitioner will be able to ascertain how to access the system successfully.

The practitioner must also be aware of the internal communication patterns followed within the organization. The type of planning methodology used within the organization will indicate how decisions are made and who has the power to effect change. There may only be downward communication or a combination of downward, upward, and lateral communication. These patterns will have a major influence on how the organization plans for progress, plans to minimize crisis, or plans for stability.

External communication patterns are also important for the organizational analysis. The marketing methodology used by the organization will indicate how its administrators wish to present the organization to consumers, third-party payers, and the community. An understanding of these concerns will be key to selecting the type of communication patterns that occupational therapy personnel will use to support the organization's efforts. The goals and philosophy of the organization are typically reflected in its marketing approach.

Lastly, the practitioner will need to consider how personnel in the inpatient unit communicate internally and externally. An objective exploration of communication in the occupational therapy department then follows. Communication patterns will suggest the political, psychosocial, and cultural forces within an organization. These forces, coupled with economic factors, will point to the critical resources and constraints within the organization that support or inhibit occupational therapy services.

Current Issues in Occupational Therapy

Besides the environmental and organizational factors mentioned above, there are equally important and influential factors within the profession of occupational therapy that shape what practitioners need to do, can do, and should do.

Occupational therapy has a culture of its own. Although we are part of a larger health care system, we have a set of values, beliefs, norms, and expectations to which we are responsible as members of the profession. The educational process, from academic preparation to field work and supervision, guides our behavior in accordance with this professional culture.

National and state associations collaborate on defining the professional culture and disseminating information about the values, beliefs, norms, and expectations to its members. Policymaking bodies (the Representative Assembly and State Executive Boards) address such concerns as the philosophical base of the profession, the definition of occupational therapy, the national stance on licensure, and responsibility for career development. The *American Journal of Occupational Therapy* and other publications of the AOTA convey the results of these policy deliberations and the direction of growth of the profession. Individual occupational therapy practitioners use this information along with their environmental and organizational understanding to decide how to provide services to patients and clients.

One example may help to illustrate the influence of the profession on practice. The occupational therapy practitioner needs to define the existing and potential roles and status of occupational therapy in the health care system and in the specific practice setting. The profession has defined uniform terminology and standards of practice, and position papers have been written on various approaches to service delivery. These describe the norms for occupational therapy nationwide. There is also another set of guidelines and expectations imposed on the practitioner by the organization and the environment. The practitioner must weigh all these many forces and determine how to present occupational therapy in a given setting.

Decision Making and Communication

Decision making and reasoning are integral elements of strategic communication. They enable the practitioner to respond to the needs and qualifications for interaction dictated by the environment, system, and profession in the same way that they enable the practitioner to respond to a patient's/client's needs and to interact with him or her effectively.

Identifying the information that needs to be communicated is a component of the environmental, organizational, and professional analysis. The practitioner isolates which economic or political factors, for example, affect the services that can be provided to each patient/client. Knowing that a patient/client is covered by Medicare, for example, dictates what needs to be communicated to ensure reimbursement. Administrators in the practice setting have additional strategies for ensuring reimbursement and designing cost-effective services; these must also be considered when defining interventions for a patient client. The occupational therapy profession also has guidelines for quality intervention which, if not followed, could result in negative consequences. All these factors are computed as the practitioner determines what to say and how to communicate with the patient/client, department personnel, organization administrators, and external agencies. They influence how the occupational therapy practitioner plans, delivers, and markets his or her services.

Disregard for the principles of decision making limits the influence that occupational therapy can have on patient/client care, the department, and the organization. Adopting and improving skills in this area gives each occupational therapy practitioner an opportunity to give better service to the patient/client population.

How to Develop Strategies for Communicating Effectively

Many skills are helpful in improving strategic communication, including listening, concept formation, organization, negotiation, and conflict resolution. The degree of skill each practitioner can gain in these areas has an impact on his or her degree of comfort in verbal and nonverbal communication.

There are numerous forms and styles of communication useful for the demands of the practice setting. The reasoning process helps practitioners decide on the best pattern choice. The following questions may help determine the content and format of strategic communication:

- What needs to be said?
- What could be said?
- What should be said?
- Who will hear it?
- Who will say it?
- When should it be communicated?
- Where should it be communicated?
- Why should it be communicated?
- How should it be communicated?
- How may it be received?
- What resistance could be anticipated?

In occupational therapy practice settings across the country, many influences affect how these questions are answered. The language of the practice setting is based on shared values, as is the conceptual model of the corporate culture. Within this culture, there are built-in patterns of communication—who talks with whom, when, where, how, and why are influenced by the value system and norms of the organization. How the patterns are

Figure 1. Strategic Communication in Practice: Budget

Issue	Environmental Resources/ Constraints	Organizational Resources/ Constraints	Goal(s) of Occupational Therapy Communication	Content of Strategic Communication	Pattern of Strategic Communication
Occupational therapy budget is limited to 5% of unit costs.	Reduced funds for mental health services in form of prospective payment system. JCAHO HCFA DRR Regional legal factors.	Budgeting process. Financial officer values constraint and compliance. Administration threatened by overspending and resistance to requests for additional funds. Financial officer influences institution director in areas of finance. Quality assurance standards for facility.	To increase budget for occupational therapy because program requires additional materials and supplies. To negotiate increase in operating budget for occupational therapy. To use information about occupational therapy to promote the department and the services offered to the organization. To use identified network of power to influence change.	Revenue-produced occupational therapy for department. Range of services provided by occupational therapy. Costs associated with various programs. Number of patients/clients seen in each type of occupational therapy service. Anticipate benefits to organization of additional expense. Survey of referral sources re satisfaction with occupational therapy.	Negotiate with unit supervisor, institution financial officer. Plan agenda and place of negotiation. Write budget. Compile survey results of patient satisfaction. Perform outcome studies. Establish reciprocal relationships and maintain informal communication. Keep up with literature to support your position.

adjusted is often the result of specific alliances that are formed between key personnel. The occupational therapy practitioner's ability to build alliances with support figures, such as the service chief, financial officer, and team members, plays a critical role in successful strategic communication.

Understanding the organization and environment enables occupational therapy personnel to integrate their services into the full range of services offered. It also has an impact on how well occupational therapy services will be funded. But understanding the system is only half of the expertise needed. The other relates to the personal communication style of the practitioner. The degree of conflict and resistance, or the support received for occupational therapy services, has a great deal to do with the practitioner's mastery of strategic communication.

Applying Strategic Communication in Practice

Figures 1 and 2 present a framework for developing the content and pattern of strategic communication within a particular practice setting and give specific examples of issues often confronted by occupational therapy personnel. The framework includes several factors, the analysis of which will increase the likelihood of achieving desired outcome(s). These factors include:

- Issue;
- Environmental Resources/Constraints;
- Organizational Resources/Constraints;
- Goal(s) of Occupational Therapy Communication;
- Content of Strategic Communication; and
- Pattern of Strategic Communication.

All kinds of issues, from management issues in the department to economic issues dictated by the environment, can be evaluated within this framework. It can be used to evaluate strategic communication in the various roles occupational therapy personnel perform in support of service delivery. The final selection of strategic communication patterns must be determined by the resources and constraints in the unique practice setting. You are urged to use this framework to analyze the factors that affect communication within your own practice setting. As with any action, it is important to assess

Figure 2. Strategic Communication in Practice: Discharge Placement

Issue	Environmental Resources/ Constraints	Organizational Resources/ Constraints	Goal(s) of Occupational Therapy Communication	Content of Strategic Communication	Pattern of Strategic Communication
Discharge placement of patient/client.	Community settings have unique culture and are affected by economic, political, legal, and social variables. Each setting is different. Management techniques differ in the same facility and between facilities.	Discharge planning is a staff team responsibility led by chief physician. Occupational therapy manages placement in school, work, volunteer job, or other prevocational/ vocational setting. Nursing staff manages placement in residential setting.	To improve reliance of physicians and nursing staff on occupational therapy assessment of functions. To negotiate expanded role of occupational therapy in self-care, work, leisure assessment and placement. To use information about patient's/ client's functional abilities to promote department and services provided. To use identified network of influence to increase team collaboration in the unit.	Survey satisfaction of patient/client and referral source with occupational therapy. Define role and contribution that occupational therapy is able to make in area of human function. Correlate outcome of occupational therapy with success of placement for previously discharged patients (length of stay in discharge placement, length of time between hospitalizations). Define patterns of coordination with other members of the treatment team.	Negotiate with unit chief, nursing staff. Write definition of role of occupational therapy in functional assessment. Survey patients/ clients, referral sources. Perform outcome studies. Establish reciprocal relationships with team members and maintain informal communication.

the results of the strategic communication and its effect on reaching desired goals. Adaptations based on assessment results will influence later communication strategies.

Resources

Bair, J., & Gray, M. (1986). *The occupational therapy manager.* Rockville, MD: American Occupational Therapy Association.

Donnelly, J., Gibson, J., & Ivanchevich, J. (1978). *Fundamentals of management.* (3rd ed.). Dallas, TX: Business Publications, Inc.

Esman, M. J. (1972). The elements of institution building. In J. Eaton (Ed.), *Institution Building and Development.* Beverly Hills, CA: Sage Publications.

Fox, E., & Wurwick, L. (1977). *Dynamic administration. The collected papers of Mary Parker Follett.* New York: Hippocrene Books, Inc.

Jacobs, K. (1987). Marketing occupational therapy. *American Journal of Occupational Therapy, 41,* 315-320.

Miyake, S., & Trostler, R. (1987). Introducing the concept of a corporate culture to a hospital setting. *American Journal of Occupational Therapy, 41,* 310-314.

Naisbitt, J., & Elkins, J. (1984). The hospital and mega-trends. *Hospital Forum,* May-June, 9-17.

Schulz, R., Peterson, R., & Greenley, J. (1984). Management, costs and quality of acute inpatient psychiatric services. *Medical Care, 21,* 911-928.

Tosi, H., & Carroll, S. (1976). *Management: Contingencies, structure, and process.* Chicago, IL: St. Clair Press.

Zaloccu, R., Joseph, W., & Doremus, H. (1984). Strategic marketing planning for hospitals. *Journal of Health Care Marketing, 4*(2), 19-28.

Section III

The Practice of Occupational Therapy Along the Mental Health Continuum of Care

Introduction

Occupational therapists in today's mental health care system have unlimited opportunities for professional growth. The current market emphasis on the development of functional living skills and increased demands for accountability in consumer-oriented treatment enable the occupational therapist to assume a leadership position in the provision of mental health services. Occupational therapy's holistic approach is highly congruent with present trends towards community integration and continuity of care. Therefore, the occupational therapist is uniquely qualified to be at the forefront of program development and treatment implementation along the entire mental health continuum of care (Baum, 1991; Fidler, 1991; Palmer, 1988).

Today's mental health care system includes a variety of treatment settings—ranging from public to private, acute to long-term, institutional to community-based—with multiple combinations possible, and a diversity of patient populations serviced (Fine, 1983; Mosey, 1986). Therefore, occupational therapists practicing in mental health have innumerable choices for their clinical settings. The opportunities for career mobility are substantial, and areas of specialization abound. The chapters in this section provide an overview of current major areas of occupational therapy practice in mental health. Additional growing areas of psychosocial occupational therapy practice will be discussed in subsequent sections. Readers are also referred to the reference list at the end of the text for resources on areas of specialization in mental health practice (i.e., substance abuse, eating disorders) that are beyond the parameters of this text.

The role of the occupational therapist on acute, inpatient psychiatric units is the focus of this section's first five chapters. Denton begins this discussion in chapter 13 by reviewing recent changes within the health care delivery system. She analyzes the impact of these trends on the provision of occupational therapy. Practical suggestions and realistic coping strategies to meet these challenges effectively and to provide relevant, quality care to persons with acute psychiatric disorders are provided.

In chapter 14 Bradlee expands this discussion of adaptive strategies for occupational therapists working on short-term inpatient units. Her primary focus is on the utilization of therapeutic groups for evaluation and intervention. Theoretical principles underlying group treatment and characteristic features of acute psychiatric units are explored to provide a foundation for the development of a relevant group program on a short-term unit. Realistic considerations for group development and constructive ideas for group modifications are supplemented by practical clinical case examples.

The efficacy of therapeutic group programs for acute, inpatient psychiatric units is further examined by Kaplan in chapter 15, on the Directive Group. In her presentation, Kaplan describes a three-level interdisciplinary group program that has a strong theoretical foundation and a well-organized program design. Primary emphasis is placed on a comprehensive description of the Directive Group. The applicability of this group approach to different treatment settings and patient populations with low functional levels is examined.

The range of functional levels among patients on a short-term psychiatric inpatient unit can be very wide; therefore, occupational therapists are often challenged to design programs to meet broad and varied functional needs. Chapters 16 and 17 describe two different program designs for acute psychiatric settings that can be utilized to meet a diversity of treatment goals. Ogren presents a living skills program, while Rider and Gramblin describe their activities approach to treatment. Patient characteristics, program goals, group format, and treatment activities are presented for each acute care program.

While short-term treatment programs can be effective in meeting the needs of many acutely ill clients, individuals with more chronic illnesses often require longer-term care. Chapters 18 through 22 focus on the delivery of extended treatment services to patients with chronic mental illness. In chapter 18 Boronow presents a comprehensive model for a long-term inpatient psychiatric rehabilitation program. Patient characteristics, treatment goals, rehabilitation principles, program activities, and behavior management techniques are described. While the therapeutic use of token economies may be questioned by some, the program Boronow presents is clearly a model for individualized treatment and the provision of comprehensive, collaborative, multidisciplinary care in a supportive, structured environment.

The relevance of supportive, structured environments in the treatment of persons with chronic mental illness is further explored in chapters 19 and 20, which address transitional residential programs. Wilberding describes a quarterway house, while Friedlob, Janis, and Deets-Aron discuss a halfway house program. In both chapters the authors use literature reviews to examine the historical development of residential care, identify principles of transitional services, and define specific residential programs. Admission criteria, resident characteristics, assessment procedures, program structure, treatment goals, intervention methods, and staff roles are described for each program. The positive effect of these programs on patient recidivism supports residential transitional living programs as effective models of intervention along the health care continuum for persons with chronic mental illness.

The need to establish treatment efficacy for approaches used in the long-term care of persons with chronic mental illness is further examined by Hayes in chapter 21. She identifies four major categories of treatment methods that have been reported in the occupational therapy literature as relevant interventions for persons with schizophrenia. A literature review of pertinent research on sensory integration, activity groups, social skills training, and living skills training is provided. The benefits and limits of these research studies, and the potential of each intervention method for the treatment of schizophrenia, are realistically analyzed.

The final chapter on long-term care in this section focuses on one of the treatment methods Hayes reviews as having potential for developing specific functional

skills. In chapter 22, Liberman, Massel, Mosk, and Wong present three models for social skills training. The rationale and implications for social skills training are explored by the authors. Each model is presented along a continuum of social skills development. Assessment methods, treatment procedures, session format, and therapists' roles are described and substantiated by clinical examples. The authors' emphasis on generalization and maintenance of skills is congruent with occupational therapy's primary goal of developing functional skills for community living.

The role of occupational therapy in developing community living skills is further explored in the chapters on community mental health. Adams initiates this discussion in chapter 23 by analyzing issues that impact the role of occupational therapy in community mental health settings. The tasks and functions of the therapist working in a community practice are identified. Adams argues that the professional philosophy and competence of occupational therapists uniquely qualifies them to provide community integration services in a collaborative and progressive manner.

The development of functional living skills for community living is explored in depth in chapter 24 by Crist. Crist reviews therapeutic models used in the treatment of patients with chronic mental illness who reside in the community. The psychoeducational model is presented as a viable form of mental health service delivery that can effectively develop community living skills. Psychoeducational concepts and principles are identified. Guidelines for program development are provided and supplemented by two program case studies. While many community mental health settings may not be able to provide "pure" psychoeducational programs, readers will find many of the psychoeducational concepts and practices described by Crist relevant to and easily implemented in a diversity of treatment programs.

In chapter 25, Coviensky and Buckley explore the role of occupational therapy in community mental health by examining day activities programming for persons with chronic mental illness. Program philosophy, structure, and goals are described. The authors emphasize that a supportive structured milieu providing consistency, concreteness, and normalization in treatment programming is essential for community integration and the maintenance of a quality life for persons with chronic mental illness.

The need for support and consistency in community mental health intervention is examined further by Moeller in chapter 26. The role of the case manager is essential to the provision of adequate services for persons with chronic mental illness. Moeller defines case management, identifies the community service needs of the chronically ill, and describes how occupational therapists can use their skills to address these needs.

The ability of the occupational therapist to coordinate effective community treatment is expanded upon in chapter 27 by Goldenberg, who describes a home-based after-care program for discharged psychiatric patients. Program goals, characteristics, format, and procedures are identified. A case study illustrates the efficacy of individualized occupational therapy in providing quality, integrative treatment, thereby ensuring continuity of care.

The need for occupational therapists to expand their role in community practice to ensure continuity of care is also explored in chapter 28 by Maynard. In her presentation, Maynard examines the role of occupational therapy in preventative and community health. She primarily focuses on the contributions occupational therapists can make to Employee Assistance Programs (EAPs). The relevance of occupational therapy evaluation and intervention principles and techniques to the promotion of health and wellness in community-based work settings is described.

Chapters 29 through 32, on vocational rehabilitation and integration for persons with mental illness, focus on the efficacy of occupational therapy in work programs. Lang and Cara begin by analyzing the reasons for poor employment among persons with mental illness. They discuss factors that can help predict clients' future vocational success and advocate the design and provision of programs that maximize these success-related factors. The authors examine occupational therapy models of practice relevant to vocational functioning and apply occupational therapy professional principles and skills to the provision of effective vocational services.

The effective provision of vocational programming is also discussed in chapter 30, by Richert, who focuses on acute care vocational rehabilitation. A literature review of the history of vocational rehabilitation is followed by a presentation of a timely and relevant vocational transition group for employed psychiatric inpatients. The philosophy, procedures, goals, and methods used in this group are presented in an extensive protocol. The efficacy of this group in assisting psychiatric inpatients who are planning to return to work after discharge is substantiated by numerous case examples that highlight a diversity of vocational concerns and therapeutic interventions.

While short-term vocational programming may be successful for many individuals, others may require more extensive, longer-term vocational services. In chapter 31, Palmer and Gatti present a comprehensive vocational program based upon sound theoretical principles. Program structure, evaluation procedures, treatment goals, activities, and tasks are described. An indepth analysis of patient characteristics, treatment concerns, and environmental considerations is well integrated with occupational therapy theory. A clinical case study highlights the relevance and efficacy of the vocational principles and methods presented.

The successful outcome of vocational rehabilitation is often dependent upon the quality of the patient's transition into competitive employment. Chapter 32, by Dulay and Steichen, describes a transitional employment program (TEP) for the chronic mentally ill. The role of the occupational therapist in the development and implementation of TEP is clearly discussed. The description of TEP screening, evaluation, and training methods is supplemented with a clear work sample and a relevant case example.

While vocational programming and the return to work often mark the endpoint of the continuum of care for many adults, the elderly person with mental illness often requires ongoing specialized care. In the final four chapters of this section, the authors explore the role of occupational therapy in psychogeriatrics. Trace and Howell begin this discussion in chapter 33 by describing the unique contributions occupational therapists can make to the mental health of elderly persons by utilizing our holistic approach. Preserving autonomy, enhancing integrity, and increasing the personal and community safety of the elderly are all viable outcomes of occupational therapy intervention. Relevant clinical issues and realistic barriers to optimal service delivery are analyzed with proactive suggestions and adaptive strategies provided to meet these challenges in psychogeriatric practice effectively.

The expansion of occupational therapy's role in psychogeriatric practice is further explored by Eilenberg in her presentation of a community-based wellness program to promote health and prevent depression in the elderly. In chapter 34 Eilenberg reviews developmental issues pertinent to aging and provides a theoretical base for the creation of this program. Needs assessment procedures, program objectives, group format, and session activities are described with realistic case vignettes supplementing the presentation. The efficacy of this wellness program is examined, with Eilenberg advocating that occupational therapists should assume an active role in health care promotion and preventative services.

While community-based services can clearly meet the needs of the "well" elderly, there is a growing necessity for institutional psychogeriatric programming to meet the specific requirements of the more severely ill elderly person. In chapter 35, Butin and Heaney describe a comprehensive psychosocial rehabilitation program used in an inpatient psychiatric setting. The program's philosophical base, assessment tools, treatment goals, and individual and group interventions are described and substantiated with practical clinical examples. The authors' emphasis on a collaborative, individualized approach to the provision of a multi-level, structured program graded according to each patient's functional abilities is consistent with occupational therapy's holistic philosophy.

The need for individualized graded treatment is also described in this section's final chapter, by Macdonald. In her presentation, Macdonald discusses the role of the occupational therapist in the evaluation and treatment of persons with dementia. The impact of dementia on cognitive and functional skills is analyzed along a developmental continuum. A multi-level activity group program, designed to meet the varying needs of dementia patients, is described. Environmental considerations and communication issues relevant to persons with dementia are also explored. Practical suggestions for activity adaptations, environmental modifications, and communication techniques are presented. A collaborative approach and a clinical emphasis on enhancing quality of life is effectively advocated by the author.

The ability of occupational therapy to enhance the quality of life for persons with mental illness is strongly supported by all the authors in this section. Whether providing effective crisis intervention, long-term care, community integration, vocational rehabilitation, or psychogeriatric services, the occupational therapist makes a significant contribution to the mental health continuum of care. Readers are encouraged to review the programs presented in this section critically, and to utilize the information to clarify the role of occupational therapy in mental health practice. However, readers are cautioned not to rely solely on clinical program descriptions for their definition of occupational therapy professional roles. A solid theoretical foundation and the ability to articulate a frame of reference for clinical practice is essential to the development of a clear professional identity. The selection of a frame of reference is a critical preliminary step in the process of providing effective occupational therapy evaluation and intervention (Bruce & Borg, 1987; Denton & Skinner, 1988: Mosey, 1986; Robertson, 1988). The relevance and value of utilizing a frame of reference to link theory to practice is strongly supported by this section's authors, who provide clear theoretical foundations for their program descriptions. While the presentation of occupational therapy frames of reference and models of practice is beyond the parameters of this text, readers are urged to utilize the excellent references provided at the end to explore further the theoretical base of occupational therapy practice.

Questions to Consider

1. What services and resources are available in your community to provide continuity of care to persons with mental illness? How can an occupational therapist advocate and network with these programs to ensure quality of care and enhance community integration for the mentally ill?

2. What were the major theoretical foundations used by the programs described in this section? Which occupational therapy frames of reference/models of practice are congruent with the different practice settings along the mental health continuum of care?

3. What are important considerations for selecting and using evaluations along the mental health continuum of care? Which evaluation methods and tools are applicable to short-term acute units? Long-term care settings? Community mental health programs? Vocational rehabilitation? Psychogeriatric programs?

4. What are the primary goals of occupational therapy along the mental health continuum of care? How can the occupational therapist facilitate functional goal attainment with the diverse patient populations seen in today's mental health care system's varied treatment programs?

5. Which occupational therapy intervention methods are most relevant to the treatment goals and patient functional levels along the mental health continuum of care (i.e., short-term acute units? long-term care settings? community mental health programs? vocational rehabilitation? psychogeriatric programs?).

6. How can therapeutic groups be employed as effective intervention methods along the mental health continuum of care? What adaptations to group structure format and activities may be needed to meet individual treatment goals and accommodate the different functional levels of clients and the varying clinical realities of different treatment settings?

7. What are the aftercare programs and support services available to clients upon completion of their treatment programs? How can the occupational therapist ensure effective referrals to maintain functional skills, community integration, and quality of life for persons with mental illness?

References

Baum, C. (1991). Professional issues in a changing environment. In C. Christiansen & C. Baum (Eds.), *Occupational therapy: Overcoming human performance deficits* (pp. 805-817). Thorofare, NJ: Slack.

Bruce, M. A., & Borg, B. (1987). *Frames of reference in psychosocial occupational therapy*. Thorofare, NJ: Slack.

Denton, P. L., & Skinner, S. T. (1988). Selecting a frame of reference/practice model. In S. C. Robertson (Ed.), *Mental health focus: Skills for assessment and treatment* (pp. I-100—1-108). Rockville, MD: American Occupational Therapy Association (AOTA).

Fidler, G. (1991). The challenge of change to occupational therapy practice. *Occupational Therapy in Mental Health, 11*(1), 1-11.

Fine, S. B. (1983). *Occupational therapy: The role of rehabilitation and purposeful activity in mental health practice*. Rockville, MD: American Occupational Therapy Association (AOTA).

Mosey, A. C. (1986). *Psychosocial components of occupational therapy*. New York: Raven Press.

Palmer, F. (1988). The present context of service delivery. In S. C. Robertson (Ed.), *Mental health focus: Skills for assessment and treatment* (pp. 1-28—1-36). Rockville, MD: American Occupational Therapy Association (AOTA).

Robertson, S. C. (1988). Assessment and treatment: The basics. In S. C. Robertson (Ed.), *Mental health focus: Skills for assessment and treatment* (pp. 1-92—1-99). Rockville, MD: American Occupational Therapy Association (AOTA).

Chapter 13

Occupational Therapy Practice in Acute Care: Changes, Challenges, and Coping Strategies

Peggy Denton, MS, OTR

This chapter was previously published in *Mental Health Special Interest Section Newsletter* (1986, March), pp. 1-4. Copyright © 1986, The American Occupational Therapy Association, Inc.

The treatment of psychiatric disorders has changed rapidly in the past few years; these advances are both exciting and overwhelming. In addition, the total health care delivery system is changing around us, creating an intense and pressured treatment environment. The following discussion will help to explain some of the system factors that currently affect occupational therapy practice in acute care.

Changes in Patient Characteristics

In recent years, there has been a drastic decrease in the length of hospitalizations. In 1982, the average length of stay for patients with depression on a psychiatric unit in a general hospital was 11.9 days (1). This represents a dramatic drop from previous years when patients often stayed 3 to 4 weeks for a depressive episode. Additionally, the reasons for hospitalization in acute care facilities are changing.

Treatment goals used to include a complete "work up," resolution of contributing "issues," and personality changes and adaptations. However, current goals are more frequently limited to resolving the immediate crisis, stabilizing the patient's symptomatology to prevent relapse after discharge, and connecting the patient to a community resource and other treatment facilities. Thorough evaluation and combinations of somatic treatments with intensive psychotherapy are common. Frequently, discharge planning begins the day of admission, and the "work" formerly done on an inpatient admission is now addressed after discharge.

These short-term admissions for crisis resolution and symptom management cause patients to attend occupational therapy during a highly acute phase of their illness. While acutely symptomatic, patients are frequently unable to sit and concentrate for long periods of time, are easily overstimulated by groups of people, and are experiencing difficulty learning through introspection or abstract symbolism. Occupational therapists once had the luxury of delaying treatment for a few days until the patient's symptoms were under control and they were better able to tolerate the environment and learn new coping skills through traditional treatment methods. However, since many patients are discharged as soon as the immediate crisis is resolved, occupational therapy may be delayed and therefore terminated.

Changes in the Health Care Industry

Although most psychiatric units have been exempted from DRGs (diagnostic related groups), some form of a prospective payment system is inevitable in the future. Restrictions on the amount of the patient's coverage is one variable that has been effective in decreasing the length of stay with Medicare patients (1). It is reasonable to expect that the prospective payment system, when applied to psychiatry, will decrease length of stay even more.

HMOs (health maintenance organizations) have provided a much more immediate influence on the length and type of available inpatient psychiatric treatment. In the HMO payment structure, physicians are strongly encouraged to save money by limiting hospital stays and dispensing with all but "essential" services. If HMO physicians refer patients to occupational therapy, it is usually for specific reasons and with a demand for accountability from the therapist for both the type of treatment provided and its effect. Physicians are under considerable pressure not to use occupational therapy services unless they believe that these services will benefit the patient. The competition between HMOs and health insurance carriers has spawned an increase in consumer choice and control in one's own health care. Customer satisfaction is gaining importance in the delivery of health care services, but this concept has some special difficulties in psychiatry, where treatment may not always be pleasant, or understood by the patient. If neither the patient nor physician has a thorough understanding and respect for occupational therapy services, continued referrals and reimbursement are unlikely.

Therapist Challenges

The occupational therapist working in acute care faces daily challenges. Scheduling becomes a major negotiation if everyone from the physician to the laboratory technician and dietician needs to see the patient in a short time. The demands are increasing for accountability in the selection or patients treated and the type and effectiveness of treatment delivered. HMOs, insurance carriers, Medicare, physicians, hospital administrators, and patients are rightfully requesting to know what we are going to do, why, and whether it will work. The statement, "I think occupational therapy would be beneficial for you," is no longer sufficient, and occupational therapy evaluation and treatment choices must be justified with logical and proven rationale. The need for frequent communication of occupational therapy eval-

uation and treatment choices and rationale with staff members is evident. We are challenged to increase efficiency, use sound clinical practices, and be accountable for our choices. The number of staff positions and size of supply budgets are often tied to the amount of money generated by the department. Therefore, fluctuations in the unit census and interruptions of evaluation and treatment for other services have potentially serious financial consequences. Overlap between the disciplines' roles, usually considered beneficial for continuity of care, also creates territorial and financial complications. At present, because occupational therapy is a reimbursable service and other expressive and recreational therapies are not, occupational therapists are experiencing pressure to bill for those other services under occupational therapy. Although this is clearly not ethical or legal practice, the pressure applied can be formidable (2). Whether occupational therapists like it or not, they are challenged to negotiate the business aspects of clinical practice.

Therapist Strategies

The following short-term coping strategies have proven useful in clinical practice on an acute psychiatric unit with an average length of stay of 8 to 10 days for most disorders.

- *Facilitate immediate and specific referral:* Prompt referrals on admission are necessary to ensure a maximum number of treatment days with each patient. A day or two lost while waiting for a referral to be written or processed results in lost treatment time and revenue. Specifying the criteria for appropriate referrals in a policy statement sent to all referral sources can help reduce the amount of time spent in responding to inappropriate referrals. Listing the reasons for referral on the referral form in a checklist may also help speed up the process.
- *Creative and flexible scheduling:* Scheduling blocks of time during the day to see patients individually or in small groups of two or three has been effective for those patients unable to tolerate a large group. Since there may not be enough people functioning at the same level or with the same needs for a particular thematic group, information can be provided to appropriate patients on an individual basis. Grouping all of the patients together and trying to find a common denominator of needs, interests, and functional level is usually ineffective. Group treatment may not be the most useful format for highly acute patients. In some instances, weekend services may be cost-effective (3).

- *Frequent communication*: Because treatment time is short, our observations of patients' performance need to be written frequently. Sending a follow-up survey (or discharge summary) to the admitting physician summarizing the patient's hospitalization from an occupational therapy perspective has been useful in ensuring that the physician uses the information provided in the charts and makes appropriate future referrals.

- *Increased accountability*: The demands for increased accountability are heard from many sources, including occupational therapists. Clinical outcome studies and research to validate both our theories and treatment techniques are currently a major focus for occupational therapy. But accountability also includes day-to-day systematic monitoring of our treatment and its effects. The single-system format promises a method of formally assessing outcome that is workable in acute care psychiatry (4).

- *Reexamine treatment models*: All of these strategies have dealt with the mechanics of providing occupational therapy services. We also need to reassess our treatment models for their clinical usefulness in today's acute care practice. Nothing is more frustrating for both the patient and the therapist than to have identified impaired areas of functioning, with the promise that those will be addressed, and to have the patient discharged before anything is accomplished. Regardless of how efficient we are, global modes of treatment that strive for some personality adaptation or change are questionable with patients hospitalized less than 2 weeks and acutely symptomatic most of that time. The cognitive disability model developed by Allen and her colleagues holds significant promise for today's acute care practice (5). She cogently articulates a concrete, specific, and relevant service that occupational therapy can provide that is minimally affected by the number of days that the patient is hospitalized. It also requires a rethinking of our current beliefs about the nature of psychiatric disorders and the role of the occupational therapist in their treatment.

The changes in acute psychiatric care require occupational therapists to adopt long-term changes and short-term coping strategies. As a profession, the time has come to evaluate and define the type of services that occupational therapy is best suited to offer in acute care. Former roles and treatment models may no longer be adequate. Our efforts may be best spent in evaluation, assisting with symptom management, and discharge planning. Acute care units in general hospitals, both medical and psychiatric, have been likened to triage units, where the patient is evaluated, stabilized, and sent to the appropriate treatment facility for continued treatment. Although we are not yet this limited, we must redefine occupational therapy's role and services if we expect to practice in this area. Some of the changes may be difficult and require a major shift in our thinking. Yet, we can be confident that occupational therapy has a viable and valuable role to play in the treatment of acute psychiatric disorders.

References

1. Taube CA, et al: Prospective payment and psychiatric discharges from general hospitals with and without psychiatric units. *Hosp Community Psychiatry* 36:754 -759, 1985

2. American Occupational Therapy Association: I'm Glad You Asked. *Occupational Therapy News* 39:6 November, 1985

3. Fogel BS, Slaby AE: Beyond gamesmanship: Strategies for coping with prospective payment. *Hosp Community Pschiatry* 36: 760-763.

4. Ottenbacher K, York J: Strategies for evaluating clinical change: Implications for practice and research. *Am J Occup Ther* 38:647-659, 1984

5. Allen CK: *Occupational Therapy for Psychiatric Diseases: Measurement and Management of Cognitive Disabilities.* Boston: Little, Brown & Co, 1985

Chapter 14

The Use of Groups in Short-Term Psychiatric Settings

Loring Bradlee, MS, OTR

This chapter was previously published in *Occupational Therapy in Mental Health, 4*(3), 47-57. Copyright © 1984, Haworth Press. Reprinted by permission.

The last two decades have witnessed significant changes in the nature and provision of occupational therapy services in psychiatric settings. Some of these changes reflect internal developments within the profession of occupational therapy while others reflect changing trends in the field of psychiatry at large. With specific regard to inpatient treatment, certainly the trend has been toward time-limited hospitalization. As stated by Crory, Sebastian and Mosey (1974), "short-term, in-hospital patient treatment is a reality brought on in part by rising hospitalization costs, more effective somatic treatment, and movement toward community-based treatment" (p. 401). This trend is based upon both clinical and fiscal considerations. In some instances, psychiatric hospitals once associated with longer-term care have dramatically shortened their average length of stay. In other instances, general hospitals have opened their own short-term psychiatric units. It has been noted that while in the 1940's there were only a few dozen such units, there are now as many as 1,700 (Sederer, 1983).

In the context of these changes, occupational therapists have been faced with the challenge of developing treatment programs that are both appropriate to short-term inpatient settings and effective in facilitating adaptive functioning. The decision to adopt a group format is often based on the therapist's own treatment philosophy, the purposes of the program, and logistical factors such as staffing patterns. Historically, occupational therapists have tended to rely upon a group orientation in the psychiatric services they provided. Consider, however, the contrast between developing a group program for a contemporary short-term unit where the average stay is a matter of weeks with a program described in a 1955 AJOT article entitled "Activity Group Therapy" in which the group membership extended for two years (Bobis, Harrison, & Traub). Additionally, there appears to be a shift away from the almost exclusively schizophrenic population reflected in this early literature to a more varied diagnostic population which often contains individuals of a higher functional level.

In developing group-oriented programs to coincide with these trends, occupational therapists have undoubtedly responded in a myriad of ways dependent in part on their own training and academic background. Some retain a traditional reliance on craft activities while others have expanded into areas of self-expression and communication skills. Some emphasize stress management while others concentrate on daily living skills. Some may stress physical modalities while others rely on cognitive strategies. Given such variation, how can one meaningfully consider such groups in terms of a larger spectrum?

To establish this broader perspective, it seems that several considerations may be necessary. First, there is the need to examine our own professional heritage in regard to the use of groups in psychiatric treatment. Secondly, there is the need to explore the specific features that are unique to the nature of inpatient units and that therefore impact on treatment programs operating within. Thirdly, there is the consequent need to look at the kinds of considerations and adaptations that may be indicated in developing group programs for short-term psychiatric settings.

The literature contains some record of efforts to conceptualize the use of groups in psychiatric occupational therapy. Shannon and Snortum (1965) proposed that "by working in a group of limited size, the patient could be provided with a more closely supervised opportunity for practicing rudimentary social skills and receive needed feedback from actual experience, thereby discovering that he is capable of handling social situations that formerly prompted his withdrawal" (p. 345). These fundamentals are expanded and elaborated by Gail Fidler in her hallmark 1969 article "The Task-Oriented Group As a Context for Treatment." In this she postulates that

> the intent of the task-oriented group is to provide a shared working experience wherein the relationship between feeling, thinking and behavior, their impact on others and task accomplishment can be viewed and explored. Task accomplishment is seen as the catalytic agent which elicits behavior and interaction, brings into focus both functional capacities and limitations, facilitates collaboration in working through problems and provides a concrete reality against which to measure learning and achievement (p. 45).

Subsequently, in her article "The Concept and Use of Developmental Groups," published in the following year, Anne Mosey outlined her developmental theory of groups which suggests that group-oriented programs should be graded so as to facilitate the acquisition of interactional skills. These skills, in mature form, endow one with "the ability to participate in a variety of groups in a manner that is satisfying for oneself and one's fellow members" (1970, p. 273). Groups designed for congruency with relative interactional skills then become arenas for developing higher level or more mature skills.

These cited authors (Shannon and Snortum; Fidler; and Mosey) point to the role of the occupational therapy group as an interactional experience which allows for the assessment and enhancement of overall social and functional skills. Other authors have described the use of particular modalities (Rothaus, Hanson, and Cleveland, 1966; Rance and Price, 1973; Angel, 1981) as well as instruction in specific functional skills within a group structure (Hughes and Mullins, 1981).

This discussion, however, will focus on the occupational therapy group as an interactional experience and on the application of such an experience within a short-term psychiatric setting where the overall goals of hospitalization are apt to be diagnostic assessment, reduction of symptomatology, and rapid reintegration into the community. In contrast to long-term outpatient or in-hospital treatment where goals are typically more ambitious in terms of personality reorganization, short-term inpatient treatment is customarily geared toward dealing with the immediate determinants of and precipitants for hospital admission. According to Leeman in his chapter in the recently published *Inpatient Psychiatry—Diagnosis and Treatment* (1983), "this requires evaluating the patient's premorbid environment, assessing the patient behavior in varied interpersonal situations, and providing opportunities to enhance the patient's responsibility and to restore optimal social functioning" (p. 223).

The short-term unit as a setting for this process tends to have certain characteristic features. The relatively brief period of hospitalization and consequent rapid patient turnover results in a continually fluctuating social situation. Physically the units are usually self-contained within a relatively small space thereby creating the potential of an intensively dynamic environment. Typically, patients have frequent, if not constant, contact throughout the day in terms of sharing a central day-room, eating in a common dining area, and participating together in various treatment programs. Most clinicians agree that patients in these settings are highly sensitive to events that occur on the unit and fluctuations in its atmosphere. Indeed, the mood of a unit is highly changeable—a volatile situation which erupts into crisis can be followed by a sense of calm resolution within a period of several hours. The patient population itself can also be highly varied in terms of diagnosis and level of function. However, despite this, patients often develop a strong sense of mutual affiliation on the basis of their shared hospitalization. In a further contribution to the dynamics of a short-term unit, individual staff members often serve in a multiplicity of roles which sometimes results in a blurring of these roles. For example, a nurse may function as both a primary therapist who meets psychotherapeutically with a patient and as a charge nurse who administers medication to that same patient.

These, then, are some of the notable features of the short-term psychiatric setting in which an occupational therapy group is developed and its objectives established. One common primary goal is assessment. The occupational therapy group can provide a cost-effective, expeditious and structured means of evaluating an individual's social-interactive skills. Occupational therapists have long identified the potential of their group-oriented programs to provide such assessment. More recently, there has been delineation of the specific aspects of social-interactive functioning that should be included in that assessment. Bloomer and Williams (1981) have described the seven parameters included in their Bay Area Functional Performance Evaluation. These are response to authority figures, verbal communication, psychomotor behavior, independence/dependence, socially appropriate behavior, ability to work with peers and participation in group/program activities. The information yielded by such an assessment is valuable in several ways. For one, it helps to determine what types of consequent treatment experiences might be indicated during hospitalization. Equally important, such assessment can suggest what kinds of treatment might be recommended for outpatient follow-up. In addition, regular participation in an occupational therapy group can provide on-going assessment data that is valuable as an overall index of progress during hospitalization. Obviously, on a short-term unit, assessment and treatment often take place concurrently and one continually impacts on the other.

The group-oriented occupational therapy program is also aimed at providing treatment. On the basis of appropriate evaluation and typically in collaboration with both patient and other staff members, a decision is made as to the advisability of involving the patient in a particular group program. Groups may differ in terms of the modalities used, the content of focus and the expectant level of participant functioning. However, one primary goal is to enhance social-interactive skills in relation to the patient's potential and the demands of the environment to which he/she will return. This overall goal is further delineated in terms of objectives which may include the reinforcement of socially acceptable behavior, the fostering of effective communication skills, the encouragement of self-awareness and self-expression, and the strengthening of interpersonal confidence. King (1978) has postulated that "we could say that occupational therapy consists of structuring the surroundings, materials and especially the demands of the environment in such a way as to call forth a specific adaptive response" (p. 16). A structured occupational therapy group can thus be seen as a setting in which more adaptive interactional skills can be identified and experienced.

In considering the feasibility of pursuing such objectives, it seems necessary to examine their compatibility with the setting in which they occur. Leeman (1983) notes that "the essence of inpatient psychiatric treatment...is that it occurs in a controlled milieu" (p. 223). Abrams (1969) has defined milieu therapy as "the means of organizing a community treatment environment so that every treatment technique can be specifically utilized to further the patient's aims of controlling symptomatic behaviors and learning appropriate psycho-social skills" (p. 559). Certainly not all short-term units subscribe to this pure model of milieu therapy; most, however, recognize the environmental aspects of inpatient psychiatry and to varying degrees use the milieu for therapeutic purposes.

There is a strong parallel between the experiential and structured nature of milieu therapy in general and the occupational therapy group in particular. As an occupational therapy group actualizes its own objectives, it also supports the overall therapeutic purpose of inpatient hospitalization. Furthermore, the capacity of the occupational therapy group to provide such catalytic experiences has particular significance in a short-term setting where time is a limited resource and treatment must be goal-oriented. Whether the purpose is to evaluate social-interactive functioning or to foster growth in specific interactional skills, the occupational therapist can actively orchestrate a group program to meet that purpose. Additionally, if comfortably skilled in group dynamics, he/she can personalize and intensify the experience for participant patients and thereby facilitate their active involvement. Therein lies the potential of the occupational therapy group to be an integrative setting in which inpatient experience can be translated into therapeutic growth.

Most therapists who work in short-term units might also add (or perhaps argue!) that the realization of this potential is hampered by the realities that characterize such units. It seems advisable, then, to outline some points to be considered in developing an occupational therapy group as well as to share specific aspects of the author's experience in doing so. Such an outline and discussion follows.

Flexibility

With as variable a population as typifies a short-term unit, occupational therapists should be prepared to be very flexible in both therapeutic approach and program content. For instance, the focus of a particular group is often determined on a day-to-day basis. Similarly, it is usually impossible to maintain a constant group membership over any extended period of time. Also, a group must be flexible so as to allow for less functional patients while at the same time provide a meaningful experience for those functioning at a higher level. The author, for instance, has developed and co-led a Communication Skills group for one short-term unit. This group met once a week for 1½ hours and averaged 5-6 members. Each group was structured to provide experiences that might increase awareness of communication patterns and encourage exploration of alternative patterns. However, the actual content differed greatly and depended upon the assessment by both the group leadership and other staff members as well as patients themselves as to how the group could be particularly helpful. Job interviewing, conversational skills, assertiveness and self-disclosure were commonly identified as issues to be worked on, and role-playing was often used to offer practice in more adaptive ways of handling such situations as they typically arise. Participants were often encouraged to further practice outside the group in hopes of maximizing the overall usefulness of their hospitalization experience.

Realistic Expectations

Time constraints create a need to be modest in setting goals for a group program. At times, assessment of interactional skills may be the primary goal. At other times, the goal may be to initiate a therapeutic process that will continue after discharge. For instance, based on an individual's participation as an inpatient, he/she might be referred to a group program on an outpatient basis. As an example of adapting expectations, the author had several years of experience being the on-going leader for a traditionally conceived verbal therapy group on a short-term unit. It became increasingly evident that the non-directive leadership and unstructured format that might be appropriate for a long-term outpatient group was not so in a short-term inpatient setting and was perhaps even counter-productive. On this basis, a model of unit-wide Community Meetings was developed for which the author provided primary leadership. These meetings were aimed at encouraging patients to address

issues occurring within the community, to exchange perceptions of their day-to-day life together and its relation to life in the community, and to directly resolve conflicts when indicated. Not only did these meetings seem to facilitate the overall functioning of the unit, but they also provided another opportunity for patients to practice social-interactive skills that have relevance to community life outside the hospital.

Understanding of Group Dynamics as Reflection of Ward Dynamics

Several authors (Levine, 1980; Kibel, 1981) have suggested the need for the therapist to be sensitive to the connection between the dynamics evident in an inpatient group and the on-going dynamics of the unit as a whole. Not only is this essential to the therapist's interpretation of the group process, but it is also key to the occupational therapy group's existence as an integrated part of the therapeutic whole. Given the previously suggested characteristics of a short-term unit, the interplay of group and ward dynamics may be particularly evident in such a setting. At one time, for instance, the author coordinated a meal preparation program in which patients of a short-term unit were expected to plan and prepare a unit-wide dinner on a weekly basis. The ability of a specified group to work cooperatively toward such a purpose was often affected by the broader dynamics of the unit at the time. An awareness of this was helpful in making the experience optimally therapeutic for those patients involved. A common case in the cooking program was that patients who were dominant figures on the unit at large often took on parallel roles in the meal preparation. This, then, could become an opportunity to allow those patients to share responsibility and to encourage other more passive patients to assert themselves. Sensitivity to the dynamics of the larger population can expedite the purposes of the occupational therapy program as well as make those purposes individually tailored. Given the limited time frame of the short-term unit, both of these aspects are significant.

Need for a System Perspective

If an occupational therapy group is to survive, let alone succeed, in a short-term unit, its role in the larger system of the unit must be considered. Klein and Kugel (1981) have noted that "it is clear that the social system of the ward—with its norms, expectations and values— plays a particularly important role in determining patient's behavior in group meetings and has a significant impact on therapeutic process" (p. 316). The identity of the group must be congruent or at least compatible with the overall treatment philosophy of the unit. Questions arising from this issue as well as others less directly related should be explored. Is the occupational therapy group sanctioned administratively and supported by other staff? Do the structure and norms of the unit reinforce regular patient attendance? Does the group reflect sensitivity to the value system of its intended participants? It has been the experience of this author, for example, that self-expressive modalities have limited relevance on a short-term unit in a Veterans' Hospital serving a rural population. This might then suggest the advisability of incorporating a task orientation into a particular group. In fact, it was found that a woodworking group that used a modality highly acceptable to a male, work-oriented population was more effective in reinforcing basic interactional skills. Similarly, this kind of group coincided with the values of the larger social system of the institution itself.

Need for Education and Collaboration

Given the interwoven dynamics and the time limitation that characterize a short-term unit, it seems particularly important that its various staff members work cooperatively. Accordingly, the occupational therapist needs to educate other staff about a particular group and its therapeutic purposes. Inservices as well as opportunities to observe and participate can facilitate staff understanding and support. Issues of professional territorialism can, however, arise and the role of the occupational therapy group may at times need to be coordinated with the efforts of other staff members. Similarly, the author has at times been integrally involved in interdisciplinary treatment programs. This has included, for example, providing co-leadership in a weekly Outward Bound treatment program for selected patients on a short-term unit. Here the role of [the] occupational therapist was to assess the social and functional levels of the participating patients, to suggest appropriate goals for the Outward Bound experience and to facilitate the group dynamics of the experience itself.

These, then, are points that an occupational therapist might consider in developing a group program for a short-term inpatient unit. He/she, however, may still experience frustration with the nature of such a unit. There is the sense of constant beginning and having to start over. The emotional drain resulting from working with individuals in a state of acute dysfunction is considerable and there is little of the satisfaction that may arise from longer-term treatment and the solidified growth that can take place there. Also, it is often difficult to delineate the specific impact of various forms of treatment in a short-term setting. However, the well-con-

ceived and sensitively executed occupational therapy group plays a vital part in the process that allows individuals to regain a sense of their ability to cope and to begin to approach their lives more adaptively. Some find a challenge within these limits—a challenge to their personal ability to adapt just as they challenge that of their patients. Occupational therapy has long proclaimed its ability to assess and enhance the interactional skills of those psychiatric populations served. With careful consideration and some modification, this strong tradition will prevail on the short-term units so prevalent today in psychiatric treatment.

References

Abroms, G. M. Defining milieu therapy. *Archives of General Psychiatry*, 1969, *21*, 553-560.

Angel, S. L. The emotion identification group. *American Journal of Occupational Therapy*, 1981, *35*, 256-262.

Bloomer, J., & Williams, S. The Bay Area Functional Performance Evaluation. In B. J. Hemphill (Ed.), *The Evaluative Process in Psychiatric Treatment*. Thorofare, NJ: Charles B. Slack, 1981.

Bobis, B., Harrison, R., & Traub, L. Activity group therapy. *American Journal of Occupational Therapy*, 1955, *IX*, 19-21.

Crory, S., Sebastian, V., & Mosey, A. C. Acute short-term treatment in psychiatry. *American Journal of Occupational Therapy*, 1974, *28*, 401-406.

Erickson, R. C. Small-group psychotherapy with patients on a short-stay ward: An opportunity for innovation. *Hospital and Community Psychiatry*, 1983, *32*, 269-272.

Fidler, G. Task-oriented group as a context for treatment. *American Journal of Occupational Therapy*, 1969, *XXIII*, 43-48.

Hughes, P. L., & Mullins, L. *Acute psychiatric care*. Thorofare, NJ: Charles B. Slack, 1981.

Kibel, H. D. A conceptual model for short-term inpatient group psychotherapy. *American Journal of Psychiatry*, 1981, *138*, 74-80.

King, L. J. Toward a science of adaptive responses. *American Journal of Occupational Therapy*, 1978, *32*, 14-22.

Klein, R. H. Inpatient group psychotherapy: Practical considerations and special problems. *International Journal of Group Psychotherapy*, 1977, *27*, 201-214.

Klein, R. H., & Kugel, B. Inpatient group psychotherapy from a systems perspective: Reflections through a glass darkly. *International Journal of Group Psychotherapy*, 1981, *31*, 311-321.

Leeman, C. P. The therapeutic milieu. In L. I. Sederer (Ed.), *Inpatient Psychiatry: Diagnosis and Treatment*. Baltimore: Williams & Wilkins, 1983.

Levine, H. B. Milieu biopsy: The place of the therapy group on the inpatient ward. *International Journal of Group Psychotherapy*, 1980, *30*, 77-93.

Llorens, L. A. Changing methods in treatment of psychosocial dysfunction. *American Journal of Occupational Therapy*, 1968, *XXII*, 26-29.

Mosey, A. C. The concept and use of developmental groups. *American Journal of Occupational Therapy*, 1970, *XXIV*, 272-275.

Rance, D., & Price, A. Poetry as a group project. *American Journal of Occupational Therapy*, 1973, 27, 252-255.

Rothaus, P., Hanson, P. G., & Cleveland, S. E. Art and group dynamics. *American Journal of Occupational Therapy*, 1966, *20*, 182-187.

Sederer, L. I. (Ed.). *Inpatient psychiatry: Diagnosis and treatment.* Baltimore: Williams & Wilkins, 1983.

Shannon, P. D., & Snortum, J. R. An activity group's role. *American Journal of Occupational Therapy*, 1965, *XIX*, 344-347.

Chapter 15

The Directive Group: Short-Term Treatment for Psychiatric Patients with a Minimal Level of Functioning

Kathy L. Kaplan, MS, OTR/L

This chapter was previously published in the *American Journal of Occupational Therapy, 40*, 474-481. Copyright © 1986, The American Occupational Therapy Association, Inc.

Patients in short-term psychiatric inpatient units function at various levels and have a wide range of functional needs; they vary greatly in terms of their age, diagnosis, and background. This diversity presents great challenges to occupational therapy programming. There are relatively few resources published that address the problems associated with treating these patients in the limited time frame of the acute care unit. In addition, many acute care units employ only one occupational therapist so that there is no daily support from similarly trained personnel. Because the health care environment stresses accountability for staff positions, reimbursement, and professional autonomy, occupational therapy must not only offer a unique service to these patients within a limited time frame, but must also find effective ways to contribute and collaborate within an interdisciplinary team.

All inpatient psychiatric units provide some form of group therapy; their structure and content vary as determined by administrative factors and philosophical values (Yalom, 1983). Brief hospitalization has accounted for improved social functioning and decreased rates of admission in some patients (Herz, Endicott, Spitzer, 1977; Decker, 1972), but the specific forms of therapy that contribute to such benefits are not clearly defined.

Based on a review of 10 years of group psychotherapy outcome studies, Parloff and Dies (1977) recommend that clinicians resolve conceptual issues before proceeding with research questions. They suggest that the highest priority is to develop explicit definitions and descriptions of specialized forms and techniques of group psychotherapy.

This advice is appropriate for our field. Occupational therapy personnel in mental health are currently competing with many other professionals who use activities and lead groups. A recent survey found that 60% of the occupational therapists sampled use groups in all areas of practice (Duncombe, 1985). Our priority should be to specify what type of occupational therapy groups are best for which patients and to examine whether changes in behavior and improved functioning are due to therapists' skills, techniques employed, duration of treatment, type of instrumentation, or theoretical assumptions.

Increasingly, short-term units are admitting more chronic psychiatric and elderly patients who, along with the acutely psychotic and organically impaired patients, are difficult to involve in the ward milieu because of their extremely disorganized, dependent, or disruptive behavior. During a brief hospitalization, these patients face the difficult task of reorganizing their behavior to learn or relearn the minimal skills necessary to perform routine daily activities.

In most settings these types of patients are treated with medication, structure, and individual therapy until they are sufficiently organized to join a psychotherapy group. Although some settings offer occupational therapy or activity groups for these patients, this kind of treatment is not usually very important within the total group program. However, based on the author's experience, occupational therapists can expand their role in mental health by developing a framework for coordinating an interdisciplinary group program and taking a leadership position in treating the most disorganized patients on the unit.

This article presents an overview of a comprehensive group program developed on a short-term inpatient psychiatric unit and describes in detail the Directive Group, a specialized form of group therapy developed by the author for patients functioning the least well.

Beginnings of the Program

The new program was developed for the 34-bed inpatient unit of The George Washington University Medical Center. The unit offers a continuum of services, including day treatment and outpatient programs. Adolescent, adult, and elderly patients are admitted for evaluation and treatment of acute emotional problems. During a 2- to 3-week stay patients participate in a wide range of therapeutic services, including individual psychotherapy, primary nursing care, psychotropic medications, family therapy, and group therapy.

Nine years ago, perceiving program fragmentation and staff isolation, several staff members revised the original program. Using a developmental approach, we reorganized the existing groups to meet the needs of the patients functioning at different levels. The Directive Group, the most innovative part of the program, was created for the patients functioning at the lowest level.

The following is a description of the program as it has evolved during the author's six years of coordinating it. Special emphasis is given to the Directive Group, which has since received public recognition (Yalom, 1983) and withstood the test of time.

Research Support

Research supports the use of group programs for the remedial treatment of the acutely ill, provided short-term treatment is part of a continuum of care. The most effective group programs and those most valued by staff members provide daily group therapy, monitor group composition, strive to decrease professional rivalry, and have an interactive focus (Yalom, 1983).

In terms of specialized approaches for the minimally functioning patient, reviews of outcome studies generally agree that there is a lack of evidence to support the value of verbal, insight-oriented group psychotherapy for psychotic and schizophrenic populations (Parloff & Dies, 1977; Bednar & Lawlis, 1971; Meltzoff & Kornreich, 1970; Stotsky & Zolik, 1965; Moriarity, 1976; May, 1976; Mosher & Keith, 1979). Groups for this population are most effective when they rely on structured activity and reality-based approaches (Bednar & Lawlis, 1971; May, 1976). In fact, groups with intense interpersonal stimulation may be harmful (Linn et al., 1976). Furthermore, groups are more effective when combined with other forms of treatment, such as psychopharmacology and individual therapy (Parloff & Dies, 1977). However, drugs and psychotherapy alone are insufficient for developing social and occupational skills (May, 1976; Keith, 1982). This finding is important for occupational therapists promoting activity-oriented groups.

Theoretical Framework

Without a theoretical framework, the clinician lacks a coherent way to organize knowledge, ascribe meaning to observations, or predict outcomes. We used the model of human occupation, which describes individuals as complex, open systems who are in constant interaction with the environment and who maintain and change their behavior through action (Kielhofner, 1985). We chose the model for several reasons. Since the model is based on general systems theory (Kielhofner, 1978; Boulding, 1956), it is congruent with interdisciplinary views. At the same time the focus on occupational behavior delineates the scope of occupational therapy services and is consistent with the short-term unit goals of improving the patient's functioning and enabling him or her to return to the community. The model allows the therapist to integrate information from other professionals pertaining to such factors as the patient's environment or support system. Finally, the model enables the therapist to specify an organized approach to the diverse patient group in acute inpatient care.

We used the model in three ways. First, the model specifies a continuum of occupational behavior represented by three levels of arousal and accomplishment: exploration, competence and achievement (Reilly, 1974; Kielhofner, 1985). Criteria for each of these levels were developed (Cubie & Kaplan, 1982) and used to organize each group in the total group program. Second, the model serves to identify the variables necessary for assessing patient behavior and specifying treatment goals (Roger & Kielhofner, 1985). Referral criteria were based on behavioral descriptions of the most typical patient problems addressed in each group and translated into the language of the model for consistency. Third, the model provides a way to conceptualize group treatment as the creation of therapeutic environments in which patients interact to learn about themselves and enact changes. The environment is created by titrating levels of arousal, enhancing internal control, stimulating interest and meaning in activities, and conveying expectations relevant to patient needs, goals, and roles (Barris, Kielhofner, Levine, Neville, 1985).

Program Design

All groups in our setting are organized by three levels of arousal and demands or performance. The exploration level groups are organized at the simplest level of challenge to help severely disorganized patients develop basic process skills, perceptual motor skills, and communication/interaction skills. The group leaders select activities and organize the treatment environment; patients are required to participate in the scheduled group meetings.

Competence level groups are appropriate for pa-tients who have basic skills but may need to integrate them into habit patterns. These groups are designed to help patients expand their skills and to identify goals, interests, and needs for meaning and action. As patients approach discharge, they begin to learn new ways to cope with problems experienced at home and in the community. Groups at the achievement level are designed to help patients integrate skills into daily life roles.

Table 1 illustrates how groups are differentiated by levels by each professional discipline. The purpose of the vertical dimension is to assure that the program has depth. Each level includes a number of groups, which are

Table 1. Program Groups Categorized by Level and Professional Discipline

Level	Professional Discipline		
	Therapeutic Recreation	Occupational Therapy	Psychiatry/ Psychology
Achievement	Leisure Awareness	Assertiveness Training	
Competence	Activity Planning Evening Activity	Task Group	Community Meeting Supportive Group
Exploration	Exercise Group	Directive Group	Directive Group

organized similarly but differ in content or focus. Therefore, groups are also planned to show variation along three horizontal dimensions (see Figure 1). The horizontal structure of the framework prompts consideration of the balance and range of groups. Together, the vertical and horizontal dimensions build a coordinated framework in which each individually designed group contributes to the group treatment program as a whole.

Figure 1. Occupational, Interpersonal, and Mind/Body Dimensions of Program Groups

Leisure	Occupational Dimensions			Work
	Leisure Awareness Evening Activities	Activity Planning Supportive Group	Assertiveness Training Task Group	
Social Interaction	Interpersonal Dimension			Intimate Relationships
	Directive Group Evening Activities	Assertiveness Training Leisure Awareness	Supportive Group Community Meeting	
Physical Capacities	Mind/Body Dimension			Cognitive Abilities
	Directive Group Exercise Group	Task Group Evening Activities	Assertiveness Training Activity Planning	

Referral Criteria

When patients are admitted to the unit, they are interviewed and evaluated by a psychiatrist and a nurse. Later, after meeting with the patients on rounds, in meetings, and informally, the interdisciplinary team members contribute to the master problem list and make referrals to groups. Each treatment group has a referral form itemizing specific referral criteria to match the patient's level of functioning with the goals of the groups. In addition, patients are referred to groups whose content is relevant. For example, a patient with depression and a workaholic lifestyle is referred to a leisure awareness group, which has an overall goal of clarifying leisure values and increasing awareness of lifestyle choices.

The occupational therapy and therapeutic recreation staff assist members of the team to think clinically about the groups and make appropriate referrals. The referral criteria serve as an individualized initial assessment of patient functioning. Identified problems are translated into short-term goals and provide a way to measure outcome. The following discussion of the Directive Group provides an example of this assessment and treatment process.

The Directive Group

The Typical Patient

The Directive Group is designed for patients with varied diagnoses whose functioning is profoundly incapacitated. The group has included patients experiencing hallucinations, paranoia, catatonia, severe depression, organicity, hyperactivity, concrete thinking, or loose associations.

The model of human occupation provides a way of conceptualizing the dysfunctions of this diverse group of patients who have extreme difficulty functioning in the most basic of tasks and roles. They feel out of control, expect failure, avoid mastery experiences, and fear exploring the environment. They typically have difficulty identifying interests and goals. Their habits of self-care and time management are markedly disrupted. Although these patients may have had adequate habits prior to the acute episode, their current situation is characterized by extremely limited interpersonal and task-oriented skills.

The Format of the Group

The term *Directive* refers to the active and supportive way in which the group leaders elicit adaptive behaviors and structure the environment to assure maximum participation of all members. The purpose of the group is to assist patients in reorganizing their behavior to a beginning level of competence. In general, patients are ready to be discharged from the group when they actively participate and can sustain minimal interaction throughout the 45-minute session.

The group, consisting of 6 to 12 members, meets 5 days a week at a routine time and place. The sessions begin and end promptly to emphasize a realistic use of and attention to time. On the average, patients attend 10 to 15 sessions, depending on the length of their hospital stay and speed of recovery. Once referred, attendance is mandatory to ensure continuity of treatment. Regular attendance depends largely on the assistance of nursing staff, since most of the patients are initially too disoriented or confused to take on this responsibility.

The relationships and activities of the Directive Group occur in a playful arena, a safe environment, which encourages risk-taking in patients who are threatened by the possibility of failure (Vandenber & Kielhofner, 1982). Patients are encouraged to move from passivity and internal preoccupation to goal-directed processes in which spontaneity and competence begin to emerge (Bertelanffy, 1966).

Content of a Typical Session

Each session of the Directive Group is complete within itself to accommodate the level of function and short stay of the patients. A session has four parts: orientation and introductions, warmup activities, selected activities and wrap-up.

The first few minutes are usually spent reviewing the purpose of the group and specific treatment goals. Members who have been in the group are relied on to explain the purpose of the group and give examples of activities they have enjoyed and found useful. Introductions are conducted to make patients realize that their presence is valued.

For example, a group session typically begins with a coleader asking a relatively experienced group member to help fill in the blanks on the blackboard. The board includes questions about the date, name of the group, its meeting time, its purpose, and the activities of the day before (or the previous weekend). Asking patients to call out the answers to the questions encourages them to focus on the activity and participate actively. This is usually followed by a balloon game in which each patient says the name of the person to whom he or she is throwing the balloon. The game is adapted by asking patients to choose a category, like cars or hobbies, and then to name items in that category.

The warm-up phase generally consists of 10 minutes of physical activity the complexity and vigor of which are based on individual capacities. Movement provides a simple, familiar, and shared experience without the stress of verbal interactions. Exercises also allow for participation in simple rule behaviors such as taking turns and following instructions. For example, in a low-energy group, members seated in a circle are told to move as little as possible. The leader slowly lifts one finger and moves it up and down. As the members imitate the movement, the leader opens and closes his or her hand. Finally, both hands are in the act. By starting slowly and matching the pace of the group, more activity is gradually elicited from the patients. Soon a member agrees to lead a simple movement while the others follow.

The major part of the group session is spent in activities especially selected for each day. These may include a series of games, each lasting a few minutes, or one long activity. For example, a regular feature of the Directive Group is the decoration of a large monthly calendar, used as a tool to help members stay oriented to the day of the week and the month. Depending on the needs and interests of the group, the sequence of events roughly proceeds from movement activities to interaction with objects to interaction with people (Robinson, 1977); the level of complexity increases from imitation to a few instructions to simple problem solving. Graded opportunities are available for leadership, decision making, expression of interests, helping others, and verbal interaction.

The last 10 minutes are spent in a verbal review of the activities and processes of the session. The leader lists on the board the patients' recall of the sequence of events, such as orientation of the board, name ball games, physical exercises, sit-down soccer, hangman, and the wrap-up. Then patients are asked to name the skills they used to perform these activities. With verbal structure, these patients are able to identify skills such as concentration, coordination, conversation, and having fun.

The wrap-up serves to attach meaning to the events of the group and provide feedback about each member's preferences and contributions. Because of the high patient turnover, group members must be helped to adjust to new members and say good-bye to old members during each session. A useful wrap-up activity is "Guess Who?" The patients answer questions like "Who was the first person in the group?" or "Who is wearing a red sweater?" or "Who laughed when we played sit-down soccer?" Such questions engage the patients' short-term memories, extend their attention, and create a supportive interactive focus.

The Coleaders' Role

The group is co-led by an occupational therapist and a psychiatrist. The leaders provide ongoing training experiences for other staff members and student coleaders.

Coleadership assures continuity of the group and consistency of meeting times. It provides security when a patient requires individual attention or assistance to leave the room in the event of out-of-control behavior. The

severity of illness necessitates the presence of at least one other leader to counteract the patients' powerful pull toward extreme passivity, disruptiveness, and disorganization. Coleaders also provide support for each other when the daily demands of the group for creative, patient, and individualized approaches become overwhelming.

Coleaders plan activities, facilitate the assumption of group roles, and modify the structure of the group to meet the changing needs of the patients. Coleaders must be flexible and able to adapt activities on the spot. For instance, based on the group's level of attention, energy and interaction on the previous day, the leaders plan a game of modified bowling. But the group shows no interest and does not respond to other alternatives offered. The leaders than engage the group in yelling "yes" and "no." Breaking the action with humor gives patients a face-saving and empathic way to get involved.

As the main providers of feedback to the patients about the effects of their actions, the coleaders encourage, cajole, limit, refocus, and challenge the group members. The main message is acceptance. There is a strong expectation that each member, when ready, will be successful and will be supported in all attempts to participate. Patients are offered choices whenever possible to enhance their sense of control and to encourage their expression of interests. The choices can be graded to offer progressively more control. For instance, patients can decide if they would rather play bean bag toss sitting or standing up; if they want to have relay races in a circle or by teams; if they would prefer one activity over another, like geography or the card game Uno; if they want to suggest an altogether different activity based on their own experiences.

Physical Environment

Space is used to emphasize the expectations of participation. The room is fairly large and has tables and chairs that can be used as needed. There is a blackboard, storage cabinets, and a sink. Attendance is made clear by a daily list, which patients check off when they enter. The environment provides cues for role behavior, orientation in time, and performance.

Materials are used to engage patients' interests and inclination toward activity. Care must be taken to select activities that are appropriate for the current low functional level of the patients but do not demean their self-esteem as adults.

Often word games allow patients to associate with the memory of more pleasant times and elicit responses that surprise everyone. For example, one day a group was playing an alphabet game in which each letter is matched with the name of a country with the corresponding first letter. When no one responded to the letter n, an elderly woman who was very depressed suddenly spoke up and said "Nepal." Her accurate response was applauded by all.

By listening to the patient's preferences during the wrap-up sessions and by observing patient responses throughout the sessions, leaders can develop a vast array of suitable resources. Other activities that have been used successfully include simple crafts (such as making a memo pad or small terrarium), parachute activities, basic food preparation, coloring adult designs, adapted common games (like balloon volleyball, or wastebasket basketball), structured communication exercises, and memory games.

Individualized Goals

The most effective way to ensure the effective use of activities and interactions within the Directive Group is to individualize each member's pattern of participation. Explicit and reasonable short-term goals are important for the patients as well as for the family members who may feel overwhelmed by the patients' level of impairment. Confusion, anxiety, and concrete thinking make it difficult for these patients to conceptualize realistic goals for themselves. The coleaders develop and review individual goals each week in staff meetings.

The Directive Group leaders identified a series of individual short-term goals that address the behaviors patients frequently exhibit in the group. The four main goals for the patients are (a) to participate in the activities of each session, (b) to interact verbally with others around the common tasks, (c) to attend the group on time and for the full 45 minutes, and (d) to initiate relevant ideas for group activities.

Specific steps have been delineated to help patients achieve these goals. For example, a withdrawn patient who has difficulty interacting verbally may first be given the goal to respond once to a question asked within the group. During the session the leader would be sure to provide the patient with an opportunity to answer a neutral question. The patient's success in engaging may again be supported by other group members during the wrap-up by identifying patients who met their goal.

Patients who are paranoid or extremely disorganized may not even tolerate attending the group. For those patients, staying in the group for 5 minutes may be a reasonable first goal. If patients have to leave, they are given support for the length of time they did stay and told they are welcome to rejoin the group as soon as they can.

A different kind of goal may be developed for an adolescent who has adequate skills to participate in group activities on a regular basis but complains about every activity, thus discouraging people from interacting with him or her. For example, a young man's negativity is first accepted and then turned into a constructive contri-

bution by giving him the goal to name at least one thing he did not like about the group during the wrap-up. It is likely that after a few days with such a paradoxical instruction (Watzlawick, 1978), the young man will ask to mention something he liked, too. At this point he has taken some initiative. The next step would be to ask him to help lead an activity or make a suggestion.

Patients generally like having personal goals. Often they are written down for them on their own cards, which they show to their nurses or post on the doors to their rooms. The leaders consider the development and presentation of goals in the same way they analyze the use of games and other activities.

The positive feedback started in the Directive Group continues in other groups on the unit and in the community. Patients who meet the four main goals of the group are given a graduation certificate and are referred to other groups in the program. Some patients do not complete the program. These are patients who initially made substantial gains, but then failed to make further progress. They are given a certificate of participation and can be assessed for readmission to the group at a later date.

Documentation and Outcome

To monitor daily functioning, the patient's performance in the Directive Group is assessed after every session using an ordinal rating scale, which corresponds to the four main goals of the group (see Table 2). A patient's longest consecutive level of attention is rated from *does not attend* (1) to *attentive throughout the entire session* (5). The extent to which a patient participates in group activities and in verbal interaction is rated separately based on the amount of structure and support the patient requires. For most patients, initiation is the hardest response. Therefore, even slight indications in this area receive a high rating.

Unit staff members are taught how to use the scale through participation in the group. By understanding the meaning of the scores, they can monitor their patients' progress and compare the individual participation of the patients in the group. In this way, small increments of change, not otherwise appreciated, can be noted. Additional information, such as monitoring effects from changes in medications or electroshock therapy, or indications of organicity based on a patient's response within the group, is reported during team meetings and documented in the problem-oriented format in the patient's chart.

Using the rating scale, outcome measures for a 6-month period indicated that out of 146 patients, 129 (88%) improved their ratings on at least one of the four measures by 1 or 2 points. Over one half of the patients improved on at least two or three of the goals. About a

Table 2. Directive Group: Key Model Variables and Clinical Characteristics

Model Variables	Patient Problems	Referral Criteria	Group Goals/ Individualized Goals[a]	Rating Scale
Performance Subsystem: Problems and Motor Skills	Passive Confused Distractible	Unable to find room or meal tray Unable to focus on a simple task for 5 min. Hyperactive or slowed activity level	Participation in Activities (showing active involvement) (focusing on activities) (following instructions)	5 Cooperates actively in all group activities without assistance 4 Needs minimal assistance to cooperate actively in group activities 3 Needs consistent support and structure to assure involvement in activities (or demonstrates hyperactive involvement) 2 Participates minimally 1 Uncooperative or resistive toward involvement in group activities
Performance Subsystem: Communication/ Interaction Skills	Isolated Aggressive Withdrawn Competitive	Speaks infrequently Monopolizes despite repeated feedback Makes inappropriate responses	Verbal Interaction (responding to question) (listening to others) (making one comment on his or her own)	5 Gives spontaneous and appropriate verbal responses to remarks and comments 4 Responds verbally and appropriately to direct questioning 3 Responds moderately to direct questioning (or monopolizes) 2 Responds minimally or offers inappropriate responses to direct questioning 1 Does not respond verbally
Habituation Subsystem: Habits	Dependent Disoriented Disorganized	Unable to stay in group for 5 min. Has difficulty performing basic self-care	Attending Group (on time) (dressed in street clothes) (for full 45 min.)	5 Attentive throughout entire session (45 min.) 4 Attends for 15 to 30 min. 3 Attends for 5 to 15 min. 2 Attends for 5 min. or less 1 Does not attend, highly distractible
Volitional Subsystem: Goals Interests Personal Causation	Unmotivated Resistant Fearful	Has difficulty identifying interests Lacks goal-directed behavior	Initiating Group Activities (helping lead activity) (explaining an instruction) (suggesting new idea)	5 Suggests, explains, or demonstrates at least one group activity (spontaneous initiation) 4 Makes suggestions (which may be inappropriate) 3 Elaborates on activity ideas with direct assistance 2 Can choose between two alternatives 1 Unable to volunteer activities on his or her own

[a] Individualized goals are shown in parentheses

quarter of the patients remained in the Directive Group until they were discharged from the hospital. These were generally the patients who required additional follow-up care in a nursing home or a day treatment program. Only a few patients (4%) appeared not to benefit from the group.

The behavior changes noted by the rating scale cannot be attributed only to the group because it is difficult to isolate the combined effects of medication, structure, and relationships. However, our clinical observation repeatedly revealed a marked difference between patient behavior in the group and elsewhere on the ward. The group is effective because it elicits and helps maintain more organized behavior.

Discussion

The comprehensive group program presented here can be the starting point for occupational therapists to analyze and reconceptualize other inpatient group programs. The systems approach integrates the special and unique contributions of each group and therefore has the potential for decreasing the professional rivalry that is typical of many inpatient group programs.

The group program gives patients an opportunity to reflect on and restructure their lives. Some patients increase their level of functioning to a new level, some return to their previous level of functioning, and some acquire enough basic skills to function in a transitional setting, such as a day treatment program, half-way house, or brief stays in the community.

A limitation of the Directive Group is that no follow-up has been done to determine, as the research suggests (Mattes, Rosen, Klein, 1977), that patients who attended the Directive Group are more likely to attend other groups because of their successful group experience. In our program, although no control group has been systematically studied, the Directive Group appears to enable patients functioning at minimal level to reorganize their lives faster than they could in other basic groups or with the help of medication only.

Conducting the group requires consistent, dedicated leaders and good cooperation with other staff members to help patients get ready for the group or to help them structure the remainder of their day. Interdisciplinary coleadership is recommended. Where this is not feasible, the alternative would be to have one identified leader and several rotating staff members or students. Based on our experiences, certain personality characteristics seem desirable in a leader. Patients respond best to leaders who are warm, enjoy being active and playful, and are not afraid of psychotic behavior. The leaders must be able to set limits in a supportive manner and be creative in developing goals and activities. It helps if at least one of the leaders is knowledgeable in group dynamics and psychopathology so that the meaning behind psychotic behavior is understood and appropriate interventions are made. The leaders have to guard against taking over and against being punitive, rigid, interpretive, or passive with patients to avoid the problems associated with countertransference.

During the author's 6 years of developing this group, certain principles emerged, which are recommended in starting a Directive Group. They are as follows:

- provide a predictable routine for patients through the organization of the group and sequence of events;
- develop realistic and individualized short-term goals for each patient;
- offer leadership and role models to patients for action, support, and collaborative interaction;
- create a playful arena which legitimizes the activities and interactions of the group and allows patients to develop skills and confidence;
- modify the physical environment and materials to foster patient participation and encourage spontaneity; and
- establish a baseline of patient group behavior, monitor daily progress, and document achievement of individual goals.

Within a supportive program, the Directive Group could be adapted to different patient settings. For instance, in a long-term facility with chronically ill patients, the group would probably need a set duration of attendance before graduation so that the many patients at the same level could eventually attend. The Directive Group has been used successfully by other occupational therapists to help patients with head injuries, stroke, mental retardation and chronic psychiatric problems, as well as for disoriented elderly patients in nursing homes. As part of a total treatment program, the Directive Group provides a first step toward self-direction.

Acknowledgements

The author thanks Marc Hertzman and Gary Kielhofner for their roles in the clinical and conceptual development of the Directive Group and Sandra Cohen and Colburn Cherney for their help in the preparation of the manuscript.

References

Barris, R., Kielhofner, G., Levine, R., & Neville, A. (1985). Occupation as interaction with the environment. In G. Kielhofner (Ed.), *A model of human occupation* (pp. 42-62). Baltimore: Williams & Wilkins.

Bednar, R., & Lawlis, G. (1971). Empirical research in group psychotherapy. In A. E. Bergen & S. L. Garfield (Eds.), *Handbook of psychotherapy and behavior change* (pp. 812-838). New York: John Wiley.

Bertelanffy, L. von. (1966). General system theory and psychiatry. In S. Arieti (Ed.), *American handbook of psychiatry* (pp. 705-721). New York: Basic Books.

Boulding, K. (1956). General systems theory—The skeleton of science. *Management Science, 2*, 197-208.

Cubie, S., & Kaplan, K. (1982). A case analysis method for the model of human occupation. *American Journal of Occupational Therapy, 36*, 645-656.

Decker, J. (1972). Crisis intervention and prevention of psychiatry disability: A follow-up study. *American Journal of Psychiatry, 129*, 25-29.

Duncombe, L. (1985). Group work in occupational therapy; A survey of practice. *American Journal of Occupational Therapy, 39*, 163-170.

Herz, M., Endicott, J., & Spitzer, R. (1977). Brief hospitalization: A two year follow-up. *American Journal of Psychiatry, 134*, 502-507.

Keith, S. (1982). Drugs: Not the only treatment. *Hospital and Community Psychiatry, 33*, 793.

Kielhofner, G. (1978). General systems theory: Implications for theory and action in occupational therapy. *American Journal of Occupational Therapy, 32*, 637-645.

Kielhofner, G. (1985). The human being as an open system. In G. Kielhofner (Ed.), *A model of human occupation* (pp. 2-11). Baltimore: Williams & Wilkins.

Kielhofner, G. (1985). Occupational function and dysfunction. In G. Kielhofner (Ed.), *A model of human occupation* (pp. 63-75). Baltimore: Williams & Wilkins.

Linn, M., Caffey, E., Klett, C., Hogarty, G., & Lamb, H. (1976). Day treatment and psychotropic drugs in the aftercare of schizophrenic patients. *Archives of General Psychiatry, 36*, 1055-1066.

Mattes, J., Rosen, B., & Klein, D. (1977). Comparison of the clinical effectiveness of "short" versus "long" stay psychiatric patients. *Journal of Nervous Mental Disease, 165*, 395-402.

May, P. (1976). When, what, and why? Psychopharmacology and other treatments in schizophrenia. *Comprehensive Psychiatry, 17*, 683-693.

Meltzoff, J., & Kornreich, M. (1970). *Research in psychotherapy*. New York: Atherton.

Moriarity, J. (1976). Combining activities and group psychotherapy in the treatment of chronic schizophrenics. *Hospital and Community Psychiatry, 27*, 574-576.

Mosher, L., & Keith, S. (1979). Research on the psychosocial treatment of schizophrenia: A summary report. *American Journal of Psychiatry, 136*, 623-631.

Parloff, M., & Dies, R. (1977). Group psychotherapy outcome research. *International Journal of Group Psychotherapy, 27*, 281-319.

Reilly, M. (1974). An explanation of play. In M. Reilly (Ed.), *Play As Exploratory Learning: Studies of curiosity behavior* (pp. 117-155). Beverly Hills, CA: Sage Publications.

Chapter 16

A Living Skills Program in an Acute Psychiatric Setting

Kristin Ogren, OTR

Training in community living skills has become recognized as one of the essential components in preventing the hospital readmission of chronic psychiatric patients by increasing their ability to cope with tasks of daily living. Traditionally, living skills programs have been a part of long-term treatment— either in preparation for re-entry to the community from state hospitals or in aftercare treatment in the community. While the area of living skills deserves attention in the acute care setting as well, time limitations imposed by a short stay and the high priority given discharge planning necessitate a different approach. This paper describes a living skills program designed to meet the needs of an acute care setting.

Setting

Located in a large metropolitan area, Overlake Hospital is a general hospital with a thirty-bed inpatient psychiatric unit. The hospital contracts with the state to provide treatment to individuals committed by the courts, which results in a diverse patient population of both private and state patients. A wide range of levels of functioning and varied diagnoses are represented. The average stay is fourteen days, and planning for disposition is usually initiated as soon as the patient is admitted. In addition to discharge planning, inpatient treatment includes medications, milieu and group therapy, and occupational and recreational therapies (OT/RT).

The OT/RT staff views the patient from the perspective of *human occupation*, or purposeful activity performed in everyday living. In the initial screening, the patient's work, leisure, and community living prior to hospitalization are considered. Based on this history and the patient's current functioning on the unit, assignment is made to appropriate groups for treatment.

Living Skills Group

Candidates for the Living Skills Group include individuals who have never lived independently or those with a history of poor adjustment in the community. Occasionally, patients who have functioned independently, but are currently clearing from acute psychosis, may be assigned to benefit from the structured, reality-based activities. Participation in the group requires that the patient be able to tolerate an hour of discussion and activity.

In response to the needs of the acute care setting, the goals of the Living Skills Group are: 1) to facilitate an appropriate and stable disposition through ongoing evaluation of the patient's living skills; 2) to promote the patient's participation in discharge planning by increasing awareness of community resources and agencies; 3) to increase independent functioning by providing information and practice of daily living skills.

The group of eight to ten patients meets daily Monday through Friday. Leadership is provided by an OTR assisted by a nursing staff member. The first three days of the week an educational format is used, with information presented through lecture, discussion and printed handouts. Skills are practiced using paper and pencil tasks, role-playing and real-life situations. Five weekly units, each consisting of three related sessions, have been developed. Each week the unit that best meets the needs of the current patient group is selected for presentation. The units, in order of increasing complexity, are:

   I. Self-Care: grooming, clothing and nutrition
   II. Health and Safety: safety, first aid and health care
   III. Community: public transportation, housing and community resources
   IV. Money Management: banking, budgeting and shopping
   V. Time Management: assessment, planning and goal setting

The group often serves to support the patient in discharge planning by providing information about local agencies and resources, i.e., the features of various half-way houses, the availability of vocational programs, etc. Patients practice decision-making and goal-setting, strengthening skills needed to develop and implement plans.

The last two days of the week the format changes to a cooperative group task. The patients plan a meal and shop for groceries one day and prepare lunch the next. Instruction is informal as they experience planning a balanced meal within a budget, shopping from a list, handling money transactions and preparing a meal. As staff and patients cook and eat together, there is an opportunity to model and reinforce basic social skills.

Living Skills Evaluation—(figure 1)

Knowledge of a patient's level of skills for community living can help assure an appropriate discharge placement. Informal assessment is done within the Living Skills Group, but in some cases there is need for a more formal evaluation. For this purpose a tool was developed that covers a broad range of skills but requires minimal time to administer. For the evaluation, information is gathered in three ways: 1) a report of the patient's functioning in self-care is obtained from nursing staff; 2) in an individual session, the patient is given a series of tasks to perform in five areas (basic skills, health and safety, transportation, money management and use of time); and 3) the patient participates in the weekly

---

Figure 1. Living Skills Evaluation

Date:

Living situation prior to hospitalization:

Independent	Needs Help	
_____	_____	*SELF CARE* (Reported by Nursing Staff)
_____	_____	Grooms self
_____	_____	Comes for medications by self
		BASIC SKILLS
_____	_____	Follows written directions
_____	_____	Can use telephone book
		HEALTH and SAFETY
_____	_____	Aware of household safety hazards
_____	_____	Knows emergency phone numbers
_____	_____	Gives proper response to emergency situations (grease fire, bleeding)
_____	_____	Knows where to obtain medical care
		TRANSPORTATION
_____	_____	Identifies independent means of transportation method
_____	_____	Knows how to use Metro Transit
		MEALS
_____	_____	Describes adequate diet
_____	_____	Able to locate and purchase food in grocery store
_____	_____	Carries out food preparation
		MONEY MANAGEMENT
_____	_____	Identifies own source of income
_____	_____	Handles cash transactions (Counts money, makes change)
_____	_____	Budgets money for food and housing
_____	_____	Knows how to use bank accounts
		USE OF TIME
_____	_____	Able to structure daily routine
_____	_____	Identifies leisure interests
_____	_____	Engages in work or is preparing to work

COMMENTS:

---

grocery shopping and meal preparation. The shopping trip affords a unique opportunity to observe behavior in the community. Performance on each task is rated "independent" or "needs help." With these observations, the therapist then recommends a type of living situation that corresponds to the skill level of the patient. Most frequently indicated are independent living, halfway house or nursing care facility.

Staff members from other disciplines, particularly those involved with placement, have responded favorably to the practical contribution of the Skills Program. A review of the discharge placements of patients whose living skills were evaluated over the past six months has shown that 91% of the actual dispositions were in accordance with the OT recommendation.

Chapter 17

An Activities Approach to Occupational Therapy in a Short-Term Acute Mental Health Unit

Barbara Burnham Rider
Julie Trapp Gramblin

This chapter was previously published in *Mental Health Special Interest Section Newsletter, 3*(4), 1-3. Copyright © 1980, The American Occupational Therapy Association, Inc.

The role of the occupational therapist in the mental health unit of a general hospital is far different from that of therapists who work in state hospitals, community mental health centers, or other long-term facilities. The primary differences relate to length of stay and chronicity of pathology. The mental health unit in a general hospital is characterized by short hospitalization and rapid turnover. Patients may be admitted in a severely disorganized state, but they usually reconstitute quite rapidly.

The short stay and rapid changes in the patient's daily status create unique problems for the occupational therapist. Occupational therapy programs tend to focus on one of two extremes. Many are craft based, relying heavily on short-term projects such as pre-poured ceramics and pre-cut kits. In other cases, the occupational therapist has become so much a part of the unit team that he or she is hardly distinguishable from the other unit staff.

These are activities of which we will give examples later. They rely heavily on traditional occupational therapy media and are based on the Task Group Model developed by Fidler and Fidler in the late '50s and expanded by Mosey in *Activities Therapy* in the early '70s. These activities are selected to fit the unique needs of the short-term psychiatric unit in the general hospital. Although many of them are group activities, they may be modified to use in individual treatment sessions as well. Each activity may be easily completed within a 45-minute period; in fact, it is often possible and even desirable to use several activities in one treatment session.

The Task Group

A Task Group is a time-limited group experience in which patients perform a task for a purpose other than the task itself. The purpose of the task may be to enhance group skills or to develop greater self-awareness or awareness of others. The tasks may be completed in one treatment session or may take one week or longer. They may be structured or there may be very little structure other than the basic rules of the institution, such as the task group method, which may be adapted for verbal, well-organized patients or for regressed patients.

On admission units, or in acute mental health units of general hospitals, the composition of the group is not stable enough to plan week-long activities. In fact, the therapist usually does not know from one day to the next who will be in the group. For this reason, activities that can be completed in one treatment session are often most successful. Since it is often impossible to assess each patient individually and plan treatment according to his or her individual needs, more general needs frequently encountered with these patients have been identified.

The activities meet broad, global goals. Some of them appear to require a high level of verbal skill and integrated thought processes; however, in our experience, these tasks have been used successfully with groups of widely varied levels of integration. Most of the activities result in some sort of product, such as a collage or drawing—representation of feelings or of self, or a group production such as a group mural. In some cases, the productions made by the patients can be useful to staff in understanding their patients, the levels of integration, and how the patients see themselves, their problems, and their assets.

Implementation

Use of the activities may present a problem of implementation to the occupational therapist. We do not recommend a sudden or total break with the old. Therefore, it is critical to have the support of the unit staff. We have found that it works best to make only a partial change initially. Our experience has been with programs that were craft based, and we continued the craft program three days a week and initiated the new Activities Program on the remaining two days. At first there was a dwindling of attendance for the new program. However, after a few weeks, the pattern reversed and the patients were skipping the craft sessions and bringing friends and new patients to the activity sessions.

When implementing the new program, the occupational therapist may encounter a lack of understanding among unit personnel. The occupational therapy group does not duplicate or replace group therapy. The mental health team on general hospital mental health units usually includes psychiatrists, psychologists, nurses, social workers, and therapists. Group treatment sessions conducted by these professionals rely almost exclusively on verbal expression. Occupational therapy is unique in the use of media as the vehicle for expression. The use of media as the primary role of expression has several distinct advantages:

1. The use of media is often less threatening to the patients than direct verbal expression.
2. The use of media is a total patient experience involving physical, mental, social, emotional,

and creative qualities of the individual.
3. Learning that occurs through the use of media is often indirect. The patient may not be immediately aware of the therapeutic outcome of the activity because the awareness is integrated at a level other than the cognitive level.
4. Learning that occurs through the use of media is fun, and is, therefore, more powerful than forced learning.

Therapy, using media, can be a partner to verbal therapy; one reinforces the other. Patients on mental health units in general hospitals participate in in-depth therapy groups in which they are often confronted with the necessity of more painful and difficult behavioral changes. Changing behavior may often be painful. Occupational therapy provides an opportunity for patients to balance the intensive, often difficult, experiences of group therapy or individual therapy with an enjoyable, creative learning experience that reinforces or supplements the learning that takes place in group therapy. Outcomes vary, depending upon the specific composition of individuals in the group and the ability of the therapist to build upon the experience. No single activity will produce the same outcome with different groups, nor will an activity produce the same results with the same group at different times. The activities listed are not presented to comprise a cookbook of time fillers. The skill of the therapist is critical to the therapeutic effectiveness of these activities. The effectiveness of the activities depends upon the knowledge of the therapist and upon a strong foundation in occupational therapy theory.

Establishing Treatment Goals

As already mentioned, in the mental health unit of a general hospital the therapist may be unable to establish individual treatment goals, and it may be necessary to establish goals that are shared by most members of the group. Some commonly shared goals are: 1) building self-esteem, 2) increasing self-awareness, 3) developing group skills, and 4) expressing feelings appropriately.

Many of the activities meet several goals. The therapist might focus on a goal that is a basic treatment goal for most of the patients in the group and select several activities that meet that goal. Or the therapist may select activities that meet a wide range of goals. In any case, it is important to determine the group goal, or goals, first and select activities to meet the goals. It is also important to balance the activities so the patients do not become bored or |feel| left out.

Determining appropriate treatment goals is critical to the therapeutic effectiveness of any activity. It is essential that the therapist have a thorough knowledge of psychology based on the firm understanding of the various theoretical approaches to occupational therapy. The manner in which the therapist defines goals and presents the activities will vary depending upon the theoretical frame of reference utilized.

Grading Activities

Occupational therapists grade activities. Traditionally, therapists move from structured activities to less structured activities, according to the group's ability to handle less structure. Groups may also be graded according to levels—for example, from a parallel group to a cooperative group. Grading group activities in this manner takes time and it is necessary to have 1) some homogeneity in the group, and 2) some assurance the constituency of the group will remain reasonably constant for an established period of time.

In the mental health unit of a general hospital, it is usually impossible to assure either of these criteria. Patients may or may not be formally referred; attendance may or may not be required; a previous evaluation of individual patients may or may not be possible; and patients may be discharged or leave the hospital with little prior notice. These factors, and many others, make traditional grading of activities impossible. While the therapist usually has a general knowledge of who group members will be on any one day, there are usually some new members or some absent members, and the therapist must be able to immediately assess the group and make a judgment about the appropriateness of the activities selected and the level at which they should be presented. In essence, the therapist grades the activity "on the spot."

In some cases, the group itself grades the activity. The activities presented are suitable for a broad range of patient abilities. They can be challenging to well-integrated patients, while at the same time offering an opportunity for participation to very regressed or acutely ill or confused patients. The therapist must be skillful in presenting the activities and guiding the discussion to include each patient at his or her optimal level.

The Importance of Discussion

The critical element in the use of these activities is the therapist. The discussions following the activities are often the most important part of each session and the most valuable therapeutically. The therapist, therefore, must be skillful in leading groups. Since therapists often have not had formal training or experience leading therapy groups, we suggest enlisting as cotherapist a social worker or psychologist or other team member who

has had experience leading therapy groups. Another occupational therapist is a good possibility. We support the use of cotherapists because one person always misses something that is going on. It is important to remember that the purpose is to enlist patient discussion, not [to present] an opportunity for therapists to lecture or theorize.

And, this raises another point. The therapist must be able to wait and tolerate silence. The group may express resistance to some of the activities—clay projects are a usual one—and be silent and totally uncommunicative when the therapist seeks discussion. The therapist must be cautious not to move in and take over, but rather to guide the group forward.

We have attempted to offer suggestions with each activity to get the discussion started. These are only suggestions, and usually something that happened in the group will provide a good starting point for discussion. The therapist must be alert to such incidents.

It is critical to keep the therapeutic goal of the activity in mind and remember that the discussion is part of the activity and also must focus on the goal. Since there are individual goals within a group activity, the needs of each group member must be addressed. Chapter 10 of *Activities Therapy* may be helpful in guiding the therapist to maximize the value of the discussion.

Precautions

As with any form of therapeutic intervention, certain precautions must be observed.

Patients on mental health units are often taking some form of medication that may influence their behavior. In many cases, motor performance and/or perceptions are distorted by drugs. It is important for therapists to understand the possible side effects of psychotropic drugs and to know the medication status of each patient. Patients usually know what medication they are taking and should be routinely asked to tell the therapist of any medication changes.

Occasionally, a patient will refuse to participate. This is more likely to occur in the early stages of the implementation of the program. Usually after the program is well established, informal communication networks serve to inform patients about what to expect, thereby eliminating the anxiety that often accompanies the unknown or the unexpected. If a patient does refuse to participate, the therapist must be able to judge the situation and determine the best action to take in the particular situation. We have found that it is often best to honor the patient's request and allow him or her to return to the unit or work on a project in another area of the clinic.

The occupational therapy group is not an intensive, in-depth, probing, analytical form of therapy. Rather, the purpose is to build patients' interaction skills, increase their understanding of themselves and others, and raise their opinions of themselves as valuable individuals and valued group members. It is not merely a diversional, pleasurable experience. The therapist must be skillful in assuring a creative and personally positive experience for each group member.

Summary

The activities presented here are designed for the occupational therapy program in a short-term mental health unit in a general hospital. They require no special equipment or materials and can be completed in one treatment session or less. They are positive building experiences designed to supplement and reinforce group therapy, and they rely heavily on traditional occupational therapy media. They are not cookbook exercises, but require the expertise and theoretical knowledge of a registered occupational therapist.

Samples from the Activity Card File include the following:

Creative Circle

Goal: Warm up
Time: Ten minutes
Setting: Room large enough for the group to form a circle
Materials: None
Group: Six or more members
Process: The group forms a circle with arms on each other's shoulders. They are then instructed to "be a creative circle" or "let's do something that no other circle has ever done." The reactions to this kind of freedom vary according to the spontaneity level of the group. There is no set way that the circle must respond. Therefore, creativity, or the lack of it, of the group at the moment is utilized.

Difficult Situation

Goal: Increase interaction skills. Raise self-esteem.
Time: Thirty minutes
Setting: Room for group members to move around freely
Materials: None
Group: Any size
Process: Group members are polled on what kinds of situations are difficult for them to handle. A member volunteers to participate and enacts his situation, using people in the group to role play if necessary. Participants are allowed to experiment with various behaviors if they desire. As closure, the group shares and offers feedback. Some common scenes are: a) returning department merchandise, b) being given a traffic ticket, c) making intro-

ductions, and d) dealing with an aggressive salesman.

Memories

Goal: Increase self-awareness
Time: Fifteen to twenty minutes
Setting: Around a table
Group: Six to ten
Materials: Large paper, crayons
Process: Instruct members to "Draw your earliest memory." Discussion may focus on what memories stand out and why; what memories will stand out about their present lives, etc.
Variation: "Draw the happiest experience of your life." "Draw the saddest experience of your life." Combine the first two variations.

Mirroring Body

Goal: To increase body awareness. Warm up.
Time: Ten minutes
Setting: An area large enough to move around without touching another person
Materials: Music
Group: Any size large enough for discussion
Process: Break up into pairs facing each other, have one partner imitate the other during music, stop the music and freeze the position. Become aware of how it feels in different positions. Imitate your partner! Share experiences in group discussion.

Sell Yourself!

Goal: Raise self-esteem. Increase self-awareness.
Time: Fifteen to twenty minutes
Setting: Around a table
Materials: Large paper, crayons, marking pens, etc.
Group: Six to ten
Process: Instruct members to "Draw a full-page advertisement selling yourself." Keep the discussion on a positive vein.
Variation: Make a collage advertisement.

References

Fidler, G. S., & Fidler, J. W. (1963). *Occupational therapy: A communication process in psychiatry.* New York: Macmillan.

Mosey, A. C. (1973). *Activities therapy.* New York: Raven Press.

Chapter 18

Rehabilitation of Chronic Schizophrenic Patients in a Long-Term Private Inpatient Setting

John J. Boronow, MD

The chronic mental patient has received much notoriety of late. News broadcasts have highlighted the problems of tardive dyskinesia and homelessness. Public television has presented an overview of the biological basis of schizophrenia in a popular series on the brain. John Talbott (1985), an authority on these patients and recent APA President, has focused both professional and policy-making attention on the obstacles to effective service delivery for this particular group (Torrey, 1983). Books demystifying and rationalizing the illness are becoming readily available in paperback at local book stores. And families, once the meek recipients of displaced contempt or rejection, have now developed effective lobbies, such as the National Alliance for the Mentally Ill.

The reasons for all this attention are varied, but perhaps the single most important factor is the manifest failure of traditional treatment programs to address the needs of these patients. In an era when rigorous experimental design is bringing conventional but unstudied treatments under scrutiny and when consumerism is at last confronting the medical profession, it is no longer sufficient to prescribe the same old approaches to patients and families uncritically. This is especially true in light of increasing scientific evidence that chronic schizophrenia has many features of a brain disease (Henn & Nasrallah, 1982). A rational response to these new forces and new data demands a reassessment of treatment programs.

Long-term inpatient care was the mainstay of therapy for chronic patients up through the 1950s. The introduction of drugs shortened hospital stays, decreased hospital censuses, and shifted the locale of psychosocial therapeutic interventions to the outpatient setting. The shortening of inpatient stays has been progressing exponentially. Even as recently as 1970, patients in New York City often stayed up to a year in a typical university teaching hospital. In contrast, today such hospitals have an average length of stay of less than a month. Long-term inpatient care for the chronic patient is now split between two extreme populations in the health care delivery system: (1) socioeconomically disadvantaged patients who have failed outpatient programs and who are often warehoused in state facilities for want of effective outpatient dispositions; and (2) upper socioeconomic patients whose families and/or insurance can pay for one of the few remaining long-term private facilities.

These latter institutions typically share a common outlook and treatment philosophy vis-à-vis chronic patients. The model tends to be psychoanalytic, either explicitly or implicitly, with emphasis on creative expression of the individual and heavy reliance on verbal transactions with staff, therapists, and peers. There is a general distrust of behaviorist or biological models as being dehumanizing or irrelevant to core unconscious conflicts. These long-term private hospitals carry on a respected and venerable tradition in American psychiatric care and offer a unique opportunity to those few patients who are lucky enough to receive it.

At present, however, there is increasing pressure from economic interests (third-party payers, federal and state governments), the research community, and patient advocacy groups for all forms of psychiatric care to justify themselves and hold themselves to the most rigorous of intellectual standards. However unfair this may at times seem (especially when compared with standards to which comparable medical disciplines are held), it is nevertheless a fact that psychiatric service providers (and especially *expensive* ones such as long-term hospitals) must provide a coherent and up-to-date rationale for their treatments. This need not be an unrealistic requirement that long-term hospital treatment "cure" patients. Indeed, there are numerous examples of expensive palliative or maintenance treatments in medicine which receive general approval (e.g., hemodialysis and various cancer therapies). But there must be a clearly stated objective, an appropriate treatment plan in keeping with the latest developments, and a rational justification of why the services need to be delivered in a long-term inpatient setting.

The Chronic Mental Patient

Who, then, are the patients that might benefit from the special environment of a long-term inpatient hospital, and what are their unique problems? It would be prudent to begin by clarifying the concept of the "chronic mental patient" (Bachrach, 1976). In general, this seems to be a euphemism for process or nuclear schizophrenics, often with an overlay of substance abuse and/or antisocial features. However, the term also includes a wide variety of other diagnostic groups, including chronic bipolar patients, schizo-affectives, mildly organic patients, and severe character disorders. Because the characteristics of such a disparate group are so diverse and their needs so different, programs must focus on a particular subgroup in order to succeed. There may be several quite different approaches to each of these diagnostic groups, each of which could justify intensive inpatient implementation in a long-term hospital. In this article, I will discuss only chronic nuclear schizophrenic patients and the problems they pose for rehabilitation.

The chronic schizophrenic patient presents us with many problems in addition to the usual psychotic symptoms (hallucinations, delusions, formal thought disorder, and impaired impulse control). These include a set of "regressed behaviors" typical of chronic deterioration, as well as a host of so-called negative symptoms such as anhedonia, poor motivation, and loss of basic self-care and social skills. Also, they often demonstrate cognitive impairments such as concreteness, inability to plan, and even grade school level reading and math skills. These patients show a degree of impairment which is so global and pervasive as to be reminiscent of the functional level of brain-injured patients, even though they are clearly different in terms of neuropathology and phenomenology. Despite such multiple deficits, many of these patients do make a successful transition to outpatient aftercare programs. However, there is a group of patients who fail modern outpatient dispositions because of fundamental incompatibilities between them and the treatment delivery system. Such patients do not get out of bed to go to their programs; they do not take their medications; they wander off and get lost or mugged; they become even more paranoid at a treatment setting, etc. The majority of these patients who fail are caught up in the so-called "revolving door" (although not necessarily in the doors of the same hospital), with little attention paid to resolving the deeper incompatibilities between the patients and the health care system. A few are ultimately kept in state hospitals for the long term. An even smaller group are referred to private long-term hospitals for more intensive treatment. It is safe to say that in 1985 almost no one with schizophrenia is referred to private long-term hospitalization as the first treatment intervention of choice. Instead, it is precisely because of *their failure* to succeed within the context of their local private or public outpatient programs that long-term hospitalization is considered as an alternative. Thus, the population is skewed towards a particularly recalcitrant subset of an already difficult diagnostic group.

It is useful to consider the specific behaviors and symptoms that cause these patients to fail in outpatient dispositions. Problems can be roughly classified into three groups: (1) the presence of overtly bizarre or odd behaviors which interfere with normal socialization in the community (positive symptoms); (2) the absence of adaptive behaviors which are normally necessary for such socialization (negative symptoms); and (3) the disorganization of basic cognitive processes. These divisions are admittedly arbitrary, but they do convey the variety of obstacles to independent functioning.

Positive symptoms lead to the most noticeable of behaviors, but they are not necessarily the most difficult to treat. They often respond to medication and are amenable to environmental manipulation. For example, *nonsense talk* (formal thought disorder) is commonly an indicator that the patient has stopped medications. It can often be reduced by restarting medications or by behavioral responses such as alternative reinforcement or simple ignoring. Episodic maladaptive behaviors such as *outbursts of yelling* or *assaults* are particularly dramatic examples of behaviors incompatible with many outpatient dispositions. These may in turn often be reduced to (or derived from) positive symptoms such as hallucinations (e.g., yelling at the "voices") or delusions (e.g., striking a person who is "attacking").

Another category of behaviors which often preclude successful outpatient aftercare can be described as bizarre or regressed. Whether these behaviors reflect positive or negative symptoms is a matter for research, but their impact on successful socialization—which is a sine qua non of outpatient care—is obvious. They include *polydipsia*, urinary and/or fecal *incontinence*, peculiar *mannerisms* (touching, rubbing, rocking, chewing, grimacing, posturing, grooming rituals), *odd appearance* (in dress, make-up, hairstyle), *hoarding, stealing, spitting, vomiting, gorging, starving, malnutritious eating*, and manifest *negativism* (i.e., predictable refusal to participate in most requested behaviors). Although such symptoms may coexist with more classic psychotic symptoms, they often spell the difference between a psychotic patient who can manage discharge in spite of his hallucinations or delusions and a patient who is functionally disabled by them. It is not the voices or the fears alone that preclude discharge, but these associated behaviors which alienate the public and require more highly supervised living situations.

Negative symptoms can often pose a more intractable, though less colorful, obstacle to successful outpatient care. Daytime *hypersomnia*, with or without a reversal of the normal nighttime sleeping pattern, leads to patients who either sit slumped in fetal position trying to sleep in the day hospital lounge chair, or who oversleep and miss the bus in the morning altogether. Disregard of *basic hygiene* can cause patients to smell strongly and look like skid-row characters. This, combined with other (related?) deficits in social skills such as *vacant facial expres-*

sions and *impoverished communications*, naturally distance patients from other people who might ordinarily be supportive and helpful. A certain *emotional emptiness* makes it hard for these patients to enjoy normally pleasurable activities, and spontaneously initiated activities of any kind are rare. They convey a sense of *not caring* by their failure to show external behaviors which are responsive to the spirit and the deeds of the outpatient program they attend. These patients' failure may be facilitated by the feelings of boredom, disgust, frustration, and rejection which they arouse in the staff. These are the patients who are so easily "lost in the woodwork," especially in systems designed to respond to acute problems on a priority basis. Few aftercare programs aggressively and actively address the negative symptom patient.

Anthony (1979) would go further and define these negative symptoms as the absence of a host of basic verbal, social, cognitive, and vocational *skills* which the patient has never learned or has forgotten. In addition to whatever apathy and emptiness which might appear intrinsic to the illness, there is also a secondary handicap of deprivation from normalizing life experiences which provide most of us with opportunities to learn age-appropriate skills. What we consider "growth" or "maturation" cannot be taken for granted as a spontaneous process. Patients whose illness has derailed them from the mainstream course of social development may appear "burnt out" in part because of never having learned alternative, adaptive, pro-social skills. This notion is a modern variation on the older concepts of institutionalism (Wing & Brown, 1970) and social breakdown syndrome (Gruenberg, 1967). Presumably there is a less bleak prospect for treating negative symptoms if such skills can be taught.

Finally, patients may be unable to achieve outpatient status because of what appear to be gross cognitive limitations. These can include such deficits as persistent functional *disorientation* to date and time, impaired *memory* for daily events, decreased ability to *learn* new material (e.g., a schedule, a bus route, or a name), specific limitations in a particular *sensory* modality (e.g., overreliance on visual, tactile, or verbal cues), *concreteness* (e.g., the inability to abstract from a route taken on foot to a map), and generally poor verbal and arithmetic skills. Such patients are forever getting lost, misplacing things, and forgetting appointments. The level of disorganization, even in the absence of prominent positive symptoms, can preclude successful outpatient management.

Thus, a composite patient who would be appropriate for long-term rehabilitation in an inpatient setting would: talk back to his voices in public; have angry outbursts; be difficult to understand; be dirty, smelly, and incontinent; appear bizarre because of some weird, repetitive behavior like neck-wringing; refuse to attend treatment; walk away when approached; not know his roommate's name or the date; not remember when his favorite activity occurred; and get lost when going from one part of the hospital to another. While this description may seem extreme, even to be a caricature of the chronic schizophrenic, it nevertheless conveys the nitty-gritty problems which the treatment team faces. Too often our professional writing, replete with jargon and abstractions (like "chronic mental patient"), tends to sanitize the patients' problems and reduce them to vacuous generalities. "Socially inappropriate" hardly conveys the feelings of the public or outpatient staff when an unshaven patient suddenly starts laughing and gesticulating wildly on a bus! And yet it is those feelings which we intuitively consider whenever we decide whether or not a patient is ready for discharge from an inpatient setting.

Goals for Inpatient Treatment

Given this rather daunting clinical picture, what might inpatient programs realistically expect to accomplish? Within a custodial framework, it would seem reasonable at the very least to halt a further progressive decline in the patient's functioning. For the patient who has gone from being an average high school student to a middle-aged mute in a state hospital who eats with his hands, it is enough to hope that he does not regress to nudity and forced feedings. Beyond mere prevention of decline, however, a custodial facility should strive to optimize functioning within the confines of the patient's and institution's limitations. Indices of such improvement would include less use of seclusion and restraint, lower doses of medications, more use of recreational opportunities off the unit, less staff turnover, and the like. These are very tangible objectives to which even seriously understaffed state facilities can aspire.

An alternative custodial arrangement exists for the very few patients who have extensive private financial resources. There are fully supervised group home arrangements, such as the Greystone House at Friends Hospital in Philadelphia, which provide 24-hour-a-day care without the trappings of a total institution. The goals are just as limited as described above, but the environment is more personal and homelike. In addition to financial resources, appropriate patients for this kind of program must have a modicum of self-care skills and no grossly disruptive behaviors. The supervision is directed more at their helplessness than at containing disturbed behavior. Although not active treatment programs, such homes provide humane alternatives to otherwise custodial inpatient care for patients who cannot succeed in higher level dispositions.

For a rehabilitation program, however, the goals are more than custodial. At the very least, the rehabilitation program strives to enable the patient *to function outside of a hospital*. To be sure, it also strives for deeper changes which allow the patient to move forward in life: to work, to marry, to achieve a measure of happiness. But in 1985, discharge criteria cannot be equated with these more long-term goals, and such further progress can be fruitfully pursued on an outpatient basis. The objective, then, is to prevent dropping out or being rehospitalized repeatedly during outpatient treatment, and that, in turn, is what we mean by "functioning outside of a hospital."

It is important to realize that the level of supervision required by our hypothetical composite patient to function outside of a hospital is still quite high, at least initially. For the chronic patient with severe handicaps, it is inconceivable that they could go directly to an unsupervised apartment (which is not a statement about schizophrenia per se, but about the skewed population that would end up in an inpatient rehabilitation program in the first place). Some patients will need a quarterway or halfway house with 24-hour-a-day counselors available. Others will require at least daily visits from staff, as in a supervised apartment setting or foster care home. The healthier ones will manage with a boarding home or bed and board, where at least the necessities are structured. All will need structured daily activities during the work day in the form of a psychosocial program, day hospitalization, volunteer work, etc.

Assuming that such aftercare, housing, and treatment facilities exist, there remains the task of actually preparing the patient to make use of them. The task is not one of "curing" the patients' symptoms or of giving them insight into their behavior. It is a functional task which identifies those behaviors incompatible with outpatient care, understands as far as possible their etiology and pathogenesis, and attempts systematic interventions at a variety of levels.

Fundamental Principles of Inpatient Rehabilitation

The private inpatient setting has unique advantages over the public sector in doing this kind of long-term, rehabilitative work. There are physical resources which make the environment less stressful (e.g., less crowding and less noise) than in most state hospitals. More important are the manpower advantages. There is a greater staff to patient ratio, which allows for more attention. Activity therapy, psychology, and psychiatry staff may be better trained. And although the patients themselves may be as sick as any in the public sector, their families are perhaps more likely to be motivated and able to be involved. This may merely reflect the obvious about characteristics of families who have this kind of health insurance.

With these advantages, it behooves the private setting to offer something special. An intensive, customized program specifically designed both to contain the extremes of behavior of the relapsed chronic patient and to rehabilitate him should be *individualized*, *thorough*, and yet *comprehensive*. By individualized, we refer to an effort at creating a unique treatment plan that caters to the specific idiosyncracies of a patient, even at the expense of program uniformity. This is more than just assigning a patient to this or that activity, or prescribing one or another medicines. That kind of specificity should be available in any treatment setting and requires little additional flexibility. The fact is that most depressives do respond to tricyclic antidepressants and support, most manics to lithium and limit-setting, most acute psychotics to neuroleptics and reality testing, etc. That is why the delivery of general psychiatry services through community general hospitals has been so successful in recent years: the needs of the vast majority of psychiatric patients can be met at a basic level through a limited number of therapeutic interventions. It is the (small) minority of "difficult" patients who have not responded to such approaches that requires more individualized treatment. Individualizing means taking the time to learn the details of a patient's history, to really get to know and feel their experience of the world, to appreciate subtle nuances of what is and is not reinforcing to them, in short, to adopt an approach that is truly unique. This may include systematically and consistently disagreeing with a success-phobic patient who says he is getting better; creating the role of "sick patient" and catering to it for a catatonic who cannot feed or toilet himself; administering unconventional doses (high or low) of medicines to patients who have not responded to conventional measures; or drastically modifying a point program to reinforce a patient who slips through the cracks of a token economy. Such modifications are usually labor intensive and take extra time. They would often be *inappropriate* for a short-term evaluation unit in a general hospital. But individualized treatment is indispensable for working with such an idiosyncratic group of patients as the refractory, chronically mentally ill.

Similarly, thoroughness is called for. When patients fail the usual therapeutic interventions, there is usually something unusual about them, and it is up to the treatment team to discover what that is. Beginning with the history, greater attention must be focused on detail than would ever be indicated in a conventional setting. Treatment failures demand reassessment: Is the patient truly unusual or was the treatment botched the first time? If it is a question of treatment failure, was it the dose of medication, the choice of medication, the diagnosis, the therapeutic alliance, the relationship with the family, etc? If the problem was within the patient, is there something organic that has gone unrecognized, does the patient have to unlearn things that stand in the way of progress, are there complicating dynamics which are misunderstood, should the family be more intensively included? This kind of review requires time: time to request and digest old records; time to interview the patient, family, past therapists, [and] employers; time to chart all the various treatments that have been tried, including doses, duration of treatment, side effects and response. The patient should be assessed drug-free, and that in itself takes up to a month.

Lastly, a comprehensive approach must be brought to bear on the refractory patient. In an era of multidisciplinary treatment plans this may seem like a truism, but with chronically regressed patients it is especially apparent. There is no area of the patient's life that is left unaffected by his illness, either "horizontally" in terms of work, leisure, friendship, and sex, or "vertically" in terms of cognition, perception, feeling, and drive. In practice this means having the flexibility to intervene with the patient at several levels and in several domains simultaneously, responding to whatever glimmering strengths the patient may demonstrate. The program should be equipped to draw from a full armamentarium of modern therapeutic interventions, including individual therapy, chemotherapy, behavior modification, social skills training, sensory integration, prevocational training, and psychoeducation. More importantly, these disparate modalities should be coordinated in a rational and flexible way. The treatment team must genuinely value the separate contributions of its component members and be able and willing to work together cohesively. This requires much less emphasis on traditional professional boundaries. Nursing may co-lead activity therapy programs, groups, and family sessions; activity therapy may supervise traditional nursing turf as with a hygiene program; medicine may join with social work in educating families; social work may coordinate education programs for the family. Ideological constraints must also defer to pragmatic considerations. Problems can be approached on many levels at the same time (biology—dynamics—behavior—family system), and practitioners must be willing to place their particular vantage points within the context of the wider biopsychosocial model.

A Model Program

The chronic schizophrenia rehabilitation program at the Sheppard and Enoch Pratt Hospital was designed to meet these needs and requirements. The program presently consists of an 18-bed inpatient unit staffed by two psychiatrists, one-half clinical psychologist, one-half postdoctoral fellow, one social worker, one activity therapist, one-third recreational therapist, and a nursing staff of four R.N.'s and 11 mental health workers. Two-thirds of the patients are male, with an average age of 31 and an average length of stay of one year. Patients are chosen on the basis of chronicity, negative symptoms, diagnosis, and previous outpatient treatment failure. The goal of the program is explicitly rehabilitative: to enable patients to learn skills and adaptive behaviors so they are capable of functioning outside of a hospital.

The centerpiece of the program is a comprehensive token economy that uses points recorded on a point card instead of actual tokens. The rationale for choosing such a system was based on several factors. Token economies have been shown to be effective treatment modalities in previous research (DiScipio, 1974). They have been found superior to milieu therapy for chronic patients in a well-designed crossover study (Paul & Lentz, 1977). Daily, indeed hourly, structure is clearly provided by such a system. Communication is clear and unambiguous. Behaviors are well-defined and concrete. Staff responses are predictable, consistent, and neutral. Lastly, the point card provides an objective record of patient behavior which can be used for clinical or research purposes.

Patients earn points for the basic activities of daily living; for hygiene (washing one's face, combing one's hair, etc.); for eating (eating with the group, eating with utensils, etc.); for participating in activities (coming, being on time, not leaving, etc.); for taking medicines (not refusing, coming promptly, discussing side effects); and for a wide variety of similar basic behaviors. Points can also be specifically tailored to the needs of an individual patient (e.g., earning five points for every four hours the patient does not steal).

Points can be exchanged at a store located on the hall for consumables such as candy, soda and cigarettes. Points can also be used to purchase special time with staff, walks off the hall, and trips into the community. Average point earnings can be used as a criterion for achieving (or losing) a particular permission level. Points also have an intrinsic value which is associated with the staff's attitude about them. Earning points is heavily praised, both individually and publicly, and patients are often very proud of their achievements, even in the absence of additional tangible reinforcers.

The point system reflects the basic principle underlying the program, namely that it is always better to reinforce positive behavior than to punish aberrancy. The design of the point program is a concrete expression of our philosophy of unconditional positive regard toward the patients. It is unconditional because the system is designed to adapt itself to the functional level of even the most regressed patient. There is no patient who cannot earn in this system. For patients who have been shown to be profoundly sensitive to perceived criticism (Vaughn, Snyder, Jones, Freeman, & Falloon, 1984) and failure, it is crucial to make everything the patient does an opportunity for success. Far from being a rigid, mechanical experience, the point card insures that every hour of every day the patient has an occasion for a positive social experience. The specific nature of the points also keeps the positive feelings from becoming overly diffuse. An emotional tone of non-critical support is thus united with a very practical set of learning objectives for behavioral change.

Daily structure is also reinforced with the use of scheduling aids. Every morning patients update a large board in the living room that lists that day's activities and times. Patients make and keep calendars in their rooms and are strongly prompted to use wristwatches. Activities are scheduled as regularly as possible to enhance routine. Indeed the patients' day is somewhat like being in school, and patients often call activities "classes." Far from cringing at this, we try and foster it. If a tightly structured setting with bells, attendance records, and monitors is accepted by us as helpful or even indispensable for 12 years of public schooling, why should such structure suddenly take on an aversive connotation when used with patients who indeed do behave like children? School it is, and the more the better (up to a point), where the curriculum is the living and coping skills needed to survive schizophrenia.

The point program provides a unifying context for all other interventions. All aspects of the patient's life and all therapeutic modalities come under the point card. Thus, points are given by psychotherapists, activity therapists, recreational therapists, occupational therapists, social workers, and even the assistant service chief and service chief. Such participation encourages better integration of the team and communicates this quite tangibly to the patient. Moreover, any and all team members can and do bring up specific issues about the point program at a weekly milieu meeting.

Medications are handled by the service chief in order to ensure consistent prescribing patterns. The service chief and the head nurse make weekly medication rounds in which drug response and side effects are discussed openly in public with individual patients. There is an emphasis on teaching patients about their medications and their symptoms. Experiences such as "voices" are demystified and treated matter-of-factly as just one of many burdens in life that one must learn to cope with effectively. Side effects are taken very seriously, and there is an attempt to give patients a large say in what, when, and how much medication they take. The object is to teach the patients how the medication can work for them, even if this takes several months of letting the patient prove to himself that he needs more or less. Patients self-administer medications under nursing supervision in their final months as they prepare for discharge. Most patients have a drug-free period of up to one month to assess tardive dyskinesia and to get a clear fix on their baseline psychopathology. Active psychopharmacological treatment includes systematic dose response neuroleptic trials, with at least one month of high dose ranges in non-responsive patients; use of neuroleptic levels; trials of depot drugs; trials of lithium, tricyclic antidepressants, monoaminoxidase inhibitors, carbamazepine, benzodiazepines (all in conjunction with neuroleptics); and occasionally reserpine and propranolol trials. Drug response is assessed by weekly Brief Psychiatric Rating Scales, which are consensus ratings done by the patient's therapist and nursing staff.

The activity program provides up to 15 hours a week of structured, hall-based activities. Many are co-directed by nursing staff. Sessions include instruction in activities of daily living, very elementary pre-vocational workshops (stapling, collating), sensory integration, dance/movement therapy, cooking, and hall trips. A recreational therapist supervises weight training, swimming, rowing, and signout planning. As patients advance, both in terms of skill development and behavioral control, they are referred to centralized activities which involve them with patients and staff from outside their hall. This involves higher level vocational training, such as work therapy, and forces the patient to confront more complex social situations. Success in dealing with such a change is an important criterion in assessing the patient's readiness for discharge, which is, of course, an even greater change.

Individual therapy is not a primary focus for the majority of patients, although it is available for all who can use it. Since many of the patients have already been in intensive psychodynamic therapy for one to seven years, true dynamic interpretive psychotherapy is reserved for those few patients who clearly seem responsive to it. The majority see their therapist for a supportive relationship which involves problem-solving and encouragement. The therapist tries to spend time with the patient in the patient's context, be it an activity, a signout, or a meal. The therapist's role is like that of a coach who knows all the players, coordinates the team, and gives helpful advice and moral support to enable the patient to live up to his potential.

The social worker's role on such a unit is quite different from other social work roles in classical psycho-analytic hospitals. There is rarely a wish to "protect" the patient and the therapist from the "sabotaging" effects of the family. Therapists, in fact, are expected to communicate treatment plans directly to the family on a monthly basis. The social worker is free instead to educate families about the illness of schizophrenia and strategies for coping with it. We have designed extensive curriculum of 20 sessions covering such things as signs and symptoms, medications and biology, genetics, natural history of the illness, expressed emotion, as well as Parent Effectiveness Training, stress reduction, and legal/community resources. Families living in other states come for two "marathon" sessions which last four days each. The social worker is available for individual family therapy as indicated, but most families need information and peer support more urgently. Family therapy, when prescribed, tends to follow a behavioral model with emphasis on clear communication, lowering expressed emotion, and clarifying the nature of the patient's deficits. The social worker also works with the family on aftercare planning, with much attention paid to the patient's explicit and detailed functional capabilities and limitations.

The nursing staff makes this multifaceted enterprise run cohesively. Chronic patients need warm, personal, supportive help with all phases of daily living. Abstract discussion, admonitions, and exhortation pale beside the clearcut effectiveness of doing things together with the patients. Staff who live and work with the patients eight hours a day, seven days a week, have enormous influence to teach and motivate. To further this, every patient has an assigned nursing coordinator. The coordinator plays a more individualized role with the patient. Most targeted interventions (e.g., special praise, special rewards, individualized projects, or limit-setting) are conveyed and carried out by this coordinator. The coordinator role insures that team decisions about a particular patient's management are implemented in a consistent way. If the plan fails, the coordinator is not held responsible, but rather serves the critical role of reporting back to the team, giving a detailed account of what went wrong and possible suggestions for correction.

Beginning with wakeup, staff are present on the hall helping patients plan their morning, do their hygiene, clean their rooms, etc. Meals are served on the hall for the lower-functioning patients, and staff join patients to role model correct manners and socialization as well as to set limits on regressed eating behavior. Staff then supervise a patient-run daily planning meeting. The doors to the patients' rooms are locked at 9:30 a.m. for all patients except those who have earned singles, and the doors are not reopened until 4:30 in the afternoon. Patients may, however, purchase rest time in their rooms with coupons earned by attending activities. Rest time is only allowed when no activities are ongoing, however.

Throughout the day, staff work with patients closely, signing point cards, problem-solving, and of course setting limits. The latter is accomplished in as neutral a fashion as possible. Quiet but consistent ignoring of provocative behavior is employed frequently. Verbal prohibitions are delivered without editorial comment about how the staff member feels about the behavior (e.g., *not* "that's disgusting when you vomit on the carpet like that!", but rather "let's clean up the vomit, shall we?"). After all, staff would not berate patients who were incontinent in a nursing home! Clearly specified behaviors such as yelling or swearing lead to clearly specified time in a Time-out room (usually 15 to 30 minutes). This is carpeted, has easy chairs and a clearly visible clock, but is otherwise bare. Fines exist for clearly specified infractions such as assault, stealing, and elopement, and are administered matter-of-factly without public shaming. Frankly, they are seldom necessary, with an average of 47 fines per month (540 patient days).

Staff also are involved in illness-education, which consists of a lengthy series of brief classes that covers the same material as is given to families. The presentation is much simplified, however, with more repetition and extensive reliance on audiovisual aids. Staff participate as well in formal social skills training groups and selected family therapy/education cases. In short, because of the extreme deficits suffered by the majority of these patients, staff have many more opportunities to take on active therapeutic responsibilities with them.

Case Example

Sandy was a 24-year-old, single, white female who developed a prominent behavioral disturbance in late adolescence characterized by loss of impulse control (multiple pregnancies, fights with family) and cognitive disorganization. She was first hospitalized only after two years of unsuccessful outpatient therapy when her behavior became grossly psychotic and she refused to take medications. Initially, she was treated on a conventional hall, where she became suicidally depressed and was treated with ECT. When she started in our program, she was no longer depressed, but demonstrated hostility, auditory hallucinations, and a gross formal thought disorder.

Medications

The patient showed no response until the dose of neuroleptic was systematically increased to approximately 3,000 Chlorpromazine equivalents. Attempts to taper the dose led to a recurrence of hallucinations and anxiety. The neuroleptic level was within normal published limits.

Addition of lithium decreased episodes of depression, which were tracked by BPRS ratings, but did not correlate with change in the thought disorder.

Behavioral Management

The patient's impulsive behavior (angry outbursts, sexual contact with peers, elopements) was gradually brought under control with a variety of interventions. Time-out was effective in controlling hostile exchanges. Linking privileges to abstinence helped contain sexual indiscretions. Elopements disappeared as the patient became more affiliated with the hall. Such affiliation was quite strong. The patient became a spokesman for those patients who favored the point card and the high degree of structure. She could openly articulate her need for rules and guidelines. We intentionally praised and encouraged her art skills by having her design the explanatory signs for the hall store, which in turn further strengthened her affiliation with the program. She began to earn more points than most of the other patients and took pride when her point card was filled.

Individual Therapy

This patient did form an alliance with a new therapist after several months of being hostile to her previous therapist on the old hall. The new therapist was able to approach the patient by focusing sessions on here-and-now issues, problem-solving, and support, with little attempt to explore unconscious material. Also, strongly affect-laden material was intentionally avoided.

Social Work

Initially, the family was very hostile, feeling the first six months on the other hall had been "a waste." Rather than fight with them, the social worker simply included them in the psychoeducation group. The family attended faithfully, asked good questions, and both supported and were supported by other families. The hostility diminished, and together with the patient they requested individual family therapy. These sessions focused on decreasing the family's high expressed emotion, especially around the topic of the patient's sexuality.

Activities

The patient went from "being on strike" with almost no participation in activities to being an eager leader who reminded others of upcoming activities. She completed hall-based activities and made a successful transition to centralized programs. She was able to get a volunteer job from the hospital with her therapist coaching her on interviewing technique. She weathered rejection by an employer without a recurrence of symptoms.

After attending our day hospital program for several weeks, she was discharged to a halfway house with a volunteer job, an individual therapist, and the day hospital as her overall treatment plan.

This case seems to have worked because the treatment met the three criteria we have been espousing above. The approach to the patient was individualized (medications, therapy, use of her innate skills), thorough (time to try different combinations of medications and doses, careful observation of which behaviors responded to which interventions) and comprehensive (wide range of modalities used coherently toward a single goal of discharge to a less structured setting).

Conclusion

In sum, we believe that there is indeed a place for long-term inpatient care of chronic schizophrenic patients. The dissatisfaction with old fashioned custodial care and even with highly thoughtful but unproven psychoanalytic treatment has led in recent years to the development of a whole variety of new approaches to this patient population. This does not mean that all of these patients can be treated as outpatients, deinstitutionalization not withstanding. The private psychiatric hospital has an obligation to lead the field of psychiatry in terms of studying what specific kinds of inpatient treatments and interventions can most effectively capitalize on the extraordinary resources which long-term inpatient care can bring to bear on a particular case. There will probably always be a need for humane custodial care of a small percentage of refractory chronic schizophrenics (Gudeman & Shore, 1984). However, some patients who might otherwise be relegated to such custodial care may be salvaged if an intensive rehabilitative approach is implemented in an inpatient setting. If the private sector can demonstrate the utility of such an approach, the public sector will have less excuse to continue its well-meaning but at times unworkable emphasis on outpatient rehabilitation. The inpatient setting should not continue to be an isolated and aberrant environment dissociated from the mainstream of outpatient aftercare. Rather, we should attempt to design comprehensive service delivery systems which do not distinguish so harshly between inpatient and outpatient, but rather ask the question, "In what setting can which interventions be most effectively applied for which patients?"

References

Anthony, W. A. (1979). *Principles of psychiatric rehabilitation.* Amherst: Human resource development press.

Bachrach, L. L. (1976). *Deinstitutionalization: An analytical review and sociological perspective.* Rockville: NIMH.

DiScipio, W. J. (Ed). (1974). *The behavioral treatment of psychotic illness.* New York: Behavioral Publications.

Gruenberg, E. M. (1967). The social breakdown syndrome—some origins. *American Journal of Psychiatry, 123*(12). 1481-1489.

Gudeman, J. E. & Shore, M. F. (1984). Beyond deinstitutionalization. A new class of facilities for the mentally ill. *New England Journal of Medicine, 311*(13), 832-836.

Henn, F. A. & Nasrallah, H. A. (1982). *Schizophrenia as a brain disease.* New York: Oxford.

Paul, G. P. & Lentz, R. J. (1977). *Psychosocial treatment of chronic mental patients.* Cambridge: Harvard University Press.

Talbott, J. A. (1985). Psychiatry's unfinished business in the 20th century. *American Journal of Psychiatry, 141*(8), 927-930.

Torrey, E. F. (1983). *Surviving schizophrenia: A family manual.* New York: Harper & Row.

Vaughn, C. E., Snyder, K. S., Jones, S., Freeman, W. B. & Falloon, I. R. (1984). Family factors in schizophrenic relapse. *Archives of General Psychiatry, 41*, 1169-1177.

Wing, J. K. & Brown, G. W. (1970). *Institutionalism and schizophrenia.* Cambridge: Cambridge University Press.

Chapter 19

The Quarterway House: More Than an Alternative of Care

Deborah Wilberding, MA, OTR/L

Rehabilitation of the chronically mentally ill encompasses a wide range of psychiatric needs that are life long. These needs are a result of severe psychiatric illnesses, such as schizophrenia, and thus involve a wide range of mental health services. For those individuals who receive their treatment in hospitals, aftercare becomes a crucial and life-saving issue for some patients and the main concern for their families and treatment providers. Aftercare means a continuation of the range of services started in a good hospital setting, but to the patient involved, aftercare can mean moving to a strange place, with totally different players and a totally different set of expectations. To begin to adjust to the community setting can be not only traumatic and fragmenting, but also a source of continual failure unless consideration is made as to what is needed to make the transition more comfortable and complete.

Residential rehabilitation is the logical and less costly next step after hospitalization for the severely and chronically mentally ill who show extensive lack of basic living skills. Myerson and Herman (1983) cited in a December 1980 report by the Department of Health and Human Services, that "the lack of adequate and stable housing opportunities linked with support services was perhaps the major unmet need of the chronically mentally ill," and noted "that increasingly large number of patients are living in board-and-care homes, single-room-occupancy residences and other settings that are generally run down and unsafe, and that offer few meaningful activities for residents" (p. 336). The report recommended transitional group homes and apartments that are rehabilitative, and homes that provided support and sustaining environments. That was ten years ago.

The following [chapter] describes one private psychiatric hospital's attempt to help meet the residential aftercare needs of its chronically mentally ill (CMI) patients through the development of a quarterway house.

Literature Review

The following literature review explores the development of residential care for the CMI in this country; [the] forces that have influenced its development or lack of development; and finally, the concept of the quarterway house and its distinctiveness from other residential care homes. Three themes seem to stand out in regard to community-based residential programs for the CMI: (1) the relatively young age in this country of community-based residential programs and the forces that influenced their development; (2) a common assumption of replacing hospital or institutional care with community-based care as opposed to utilizing the hospital as part of the criteria, and policies distinguishing one type of residential program from another. The following explores these themes.

Historical Development of Residential Care

Arce and Vergare (1985) state that "a current pressing need to examine the role and utilization of community-based residential facilities for the mentally ill" exists and is the "result of significant changes in the mental health delivery system over the past three decades" (p. 423). They attribute these changes to "powerful medical, social, legal, and economic factors," and view the changes historically. They cite the 1950's as the period when social and psychopharmacological forces influenced the shift from hospital care to community care. This was the beginning of an "explosive increase in the types and number of residences for the mentally disabled," (pp. 423-424). According to the authors, when the federally funded community mental health centers began, transitional housing was one of the many services mandated to reduce the need for hospitalization. The number of such facilities had grown from ten in 1960 to 128 in 1969. Subsequently, legal forces influenced change in the 1970's when, beginning with Wyatt v. Stickney (1971), the courts "repeatedly affirmed a constitutional right to treatment," affirming protection from involuntary hospitalization, and care and treatment under the least restrictive conditions (pp. 424-425). In the last decade, economic factors have impinged on hospital care even more forcefully, leaving the CMI with less hospitalization coverage, both in the private and public sectors and have forced the CMI into more vulnerable, often homeless situations.

As a result of all of these forces, Arce and Vergare maintain that "serious conceptual and operational deficiencies" characterize alternative programs, and the "lack

of planning for alternative housing facilities at different levels of care to form a continuum for the patient population" is a prime example (p. 425). In addition, they claim that "local communities" and the "free enterprise system" influence the housing alternatives rather than the meeting of the needs of a "diverse patient population" (p. 425).

A Relationship to Hospital Care

Again as a result of social, economic, political, and medical forces, change has come about in the delivery of care systems. However, the patient's clinical needs and realities, based on the research and further understanding of the illness itself, are still left in question and are given last priority. According to Mechanic (1986), "The community mental health movement was a blend of idealism, optimism, opportunism, and naivety," and that "developing integrated systems of community care for chronic patients is limited less by inadequate knowledge than by organizational, political, economic, and professional barriers" (pp. 893-894).

Myerson and Herman (1983) maintain that what exists are "substantial barriers to the development of housing arrangements, such as community opposition, lack of funding for suitable and affordable facilities," and, an important one for this paper, "the lack of involvement of the private sector" (p. 337). Among their conclusions, justified by several studies made on the effect of community programs, was that the "effectiveness of the programs is enhanced by thorough integration with the original referring inpatient service" (p. 340). This leads into the second common theme or observation in this literature review, the assumption that community programs replace hospitalization.

As stated above, integration with the original referring inpatient service implies use of the hospital as the professional referral service and as part of the continuum of care as opposed to the "costly enemy" of effective treatment. Mechanic (1986) pointed out that the movement away from hospital care to the community was greatly influenced not only by cost benefits but by an ideology based on scientific research demonstrating "secondary disabilities associated with custodial hospital care and inactivity." No recognition was made for good hospital care nor possibly some patients benefiting from asylum (p. 893). Hospital level care is needed, and must remain a part of the whole continuum of care. It is the logical resource for safe psychiatric treatment of the CMI when warranted, but always in preparation for and toward the sustaining of a patient's illness management and skill learning beyond its walls in various levels of community care. According to Wilberding (1987), "the goal of in-hospital treatment does not necessarily lead to complete independence but rather to an ability to successfully participate in outpatient programs and break the cycle of more costly rehospitalization" (p. 46). According to Hefmeister, Weiler, and Scherson (1989), the private sector "has been reluctant to develop residential programs because of a lack of replicable models, limited outcome data, and uncertain third-party reimbursement" (p. 927).

Toward a Definition

The third theme found throughout the literature was the lack of definitional criteria, program standards, and policies for residential programming. Rarely mentioned was the concept of quarterway group homes. A definition of types of community residences is important to establish because it lends to their effectiveness and efficiency, and also serves to recognize and clarify the effect that facility characteristics play on the management of illness factors. According to Arce and Vergare (1985), the lack of "unifying policy, program standards, or precise definitional criteria" contributes to "confusing communication between professionals and across jurisdictions" (p. 426). Names, such as halfway house, transitional facility, board and care home, [and] quarterway house have become commonplace, but are used imprecisely—identical labels applied to dissimilar settings.

Arce and Vergare (1985) cited a 1982 task force of the American Psychiatric Association that surveyed existing residences of all 50 states and found them named under 100 different labels. They recommended a uniform typology consisting of seven types of possible residential settings for the CMI based on programmatic factors. These progressed from most restrictive and intensive to least restrictive and intensive and were as follows:

1. Nursing facility (both skilled and intermediate care);
2. Group home;
3. Personal care home;
4. Foster care;
5. Natural family placement;
6. Satellite housing (supervised apartments); and
7. Independent living (p. 497).

This typology described the full range of residential facilities used as alternatives to hospitalization and again was based on a series of programmatic criteria. The group home category included a variety of program names, i.e., halfway houses, transitional living facilities, group care homes, hostels, [and] residential homes. (This category came the closest in definitive criteria to include the quarterway house concept, but it was not mentioned in this particular study.) The category was still broad in definition. The definitive criteria covered a wide range of populations, age groups, [and] lengths of stay, but was very focused in its criteria in regards to purpose, licensure, and staffing. The program goal in the group home category was psychosocial rehabilitation within a group of eight to 15 clients through use of a milieu, utilizing a 24-hour, full-time staff (professionals and paraprofessionals), and served mostly mildly to moderately disabled. The severely disabled were mentioned as being appropriate for the group home category, if appropriate staffing and support services were available. (This also would include the quarterway house concept because this type of program serves [the] severely disabled, as will be described later.) What broadened the definition of this category even further, was the described range of uses of group homes. They were as follows:

1. Alternative to acute hospitalization;
2. Shorten inpatient length of stay;
3. Transition from hospital to community;
4. Permanent placement; [and]
5. Respite care (p. 432).

However broad and general in description, the group home category at least was a start toward a formal definition of residential group homes, including quarterway homes.

Assuming community integration is the goal, when further definition is made of the characteristics of the facility (and program), the community in which the facility is located, and the clients themselves, the differences between the various programs considered "group homes" becomes even more apparent. A study was done by Kruzich (1985) to identify not only client characteristics, but also facility and community characteristics. Their impact was shown to influence community integration of 87 former state hospital patients residing in residential facilities. Kruzich found that "as the number of daily living skills programmed in the facility increases, so too does the residents' level of participation in the larger community" (p. 557). Other characteristics cited as important were:

1. Level of personal, individualized care;
2. City size and availability of community resources;
3. Discharge planning in regards to matching client needs and environmental (program) demands;
4. View of the clients themselves regarding suitability of facilities' environments; [and]
5. Staff attitudes and involvement.

Kruzich emphasized the importance of management practices in determining residents' community integration through staff and administrators' explicit and implicit expectations (p. 562). Kruzich concludes, "These findings point to the importance of residential care administrators articulating a philosophy through their programming, physical environment, and emotional climate that supports clients' attempts to become part of the larger community" (p. 562).

The term "quarterway" used to describe a type of group home, was cited in only a few articles, and was usually a part of a continuum of residential care. Gudeman, Dickey, Rood, Hellman, and Grinspoon (1981) describe the Quarterway House of the Massachusetts Mental Health Center, founded in 1978. It is located in a refurbished unit of a public psychiatric hospital, and designed for "unplaceable" psychiatric patients with both behavioral problems and lack of basic living skills. Mann (1976) describes a quarterway house set up in a building on the grounds of Harlem Valley Psychiatric Center in New York for both acute and chronic patients with psychiatric illnesses. This is the earliest recorded quarterway house found in the literature, but has dissolved after the center's inpatient census shrunk. A third quarterway house program was cited in an article by Purnell, Jackson, and Wallace (1982) for chronic patients in New Jersey. They described a three bedroom house on a state hospital grounds, with the program supported by the then federally funded CETA program (Comprehensive Employment Training Act). The program terminated when funds expired. A fourth, and most recent quarterway house program is described by Ranz (1989). Located in a separate building on the campus of Rockland Psychiatric Center, the 16-bed facility is part of a well developed series of supervised residences on Rockland's state hospital campus, and is designed as the first step of their continuum of residential care. It is important to note that many articles were reviewed describing residential programs that have some elements of "quarterway" level of programming, but were referred to as "halfway," "transitional," or "shelter care" homes. Again, the importance of a precise nomenclature is a focus of this paper, therefore these programs were not included here.

A Proposed Definition

To summarize then, a quarterway house can be defined as a group home, transitional in nature, and the first step after hospitalization in preparation for community placement. The quarterway house serves the most disabled and chronic psychiatric patients, whose only alternative is long term institutional care. Its focus is psychiatric rehabilitation, specifically designed to teach and to promote the learning of basic living skills in the areas of work, self-care, and leisure through a daily, structured program within a home environment. Its location is usually on or near a hospital setting, which serves as both a referral source and clinical support when necessary. Its thrust, however, is to promote its residents toward integration in the larger community by utilizing a wide variety of community resources. A quarterway house provides a high staff to patient ratio, 24-hour coverage, and is comprised of both professionals and paraprofessionals trained in the philosophy, purpose, and methods of the program.

Its methods are well defined and behavioral in orientation. It provides clear, reasonable expectations, rules,

and standards of behavior that are both socially acceptable and promote stabilization, and, finally, a quarterway house promotes illness management through use of medications and formal education.

The following is a description of the Mt. Airy House, a quarterway house program that was designed to meet the needs of moderately to severely disabled patients, based on the psychiatric reality of a life-long illness and thus life-long dependence on some level.

The Program Components

The Mt. Airy House is a free-standing, two-story, Tudor-style home, on the campus of The Sheppard and Enoch Pratt Hospital [SEPH] in Baltimore, Maryland. Licensed by the state of Maryland as a group home for 16 mentally ill adults, Mt. Airy is part of the range of outpatient services in the Ambulatory Division of the hospital. The facility, from its inception, was specifically designed to rehabilitate the CMI.

The Resident

Patients with severe mental disorders often share common characteristics. The Mt. Airy House was designed for certain diagnoses within the CMI population, i.e., schizophrenia, schizo-affective disorder, major affective disorder, and mild organic brain syndrome.

These diagnoses were selected due to [the] homogeneity of their characteristics, and this selection provided for a certain amount of specialization in assessment and treatment. Those characteristics are as follows:

1. Ongoing psychotic symptoms not likely to remit.
2. Cognitive deficits apart from psychotic symptoms.
3. High vulnerability to stress.
4. Extreme dependency.
5. Difficulty sustaining activities.
6. Difficulty in establishing interpersonal relationships.

Admission criteria were developed based on these characteristics to help assess appropriateness of placement. Some of the criteria also describe the patient's behavioral problems and strengths. They are as follows:

1. Be between the ages of 18-65 years old.
2. Seek voluntary admission.
3. Have the ability to comprehend rules of the home and be willing to sign a contract agreeing to comply with house rules.
4. Have been previously hospitalized for a psychiatric disorder such as schizophrenia, major affective disorder or organic brain syndrome. Sociopathic, borderline disorders, severe brain damage, or a diagnosis of mental retardation

without psychotic features are not appropriate.

5. Have demonstrated the absence of alcohol/drug abuse for 90 days prior to admission. Not have a primary diagnosis of alcoholism or drug abuse.
6. Have minimal physical disabilities.
7. Be stable on a medication regime and be willing to take medications under supervision.
8. Not be actively suicidal, homicidal, or destructive of property, and not exhibit current violent or seriously disruptive behavior (hitting others, throwing things, verbal threats, loud yelling, stealing consumable items, dangerous smoking, fire setting, elopement) for a period of at least 30 days.
9. Be able to tolerate the presence of others, follow simple instructions, observe basic hygiene principles, and have a minimum of regressed behaviors such as vomiting or incontinence.
10. Be able to take appropriate action for self-preservation under emergency conditions.
11. Be able to take care of own possessions and laundry with minimum supervision.
12. Furnish proof of freedom from or control of communicable disease, such as tuberculosis.
13. Be able to remain in the program for a minimum of six months.

Another descriptive source of the residents' characteristics is in the behavioral assessment used at Mt. Airy. Behavioral problems, as a result of the disease process and maladaption to the environment, can be a serious impediment to a patient ever discharging from the hospital, and some maladaptive behaviors are described in the criteria just mentioned. Once a resident is accepted into the program, a careful assessment of his/her behaviors is made. These behaviors are considered either behavioral deficits (absence of adaptive behaviors); excesses (acting out, bizarre, or odd behaviors); or behaviors present or absent in functional skill areas.

Two sources used for assessing these behaviors are the formal assessment (see Figure 1), which is done after a resident is in the house for two weeks; and an assessment based on the "excessive behavior" list (see Figure 2), which is also used to determine readiness for progressing in the tier system of the program. The list of excessive behaviors was developed by the residents themselves during a formal group meeting after the first year of operation. Once a resident is assessed by these tools, a clearer description of his/her behavior and individual characteristics is attained. Often, recognition of these behaviors by the residents themselves is the first positive step toward managing them.

The Community

The Mt. Airy House is on the 110-acre campus of SEPH located in a suburb of Baltimore, Maryland. The integration into the community from a psychiatric hospital campus is a challenge for both the staff and residents of Mt. Airy, and is done in a variety of ways.

The dependency that usually develops between the patient and the hospital, both practically and emotionally is discussed with the new resident. It is made clear that after discharge these ties will change and most of the resident's needs will be met in the community. This is usually stated periodically, and then experienced immediately and routinely through the weekly schedule of activities. Medications are purchased at the local pharmacy; medical and dental needs are met through local doctor and dental offices; groceries are purchased at the local grocery; a passbook savings account is set up at the local bank where the resident is welcomed and introduced to the bank's services by the manager; a library card is applied for at the local library; a mall trip or movie or bowling trip is planned in the afternoons or evenings; and the Sunday trip to some event in the city is organized.

After the initial month, usually the new resident has established him or herself into both the house program and the community by participation on a supervised group level. A more independent and individualized level comes about much later depending on behaviors and skills.

The community resources used (grocery, pharmacy, bank, library, etc.) have been exceptional in providing the attention, acceptance, and care for the residents' situation. It was however important to recognize that both incentives and information were needed and given to the grocery, pharmacy, and bank to establish the relationships. Initially, they were formally asked if they would be willing to participate in the Mt. Airy experiment. Social responsibility appeared to be as important as increased business to the managers. All were somewhat familiar with severe mental illness at some level, and were clinically curious, asking good questions to make themselves more informed. Were these exceptional people or is the public becoming more informed? This is hard to assess, but trust has been established both through the reputable name of the hospital, and the fact that the Mt. Airy staff have been clear to the managers and personnel that they would provide supervision and behavioral limits for the residents. After a year in operation, the grocery manager commented on how well residents behaved. This was after a year not free of incidents, but was a year of incidents properly handled.

The second source of community integration is through community programs. A psychosocial program, funded by both the state and SEPH, is well utilized and has a very active recreational and vocational component that uses a wide variety of community resources. The Adult Day Hospital of SEPH is also used, as well as an

Figure 1. Formal Assessment

Mt. Airy House
RESIDENT ASSESSMENT

Resident's Name: _____ Date: _____

Person Filling Out Form: _____

SCALE:
1. Good Functioning or Not a Behavior Problem
2. Mildly Impaired Functioning or Mild/Infrequent Behavior Problem
3. Moderately Impaired Functioning or Moderate Behavior Problem
4. Seriously Impaired Functioning or Serious/Frequent Behavior Problem

Content areas below contain both functional behaviors and problem behaviors.

		1	2	3	4
I. EATING					
1.	Eats and drinks neatly	☐	☐	☐	☐
2.	Chooses a well-balanced diet	☐	☐	☐	☐
3.	Eats or drinks too much	☐	☐	☐	☐
4.	Eats or drinks too fast	☐	☐	☐	☐
5.	Refuses regular meals	☐	☐	☐	☐
6.	Takes food or drink that has been discarded or that belongs to another	☐	☐	☐	☐
II. HYGIENE					
7.	Bathes or showers using soap daily	☐	☐	☐	☐
8.	Brushes or combs hair daily	☐	☐	☐	☐
9.	For males, shaves as needed or keeps beard neat	☐	☐	☐	☐
10.	Takes care of nails	☐	☐	☐	☐
11.	Brushes teeth at least once a day	☐	☐	☐	☐
12.	Changes clothes daily	☐	☐	☐	☐
13.	Wears appropriate clothing	☐	☐	☐	☐
14.	Has noticable body odor	☐	☐	☐	☐
15.	For females, wears excessive or bizarre make-up	☐	☐	☐	☐
16.	Changes clothes excessively	☐	☐	☐	☐
17.	Disrobes publicly or exposes self	☐	☐	☐	☐
III. PERSONAL DOMESTIC ACTIVITIES					
18.	Gets up in a.m. on time	☐	☐	☐	☐
19.	Makes bed daily	☐	☐	☐	☐
20.	Keeps room neat and clean	☐	☐	☐	☐
21.	Changes bed linens as needed	☐	☐	☐	☐
22.	Stores soiled clothing for washing	☐	☐	☐	☐
23.	Does personal laundry	☐	☐	☐	☐
24.	Puts clean clothes away	☐	☐	☐	☐
25.	Prepares lunch and snack food for self safely	☐	☐	☐	☐
26.	Uses smoking materials safely and smokes only in designated areas	☐	☐	☐	☐
27.	Sleeps excessively	☐	☐	☐	☐
28.	Bedroom has noticable odor	☐	☐	☐	☐
29.	Is incontinent	☐	☐	☐	☐
IV. HOUSEHOLD DOMESTIC ACTIVITIES AND JOB READINESS					
30.	Follows requests and directions	☐	☐	☐	☐
31.	Follows through on tasks started	☐	☐	☐	☐
32.	Starts and completes tasks promptly, neither too fast nor too slow	☐	☐	☐	☐
33.	Able to work independently	☐	☐	☐	☐
34.	Cooperative with others in completing tasks	☐	☐	☐	☐
35.	Consistent in work performance	☐	☐	☐	☐
36.	Has adequate duration of attention and ability to focus on tasks	☐	☐	☐	☐
37.	Maintains own schedule throughout day without being reminded	☐	☐	☐	☐
38.	Participates in shopping for, and stocking, house supplies	☐	☐	☐	☐

Psychosocial Occupational Therapy: Proactive Approaches

Figure 1. (continued)

	1	2	3	4
39. Performs household cleaning tasks	☐	☐	☐	☐
40. Prepares meals adequately and safely for house	☐	☐	☐	☐
41. Cleans up after house meals	☐	☐	☐	☐
42. Performs other household chores as assigned or needed	☐	☐	☐	☐

V. INTERPERSONAL SKILLS

	1	2	3	4
43. Speaks up in community meetings appropriately	☐	☐	☐	☐
44. Initiates conversations with others	☐	☐	☐	☐
45. Establishes relationship with resident advisor	☐	☐	☐	☐
46. Maintains relationship with family/significant others	☐	☐	☐	☐
47. Able to express positive feelings	☐	☐	☐	☐
48. Able to express negative feelings	☐	☐	☐	☐
49. Able to respond constructively to anger and/or criticism	☐	☐	☐	☐
50. Goes on staff-accompanied group outings	☐	☐	☐	☐
51. Uses telephone appropriately	☐	☐	☐	☐
52. Threatens others	☐	☐	☐	☐
53. Makes hostile, vulgar, rude comments	☐	☐	☐	☐
54. Shouts or yells	☐	☐	☐	☐
55. Talks too much	☐	☐	☐	☐
56. Intrudes on others	☐	☐	☐	☐
57. Talks to self	☐	☐	☐	☐
58. Engages in inappropriate sexual behavior	☐	☐	☐	☐
59. Is uncommunicative or withdrawn	☐	☐	☐	☐
60. Hits others or throws things	☐	☐	☐	☐
61. Steals or takes things from others	☐	☐	☐	☐

VI. HEALTH

	1	2	3	4
62. Able to identify psychiatric problems/symptoms	☐	☐	☐	☐
63. Understands nature of psychiatric illness and need for treatment	☐	☐	☐	☐
64. Reports physical problems appropriately to house staff and/or doctor	☐	☐	☐	☐
65. Follows through on advice from doctor or nurse	☐	☐	☐	☐
66. Treats own minor physical problems appropriately	☐	☐	☐	☐
67. Cooperates with person who dispenses medication	☐	☐	☐	☐
68. Can reliably self-administer medication	☐	☐	☐	☐

VII. MONEY MANAGEMENT

	1	2	3	4
69. Buys own clothes	☐	☐	☐	☐
70. Purchases own personal items	☐	☐	☐	☐
71. Budgets money for day/week	☐	☐	☐	☐
72. Makes deposits/withdrawals at bank as needed	☐	☐	☐	☐
73. Counts change in store	☐	☐	☐	☐
74. Behaves inappropriately at store	☐	☐	☐	☐

VIII. TRANSPORTATION

	1	2	3	4
75. Cooperative on van trips	☐	☐	☐	☐
76. Walks to places on grounds and in Towson	☐	☐	☐	☐
77. Follows pedestrian rules	☐	☐	☐	☐

IX. LEISURE

	1	2	3	4
78. Works regularly on a hobby	☐	☐	☐	☐
79. Takes walks outside	☐	☐	☐	☐
80. Works in the garden or yard	☐	☐	☐	☐
81. Listens to the radio or watches tv appropriately	☐	☐	☐	☐
82. Goes to the movies or sporting events	☐	☐	☐	☐
83. Plays sports or table games	☐	☐	☐	☐
84. Reads the newspaper, books, or magazines	☐	☐	☐	☐

X. COMMENTS: _____
_____
_____
_____

outpatient vocational service supported by both SEPH and the State Department of Vocation Rehabilitation.

Figure 2. Excessive Behavior List

This is what we mean by "excessive behaviors":

1. Impulsivity
   a. money
   b. massive consumption of anything
   c. splitting (running away)
   d. shoplifting
   e. substance abuse
   f. self-destruction
   g. threatening others
   h. destruction of property
2. Poor Boundaries
   a. asking for things beyond what is reasonable
   b. acting in an intrusive manner toward others
   c. wandering off
3. *Socially Inappropriate Behavior
   a. vulgar and rude comments to others
   b. talking and/or laughing to yourself while out and about
   c. dressing in bizarre ways
   d. poor hygiene
   e. inappropriate sexual behavior

*This means behaving in ways that would embarrass someone else, make someone else nervous, or make people look at you funny.

4. Angry outbursts
5. Dangerous smoking
6. Inability or unwillingness to respond to limits or requests

The Facility

Architecture and the decor were very important in the design of Mt. Airy. For example, the organization of the kitchen was designed to provide space as well as ease of use; comfortable but durable and nonreclining furniture was bought; the color scheme and decor was chosen not only to look coordinated and pleasing to the eye, but also to create a soothing, less stressful environment; ample space was provided for self-care and storage of personal belongings.

The house supports 16 residents with ample space and substantial supplies and equipment to allow for resident participation in all the cooking and cleaning chores, as well as recreational and formal learning activities. Of most importance is the home-like atmosphere and the first impression the facility makes on the incoming new resident—an impression of self-worth.

Program Components

The Mt. Airy House is a 16-bed residential rehabilitation program, with an aim toward providing chronically hospitalized patients with the next step in transition between hospital and community placement. The goal is to enable each resident to become a community participant rather than a community dependent.

The philosophy of the Mt. Airy House is based on the belief that successful adjustment to community life requires understanding the specific and unique problems of each resident. This understanding, coupled with the value of a meaningful, less isolated, and more rewarding life, is the cornerstone of the Mt. Airy House. In order for the resident to learn new and more adaptive skills and behaviors, the program model is based on behavioral rehabilitation principles.

The program objectives are to:
1. Provide an atmosphere for the learning and maintenance of the highest attainable levels of functioning.
2. Focus on building social skills, daily living skills for community participation.
3. Reduce loneliness, isolation, and lack of meaningful activity.
4. Provide emotional and practical support.
5. Set expectations at levels within which the resident is able to function.
6. Assist in arranging placement for residents at time of discharge from the program.

These objectives are reflected in the focused areas of rehabilitation, the rehabilitation characteristics and strategies, and the rehabilitation goals. The nine components of rehabilitation constitute the assessment areas: eating, hygiene, personal domestic activities, household domestic activities/job readiness, interpersonal skills, health, money management, transportation, and leisure (see Figure 1). The program is based on the self-care-work-leisure model, adapted from the work-play-rest model proposed by Reilly (1966) [sic], rest being considered part of self-care. Rehabilitation strategies are characterized by the structure and routine provided, the kind of support given by the staff, the contained emotional environment maintained, behavioral contingencies, and use of community resources.

The daily schedule begins with the morning wake-up call, encouraging the resident to use an alarm clock when ready. The morning routine, i.e., completing hygiene, room care, breakfast, and obtaining morning medications, is expected to be completed by the time of the Planning Meeting. The Planning Meeting is used to give the schedule for the day on both a collective and individual basis; at this time, residents obtain their credits for the previous day's work accomplishments. Each resident possesses a folder containing their credit card and Budget Sheet that they are responsible for bringing to the meeting. Some residents have personalized their folders, reminding the staff of how much like a school it becomes, [which] also is a good sign of self-identity forming. The weekly schedule includes activities in all the nine focused areas mentioned, and is followed both routinely and repetitively (see Figure 3). It is also balanced and scheduled so as not to overwhelm the residents.

Staff are trained in providing both emotional support, task assistance, and active involvement of a process quoted from Fidler (Wilberding, 1987) of "learning by doing." Techniques used are in the forms of behavioral reinforcements (verbal praise and encouragement, credits/money earned, privileges earned) and are constantly being individualized. Problem behaviors are contained within the expectations and limits well known by both staff and residents through the house rules. The staff are very firm, and try to remain neutral in their approach. Written Behavioral Contracts are used to formalize and make clear the steps toward eventual gain of behavioral control. Skills are learned through active participation and are taught by the use of demonstration, redirection, written instruction and check lists developed by task analysis. Independence from staff is gained by eventual use of only the written instruction

Figure 3. Mt. Airy Weekly Schedule

MT. AIRY HOUSE
WEEKDAY SCHEDULE FOR RESIDENTS

7:30 a.m.	WAKE-UP CALL
	BREAKFAST PREPARATION (DUTY ROTATES)
8:00 a.m.	BREAKFAST SERVED
8:30 a.m.	BREAKFAST CLEAN-UP (DUTY ROTATES)
	MORNING MEDS
9:00 a.m.	DAILY PLANNING MEETING
9:30 a.m.	DAILY EXERCISE GROUP (REQUIRED)
10:00-11:30 a.m.	MORNING ACTIVITIES

- Monday—menu planning, inventory, grocery list, healthy eating group
- Tuesday—communications group, gardening
- Wednesday—house cleaning, budgeting
- Thursday—personal shopping, banking
- Friday—health workshop, community outing

12:00 p.m.	LUNCH
1:00 p.m.	LUNCH CLEAN-UP (DUTY ROTATES)
1:30-3:00 p.m.	AFTERNOON ACTIVITIES

- Monday—grocery shopping
- Tuesday—recreation (structured)
- Wednesday—beachball (volleyball)
- Thursday—leisure planning, video
- Friday—gardening, recreation

3:00-4:00 p.m.	AFTERNOON BREAK
4:00 p.m.	DINNER PREPARATION (DUTY ROTATES)
	• Monday—pharmacy
6:00 p.m.	DINNER
6:30 p.m.	DINNER CLEAN-UP (DUTY ROTATES)
7:30 p.m.	EVENING ACTIVITIES

- Monday—library
- Tuesday—double trouble group, games
- Wednesday—communications/movie, budgeting
- Thursday—personal & grocery shopping
- Friday—mall night

8:30 p.m.	EVENING MEDS

Figure 4. House Chore Written Instruction Based On Task Analysis

Dinner and Clean-up Crew Responsibilities

Cook 1	Cook 2
Start at 4:00 p.m.	Start at 4:00 p.m.
Main dish	Salad—if none, then vegetable.
Vegetable	Set the table, including
Side dish	condiments and 2 jugs of milk and 2 pitchers of ice water. Wash prep dishes, including any leftover dishes from the day. Make coffee.

Clean-Up 1	Clean-Up 2
Start immediately after dinner	Start immediately after dinner
Clear the table	Put away clean prep dishes (in drainer & dishwasher).
Put food away	Scrape and rinse dishes.
Wipe off and put away placemats	Wipe off all counters.
Vacuum the dining room if needed	Empty and clean the coffee pot.
Take out trash & replace bag.	

Clean-Up 3	Snack Person
Start immediately after dinner	Start at 8:00 p.m.
Scrape, then wash pots, pans, utensils (in sink by window).	Take out snack and place in activity room.
Sweep the floor.	Fill blue cooler with ice.
Put dishes away by 7:30 p.m.	Fill bowl 1/2 way with ice
Straighten utensil drawers to insure neatness	Place jug of milk inside and take to act. room. Place cups in activity room.

	Snack Clean Up
	Start at 9:00 p.m.
	Put away milk and snack. Wipe counters, tables, and ashtrays. Empty trash and replace bag. Load all dishes into dishwasher. Sweep the floor.

and checklists (see Figures 4 and 5).

The overall treatment goals of the Mt. Airy Program are in four areas: maintaining the management of the illness itself (taking meds, keeping therapists' appointments, symptom control); the learning and maintenance of daily leaving skills; the acquisition of a place to work; and the acquisition of a place to live. Discharge planning is based on these four areas. In order to reach these goals, the program is designed for a minimum of six months to a maximum of four-year stay. Within this time, a resident can learn the skills needed to meet expectations, but is set within a three-tier system (see Figure 6). Movement from one tier to another is based on meeting expectations, and attaining behavioral control of any excessive behaviors (see Figure 2).

The Staff

The characteristics of the resident population described at Mt. Airy House warrant a high staff-resident ratio for several reasons: lack of motivation coupled with

---

Figure 5. House Chore Checklist

Date: _____

Dinner Prep 1 _____   Dinner Prep 2 _____

	You check when done	Staff check
Clean-Up Person #1 Checklist		
1. Table cleared	☐	☐
2. Cond., milk, & water put away	☐	☐
3. Placemats wiped off and put away	☐	☐
4. Table wiped off	☐	☐
5. Dining room vacuumed	☐	☐
6. Trash taken out, new bag put in	☐	☐
Clean-Up Person #2 Checklist		
1. Prep dishes put away	☐	☐
2. Dishes scraped and rinsed	☐	☐
3. Dishes washed	☐	☐
4. Counters wiped off—including pantry	☐	☐
5. Empty and clean coffee pot	☐	☐
6. All clean dishes put away	☐	☐
Clean-Up Person #3 Checklist		
1. Pots, Pans, and Utensils washed—2nd sink	☐	☐
2. Sweep the floor	☐	☐
3. Put clean pots, pans, and utensils away	☐	☐
4. Straighten utensil drawer to insure neatness	☐	☐
Snack Person Checklist		
1. Take out snack and place in activity room	☐	☐
2. Fill blue cooler with ice	☐	☐
3. Fill bowl 1/2 way with ice—place milk in bowl, take to activity room	☐	☐
4. Place cups in activity room	☐	☐
Snack Clean-up Checklist		
1. Put milk and all food away	☐	☐
2. Wipe all counters, tables, and ashtrays	☐	☐
3. Empty all trash and replace bag	☐	☐
4. Load all activity room dishes into dishwasher	☐	☐
5. Sweep the activity room floor	☐	☐

Figure 6. The Tier System (I, II, III)

TIER I

1. Participate in the daily House program.
2. *Earn at least 70% of your credits on a regular basis.
3. Follow the Basic House Rule.
4. Comply with any contracts that have been designed for you.
5. Take your meds consistently.

*On Tier I you can earn a maximum of $30.00 per week so that:

90 - 100%	=	$30.00
80 - 90%	=	$25.00
70 - 80%	=	$20.00

To move to Tier II you must "present your case" and the reasons why you should be able to move with your resident advisor to the rest of the staff.

TIER II - TRANSITIONAL

1. Earn 90-100% of your credits consistently (3 out of 4 weeks)
2. Consistently do your hygiene (showering, laundry) without being reminded.
3. Take your meds without being reminded.
4. Attend your regularly scheduled appointments without being reminded after planning meeting (i.e., therapy).
5. Use cabs, the bus or walk to where you need to go.
6. Own and use an alarm clock to get up—you may have one wake-up call after the alarm.
7. Can responsibly budget $40 per week.
8. Participate in movie and/or mall trips.

To move to Tier III you must "present your case" and the reasons why you should move with your resident advisor to the rest of the staff.

TIER III

1. Can maintain a weekly schedule (instead of a daily schedule) that you work out with your resident advisor. This includes getting yourself up.
2. Can get yourself wherever you need to go—i.e., find and use your own means of transportation.
3. Can make and keep all of your own appointments— i.e., doctor, dentist, therapist.
4. Can take your meds and take care of your prescriptions on your own.
5. Have an overall absence of "excessive behaviors."
6. Can budget on your own and keep up without being on the credit system.

problem behaviors; the complex and often stressful level of individual needs; and the coordination and execution of the wide variety of daily tasks involved in maintaining the program and facility. The House opened in September 1988 with a skeletal program. The staff developed and refined most of the structure, the related forms, protocols, and organization of the program, and thus have become dedicated and invested in seeing that it runs according to the guiding philosophy and principles.

The staff consists of the following: the Director (a master's level occupational therapist); The Psychologist Consultant; the Program Nurse (master's level); six full-time Rehabilitation Workers; two part-time Rehabilitation Workers; and five 16-hour per week Rehabilitation Workers for weekends. The staffing pattern provides for both the Director and the Program Nurse to be available for day shifts and some evening shifts. Team Meetings are held daily during shift change to include the total staff. Day staff consists of two Rehabilitation Workers, whereas evening staff consists of three full-time plus one part-time Rehabilitation Workers. Weekends are separately staffed with the 16-hour Rehabilitation Workers. These are ideal positions for students in psychology or related fields. The majority of rehabilitation workers, even though considered paraprofessionals, come to the program with various levels of experience, [and] expertise, and some with degrees in a related field.

The Program Nurse serves not only as part of the day shift, assisting in all the daily tasks of the program for the residents, but also serves as the primary liaison to all of the doctors involved. Each resident has his or her own private psychiatrist. The Nurse oversees all medications which are prescribed by physicians. The medical needs of the residents are extensive, partly due to somatic complications and complaints that are part of the illness. The Nurse provides management of these needs, conducts a health workshop for residents, and also is a good resource for overseeing the menu and daily diet of the residents and providing state of the art education for both residents and staff in healthier ways of eating. The Program Nurse is in charge in the absence of the Director.

The Psychologist Consultant not only serves as a primary consultant to the program, but also is the Assistant Service Chief of the Chronic Schizophrenic Research Unit, and is the primary liaison between the House and Inpatient Division. The Psychologist Consultant, with the Director, screens all applicants as well as mediates when problems arise, consults in treatment, and educates staff.

The Director is in charge of the overall administration of the program, providing staff supervision, direction, and consultation to overall policies, procedures, licensure, and program development and is on 24-hour call. The Director is also the primary liaison between the program and third party reimbursement case managers. Presently 70 percent of the residents are funded by private insurance.

Each staff member has two residents for whom he/she is responsible, as both a case manager and a resident advisor. The role of a case manager at Mt. Airy is to:

1. Provide all necessary documentation.
2. Conduct team meetings for establishing the residents' Rehabilitation Plans and monthly reviews.
3. Serve as a liaison to families, therapists, and community programs regarding residents' status.
4. Assure information regarding entitlements is procured.

The role and function of a resident advisor at Mt. Airy is to:

1. Serve as the primary advocate for his/her resident.
2. Give both practical and emotional support.
3. Meet weekly with the resident for budgeting and planning.
4. Assist the resident in establishing goals in response to problem areas.
5. Assist the resident in [his or her] formal presentation to staff for Tier promotion.
6. Draft behavioral contracts in response to problem behaviors and promote cooperation.

Summary

The Mt. Airy House is a model based on a formal definition of a quarterway house. This definition was drawn from years of experimentation and research in the mental health field toward meeting the residential after care needs of the CMI. It represents one step within a needed spectrum of housing particularly suited for the CMI, and fully acknowledges the need for a network of support services in conjunction with housing.

According to Fine (1983), "Both rehabilitation and traditional treatment models have been guilty of addressing their efforts to the healthiest sectors of the patient population. Successful outcome with a chronic population should not be measured by the same yardstick used for the acutely ill and less disabled" (p. 12). [She adds] that important determinants of outcome in all rehabilitation efforts are: repetition and frequency of practice in skill learning, appropriate performance expectations, supportive staff attitudes, movement into more normative settings with social supports, and appropriate length of time allotted to such an effort. Based on this premise, Mt. Airy House represents a good model and first step in a crucial continuum.

Mt. Airy House is approaching its third year of oper-

ation. To date, the program is operating to capacity, of which nine out of the 16 residents are approaching their second and third years in the program. The future of these residents depends on continuing to explore and creatively provide even more normative housing arrangements in the effort toward better community integration. For some residents, there is evidence that a supervised apartment would be suitable as the next step after Mt. Airy, if given enough social supports. For others, there is beginning evidence that a permanent group home setting is warranted. What is clear however, is the need for a system that is available and open to the fluctuating needs of the CMI, and according to Crowel (1988), "enable patients to view housing changes as routine and normal, and not a sign of failure" (p. 66).

References

Arce, A. & Vergare, M. (1985), An Overview of Community Residences as Alternatives to Hospitalization. *Psychiatric Clinics of North America, 8,* 423-436.

Crowel, R. L. (1988), The Integrated Clinically Managed Housing Network, *New Directions for Mental Health Services,* No. 40, 59-64.

Fine, S. B. (1983), Psychiatric Treatment and Rehabilitation: What's in a Name? *NAPPH Journal, 11,* 5, 8-13.

Gudeman, J. E., Dickey, B., Rood, Laura, Hellman, S., Grinspoon, L. (1981), Alternative to the Back Ward: A Quarterway House, *Hospital and Community Psychiatry, 32,* 359-363.

Hofmeister, J. F., Weiler, V. E., Ackerson, L. M. (1989). Treatment Outcome in a Private-Sector Residential Care Program, *Hospital and Community Psychiatry, 40,* 927-932.

Kruzich, Jean M. (1985), Community Integration of the Mentally Ill in Residential Facilities, *American Journal of Community Psychology, 13,* 553-564.

Mann, William C. (1976), A Quarterway House for Adult Psychiatric Patients, *The American Journal of Occupational Therapy, 30,* 646-647.

Mechanic, Ph.D. (1986), The Challenge of Chronic Mental Illness: A Retrospective and Prospective View, *Hospital and Community Psychiatry, 37,* 891-896.

Myerson, A. T. & Herman, G. S. (1983), What's New in Aftercare? A Review of Recent Literature, *Hospital and Community Psychiatry, 34,* 333-342.

Purnell, T. L., Jackson, S. M., Wallace, E. C., (1982), A Quarterway House Program for Hospitalized Chronic Patients, *Hospital and Community Psychiatry, 33,* 941-942.

Ranz, J. M. (1989), Home II: Preparing Chronic Mental Patients for On-campus Living, *Hospital and Community Psychiatry, 40,* 1190-1191.

Wilberding, D. (1987), Rehabilitation Through Activities For the Chronic Schizophrenic Patient, *The Chronically Mentally Ill: Issues in 0. T. Intervention, Proceedings,* AOTA, Inc., pp. 37-47.

Chapter 20

A Hospital-Connected Halfway House Program for Individuals with Long-Term Neuropsychiatric Disabilities

Sally A. Friedlob, MSW, OTR
Gloria A. Janis, OTR
Carole Deets-Aron, MS

The life pattern of many chronic psychiatric patients is characterized by poor community adjustment, which leads to numerous rehospitalizations within short time periods. A major factor in this pattern is a deficiency and/or low confidence in performing day-to-day living skills. Inpatient treatment tends to focus on alleviating symptoms or resolving problems such as financial difficulties. Consequently, these patients are not prepared to handle the social isolation and the responsibilities they often face upon reentry into the community (1). Thus their symptoms may quickly recur, and they may return to the hospital, engaging in a "revolving door" cycle of admission and discharge. Recognizing that hospital-based occupational therapy often does not provide patients with opportunities for learning and practicing living skills in the community, the occupational therapists at Sepulveda Veterans Administration Medical Center (SVAMC) developed a halfway house program located outside the hospital grounds that provides supportive training for the acquisition of community living skills.

This [chapter] describes the hospital-connected halfway house program and examines the impact such a program can have on the community adjustment of neuropsychiatric clients based on a 5-year follow-up study of the participating residents.

Literature Review

A halfway house is defined as a transitional residence for people with various disabilities, people who need not be confined to an institution but are not ready to cope with family and community life (2). The halfway house idea was in part a reaction to the negative effects of the closed, jail-like hospitals to which most mental patients were confined during the first part of this century. Early halfway house proponents viewed people with emotional illness neither as criminals who needed to be jailed nor as patients who needed to be hospitalized. They viewed them as troubled, anxious, often frightened people, who are in need of support, understanding, and a low-stress, homelike atmosphere in which to work through difficulties, develop self-esteem, and face challenges gradually (3).

The term *halfway house* appeared in the literature in 1953 (2). In 1960, seven urban halfway houses and three rural "work camp houses" were in operation. In 1963, the number had increased to at least 40; in 1965, 100 houses were functioning. By 1978, a National Institute of Mental Health survey (4) identified 20,385 halfway houses. Of these, 26% provided treatment for individuals with a mental illness, and 46% provided treatment for individuals with alcohol problems.

Factors that promoted the rapid increase of halfway houses included the following: (a) the emphasis on maintaining patients as close as possible to the community; (b) an awareness and recognition of the monetary and psychological costs of institutionalization; (c) the growing awareness of the shared responsibility of family and society for the onset and treatment of emotional disorders; (d) the development of the concepts of therapeutic community, the open ward, and community psychiatry; (e) the reliance on the use of psychotropic drugs; and (f) the development of aftercare services adapted to the needs of different groups at different stages of rehabilitation (e.g., day and night hospitals, expatient clubs, sheltered workshops).

Some of the successful early transitional living programs have been reviewed by Greenblatt and Budson (5), including the Fort Logan Mental Health Center in Denver, Colorado; Training in Community Living Program, Mendota Mental Health Institute, Dana County, Wisconsin; the Southern Arizona Mental Health Center, Tucson; Berkeley House in Boston; and Soteria in San Francisco. These programs ranged from family and home care to halfway houses. In general, patients appeared to make gains in socialization and ability to work and functioned satisfactorily without burdening their families. The authors concluded that approximately 80% of patients discharged from halfway house programs made a successful transition to community life and had lower rehospitalization rates than expected.

Halfway houses use one of two approaches: the "nurturing" or the "high-expectation" approach. In the nurturing approach, the staff assumes responsibility for running the house, recognizes the illness of the resident, acknowledges that progress toward health takes time, and sees the halfway house as a good place in which to make such progress. In the high-expectation approach, the health of residents is emphasized; residents are expected to take on responsibilities and deal with pressures to hasten a move toward independence.

In both approaches, halfway houses deemphasize the patient role, minimize distance between staff and residents, and encourage residents to help each other. The sharing of essential work makes each member an important part of the community.

Unlike a hospital, the halfway house encourages people to become less dependent on others and expect more of themselves. It provides a bridge between the hospital and the community via a therapeutic milieu designed to prepare residents for resuming their roles in society. It encourages normal patterns of living, offers support, and supplies opportunities for trying different roles and behaviors in a safe environment.

A halfway house seemed to be the ideal program to meet patient needs at SVAMC. Rose and associates (6) found that 79% of the applicants for psychiatric inpatient status at SVAMC were "revolving door" patients. Of these, 80% had been discharged within the past year, 50% within the preceding five months, and 32% within the last month. Gross (7) showed that problems of both Vietnam-era veterans and older veterans at the Los Angeles Outpatient Clinic could be classified as living skills deficits related to self-maintenance. The aim of the SVAMC halfway house program was to reduce the rate of rehospitalization by remediating the observed life skills deficiencies.

Method

Subjects

A screening team to select applicants for the program comprised occupational therapists, a resident in psychiatry, and representatives from the nursing service. The following criteria were established for program eligibility: (a) applicants must be capable of and interested in moving to independent community life; (b) applicants must be between 20 [and] 50 years old; (c) applicants must not have substance abuse problems; (d) applicants must be responsible for self-medication; and (e) applicants must be employable, employed, attending school, or participate in other occupational activity (i.e., sheltered workshop or volunteer work).

Applicants approved for the program agreed by signed contract to participate in all aspects of the program, abide by the existing policies, set aside funds for community living, and take part in an alumni group so that they could serve as models for future residents.

A total of 21 inpatients met the criteria for the program. The group included inpatients with the following disorders: eleven with chronic schizophrenia, two with manic depression, three with depression, three with a personality disorder, and two with an anxiety neurosis. Of these inpatients, two were released after a short time in the program for failure to maintain program requirements. The remaining 19 patients ranged in age from 22 to 42 years; the average age was 30. More than half of the participants experienced three or more hospitalizations in a 5-year period.

Halfway house staff (e.g., two occupational therapists) agreed by signed contract to provide learning experiences, counseling, and consultation in daily living skills; provide a graded program according to participants' needs (i.e., varied supervision and learning experiences); assist participants in making concrete discharge plans; and provide appropriate follow-up in the community.

Procedures

The two occupational therapists were the sole permanent staff members responsible for program development, which included planning, coordination, implementation, and supervision. Dietitians, nurses, medical residents, physician's assistants, psychologists, and social workers were called on periodically to consult with the residents for an in-service training program. Selected students from these fields also participated in the halfway house program as part of their clinical training.

The halfway house setting provided a homelike atmosphere in a single-story dwelling with wood paneling and a fireplace, two bedrooms, one bathroom, a separate dining room, kitchen, and large lawns in the front and rear of the house. The house was located outside the gates of the SVAMC grounds and was connected with the hospital only through a telephone system that was used primarily for reporting emergencies. The neuropsychiatric officer of the day (i.e., the doctor on call) was available in the evening for emergencies. A pay phone was installed for personal calls.

Residents were introduced into the house in groups of four for a 3-month treatment period. The residents were patients selected from the SVAMC inpatient program who were ready for discharge into the community. During the 3 months in the halfway house program, concrete discharge plans were made and assessed according to each resident's capabilities (e.g., plans to go home, into own apartment, to find board and care, or arrange for cooperative housing). The inpatient staff agreed to accept a resident on the inpatient ward in the event that a resident required rehospitalization. Residents rotated through the program only once. However, if a resident required rehospitalization for a few days, he or she was returned to the program.

The program focused on developing competence in daily living skills in the following areas: health and hygiene, nutrition, household management, budgeting, interpersonal relationships, community resources and leisure activities, and occupational (vocational and avocational) training.

Each four-person resident group, with the help of the two occupational therapists, set goals according to the group members' perceived assets and liabilities. These goals were reassessed weekly and modified according to each individual's level of competence and immediate needs. In addition, to receive some help with individual concerns and self-development, each resident was assigned a counselor. It was generally the occupational therapists and the occupational therapy students who assumed the role of counselor.

The program was divided into three segments of four weeks. Ongoing education in each of the areas listed earlier was provided throughout the program. Priorities were set during each segment, and supervision was graded.

The first segment focused on nutrition. The activities of planning balanced meals, marketing and properly storing food, and preparing meals involve good problem solving and decision making, and results are seen immediately. Sharing meals increases interpersonal interaction, creates trust, and provides a relaxed atmosphere. As relationships began to build, residents were introduced to a 12-week course in interpersonal skills that incorporated assertiveness and empathy training. Additionally, activities such as housekeeping tasks, laundry, and basic clothing repair were planned. Weekly sessions on finance included basic arithmetic necessary for making change, and performing and managing the previously discussed activities. The two therapists provided 4 to 6 hours of supervision daily.

During the second segment of the program, residents were more independent. Emphasis shifted to vocational training and the effective use of leisure time and community resources. Using the skills they had learned in interpersonal relationships training, the residents explored the community's agencies and resources for recreation and other services. Problem solving, decision making, and follow-through skills were expanded. The weekly sessions on finance were expanded to include payment schedules, budgets, and the handling of a bank account. Residents identified interests, planned activities, and followed through on scheduled and spontaneously initiated activities.

The second segment was more difficult for the residents because they began to realize that discharge into the community was imminent. Awareness of the cost of living with little left over for leisure activities produced mild to high anxiety. The therapists were prepared to deal with more intense clinical issues and provide support and acceptance for residents (especially for those who began to regress).

During the third segment, supervision was minimal. Residents were involved in work, school, and/or volunteer programs (finding their own placements), or in problem solving during individual sessions with their assigned counselor. They were responsible for managing and balancing their day. Weekly assessment, weekend planning groups, and leisure and social network groups were maintained. Emphasis was placed on finding adequate living arrangements in the community, including selecting a community, being aware of community resources, and planning for individual or shared living. Residents who wished to start a cooperative (i.e., a house or apartment in which a group lives and shares household responsibilities and finances) were assisted by the social work staff.

After completing the program, each resident returned one evening per month for alumni meetings to share experiences and obtain guidance and support. When feasible, alumni members assisted the current resident group in programming and served as role models. When indicated or requested, the staff visited alumni members in the community for consultation.

Results

Five years following treatment, 63% of the 19 patients who completed the halfway house program remained in the community. The halfway house program produced significant changes in rehospitalization rate, length of rehospitalization, living environment, and occupational behavior (i.e., vocational and avocational activities).

Table 1 shows the recidivism rate for this group before and after treatment. For example, eight patients had no rehospitalizations, and four patients had multiple hospitalizations. In two of these four patients, the duration of hospitalization markedly decreased (from a 3- to 6-month period to a 2- to 4-week period).

Table 2 illustrates the participants' living patterns before and after treatment. Major environmental changes were made by 13 patients. Twelve patients who had lived with their parents before treatment moved to independent living in an apartment, home, or in cooperative housing after treatment, and one patient moved into a Veterans Administration-sponsored cooperative. Eleven of these 13 patients moved into their own apartments. Of these eleven, two returned briefly to their parents and then moved into an apartment; two married shortly after

moving to their own apartment and then bought homes through the GI Bill; two moved in with a female roommate. Three patients, each of whom had lived previously in an apartment or at home with a spouse, returned to their previous living situations. Four patients returned to their families.

The occupational behavior of 17 patients was altered. (Nothing was known about the occupational behavior of two of them.) Including those displaying job stability, 13 expressed discontent with their vocational choice and changed vocations through formal or on-the-job training. Five patients changed jobs. Nine working at a vocation and/or odd jobs terminated employment to prepare for a new career; six attended junior college, three attended a trade school. Three patients experiencing difficulty in balancing avocational activities began attending a Veterans Administration Satellite Center (a community-based outpatient treatment center) and participated in an outpatient social club and support group. Two had previously participated in little or no daily activities; one had poor work adjustment and social skills on the job. One patient who had previously attended college was able to continue with his vocational goals. One patient with a master's degree accepted menial jobs but remained unhospitalized and is currently working consistently as a waiter.

Although the comparison of progress between the nine patients with schizophrenia and the ten with other psychiatric disorders was not the major focus of this study, the similar outcomes of the two diagnostic groups is interesting. Of the patients with schizophrenia, four had no rehospitalizations, and two had one rehospitalization within 2 years following treatment. Prior to treatment, five of these six had at least one hospitalization for approximately 1 year. Seven living with parents moved to independent living; six made major vocational changes. Of those with other psychiatric disorders, three had no rehospitalizations, and two were rehospitalized for about 1 month. For two patients with multiple rehospitalizations the duration of each rehospitalization decreased after treatment. Five who were living with parents moved to independent living, and six made major occupational changes.

Discussion

All of the 19 participants in the halfway house program had multiple rehospitalization histories, which characterizes them as a chronic group. They are representative of veterans requiring psychiatric treatment at SVAMC. The rate of rehospitalization as a measure of chronicity is the most common statistic cited for a schizophrenic population. In Great Britain, Todd and associates (8) studied a group of patients who had "hard

Table 1. Recidivism: Pre- and Posttreatment

Diagnosis	Age	Number of Hospitalizations 5 years prior to Treatment	Duration of Hospitalizations in Months	Number of Hospitalizations at 5-year Follow-up	Duration of Hospitalizations in Months
1. Schizophrenia, paranoid	28	3+*	2-6	1	1
2. Depression	28	2	3	1	1
3. Anxiety neurosis	28	1	6	0	0
4. Schizophrenia, acute	24	4	unknown	0	0
5. Schizophrenia, chronic	26	4+*	unknown	3	1
6. Inadequate personality	41	1	2	0	0
7. Schizophrenia, chronic	24	4+*	3-5	5	2 (3 for 1 wk)
8. Schizophrenia, chronic	23	4+*	1-7	0	0
9. Manic depression	41	3+*	4-6	2	1, 4
10. Schizophrenia, chronic	26	3	4-12	1	1
11. Manic depression	29	4+*	3-5	2	5
12. Schizophrenia, paranoid	26	3	12	0	0
13. Manic depression	28	4+*	unknown	1	1
14. Inadequate personality	22	2	1, 5	3	2, 10 (1 for 1 day)
15. Personality disorder	36	4+*	unknown	0	0
16. Inadequate personality	46	1	2	0	0
17. Schizophrenic, paranoid	21	3	6	4	2 (3-9 days each)
18. Schizophrenia	21	2	7, 12	0	0
19. Schizophrenia, paranoid	36	5+*	unknown	unknown	unknown

*The veteran had multiple hospitalizations at other facilities, the exact number and length of which is unknown.

core" chronic schizophrenia and found them to have an average of 3.3 previous admissions and 15 years of illness. Studies in the United States show a shorter readmission period (1).

For the majority of the chronic patients in these studies (1, 8), the quality of community life improved in terms of duration in the community, length of rehospitalization, living environment, and occupational behav-

Table 2. Living Pattern: Pre- and Posttreatment

Living Pattern	Pretreatment	Posttreatment
Transient	2	0
With parents or sibling, or board and care	15	3
Cooperative housing	0	1
With wife and children, or with female roommate	1	2
Independent	1	9
Unknown	0	1

ior. An outcome of 63% avoiding rehospitalization was superior to the findings of at least two earlier studies. Mosher (9) and Talbot (10) demonstrated that 50% to 60% of patients with schizophrenia who are released into the community cannot sustain a successful rehospitalization outcome for 2 years. In another study (11), 45% were readmitted within 6 months of discharge.

In this study, 86% of the halfway house patients requiring rehospitalization increased the duration of their stay in the community and required a shorter rehospitalization. In addition, 57% of these patients were able to maintain and return to apartments and jobs.

These findings suggest that in the long term some chronic patients may be highly vulnerable to stress and have difficulty coping with the demands of daily living despite intensive life skills treatment. Three of the six patients who required multiple rehospitalizations after treatment were manic depressives. Their recidivism may have been a result of the cyclical nature of the illness or the possibility that the halfway house program may not be the treatment of choice for this type of patient.

Three of the four patients who returned to their families showed high recidivism rates after treatment. Records and an interview with one patient showed that a major problem was family conflict. Studies in London (12) and in the United States (13) concluded that, in addition to life skills deficits, the most powerful predictor of symptomatic relapse among schizophrenics is the return to relatives where there is negative "expressed emotion" in terms of criticism and overinvolvement. This finding suggests that family therapy may be indicated as an additional treatment modality.

In running a program that provided structured training in self-help and independent living skills for a population of chronic, hospitalized, mental health patients, Tyler (14) found a greater portion of those with schizophrenia completed treatment than of those with other personality disorders. These findings are at odds with this study in that both groups had similar treatment outcomes. Although the nonschizophrenic participants had great difficulty maintaining themselves in the community and consistently holding jobs, they entered the program at a higher level of functioning: 89% already had vocational skills and 40% already had experienced living independently. The schizophrenic participants, as a group, entered the program at a lower level of functioning and demonstrated a greater range of improvement from their baseline. Of great significance is the fact that five of those with schizophrenia had at least one hospitalization of approximately 1 year prior to treatment, whereas 5 years after treatment only two of these required rehospitalization and for only 1 month. Thus, both groups demonstrated an ability to learn and use a variety of living skills.

Implications for Future Programming

The positive results of the halfway house program for individuals with chronic schizophrenia have generated interest in further program development and formal research from the Veterans Administration Psychiatry Service. Interest arose because the chronic schizophrenic patient is the most visible of the psychiatric population and because there are few reports that focus on the training of daily living skills with schizophrenic patients. Additionally, it would seem that occupational therapy treatment modalities need to be validated.

For these reasons, a standardized life skills training program and research project for an exclusively schizophrenic population was developed by the occupational therapy staff in collaboration with staff in the Department of Psychiatry, Behavioral and Mental Health Research and Education Section, UCLA/SVAMC.

Conclusion

Follow-up data on 19 veterans suggests that a hospital-based halfway house intervention as a transition between the hospital and the community can have a significant impact on the length and the quality of community life for the patient with a chronic neuropsychiatric disorder and that it may be particularly beneficial for individuals with chronic schizophrenia.

References

1. Brown, MA: Maintenance and generalization issues in skills training with chronic schizophrenics. Read before the Symposium on Social Competence and Psychiatric Disorder: Therapy and Practice, Provider, VAMC, Providence, RI, March 20, 1980.

2. Raish HL, Rog D: Psychiatric halfway house, "How is it measuring up?" *Community Ment Health J* 11(12):310-317, 1975.

3. Serban, G, Gidynski C, Melnick E: Social performance and readmission in acute and chronic schizophrenics: Comparison of two approaches. *Behavioral Neuropsychiatry* F:6-12, 1975.

4. Greenblatt M: *Psychopolitics.* New York: Grune & Stratton, 1978.

5. Greenblatt M, Budson RA (Eds.): Symposium, follow-up studies of community care, *Am J Psychiatry* 133(8):916-921, 1976.

6. Rose S, Hawkins J, Apodaca L: The decision to admit: Criteria for admission and readmission at a V.A. hospital. *Arch Gen Psychiatry* 34:418-421, 1977.

7. Gross C: Characteristics and problems of a veteran outpatient population. Prepared for the Veteran Need Identification Project, Los Angeles Outpatient Clinic, Los Angeles, CA, January 1975.

8. Todd N, Bennie EH, Carlisle JM: Some features of "new long-stay" male schizophrenics. *Brit J Psychiatry* 129:424-427, 1976.

9. Mosher LR: Madness in the community. *Attitude* 1:2-21, 1971.

10. Talbot JA: Stop the revolving door: A study of recidivism to a state hospital. *Psychiatric Quart* 48:159-167, 1974.

11. Evans JR, Goldstein MJ, and Rodnick EH: Premorbid adjustment, paranoid status, and patterns of response to phenothiazine in acute schizophrenia. *Schizophr Bull* 3:24-37, 1970.

12. Vaughn C, Leff JP: The influence of family and social factors on the course of psychiatric illness: A comparison of schizophrenic and depressed neurotic patients. *Brit J Psychiatry* 129:125-137, 1976.

13. Liberman RP, Wallace CJ, Vaughn CE, Snyder KL: Social and family factors in the course of schizophrenia: Towards an interpersonal problem solving therapy for schizophrenics and their families. Read before the Conference on Psychotherapy of Schizophrenia: Current Status and New Directions, Yale University School of Medicine, New Haven, CT, April 9, 1979.

14. Tyler RM: Psychiatric diagnosis and behavior therapy. *The Behavior Therapist* 3:4-9, 1980.

Chapter 21

Occupational Therapy in the Treatment of Schizophrenia

R. Hayes

The high relapse rates and poor social and community functioning of adequately medicated schizophrenic patients has prompted health professionals who work with them to assess the influence of psychosocial treatment on the course of schizophrenia (Anthony & Liberman, 1986).

A large percentage of studies evaluating the impact of different treatment media on schizophrenic patients have methodological deficits which severely limit the interpretation and application of their results. The major deficits are lack of specific diagnostic criteria, no control of degree of patient pathology or level of chronicity and no control of medication. These are particularly important because it has been suggested that schizophrenic patients' receptivity to psychosocial intervention is influenced by their current level of psychopathology or by the particular subtype of schizophrenia they belong to (May, 1976). Patients with the more acute subtype of schizophrenia are thought to be more likely to respond to psychosocial intervention than those with a chronic condition characterized by high levels of negative symptoms such as avolition, apathy, anhedonia, alogia, social withdrawal and affective flattening (Crow, 1985).

Occupational therapy journals from a number of countries, the *American Journal of Occupational Therapy*, the *Australian Occupational Therapy Journal*, *The British Occupational Therapy Journal*, the *Canadian Journal of Occupational Therapy*, the *New Zealand Journal of Occupational Therapy*, the *Occupational Therapy Journal of Research* and *Occupational Therapy in Mental Health*, were scrutinized to identify treatment media used with schizophrenic patients. The treatment methods found fit into four loosely defined, often overlapping categories: sensory integration, activity group therapy, social skills training and living skills training. This article reviews the four treatment methods.

Sensory Integration

The theory of sensory integration was developed by Ayres in the 1950s for use with neurologically disabled children (Ayres, 1974). According to Ayres (1981) the taking in and organization of sensory information for use in relating to the environment is called sensory integration. Sensory integrative dysfunction hinders an individual's ability to interact effectively with the environment and perform normal day to day tasks. Ayres (1974) stated that by providing the individual with controlled sensory input via the vestibular system, muscles, joints and skin [he or she] will spontaneously make adaptive responses that interpret those sensations.

Ayres has recommended numerous activities to provide tactile, proprioceptive and vestibular input. These include direct sensory stimulation such as brushing, rubbing and vibration of the skin as well as games using equipment such as scooter boards, net hammocks, bolster swings and suspended inner tubes (Ayres, 1981).

King (1974) hypothesized that many of the deficits found in schizophrenic patients, such as perceptual dysfunction, abnormal posture and poor body image and motor planning, are the result of poor sensory integration and contribute to severe emotional stress and a predisposition to hallucinations. King (1974) drawing on the work of Ayres published the first of many articles by occupational therapists on sensory integration in schizophrenia. In this early study, 15 hospitalized chronic schizophrenic patients participated in noncompetitive activities such as ball games, jumping and marching. This was congruent with the treatment principles recommended by Ayres. After two to three weeks of treatment, the therapists subjectively evaluated the participants as having increased their levels of vocalization, smiling and grooming. This study was, however, exploratory and based on unsubstantiated theories.

Sturgess and Clancy (1981) conducted a thorough evaluation of the scientific basis for King's hypothesis and reviewed related experimental studies. From this they concluded that, "...there is no theoretical justification for the use of Sensory Integration Therapy with adult schizophrenic clients" (p. 184), and "...there is no experimental evidence to support claims for the effective use of sensory integration therapy and significant postural behaviour change in adults diagnosed as process schizophrenia" (p. 185). Since Sturgess and Clancy's (1981) review, other intervention studies using sensory integration in schizophrenia have been published. The later results are no more promising than those reviewed earlier (Crist, Thomas & Stone, 1984; Hixson & Mathews, 1984). Crist, Thomas and Stone (1984) compared the sensory integration approach with prevocational training. Prevocational training using group discussion and pencil and paper tasks proved to be superior to the sensory integration treatment on 53 of the 54 measures of cognitive, work, motor and psychological performance. A study by Blakeny, Strickland and Wilkinson (1983) provided more optimistic results comparing sensory integration with "sedentary" occupational therapy but their findings were based heavily on subjective observation. It was not stated whether the raters were blind to the treatment distribution of the subjects.

Reports of positive feedback from subjective observations of participants in sensory integration programs are prevalent. Schizophrenic patients, following sensory integration treatment, have been observed to be more relaxed (Rider, 1978), smile more (Crist, 1979; Rider, 1978), verbalize more (Leveille, 1981) and behave more positively about treatment (Crist 1979; Leveille, 1981; Levine, O'Connor & Stacey, 1977; Rider, 1978). Very similar behavior changes were noted by Ross (1977) who conducted a "physical activation" program with young chronic psychiatric patients. The program involved a gym workout, team games and races and relaxation in a hydrotherapy pool. The gross-motor activities and games resembled sensory integration treatment but the competitive element is contraindicated in the sensory integration approach.

Sturgess and Clancy (1981) suggest four possible reasons for the observed behavior changes following sensory integration treatment. One is that sensory integration programs do have some as yet unexplained impact on the central nervous system. Another possibility is the existence of a Hawthorne effect; that is, patients respond to the increased attention they receive from participating in the study. A third possibility is that patients respond to the social context of treatment. Sturgess and Clancy (1981) also suggested that change could result from the demands for attention made within treatment. By being required to attend, patients could possibly experience an improved attention structure. The concept of altering attention or training schizophrenic patients using attention focusing techniques has been used recently by Wong, Massel, Mosk and Liberman (1986) in social skills training with some degree of success.

Although sensory integration treatment appears to have no impact on the sensory integrative functioning of adult schizophrenic patients, it has been found to have some impact on behaviors such as increased motivation to participate in specific tasks and more positive affect. These are important factors in a rehabilitation program but this change is not enough on its own to restore function and increase independence. It is also possible that nonsensory integration programs with similar levels of staff attention and physical exercise could have the same impact on participants.

Activity Groups

Activity groups are regarded as one of the legitimate tools of Occupational Therapy (Mosey, 1986). According to Hopkins, Smith and Tiffany (1983) for human beings activities "... provide a bridge between their inner reality and their external world." For the purpose of this review "activity groups" are defined as aggregates of people participating in the same or related purposeful activities. The participants may be working cooperatively or in parallel. The role of the therapist in an activity group is as a facilitator of behaviors such as social interaction, discussion and problem solving rather than as an instructor. Groups for training specific skills will be covered under living skills training and social skills training.

Many studies report the involvement of schizophrenic patients in specific activity groups. The activities have included arts and crafts, current events, gym (Gautier, 1980), remedial drama (Spencer, Gillespie & Ekisa, 1983), photography (Phillips, 1986), personal care and beauty groups, word games, quizzes, music and play reading (Gan & Pullen, 1984) to name a few.

Some studies with schizophrenic populations provide support for the use of object focused activity (Liberman et al., 1986; Linn, Caffey, Klett, Hogarty & Lamb, 1978 [sic]). Linn et al. (1978) [sic] on analyzing the outcome of schizophrenic patients from 10 day centers concluded that successful outcome centers were characterized by more occupational and recreational therapy. The content of therapy was not specified. It has been consistently found across a variety of settings, board and care homes, hospitals and mental health centers that there is an inverse relationship between the amount of structured programing and bizarre behavior of schizophrenic patients (Liberman et al., 1986). Wong, Massel, Mosk, and Liberman (1986) found that when patients were engaged in structured recreational activities such as crafts, card games and music, there was a significant reduction in bizarre behaviors such as inappropriate laughter, mumbling to self, obsessive-compulsive ruminations and posturing.

The relative impact of different activities on the individual's acquisition of specific skills and ability to function in the community is unclear. For occupational therapists to identify optimal treatment for schizophrenic patients, they must evaluate what impact different activities and their method of presentation have on participants.

Some studies have compared the impact of different group variables on schizophrenic patients. An important area of investigation is the impact of therapist behavior. Turvey, Main and McCartney (1985) found that participants in a card game were more likely to prompt each other if the therapist delayed prompting for 10 to 15 seconds. A similar trend was found by Odhner (1970). In his study, subjects from groups whose leaders initiated the most statements initiated fewer statements with each other and more with the leader.

Odhner (1970) also assessed the relative impact of activity and verbal groups. He found, contrary to his hypothesis, that subjects spoke significantly less during a group construction task than a verbal activity. Information processing and attentional deficits prevalent in schizophrenic patients (George & Neufeld, 1985) possibly limit their ability to concentrate on a task and converse with other patients at the same time. The construction task group, however, spoke to each other 60 percent more than the verbal groups in the discussion following the task. It is possible that the cooperative activity provided the activity group with a mutual nonthreatening concrete interest that members could talk more easily with each other about.

DeCarlo and Mann (1985) also compared the effectiveness of verbal and activity groups. Schizophrenic and depressed participants of an activity group improved in their subjective perception of their communication skills, but not significantly. The discussion group deteriorated, but not significantly. There was no objective measure of actual skill levels. It should be noted that the activity group was actually a discussion and activity group. The activities had a structured discussion component within them in contrast to the relatively unstructured discussion in the verbal groups. It is possible that the different responses of the two groups were related to factors such as degree of structure and opportunity for introspection rather than the activity/verbal components of the content. In a review of inpatient psychosocial treatment of schizophrenia, Drake and Sederer (1986) concluded that therapy which highlights self-disclosure, expression of strong negative affects and insight oriented techniques is potentially toxic to the participants, whereas groups with active leadership, structure, support, practical advice, reality testing, and opportunities for skill enhancement have been found to be helpful.

Group discussion has also been compared with remedial drama and role play based social skills training (Spencer, Gillespie & Ekisa, 1983). Both social skills training and remedial drama groups exhibited increases in ward social interaction. Only social skills training produced significant improvement of conversation skills measured in a role play test.

The provision of structured activity programs in inpatient, day care and residential settings appears to reduce the incidence of bizarre behavior in schizophrenic patients. In day centers it has been found to correlate with more successful outcome. From a limited number of studies it appears that by manipulating group variables, such as therapist interaction style and activity content and structure, it is possible to make an impact on the quantity and quality of communication during that group and in some instances immediately after. It is possible that responses vary according to a number of variables, such as patients' characteristics, the chosen activity, degree of structure within the activity, group size and even the environment. It has still to be established whether activity groups have any impact on factors such as negative symptomatology, self-esteem, the establishment of social networks, community tenure or quality of life.

Social Skills Training

The schizophrenic population is characterized by substantial deficits in community and interpersonal functioning (Wallace, 1984). In a recent survey of clients with "a psychotic condition," Orford (1986) found that making friends and meeting people was the most frequently expressed desire. The absence of social and life skills has been attributed to understimulating and unstructured environments (Glynn & Mueser, 1986), |or| disuse of skills through long term psychiatric illness, cognitive disturbance, high levels of anxiety or from never having learned them in childhood (Curran, Monti & Corriveau, 1982).

Anthony and Liberman (1986) define social skills as the skills an individual uses to: "Promote problem solving, engage others in successful affiliative and instrumental relationships, mobilize supportive networks and engage in work" (p. 544). Wallace et al. (1980) have outlined the four major elements of definitions of social skill: (1) patients' internal states, i.e., their feelings, attitudes and perceptions of interpersonal contexts; (2) the topography of patients' behaviors—the rates of behaviors such as eye contact, hand gestures, body posture, speech disfluencies, voice volume, and speech latency; (3) the outcomes of interactions, as reflected in the achievement of patients' goals; and (4) the outcomes of interactions as reflected in the attitudes, feelings, behaviors and goals of other participants.

Social skills intervention studies generally use a highly structured behavioral approach (Liberman et al., 1985 [sic]). A typical training session would begin with the systematic assessment and identification of social skills deficits. This would be followed by instruction in, and modeling of specific changes the participant could make to |his or her| interpersonal behavior. The patient would then role-play the new behaviors and receive positive feedback for appropriate behavior. Specific feedback is also given about those behaviors that need changing. Representative examples of social skills training programs have been described by Beidel, Bellack, Turner, Hersen and Luber (1981), Trower, Bryant and Argyle (1978) and Wallace (1982) [sic].

Social skills training (SST) has been used with schizophrenic patients for over two decades as a method of remediating problems in social functioning (Wallace et al., 1980). Occupational Therapists perceive the importance of SST with schizophrenic patients (Hewitt, Wishart & Lambert, 1981; Drouet, 1986) but have contributed

little to the literature in this area. Of those studies which do exist, methodological flaws limit their interpretation (Denton, 1983 [sic]; Drouet, 1986).

Drouet (1986) described in detail a SST program with long term schizophrenic patients in which participants were subjectively perceived to have improved. As SST was only one of many interventions used concurrently with this group, it was impossible to assess the impact of any one intervention from another. Hewitt et al. (1981) compared SST with an unspecified control condition. Just over half the patients had a diagnosis of schizophrenia. Only the SST group improved significantly on a scale of social behavior. There were also anecdotal reports of generalization of skills to other settings within the hospital. Neither of these occupational therapy intervention studies considered their impact on the longer term outcome and community functioning of the subjects.

Denton (1983) used an innovative approach comparing standard SST with a task oriented group. The task was making a videotape of SST. Although no group obtained a statistically significant effect, the video group was observed to display more enthusiasm and active participation. The author felt that the video had been a motivating factor. The study's design limited the likelihood of either treatment obtaining significant improvement. The SST group received a total of three hours and fifteen minutes |of| treatment compared with seven and a half hours for the task oriented group. Also, with small sample sizes of four and five respectively only a dramatic change could have been detected.

Most research in the area of SST in schizophrenia comes from the discipline of psychology. The psychosocial model used by psychologists working in the field is the "vulnerability-stress-coping-competence model" of major mental disorders (Anthony & Liberman, 1986). According to this model, individuals with a psychobiological predisposition to schizophrenia are more likely to remain functioning in the community if they have antipsychotic medication to protect against biological stress and skill building programs such as SST and life skills training to enhance personal coping.

Previous reviews of research on SST and schizophrenia (Curran et al., 1982; Hersen, 1979; Wallace et al., 1980), generally agree that SST increases participants' feelings of ability and comfort in social situations. Reviewers also agreed that evidence of improved topographical elements such as eye contact, posture, response duration and response latency, were not so promising. Topographical improvement usually only occurred when the assessment format, usually a type of role play, was similar to that of the training session. When these changes were measured using evaluation tools which were dissimilar, treatment results were inconsistent.

There are five recent well controlled group comparison studies of SST with schizophrenic patients (Bellack, Turner, Hersen & Luber, 1984; Brown & Munford, 1983; Hogarty et al., 1986; Liberman, Mueser & Wallace, 1986; Spencer et al., 1983). These five studies demonstrate a wide variation in what constitutes SST. All groups used some form of behavioral SST with instruction, modelling, rehearsal and feedback. Two also used a family education component and a social problem solving approach in which subjects were trained in the receiving, processing and sending skills of communication (Hogarty et al., 1986; Liberman et al., 1986). Brown and Munford (1983) trained interpersonal skills as just one part of a six module life skills program.

In two of the three studies which evaluated positive symptomatology (Bellack et al., 1984; Hogarty et al., 1986; Liberman et al., 1986) SST made significantly more impact than the control group. In Bellack et al's. (1984) study, an SST group superimposed on a day hospital program and day hospital only control groups improved equally on positive symptomatology. As stated earlier, structured activity programs can reduce psychotic behavior in schizophrenic patients (Wong et al., 1986). It is likely that the decrease in positive symptoms for both groups was the result of a highly structured day hospital activity program.

No study measured negative symptomatology. Brown and Munford (1983), however, found significant improvements in optimism for the future and on a depression scale with SST. SST produced significant improvements in the four studies which measured specific social skills (Bellack et al., 1984; Brown & Munford, 1983; Liberman et al., 1986; Spencer et al., 1983). Generalization of social skills to a naturalistic, noninstitutional setting was only assessed by Liberman et al. (1986) whose SST group subjects were significantly more successful conversing with a stranger and more likely to retain new skills than the control group. Only in the Hogarty et al. (1986) study were the relapse rates for [the] SST group significantly lower than the control. There was a trend in this direction in the Liberman et al. (1986) study, but not in the Bellack et al. (1984) study. At 12 months post-discharge in the Hogarty et al. (1986) study relapse rates were 41% of the medication only controls, 20% of the SST only group, 19% of the family treatment only group and 0% of the SST + family treatment group. In this study there appears to be a positive cumulative effect with the two treatment modalities.

It is likely that staff and group support are responsible for at least some of the change experienced in both treatment and control groups. In future research, comparison conditions and SST subjects should receive comparable amounts of time spent with staff expressing care and concern, to control for nonspecific treatment factors.

It has been suggested that because of the heterogeneity of patients' responses to SST, training would be best tailored to meet the needs of individual clients (Liberman et al., 1985 [sic]). Liberman et al. (1985) [sic] are now advocating three levels of social skills training. At the most basic level, patients who have severe attentional deficits are trained using an attention-focusing procedure in which very specific skills are trained in a highly repetitious manner. On the next level, patients are trained using the modelling, role play, feedback model. At the highest level schizophrenic patients with higher cognitive functioning are trained in problem solving strategies.

SST shows potential to help schizophrenic individuals cope more effectively in the community. There needs to be further investigation to clarify which patients respond to what particular forms of treatment, what behaviors and symptoms can be changed and whether specifically trained skills generalize to the home, and the community.

Living Skills Training

Living skills are those skills required to function independently in the community. The living skills area of schizophrenia has received considerable attention from occupational therapists, and now some of the major psychological proponents of SST are incorporating more life skills into their programs (Liberman et al., 1986). A typical living skills program is described by Wallace, Boone, Donohue and Foy (1985). Their program contained 10 training modules: conversational skills, vocational rehabilitation, medication management, self-care skills, personal information, home finding and maintenance skills, leisure/recreational skills, food preparation, public transportation and money management. As with SST, instruction, demonstration, practice, feedback, reinforcement, and homework were used to train skills in each area. In conjunction with laboratory training, participants typically practice their new skills in the natural environment. For example, participants might plan a menu, shop for groceries and prepare a meal as in vivo practice for food preparation, public transportation and money management training modules.

Life skills have been taught as part of the daily routine of specialized treatment wards (Drouet, 1983), as community living preparation units within a standard program, or as single components such as money management training (Kaseman, 1980) or prevocational groups (Kramer & Beidel, 1982).

Some very impressive results, particularly in increasing community tenure, have been achieved by training life skills with long stay schizophrenic patients within a token economy program (Paul & Lentz, 1977; Drouet, 1986). Despite these positive results, most occupational therapists are not in the position to transform their working environments into total token economy systems and must rely on less comprehensive treatment.

Several occupational therapists report living skills programs conducted without the background of a token economy or milieu therapy (Campbell & McCreadie, 1983; Durham, 1982; Friedlob, Janis & Deets-Aron, 1986; Johnson, Vinnicomb & Merrill, 1980 [sic]). Unfortunately the majority of these studies evaluated their programs subjectively. Only Campbell & McCreadie (1983) and Friedlob et al. (1986) presented their results in a statistical mode. Both found statistically significant support for the use of living skills training with schizophrenic patients.

Friedlob et al. (1986) studied clients in a halfway house. This study is particularly important because of their considerable five year follow-up period. Results indicated that patients were able to transfer and maintain their new skills within the community. The program's existence within the community rather than a hospital enhanced the generalization of new skills. Brown (1983) has described strategies for the generalization of skills treatment with chronic schizophrenic patients. They are: involvement in the real world, and involvement of patients in goal setting and choice of treatment. All [are] featured in Friedlob et al.'s (1986) program.

Prevocational Skills Training

Employment rates for schizophrenic patients one to five years post discharge have been estimated to be as low as ten to 15 percent (Anthony & Liberman, 1986). This has been attributed to factors such as poor presentation at job interviews and patients' social deficits such as inability to ask for assistance and accept criticism (Anthony & Liberman, 1986).

Prevocational training programs include such topics as approaching the job market, writing job applications and role playing job interviews (Kramer & Beidel, 1982; Liberman et al., 1986; Mauras-Corsino, Daniavicz & Swan, 1985 [sic]).

Kramer and Beidel (1982) involved 44 patients (26 of whom had schizophrenia) in a 10 week job seeking skills group for two hours per week. After one year, one-third of the participants were "gainfully employed" and this included patients in other training programs and voluntary employment. Jacobs, Kardashian, Kreinbring, Ponder and Simpson (1984) obtained more promising results with a job finding club with a much more intensive program. Sixty-five percent of the 300 referred patients (the majority of whom had schizophrenia) entered full-time vocational education or obtained paid employment. Unlike Kramer and Beidel's (1982) structured ten session program, Jacobs et al.'s (1984) program was individualized with patients guided step by step through each stage of the job finding process.

Specific Life Skills

Occupational therapists have trained specific life skills such as mathematics and money management with mixed results. Miller and McCreadie (1978) tutored eight schizophrenic patients in basic arithmetic. Only three subjects improved, and only two of these have retained their skills at a six month follow-up. Kaseman's (1981) [sic] course in money management achieved positive trends at post treatment evaluation but the durability and generalization of the skills were not considered.

Training [in] mathematical calculation and money management is likely to be demanding for schizophrenic patients who are more likely to have generalized deficits in intelligence (Aylward, 1984), information processing and attention (George & Neufeld, 1985). Teaching these skills is likely to need to go beyond standard tuition. It is possible that techniques such as attention focusing, structured behavioral training with rewards, and the use of generalization techniques, such as overtraining through large numbers of treatment sessions, would be more effective with some schizophrenic patients (Brown, 1983).

Successful life skills programs generally have the common characteristics of intensive treatment and training within a real life context, be it in the day to day tasks of an inpatient setting (Drouet, 1983; Paul & Lentz, 1977), a halfway house or [a] prevocational program targeting skills for actual jobs (Jacobs et al., 1984).

Discussion

Occupational therapists are evaluating the effectiveness of the treatment tools they use with schizophrenic patients. In some areas evidence is fairly conclusive while in others it has only just begun to be gathered.

To properly assess the value of Occupational Therapy for schizophrenic patients, researchers must establish appropriate criteria for successful treatment. There is little consensus within the four treatment approaches discussed on what are desirable outcomes. Molecular measures such as grip strength, gait, psychomotor retardation (Blakeney, Strickland & Wilkinson, 1983), eye contact, asking and responding to questions (Denton, 1983 [sic]) and specific life skills assessed in a hospital context (Campbell & McCreadie, 1983) have limited value unless they contribute to more molar [sic] performance.

If treatment is able to make a durable impact on positive and negative symptomatology and community tenure, schizophrenic individuals will benefit from an improved quality of life and the community will benefit from the decreased cost of hospitalization.

From the available data it is possible to say that, for schizophrenic patients, sensory integration appears to have a positive impact on mood and expressed interest,

152

structured activity programs have been found to contribute to a reduction in positive symptomatology, [and] SST and life skills training show potential to improve specific skills and extend community tenure. It also appears likely that schizophrenic patients with different levels of functioning and symptomatology respond differently to the various types of treatment. If this is so, a major role of future work in the area is to identify who responds to what treatment under which conditions.

References

Aylward, E., Walker, E., & Bettes, B. (1984). Intelligence in schizophrenia: Meta-analysis of the research. *Schizophrenia Bulletin, 10,* 430-459.

Ayres, A. J. (1974). *Sensory integration and learning disorders.* Los Angeles: Western Psychological Services.

Ayres, A. J. (1981). *Sensory integration and the child.* Los Angeles: Western Psychological Services.

Anthony, W. A., & Liberman, R. P. (1986). The practice of psychiatric rehabilitation: Historical, conceptual, and research base. *Schizophrenia Bulletin, 12,* 542-559.

Bellack, A. S., Turner, S. M., Hersen, M., & Luber, R. F. (1984). An examination of the efficacy of social skills training for chronic schizophrenic patients. *Hospital and Community Psychiatry, 35,* 1023-1028.

Blakeny, A. B., Strickland, L. R., & Wilkinson, J. H. (1983). Exploring sensory integrative dysfunction in process schizophrenia. *American Journal of Occupational Therapy, 37,* 399-406.

Brady, J. P. (1984). Social skills training for psychiatric patients, II: Clinical outcome studies. *American Journal of Psychiatry, 141,* 491-498.

Brown, M. (]983). Maintenance and generalization issues in skills training with chronic schizophrenics. In J. P. Curran & P. M. Monti (Eds.), *Social skills training: A practical handbook for assessment and treatment.* (pp. 90-116). New York: Guilford Press.

Brown, M. A., & Munford, A. M. (1983). Life skills training for chronic schizophrenics. *The Journal of Nervous and Mental Disease, 171,* 466-470.

Campbell, A., & McCreadie, R. G. (1983). Occupational therapy is effective for chronic schizophrenic day patients. *The British Journal of Occupational Therapy, 46,* 327-328.

Crist, P. A. H. (1979). Body image changes in chronic, nonparanoid schizophrenics. *The Canadian Journal of Occupational Therapy, 46,* 61-65.

Crist, P. A. H., Thomas, P. P., & Stone, B. L. (1984). Pre-vocational and sensorimotor training in chronic schizophrenia. *Occupational Therapy in Mental Health, 4,* 23-37.

Crow, T. (1985). The two-syndrome concept: Origins and current status. *Schizophrenia Bulletin, 11,* 471-485.

Curran, J. P., Monti, P. M., & Corriveau, D. P. (1982). *International handbook of behavior modification and therapy.* New York: Plenum Press.

DeCarlo, J. J., & Mann, W. C. (1985). The effectiveness of verbal versus activity groups in improving self-perceptions of interpersonal communication skills. *American Journal of Occupational Therapy, 39,* 20-27.

Denton, P. L. (1982). Teaching interpersonal skills with videotape. *Occupational Therapy in Mental Health, 2,* 17-34.

Drake, R. E., & Sederer, L. I. (1986). Inpatient psychosocial treatment of chronic schizophrenia: Negative effects and current guidelines. *Hospital and Community Psychiatry, 37,* 897-901.

Drouet, V. M. (1983). Behaviour modification research project occupational therapy involvement. *The British Journal of Occupational Therapy, 46,* 137-140.

Drouet, V. M. (1986). Individual behavioral programme planning with long-stay patients part 1: Programmes planned and followed in an occupational therapy department. Part 2: Social skills training. *The British Journal of Occupational Therapy, 49,* 227-232.

Durham, T. M. (1982). Community living skills training in psychiatric rehabilitation. *The British Journal of Occupational Therapy, 45,* 233-235.

Friedlob, S. A., Janis, G. A., & Deets-Aron, C. (1986). A hospital connected half-way house program for individuals with long-term neuropsychiatric disabilities. *American Journal of Occupational Therapy, 40,* 271-277.

Gan, S., & Pullen, G. P. (1984). The unicentre: An activity centre for the mentally ill. The first two years. *The British Journal of Occupational Therapy, 47,* 216-218.

Gautier, M. (1980). The alternate program: An alternative for chronic care. *Canadian Journal of Occupational Therapy, 47,* 211-215.

George, L., & Neufeld, R. W. J. (1985). Cognition and symptomatology in schizophrenia. *Schizophrenia Bulletin, 11,* 264-285.

Glynn, S., & Mueser, K. T. (1986). Social learning for chronic mental patients. *Schizophrenia Bulletin, 12,* 648-668.

Hersen, M. (1979). Modification of skill deficits in psychiatric patients. In A. S. Bellack & M. Hersen (Eds.), *Research and practice in social skills training* (pp. 189-236). New York: Plenum Press.

Hewitt, K., Wishart, C., & Lambert, R. (1981). Social skills training with chronic psychiatric patients. *The British Journal of Occupational Therapy, 44,* 284-285.

Hixson, V. J., & Mathews, A. W. (1984). Sensory integration and chronic schizophrenia: Past, present and future. *The Canadian Journal of Occupational Therapy, 51,* 19-24.

Hogarty, G. E., Anderson, C. M., Reiss, D. J., Kornblith, S. J., Greenwald, D. P., Javna, C. D., & Madonia, M. J. (1986). Family psychoeducation, social skills training and maintenance chemotherapy in the aftercare treatment of schizophrenia. *Archives of General Psychiatry, 43,* 633-642.

Hopkins, H. L., Smith, H. S., & Tiffany, E. G. (1983). Therapeutic application of activity. In H. L. Hopkins & H. D. Smith (Eds.), *Occupational Therapy* (6th., pp. 223-229). Philadelphia: J. B. Lippincott.

Jacobs, H. E., Kardashian, S., Kreinbring, R. K., Ponder, R., & Simpson, A. R. (1984). A skills-oriented model for facilitating employment among psychiatrically disabled persons. *Rehabilitation Counseling Bulletin, 28,* 87-96.

Kaseman, G. M. (1980). Teaching money management skills to psychiatric outpatients. *Occupational Therapy in Mental Health, 1*, 59-71.

King, L. J. (1974). A sensory-integrative approach to schizophrenia. *American Journal of Occupational Therapy, 28*, 529-536.

Kramer, L. W., & Beidel, D. C. (1982). Job seeking groups: A review and application to a chronic psychiatric population. *Occupational Therapy in Mental Health, 2*, 37-44.

Leveille, J. (1981). Outline of a sensory integrative approach with a chronic tactile defensive schizophrenic. *The British Journal of Occupational Therapy, 44*, 160-162.

Levine, I., O'Connor, H., & Stacey, B. (1977). Sensory Integration with chronic schizophrenics: A pilot study. *The Canadian Journal of Occupational Therapy, 44*, 17-21.

——. (1985). Social skills training for chronic mental patients. *Hospital and Community Psychiatry, 36*, 396-403.

Liberman, R. P., Mueser, K. T., & Wallace, C. J. (1986). Social skills training for schizophrenic individuals at risk for relapse. *American Journal of Psychiatry, 143*, 523-526.

Liberman, R. P., Mueser, K. T., Wallace, C. J., Jacobs, H. E., Eckman, T., & Massel, H. K. (1986). Training skills in psychiatrically disabled: Learning coping and competence. *Schizophrenia Bulletin, 12*, 631-647.

Linn, M. W., Caffey, E. M., Klett, C. J., Hogarty, G. E., & Lamb, H. R. (1980). Day treatment and psychotic drugs in the aftercare of schizophrenic patients. *Occupational Therapy in Mental Health, 1*, 77-106.

May, P. R. A. (1976). When, what and why? Psychotherapy and other treatments in schizophrenia. *Comprehensive Psychiatry, 17*, 683-693.

Miller, A., & McCreadie, R. C. (1978). Basic numeracy in chronic schizophrenia. *The British Journal of Occupational Therapy, 41*, 339-342.

Mosey, A. C. (1986). *Psychosocial components of occupational therapy.* New York: Raven Press.

Odhner, F. (1970). A study of group tasks as facilitators of verbalization among hospitalized schizophrenic patients. *American Journal of Occupational Therapy, 24*, 7-12.

Orford, J. (1986). Long-term mental health disability: Going to the consumers to assess need in the community. *The British Journal of Occupational Therapy, 49*, 357-361.

Paul, G. L., & Lentz, R. J. (1977). *Psychosocial treatment of chronic mental patients: Milieu versus social learning programs.* Cambridge, MA: Harvard University Press.

Phillips, D. (1986). Photography as a metaphor of self with stabilized schizophrenic patients. *The Arts in Psychotherapy, 13*, 9-16.

Rider, B. A. (1978). Sensorimotor treatment of chronic schizophrenics. *American Journal of Occupational Therapy, 32*, 451-466.

Ross, C. R. (1977). Physical activation as a specific treatment for young, chronic, psychiatric patients. *The New Zealand Journal of Occupational Therapy, 28*, 30-31.

Spencer, P. G., Gillespie, C. R., & Ekisa, E. G. (1983). A controlled comparison of the effects of social skills training and remedial drama on the conversational skills of chronic schizophrenic inpatients. *British Journal of Psychiatry, 143*, 165-172.

Sturgess, J., & Clancy, H. (1981). The case for a sensory-integrative approach to schizophrenia: An evaluative review. *The British Journal of Occupational Therapy, 44*, 182-186.

Turvey, A. A., Main, C. J., & McCartney, A. (1985). Social activity groups with chronic schizophrenics: The influence of therapists behaviour. *The British Journal of Occupational Therapy, 48*, 302-304.

Wallace, C. J. (1984). Community and interpersonal functioning in the course of schizophrenic disorders. *Schizophrenia Bulletin, 10*, 233-257.

Wallace, C. J., Boone, S. E., Donohue, C. P., & Foy, D. W. (1985). The chronically mentally disabled: Independent living skills training. In D. Barlow (Ed.) *Clinical handbook of psychological disorders* (pp. 462-501). New York: Guilford.

Wallace, C. J., Nelson, C. J., Liberman, R. P., Aitchison, R. A., Lukoff, D., Elder, J. P., & Ferris, C. (1980). A review and critique of social skills training with schizophrenic patients. *Schizophrenia Bulletin, 6*, 42-63.

Wong, S. E., Massel, H. K., Mosk, M. D., & Liberman, R. P. (1986). Behavioral approaches to the treatment of schizophrenia. In D. Burrows, T. R. Norman, & G. Rubenstein (Eds.), *Handbook of studies on schizophrenia* (pp. 79-99). Amsterdam: Elsevier Science Publishers.

Chapter 22

Social Skills Training for Chronic Mental Patients

Robert P. Liberman, MD

H. Keith Massel, MA

Mark D. Mosk, PhD

Stephen E. Wong, PhD

This chapter was previously published in *Hospital and Community Psychiatry*, *36*, 396-403. Copyright © 1985, the American Psychiatric Association. Reprinted by permission.

The care and treatment of chronic mental patients in the United States represents a public health problem of major proportions. Whether chronic patients reside in community back streets or institutional back wards, their adaptation is hampered by behavioral deviance and symptoms such as delusions, hallucinations, and agitation. They are also frequently deficient in many areas of basic human functioning, such as socialization, grooming, and personal hygiene.

Psychotic symptoms and their accompanying behavioral disabilities emerge or exacerbate when environmental, behavioral, or biological stressors impinge on an individual with an underlying and enduring biobehavioral vulnerability (1). This vulnerability is manifested by neurotransmitter abnormalities, poor premorbid social adjustment, and cognitive and attentional deficiencies.

Characteristic schizophrenic symptoms or impairments may appear or intensify in response to a number of situations. Abuse of alcohol or street drugs may increase physiological stress and heighten underlying biological vulnerability. Stressful life events or daily levels of tension may overwhelm the individual's coping mechanisms. An individual's social or professional support network may be weakened or diminished by the death of a family member, the termination of a therapist, or a move out of the family home. Social problem-solving skills previously possessed by the patient may atrophy as a result of disuse, reinforcement of a sick role, or loss of motivation.

The symptomatic and social status of a person with the biological vulnerability for schizophrenia depends on the way in which he and his social support network are able to modulate the impact of interpersonal, financial, and biological stressors. Too much environmental change or too many stressors can lead to breakdown and exacerbation of symptoms, as can deficiencies in coping skills and social support.

The significance of this bidirectional model of symptom formulation and adaptation is that the patient's coping skills and support system play an active role in promoting favorable outcomes. The interactional nature of the model also clearly targets therapeutic objectives and modalities for interventions. The clinician may prescribe neuroleptic drugs to reduce the individual's underlying biobehavioral vulnerability. The environment may be modified to ameliorate the impact of the stressors. Structured, community-based aftercare environments like Fountain House, day treatment centers, and foster and board-and-care homes have been effective in providing patients with support to compensate for deficiencies in community living skills. Alternatively, psychosocial rehabilitation approaches involving family and group therapy can focus on strengthening the patient's social support network.

Neuroleptic drugs are effective in reducing positive symptoms of schizophrenia, such as delusions and hallucinations, but some patients do not respond to drugs or continue to have social and vocational handicaps even with symptomatic improvement. The negative symptoms of schizophrenia, which include social withdrawal, apathy, anergy, slovenliness, and anhedonia, do not respond well to drugs. The most effective treatment for schizophrenic patients combines the use of drugs, which ameliorate and prevent symptoms, with psychosocial interventions aimed at building skills and coping capacities. One type of psychosocial treatment that has proven to be effective with chronic mental patients is social skills training.

Rationale for Social Skills Training

Three sources of empirical data support the use of social skills training as a means of improving patients' competence and ability to cope with stressors. First, many studies have highlighted the importance of premorbid and postmorbid social competence as a predictor of outcome in major psychiatric disorders (1-3). This finding suggests that social skills training might improve the long-term prognosis by upgrading the postmorbid social competence of chronic patients.

Second, the magnitude of deficits in social and living skills has been well documented in chronic psychiatric patients. For example, one study found that more than 50 percent of a sample of chronic psychiatric patients had major functional deficits in social and personal areas (4). A multihospital study of schizophrenic patients placed in foster homes after relatively brief hospitalizations found that relapse rates at one year after discharge were significantly higher among patients who had prerelease deficiencies in social skills (5). In another large-scale study in which depressed patients and normal subjects were compared, social introversion and interpersonal dependency were the most significant premorbid personal characteristics associated with the patient sample (2).

Third, certain types of family interaction patterns have been implicated in the course of schizophrenia and depression (6,7). Four studies conducted in London and Los Angeles over a ten-year period have shown that criticism and emotional overinvolvement by relatives significantly increase the probability of relapse. These findings suggest that improving the problem-solving and communication skills of family members, as well as the social and independent living skills of patients, might have a beneficial impact on relapse, family burden, and social adjustment.

Social Skills Training Defined

Social skills training is designed to train individuals in specific interpersonal skills and to promote the generalization and maintenance of these skills. The procedures, which are based on principles of human learning, have been empirically tested and packaged for ready use by practitioners.

While many psychosocial programs are described as social skills training, it is important to distinguish between nonspecific group activities that engage patients in socialization and methods that deliberately and systematically utilize behavioral learning techniques in a structured approach to skills building. Socialization activities can lead to acquisition of skills through incidental learning during spontaneous social interactions (8). In the remainder of this article, we shall limit our definition of social skills training to methods that incorporate the specific principles of human learning to promote the acquisition, generalization, and durability of skills needed in interpersonal situations (9).

The learning disabilities experienced by many chronic psychiatric patients require the use of highly directive behavioral techniques for training social skills. For example, most chronic patients have attentional and information-processing deficits. They show hyperarousal or underarousal in psychophysiological testing, and they experience overstimulation from emotional stressors or even from therapy sessions that are not carefully structured and modulated.

Chronic patients often fail to be motivated by the customary forms of social and tangible rewards available in traditional therapy. In addition, they generally lack conversational ability, a basic building block for social competence. Schizophrenic patients, in particular, are deficient in social perception and have difficulty finding alternative ways of coping with everyday problems, such as missing a bus, making an appointment, or getting help with bothersome drug side effects. Schizophrenic patients tend to make less eye contact, are less fluent verbally, and use less vocal intonation, all of which may impair social learning.

It is important to tailor social skills training procedures to the needs of the individual patient, since all patients present different constellations of social abilities and deficiencies. Several training models are currently available to the clinician. Longest in use is a basic treatment package that calls for the therapist to demonstrate appropriate use of the skills to the patient, for the patient to role-play interpersonal situations, and for the therapist to provide reinforcement and corrective feedback.

Recently training within an information-processing framework has been shown to be effective for patients capable of learning problem-solving strategies (10). Patients are taught to improve their perception of information in immediate interpersonal situations, to process that information and choose a response, and to send a response back to the other person. However, both the basic training model and the problem-solving model are ineffective for patients with severe attentional deficiencies. A model using attention-focusing procedures that simplify the learning of complex skills has been effective in training some seriously regressed chronic patients in conversational skills. These three models will be described in more detail in the following sections.

The Basic Model of Social Skills Training

In the basic model, social skills training is generally conducted in a training room with either individual patients or groups of patients. Additional training sometimes takes place in natural settings such as the patient's home, hospital ward, or community facility to increase the generalization of treatment effects. The therapeutic process is designed to gradually shape the patient's behavior by reinforcing successive approximations of the appropriate skill.

Researchers and clinicians have been successful in training patients in a full range of verbal and nonverbal social skills. They include assertive responses (11, 12), nonverbal behaviors like eye contact and smiles (13, 14), paralinguistic behaviors like voice volume or speech duration (15, 16), conversational skills such as asking questions and giving compliments (17, 18), community-based instrumental skills (19), and job interview skills (20, 21).

The procedures used for assessing deficiencies in social skills are of paramount importance in the behavioral approach. Assessment determines the initial extent of the patient's deficiencies, sets the scope and goals of treatment, and enables ongoing monitoring of progress throughout the course of treatment. A wide variety of measures have been used, including self-report inventories, subjective ratings on improvement in skill levels and interpersonal comfort, global measures of social skills or social anxiety, physiological measures of social anxiety, and direct observations of interpersonal behavior.

Direct observation of patients' interactions in natural settings, while ideal for assessment, is not always practical. Many interpersonal situations occur infrequently, like interacting with a rude waitress or interviewing for a job; others are essentially private in nature, such as asking someone for a date. Therefore, a variety of contrived "naturalistic" procedures and role-play simulations have been designed to assess social skills. Assessments are usually made before, during, and at the end of therapy.

Like any form of therapy, to be effective social skills training should be conducted within a warm and trusting therapeutic environment. The patient and therapist work in collaboration to define problems, select goals, and formulate solutions. The trainer takes a directive role in monitoring the patient's performance as well as in helping to maintain the patient's motivation. Training utilizes a package of treatment components, including role-playing, modeling, prompting, feedback, reinforcement, and shaping.

In a typical session the patient is asked to role-play a problematic interpersonal situation with another patient or the trainer. Formulation of a scene that simulates the problem may be aided by determining the goal of the interaction, the most effective way to achieve the goal, and with whom and in what situations the problem occurs. Ideally, the scenes should mirror, as much as possible, real and significant life events, although standard role-play scenes are used in many programs.

The following is an example of training using the basic social skills model. Bob, a 32-year-old chronic schizophrenic patient who has had multiple admissions to psychiatric hospitals over the past ten years, has difficulty conversing with people. Training focuses on helping Bob feel more comfortable and be more effective in casual conversation. At an early stage of training, the therapist works with Bob on asking questions of others and on making appropriate self-disclosures so friendships might develop. Nonverbal behaviors—like eye contact and expressing appropriate affect—will be targeted for later stages of training.

> Therapist: All right, Bob, I want you to practice having a conversation with Jim [another patient in the group]. Talk to Jim for a few minutes about whatever you want, but remember to ask him questions and tell him about yourself. Do you understand, Bob?
> Bob: Yes, I understand but I don't think I can do it.
> Therapist: I'd like you to try. Just do the best you can.
> Bob: Okay, I'll try.
> Therapist: Good. Jim, you start the conversation off.
> Jim: Okay. Hi, Bob. How are you today?
> Bob: I'm fine, Jim. How are you?
> Jim: Very well, Bob. Thanks for asking.
> Bob: What have you been doing today?

Jim: I've been working hard. Later today I'm going to the beach with a friend.

Bob: That sounds like fun. Do you go to the beach often?

Jim: Yes, I do. I really enjoy the ocean.

Bob: What else do you like to do?

Jim: I like to go to movies.

Bob: Have you seen any good movies lately?

Jim: No, I haven't been able to afford the movies lately.

Therapist: Okay. That's fine. Let's review your performance, Bob.

At the conclusion of the scene the therapist gives feedback to the patient. Positive aspects of the performance are emphasized, along with areas that need improvement. Feedback is often accompanied by a videotaped playback of positive segments of the patient's performance.

Therapist: Let's look at the videotape, Bob, to see how well you did. In general, you asked a lot of good questions. When Jim said he likes to go to the beach, you asked, "Do you go to the beach often?" Then when he said he likes to go to movies, you asked if he has seen any good movies lately. Those are excellent questions, Bob. You are making great progress in asking questions to get to know others better.

Two points need to be made about this positive feedback. First, it is very specific. The trainer noted exact instances when the skill was appropriately applied. Second, the patient was praised or reinforced for using the skill correctly. Next, the therapist points out ways in which the patient may improve his performance.

Therapist: Bob, you asked some good questions, but you did not make any self-disclosures. For example when Jim said he enjoys the beach you could have said, "I like the beach too" instead of asking him what else he likes to do. Telling people about yourself is very important because people will get to know you better and maybe make friends with you.

Again, the corrective feedback is very specific and constructive, to help the patient know exactly how he could have improved. A brief rationale for using the skill is also usually given. The next step in training might involve the trainer's modeling the correct skills while the patient observes closely.

Therapist: Bob, you have been making great progress in asking questions, but you still need to work on making self-disclosures. Pay close attention now. I am going to have a conversation with Jim. I will ask him questions and tell him some things about myself. Listen carefully so you can learn how to have better conversations.

Following the modeling scene the patient would be asked to repeat the role-play scene. Feedback is provided after the scene, and then the session is terminated.

Progress is usually measured by assessments made each day of training. Role-play conversations are often used to assess changes in the targeted skills. Sometimes the role-plays during training are used for assessment purposes; other times assessments are made after training. Training usually continues until a criterion for adequate performance is met. One clinically sound criterion is the completion of a homework assignment in a natural setting linked to the practiced skill.

Most studies of social skills training with chronic psychiatric patients, using variations of the basic training model, have reported positive results (22-24). However, some patients do not show improvement with training in the basic model (25, 26), and the generalizability and durability of treatment gains tend to be limited (27).

Positive changes in the social skills levels of patients must eventually be maintained in the natural environment; otherwise the patient's newly acquired skills will deteriorate. One means for enhancing transfer of skills to other environments is by training the patients in general strategies for dealing with a variety of social situations. A training model based on a problem-solving strategy is presented next.

A Problem-Solving Model for Skills Training

Inadequate performance in social situations may result partly from deficits in cognitive problem-solving abilities. Chronic psychiatric patients have been found to be deficient in basic problem-solving skills (28-30). In this social skills model, training focuses on components of problem-solving.

Interpersonal communication is viewed as a three-stage process, requiring three types of skills. They are receiving skills, attending to and accurately perceiving cues and contextual elements of interpersonal situations; processing skills, generating response alternatives, weighing the consequences of each alternative, and selecting optimal options; and sending skills, using the chosen option for an effective social response that integrates both verbal and nonverbal skills.

As in the basic training model, an interpersonal scene is role-played and videotaped. After the role-play the therapist asks specific questions to assess the patient's receiving skills. The following example illustrates the technique.

Jim, age 38, is a chronic schizophrenic patient who has been hospitalized on several occasions but is currently an outpatient. Jim has just become part of a social skills training group, with a focus on heterosocial or dating skills. A role-play conversation between Jim and Trudy, another patient, has just been completed.

Therapist: That was good, Jim. You participated well in the conversation with Trudy. I think this will be a good start for training. I want to ask you a few questions first, though. Jim, what was Trudy talking about?

Jim: She was talking about walking on the beach and enjoying sunsets and cool drives.

Therapist: How did she feel?

Jim: I think she felt relaxed. She seemed comfortable with me.

Therapist: Very good. What was your goal in this interaction, Jim?

Jim: I think it was to get to know Trudy better.

Therapist: That is right. You want to get to know Trudy better and to feel comfortable enough to ask her for a date. You are doing very well so far, Jim. You are paying attention, and you have a good idea of what you need to work on.

The therapist asked Jim specific questions to see if his perception of the situation was accurate. After the receiving skills stage is completed, processing skills are assessed and training is given if necessary. This stage involves generating response options and identifying positive and negative consequences of the potential options. The patient again role-plays a conversation with the trainer or another patient and is asked another series of questions following the scene.

Jim has just completed a role-play conversation with Trudy, in which he asked her for a date. In the following sequence Jim's processing skills are assessed.

Therapist: That was a very good conversation, Jim. You seemed relaxed for the most part. What could you have done when Trudy said she already had plans for Saturday night?

Jim: I'm not sure. I guess she didn't want to go out with me.

Therapist: That may not be right, Jim. What could you have done to check that out?

Jim: Maybe I could have asked her out for another night.

Therapist: Exactly. How do you think Trudy would have felt if you had asked her out for another night?

Jim: That I am too interested in her, I guess.

Therapist: Possibly, but more than likely she would have been flattered that you were really interested in her. What could she have done if she was interested in going out with you?

Jim: She could have said that she was busy for that night but she would like to go out with me another time.

Therapist: Very good. How could you have achieved your goal of making a date with her?

Jim: I guess by being more persistent and not feeling rejected when she said she was busy.

Therapist: Exactly right, Jim.

The therapist asked specific questions to gauge Jim's processing abilities and prompted alternative respons-es within his repertoire of skills. The next step is to assess the patient's sending skills. The therapist and patient view the videotaped playback of the role-play and the patient is asked to assess his performance in response to the therapist's questions.

Therapist: I want to ask you some more questions now, regarding the conversation you just had with Trudy. How was your voice volume, Jim?

Jim: It was all right. Maybe it was too soft.

Therapist: Good. I think you could have spoken a little louder also. That's something we can work on later. How was your facial expression?

Jim: I think it was good. I looked interested in Trudy and I was smiling quite a bit.

Therapist: Right. Maybe you felt a little nervous but your face showed relaxation. What about your posture?

Jim: It looked all right to me.

Therapist: Well, maybe you could have leaned closer to her. That would show interest Do you think you made enough eye contact?

Jim: I guess I was looking down a bit too much, but I did make some eye contact.

Therapist: You did make some good eye contact. We can work on increasing the contact that you make. Jim, basically you are able to look at yourself on the screen and have a good idea of your strengths and weaknesses. That is a very good start.

The therapist again asked specific questions to determine how the patient perceives his sending skills. As in all stages of social skills training, reinforcement is given for responding appropriately. In all three stages of this model, the therapist may prompt or model correct responses or ask that the scene be role-played again. When the patient performs the sending skills at an acceptable level, assessment and training continue with a new scene.

In subsequent development of this problem-solving model, the approach has been expanded to areas of social and independent living other than conversational skills (10). Training modules are being developed on leisure and relaxation, medication management, and money management, among other areas. The modules are constructed to teach the patient specific functional skills, to train the patient to solve problems that may be encountered while attempting to employ these new skills, and to give the patient a chance to practice the skills in vivo. This model offers considerable promise for patients able to learn strategies for engaging in social skills.

The Attention-Focusing Skills Training Model

A patient's ability to attend to relevant features of the training situation for periods of 30 to 90 minutes is assumed in both the basic and problem-solving training models. However, a significant number of chronic psychiatric patients have such severe cognitive, memory, and attentional impairments that they cannot participate collaboratively in a group-based training procedure. The Camarillo/UCLA Clinical Research Center has recently developed a method for training in social skills that helps focus the patient's attention on relevant training materials while minimizing demands on cognitive abilities (31).

The attention-focusing procedure is characterized by multiple, discrete, relatively short training trials. A closely secured training situation minimizes distractibility by carefully manipulating the teaching components in each trial. This procedure has been used to train highly distractible institutionalized chronic schizophrenic patients in conversational skills.

While role-playing, corrective feedback, modeling, prompting, and reinforcement are important elements, the attention-focusing model is distinguished by the controlled and sequential presentation of the training components. The trainer initiates a conversation with the patient by making a statement. If the patient makes a correct response, he is praised, and the response is sometimes reinforced with something to eat or drink. If a correct response is not forthcoming, the trainer implements a prompt sequence. The patient is praised if he responds appropriately. The trainer presents the same statement to the patient until he responds correctly several times in succession. Then the patient is trained in responses to new conversational statements.

The following is an example of attention focusing with a chronic schizophrenic patient named Sue who has been hospitalized continuously for 15 years. She has been described as socially isolated and highly distractible. In an individual session a therapist and an aide named Tom are training Sue in how to compliment others.

> Tom: I just bought this shirt yesterday.
> Sue: (no response)
> Therapist: Sue, give Tom a compliment.
> Sue: (no response)
> Therapist: One compliment you can give is "That's a nice shirt."
> Sue: (no response)
> Tom: I just bought this shirt yesterday.
> Sue: (no response)
> Therapist: Sue, give Tom a compliment.
> Sue: (no response)
> Therapist: One compliment you can give is "That's a nice shirt."
> Sue: That's a nice shirt.
> Tom: Thank you very much.
> Therapist: Very good, Sue, that is a nice compliment.
> Tom: I just bought this shirt yesterday.
> Sue: (no response)

> Therapist: Sue, give Tom a compliment.
> Sue: I like your shirt.
> Tom: I'm glad you like it.
> Therapist: That is a very good compliment, Sue.
> Tom: I just bought this shirt yesterday.
> Sue: That is a nice shirt.
> Tom: Oh, thank you, Sue.
> Therapist: Excellent, Sue. That's a nice compliment. Have a little soda.
> Tom: I just bought this shirt yesterday.
> Sue: That is a nice shirt.
> Tom: Thank you, Sue.
> Therapist: Very, very good, Sue. Now you are making nice compliments.

Typically patients are taught to make eight to 12 alternative responses, or exemplars, in each domain of conversational skills. Steps are then taken to promote transfer of training to other appropriate situations if generalization does not occur spontaneously. This model is in the process of being validated by training a group of patients in three conversational skills—asking questions, giving compliments, and making requests to engage in activities with others. Results indicate this highly structured procedure is effective for providing training in social skills to withdrawn, low-functioning, chronic psychiatric patients.

Generalization and Maintenance

Social skills training is generally conducted in a setting, such as a clinic or inpatient facility, that is removed from the patient's natural environment. However, for an intervention to be considered clinically significant, generalization to other situations and to more natural settings is important. While social skills training has made considerable progress in enhancing skill levels of psychiatric patients, more work is needed in assessing and promoting generalization and long-term change.

Transfer of training effects to interpersonal situations for which the patient has not received training, known as response generalization, is routinely assessed as part of social skills training. For instance, an unassertive individual might be trained in effective ways to deal with an incompetent waitress or a rude stranger. Generalization might be tested by a scene involving a pushy door-to-door salesman. The clinical validity of training is enhanced if the patient is able to respond appropriately to these novel situations because it demonstrates that the patient has learned more than simple responses to standard situations.

Response generalization has been assessed in many clinical studies. The results, ranging from moderate to substantial generalization of responses to novel scenes and items, have been overwhelmingly positive (26, 27, 32, 33). The success of response generalization may lie in the unintentional strengthening of classes of responses as a by-product of providing training in numerous related behaviors.

In social skills training a number of different role-play scenes and responses are practiced, which prompts and reinforces various forms of the target skill. For instance, an unassertive patient might practice sending burnt food back in a restaurant, confronting a person who cut in front of him in line, and saying no to unreasonable requests. In the attention-focusing model, a patient may be trained to ask questions of his conversational partner when presented with statements like "I went to a movie last night," "I like to fly in planes," and "Baseball is my favorite sport." This method of training, which emphasizes a variety of uses of a particular skill, has been recommended as a way to establish generalized responses (34).

Assessments of generalization from a clinical training milieu to more natural settings have ranged from naturalistic observations to contrived encounters with confederates presenting opportunities to apply skills. For instance, in two studies patients who were taught interactive skills exhibited little or no generalization of these skills when observed during mealtimes, although they were rated slightly higher on subjective ratings of social interaction than control group patients (35, 36). While not uniformly generalizable, the effects of conversational skills training have often carried over to interactions with unfamiliar confederates (17, 18, 27, 33, 37). For the most part, the presence or absence of generalization has been a function of the assessment method used as well as of the type of skill for which training is offered and the initiative required of the patient

With schizophrenic and other severely impaired patient populations, generalization is usually limited if efforts are not made to promote use of the skills in settings outside therapy. For instance, a patient may be well trained in skills that are important to a good conversation, such as making appropriate self-disclosures and asking good questions. However, generalization may be impeded because factors present in the training situation, such as attentiveness, responsiveness, reinforcement, and feedback, may not be available in the natural environment.

It may be expecting too much of the patient to use his newly learned skills in other environments and with people who are not always attentive and responsive. In natural situations praise or rewards are rarely provided for asking questions or making self-disclosures. Usually inappropriate responses are not corrected; rather, people tend to cut a conversation short if inappropriate things are said. Ideally, the skills would be maintained in other settings by the reinforcement qualities of engaging in interesting conversations. However, this is usually not achieved without active programming.

One way to establish a solid link between the training setting and extratherapy settings is by issuing homework assignments to use the new skills in other settings and with other individuals. A number of clinical researchers have used such assignments with positive results (16, 27, 38, 39). This tactic has proven to be more effective when accompanied by prompts and reinforcement in the other setting (38). Friends, family members, nursing personnel, and peers can aid in this process by prompting and reinforcing new social behaviors until they are established (16, 40).

Once the trained skills are well established and maintained by natural reinforcements in the environment, prompts and external reinforcement may be withdrawn. Gradually delaying reinforcement and making its delivery more variable will minimize the likelihood that newly learned patterns of behavior will be disrupted (34, 41).

Training should not be separated from the patient's everyday world but, rather, fully integrated with it. Whenever possible, therapy should be taken out of the clinician's office and practiced in homes, wards, schools, stores, restaurants, and other environments where it is desirable to perform the target behaviors. Potent reinforcers such as praise, money, edibles, and privileges should be initially tied to successful performance of the behavior; only after the behavior is thoroughly ingrained and under the control of natural contingencies should prosthetic reinforcement be removed.

Validation of Treatment Effects

Clinicians and researchers are becoming increasingly concerned that improvements in patients' social skills are clinically relevant. The results of training are being subjected to independent validation by other clinicians or individuals working with the patients. If individuals not involved in treatment view patients more positively on global measures of social appropriateness after social skills training than before, that is an indication of the clinical significance, or social validity, of the training.

Studies have established the clinical relevance of conversational skills training with chronic psychiatric patients (17, 18, 33). Training in other social skills, such as job interviewing (20, 21) and anger control (14), have also been shown to be clinically relevant with psychiatric patients. These studies reflect successful attempts to establish the clinical significance of social skills training with chronic psychiatric patients.

While it has been amply demonstrated that behavioral training produces incremental improvement in social competence, the data are far less convincing that such interpersonal strengthening actually reduces the probability of relapse or symptom exacerbation. Skills training imbedded within a family therapy context may prove to have greater impact on the long-term clinical status of chronic patients, such as in preventing relapse (42, 43).

Conclusions

We have attempted to highlight some of the salient issues in social skills training for the clinician working with chronic psychiatric patients. While the technology for social skills training has matured and the empirical validation for its efficacy has grown over the past ten years, its use is still limited to a relatively small number of behaviorally oriented practitioners. Many institutions and clinics offer socialization groups and experiences for chronically mentally ill patients, but very few offer structured and systematic social skills training. A major challenge in the field is how to promote wider dissemination and faithful replication of social skills training.

The importance of carefully selecting the type of training model to fit the needs of individual patients is increasingly clear. Many patients may benefit from basic social skills training conducted in a role-playing format. However, patients who are functioning at a higher social level may derive more benefit from a format that emphasizes cognitive problem-solving strategies. Alternatively, highly withdrawn and distractible chronic patients may need a more structured type of training based on attention-focusing procedures.

Generalization and maintenance are of critical importance to the success of any social skills training program. One promising strategy for maintaining social skills in natural living environments is to follow the intensive training in a clinic or hospital with booster sessions in the aftercare period.

Recent studies have shown that patients who have undergone social skills training are viewed as more socially adept by individuals in the community. However, we are only beginning to document the extent to which social skills training leads to improved and durable social functioning, quality of life, and clinical remissions.

References

1. Liberman RP: Social factors in the etiology of the schizophrenic disorders, in Psychiatry 1982: The American Psychiatric Association Annual Review. Edited by Grinspoon L. Washington DC, American Psychiatric Press, 1982

2. Hirschfeld RMA, Klerman GL, Clayton PJ, et al: Assessing personality: effects of the depressive state on trait measurement. American Journal of Psychiatry 140:695-699, 1983

3. Presly AS, Grubb AB, Semple D: Predictors of successful rehabilitation in long-stay patients. Acta Psychiatrica Scandinavica 66:83-88, 1982.

4. Sylph JA, Ross HE, Kedward HB: Social disability in chronic psychiatric patients, American Journal of Psychiatry 134:1391-1394, 1978

5. Linn MW, Klett J, Caffey FM: Foster home characteristics and psychiatric patient outcome. Archives of General Psychiatry 37:129-132, 1980

6. Vaughn CE, Leff JP: The influence of family and social factors on the course of psychiatric illness. British Journal of Psychiatry 129:125-137, 1976

7. Vaughn CE, Snyder KS, Freeman W, et al: Family factors in schizophrenic relapse: a replication. Schizophrenia Bulletin 8:425-426, 1982

8. Test MA, Stein LI: Special living arrangements: a model for decision-making. Hospital and Community Psychiatry 28:608-610, 1977

9. Liberman RP, King LW, DeRisi WJ, et al: Personal Effectiveness: Guiding People to Assert Themselves and Improve Their Social Skills. New York, Plenum, 1975

10. Foy DW, Wallace CJ, Liberman RP: Advances in social skills training for chronic mental patients, in Advances in Clinical Behavior Therapy. Edited by Craig KD, McMahon RJ. New York, Brunner/Mazel, 1983

11. Eisler RM, Blanchard EB, Fitts H, et al: Social skill training with and without modeling in schizophrenic and nonpsychotic hospitalized psychiatric patients. Behavior Modification 2:147-172, 1978

12. Hersen M, Bellack AS, Turner SM: Assessment of assertiveness in female psychiatric patients: motor and autonomic measures. Journal of Behavior Therapy and Experimental Psychiatry 9:11-16, 1978

13. Edelstein BA, Eisler RM: Effects of modeling and modeling with instructions and feedback on the behavioral components of social skills. Behavior Therapy 7:382-389, 1976

14. Kolko DJ, Dorsett PG, Milan MA: A total-assessment approach to the evaluation of social skills training: the effectiveness of an anger control program for adolescent psychiatric patients. Behavioral Assessment 3:383-402, 1981

15. Eisler RM, Hersen M, Miller PM: Effects of modeling on components of assertive behavior. Journal of Behavior Therapy and Experimental Psychiatry 4:1-6, 1973

16. Finch BE, Wallace CJ: Successful interpersonal skills training with schizophrenic inpatients. Journal of Consulting and Clinical Psychology 45:885-890, 1977

17. Holmes MR, Hansen DJ, St Lawrence JS: Conversational skills training with aftercare patients in the community: social validation and generalization. Behavior Therapy (in press)

18. Urey JR, Laughlin C, Kelly JA: Teaching heterosocial conversational skills to male psychiatric inpatients. Journal of Behavior Therapy and Experimental Psychiatry 10:323-328, 1979

19. King LW, Liberman RP, Roberts J, et al.: Personal effectiveness: a structured therapy for improving social and emotional skills. European Journal of Behaviour Analysis and Modification 2:82-91, 1977

20. Furman W, Geller M, Simon SJ, et al.: The use of a behavioral rehearsal procedure for teaching job-interviewing skills to psychiatric patients. Behavior Therapy 10:157-167, 1979

21. Kelly JA, Laughlin C, Claiborne M, et al.: A group procedure for teaching job interviewing skills to formerly hospitalized psychiatric patients. Behavior Therapy 10:299-310, 1979

22. Christoff KA, Kelly JA: Social skills training with psychiatric patients, in Handbook of Social Skills Training. Edited by Milan M, L'Abate L. New York, Wiley (in press)

23. McFall RM: A review and reformulation of the concept of social skills. Behavioral Assessment 4:1-33, 1982

24. Wallace CJ, Nelson CJ, Liberman RP, et al.: Social skills training with schizophrenic patients. Schizophrenia Bulletin 6:42-63, 1980

25. Argyle M, Trower P, Bryant B: Explorations in the treatment of personality disorders and neuroses by social skills training. British Journal of Medical Psychology 47:63-72, 1974

26. Bellack AS, Hersen M, Turner SM: Generalization effects of social skills training in chronic schizophrenics: an experimental analysis. Behavioural Research and Therapy 14:391-398, 1976

27. Liberman RP, Lillie F, Falloon IRH, et al: Social skills training with relapsing schizophrenics. Behavior Modification 8:155-179, 1984

28. Platt JJ, Spivack G: Problem solving thinking of psychiatric patients. Journal of Consulting and Clinical Psychology 39:148-151, 1972

29. Platt JJ, Spivack G: Social competence and effective problem solving thinking in psychiatric patients. Journal of Clinical Psychology 28:3-5, 1972

30. Edelstein BA, Couture E, Cray M, et al: Group training of problem solving with psychiatric patients, in Behavioral Group Therapy: An Annual Review, vol 2. Edited by Upper D, Ross SM. Champaign, Ill, Research Press, 1980

31. Mosk MD, Wong SE, Massel HK, et al: Graduated and traditional procedures for teaching social skills to chronic low-functioning schizophrenics. Presented at the American Psychological Association annual meeting, Anaheim, Calif, Aug 1983

32. Goldsmith JB, McFall RM: Development and evaluation of an interpersonal skill-training program for psychiatric patients. Journal of Abnormal Psychology 84:51-58, 1975

33. Kelly JA, Urey JR, Paterson JT: Improving heterosocial conversational skills of male psychiatric patients through a small group training procedure. Behavior Therapy 11:179-183, 1980

34. Stokes TF, Baer DM: An implicit technology of generalization. Journal of Applied Behavior Analysis 10:349-369, 1977

35. Gutride ME, Goldstein AP, Hunter GF: The use of modeling and role playing to increase social interaction among asocial psychiatric patients. Journal of Consulting and Clinical Psychology 40:408-415, 1973

36. Jaffe PG, Carlson PM: Relative efficacy of modeling and instructions in eliciting social behavior from chronic psychiatric patients. Journal of Consulting and Clinical Psychology 44:200-207, 1976

37. Hersen M, Eisler RM, Miller PM: An experimental analysis of generalization in assertive training. Behaviour Research and Therapy 12:295-310, 1974

38. Martinez-Diaz JA, Massel HK, Wong SE, et a.l: Training and generalization of conversational skills in chronic schizophrenics. Presented at the World Congress of Behavior Therapy, Washington, DC, Dec 1983

39. McGovern KB, Burkhard J: Initiating social contact with the opposite sex, in Counseling Methods. Edited by Krumboltz JD, Thoresen CE. New York, Holt, Rinehart & Winston, 1976

40. Azrin NH, Flores T, Kaplan SJ: Job-finding club: a group-assisted program for obtaining employment. Behaviour Research and Therapy 13:17-27, 1975

41. Kazdin AE: Behavior modification in applied settings. Homewood, Ill, Dorsey, 1975

42. Liberman RP, Falloon IRH, Wallace CJ: Drug and psychosocial interactions in the treatment of schizophrenia, in The Chronically Mentally Ill. Edited by Mirabi M. New York, SP Medical & Scientific Books, 1984

43. Falloon IRH, Boyd JL, McGill CW, et al.: Family management in the prevention or exacerbations of schizophrenia: a controlled study. New England Journal of Medicine 306:1437-1440, 1982

Chapter 23

The Role of Occupational Therapists in Community Mental Health

Ralph Adams, MS, OTR/L

This chapter was previously published in *Mental Health Special Interest Section Newsletter* (1990, March), pp. 1-2. Copyright © 1990, The American Occupational Therapy Association, Inc.

Occupational therapists working in the area of mental health serve primarily in hospital settings, yet the majority of mentally ill persons are not in psychiatric hospitals. As many as 500,000 of these people may currently reside in shelter-care homes that provide varying degrees of attention. About 16% of nursing home residents have a primary diagnosis of chronic mental illness, and more than 5% of jail and prison inmates are mentally ill. The number of homeless Americans with schizophrenia is greater than the number of persons hospitalized with that diagnosis! There is no irrefutable information about the number of mentally ill persons living alone or with relatives, but one recent estimate suggested that persons with schizophrenia alone in this category number more than 500,000 (Torrey, 1988). These estimates may well be conservative. Given this distribution of clients, the distribution of occupational therapists in various work settings would seem to be more than a little out of proportion.

Nonetheless, occupational therapy is imbued with a dynamic holistic philosophy. It possesses a solid theoretical foundation and a comprehensive body of knowledge. On this basis, one could affirm that the practice of occupational therapy is as appropriate to community-based settings as it is to hospitals—even more so. This awareness is particularly significant at a time when social advocacy on behalf of people with mental illness is gaining momentum, and when legislation is creating new opportunities for both the profession and for individual therapists. Within this context, the author suggests two possible explanations for the underrepresentation of occupational therapists in community-based settings. First, it would appear that the role of therapists in community settings has not been as clearly defined as the role of their colleagues in hospital practice. Second, it is also evident that opportunities inherent in community settings have not received sufficient attention. These opportunities are of two types: opportunities to establish the profession as an essential discipline in community mental health, and opportunities for career enhancement and development by individual therapists.

The role of an occupational therapist in a community mental health setting includes both traditional and nontraditional components. Based on his experience as a therapist in a community setting, the author identifies three major functions as characteristic of that role: program planning, evaluation, and implementation; collaboration with other community-based professionals; and interfacing with other service providers, with relatives, and with the public.

Planning programs and providing direct service to clients are functions common to both community-based therapists and their hospital counterparts. Service provision in community mental health, however, requires an orientation and approach all its own. This is particularly evident in the areas of work readiness training and independent living skills training. From the outset, the therapist must acquire knowledge and expertise that the academic curriculum never provided. To help a client deal with his or her environment, the therapist must also be familiar with that environment. Within that environment, the client's resources and abilities are limited by hard socioeconomic realities defined by bureaucratic jargon: Social Security Supplemental Income, Social Security Disability Insurance, "fair share allotment," "trial work period," "eligibility review," and so on. In addition, there are applications or forms in triplicate, accompanied by the implicit threat of denial of benefits. Assuming that a client's income remains intact, other components of independent living may then be addressed. The only remaining constraint is the actual level of income. Teaching a client to live on a budget of $357 a month forces the therapist to acquire a few new skills of his or her own.

Therapists in community settings also collaborate with other professionals. Traditional team conferencing is one aspect of this collaboration; service development based on needs analysis is another. In our agency, occupational therapists have often worked on requests for proposals, both as sole contributors and as part of a committee; we have also handled a number of referrals for consultation, assessment, and treatment, including many for mentally ill persons with physical disabilities. These are all examples of ways that occupational therapists can collaborate with other community-based professionals.

Perhaps the most nontraditional role of a therapist in a community setting is that of a "boundary spanner"—one who interfaces with others to bridge gaps in service provision. Treatment-related interface must be maintained with other service providers, with relatives, and with the public. This interface activity is necessitated by commitment to systematic treatment. In the current health care arena, systematic treatment is a practical aspect of holism.

Interface begins with the initial receipt of a referral. By establishing and maintaining contact with referral sources, it is possible for the therapist to assess the client's appropriateness for services and current level of function while the client is still hospitalized or still participating in another program. The therapist is then able to make recommendations to both the discharge planner and the receiving program coordinator. Continuing liaison with hospital caregivers maintains continuity should rehospitalization occur, and provides for a more comfortable transition at discharge. During treatment, the therapist familiar with legal services, mutual help and self-help groups, food cooperatives, and so on is in a position to make recommendations to clients in psychosocial rehabilitation programs, and to incorporate participation in outside activities as treatment objectives. Being able to provide a client with the name of a contact person goes a long way toward relieving suspicion or apprehension. Helping with telephone contact and demonstrating easy familiarity with the contact person goes even further. Occupational therapists have the credentials to serve as discharge planners when program objectives have been met. For realistic discharge planning, thorough knowledge of the client's abilities and interests provides half the equation for success. The other half consists of knowing which available services or programs will genuinely benefit the client. Collaboration with the receiving agency while the client is still involved in home agency programs makes the transition smoother.

Liaison with family members is another area of interface. This interaction extends beyond family cooperation and involvement in treatment into areas of education and support. Family members need the expertise of the therapist as much as the client does, because they are frequently caught up with the client in the bureaucratic morass and share in the client's social and cultural disenfranchisement. Establishing and coordinating a support and education group for relatives is one way to interface in this area. Our professional philosophy provides a healthy climate for a relatives' support group. Occupational therapy's professional philosophy, rooted in the concept of wellness, inculcates in therapists an attitude toward people with mental illness that stands in sharp contrast to prevailing social perception. The prevailing opinion is that mental illness is incurable. This is what many patients and relatives have been told. They may not have been told that to be well and to be cured are not synonymous, and that one may experience wellness and quality of life in the face of an incurable illness.

Another area of interface is with the public at large. The ultimate goal of community treatment is community reintegration. In order to accomplish this, it is necessary for a community agency or group of agencies to provide a broad array of services, such as residential group homes, scattered-site apartment programs, supported employment, job coaching, and other services that are conducted in the community at large. The public has received its education about mental illness from the media, so tactful reeducation of potential landlords, employers, neighbors, and others becomes the responsibility of the therapist who is coordinating, supervising, or participating in these programs.

Finally, aside from functioning as a therapist in a community setting, there are numerous opportunities for occupational therapists in other areas of community mental health. The Omnibus Budget Reconciliation Act (1981) has mobilized individual states to rechannel resources and develop new approaches to mental health care. These changes, coupled with the results of advocacy action, have led to new employment categories and classifications. Occupational therapists, by training and experience, are qualified to pursue many of these opportunities.

References

Omnibus Budget Reconciliation Act of 1981 (Public Law 97-35).

Torrey, E. F. (1988). *Surviving schizophrenia: A family manual.* New York: Harper & Row.

Chapter 24

Community Living Skills: A Psychoeducational Community-Based Program

Patricia Hickerson Crist, MS, OTR, FAOTA

Persons with chronic mental health problems are frequently found residing in the community, participating in various support systems and living at varying quality of life levels. This variety is related to the development of community resources, the accessibility of services and the needs of persons being served. Most communities have developed crisis, acute and long-term partial care facilities in response to the Community Mental Health Act of 1963 (P.L. 88-164) and its revisions. Though rehabilitation programs are suitable for patients with acute or initial exacerbations of mental health pathology, these programs alone are necessary but not sufficient to meet the long-term needs of the chronic person.

Long-term reliance on biomedically-based rehabilitation produces dependence on the system and maintains reliance on the "sick role." A major problem among persons with chronic mental health problems results from the ambivalence created between being dependent on a biomedical rehabilitation service delivery system versus independence in community life; the latter having greater social value. To close the gap between dependence-inducing models and client desires for independence with minimal labeling, psychoeducation emerges as a potential alternative.

Occupational therapists have indirectly been led in this direction for several years. Lorna Jean King (1978) provided a salient example when she stated that:

> "Mental health is achieved through the *learning* of new adaptive behaviors and/or the *unlearning* of old maladaptive patterns."

One way to learn new adaptive behaviors is through the teaching-learning process where the student (person with a chronic mental health problem) is taught new information and given [the] opportunity to explore and practice new living skills. Psychoeducation can be supportive of one of occupational therapy's central philosophical tenets—"to learn by doing" (Lillie & Armstrong

1982). By using an educational model, new living skills which have been acquired can assist in an increased independence in independent living skills among persons with chronic mental health problems which in turn should enhance their quality of life.

Mental Health Service Delivery

In 1975, 50 million Americans were considered to be peripherally or socially marginal due to chronic mental health problems (Spiegler & Agigian, 1977). This was attributed to skill deficits, maladaptive behavior or stresses and deficiencies in one's social environment. Neither the environment nor personal interactions alone can account for the variations or dysfunctions in human performance but a person-environment, interaction-based, service delivery model could offer solutions to this complex problem (Short & Pagliaro, 1981).

Skill training programs which teach new methods of effective interpersonal interaction through appropriate object use and adaptive task performance are likely to be effective (Lillie & Armstrong, 1982). The authors further state that if mental disorders are reclassified as problematic behaviors in community living then symptom alleviation is not the primary focus but the replacement of skill deficiencies through skill training experiences. In the past, this training has been couched in the current service delivery system or environment and consequently, the processes and outcomes of skill training have reflected the central philosophies or beliefs of the selected service delivery model which are not always matched to the essential needs of the clients.

Early mental health paradigms promoted dependency among service recipients (Lillie & Armstrong, 1982). The primary stimuli for the dependency was three-fold: reliance on the medical model which gave authority to the medical personnel and reinforced submission by the recipient, labeling and pharmacologic intervention (Berkell, 1982; Lamb, 1976). In a system where authority is prescribed to select individuals, usually a physician, due to education and/or power, dependency of the recipient on the authoritarian figure is expected and reinforced. With skills training, the recipient must wait for the prescription and then follow the treatment regimen as deemed by others to be appropriate. Labeling has also generated dependency in that it reinforces that the recipient is sick, ill or stereotypically unable to care for [him or herself]. Further, due to diagnostic labeling, persons with mental health problems are not expected to be responsible for their activities. A case in point is the legal system and its allowance for the plea of "not guilty by reason of insanity," which indicates social belief that a person who is mentally ill is not accountable or respon-

sible for [his or her] actions. Skill training is hampered by these lowered expectations for responsible performance associated with mental health problems. At one point pharmacology was perceived as the panacea or answer. Pharmacology must not be underestimated, as it permits clients previously too disturbed to benefit from therapy or the opportunity to participate in skill training. Pharmacologic intervention only alleviated symptoms and skill dependency remained, creating problems for community adjustment.

Milieu and social learning therapies were alternatives to programs which reinforced dependency issues. Milieu or therapeutic communities created environments where group pressure and confrontation were used to promote responsible behavior. The underlying assumption for most of these programs was that the clients possessed the requisite social behavior in their current repertoire, which was seldom the case (Berkell, 1982). Token economies created a similar atmosphere. Social learning therapies eliminated the problems of token and milieu therapies by providing modeling, positive expectancy and reinforced rehearsal to learn new skills (Hersen & Bellack, 1976; Falloon, Lindley, McDonald & Marks, 1977; Lillie & Armstrong, 1982). The problem with these therapies is that the usual focus was on interpersonal communication and not task development in functional living skills. Occupational therapists' major contribution to mental health services, besides understanding the implications of physical disabilities on mental health, has been to provide services not simply based on "talking" but on "doing." This active process is central to occupational therapy, and chronic mental health problems and other therapies, such as psychology, counseling and nursing, are increasingly reporting in their literature this core concept of occupational therapy as important to individual and overall program gains.

At the same time that these two models were popular in addressing the problems of the chronically mentally ill, several socio-political events were occurring which changed the mental health environment: (1) deinstitutionalization became a central focus but frequently occurred without adequate development of community living resources for the special population released; (2) the biomedical model became less desirable and efficient as mental health care values changed and the perceived pressure of deinstitutionalization was felt; (3) community mental health services were proposed and federally funded; and, (4) quality of life issues became prime movers in health care service delivery. Dissatisfaction with the medical approach to mental health problems and its reductionistic dependence on disease, symptoms, and diagnosis was emerging. Trends toward enhanced moral or humanistic treatment in community settings were promoted. Holism coupled with self-responsibility were values for recipients of healthcare in the future. A comprehensive review of this movement is provided by Schulberg and Killilea (1982) in their edited book on community mental health.

Psychoeducation

With the advent of community mental health in the '60s and '70s, when mental disorders were defined in more functional modes, occupational therapy philosophy was closely allied with the new system. Mental disorders were seen as problematic behaviors which resulted in skill deficiencies. The interaction of the environment and human performance abilities was central in analyzing skilled performance or action. The pressure to assume self-responsibility for one's action was advocated. Fidler (1984) stated basic goals for occupational therapy in mental health: (1) to create a performance skill learning and practice environment so that skills become habitual patterns of behavior; (2) to provide acting-doing experiences that enable clients to acquire a repertoire of self-care, work, and leisure skills in order to achieve maximum independence, develop appropriate socio-cultural role expectations, and experience self-satisfaction and self-worth; (3) to alter the role orientation from passive recipient to self agent in order to develop a sense of being able to influence and have some control over daily life; and, (4) to reduce dependency on external motivational forces and increase self-initiating behavior. All four goals can be facilitated through occupational therapy as part of a community-based psychoeducational program while addressing limitations of the other service delivery models as noted earlier.

Psychoeducation is a mental health service delivery model which is closely allied to community mental health but yet sufficiently different in practice. Both psychoeducation and community mental health have major differences with the biomedical model, which can be seen in Table 1. Psychoeducation advocates for the learning process through an educational system, which is different than the biomedical service delivery system. The therapist becomes teacher; patient or client becomes student; and the clinic becomes a classroom. The treatment plan is replaced by the course syllabus and treatment takes the form of educational courses. Medical diagnosis is not the admission ticket to service but voluntary motivation to acquire new living skills. Reviews of several psychoeducational programs are available (Bakker & Armstrong, 1976; Berkell, 1982; Hewett, 1967; Lamb, 1976; Lillie & Armstrong, 1982; Short & Pagliaro, 1981; Speigler & Agigian, 1977 and Stern & Minkoff, 1979). These reviews explore programs offered for students with chronic mental health problems who have problems with living skills. Training living skills is a high priority among the domains of concern for occupational therapy. In an educational model, occupational therapists can contribute their skills in analyzing and teaching the basic, non-academic skills of independent learning when coupled with mental health problems. This is essential when aware, as stated earlier, that many of the problems seen among persons with chronic mental health problems begin with the basic skills of living or survival. Though seldom mentioned, it is apparent the relevance of occupational therapy to these programs is self-evident.

The philosophy and values of occupational therapy can be implemented in a psychoeducationally-oriented setting as it seeks to create a learning environment to foster learner independence and provide maximal control over ones's life (Bakker & Armstrong, 1976). Educationally, the goal is to teach the student to set attainable goals for personal change and to develop skills required for reaching them. The occupational therapist will introduce positive expectancy in a more normalized environment such as a classroom, community center or vocational/trade school which enhances the students' self-esteem and self-confidence as [the therapist] mobilizes to meet the needs of persons with chronic mental health problems (Lamb, 1976). Through the voluntary practice of new skills in a safe environment, community survival and enhancement skills are learned and practiced. Since the students elect which courses to enroll in, the expectation is that motivation for new learning will be great as content will be student-specific, desired by the student and, thus, habitually practiced outside the classroom. The last major component is time orientation as these programs are time-limited. This may increase the student's sense of urgency to acquire the new skills.

Many chronic mental health clients who live in the community desire normalization through acquisition of socially appropriate skills and behaviors. A model based on educational premises teaches new skills while decreasing the dependence on the day-care programs so frequently used in community mental health as management or maintenance programs. The dependence on and reinforcement of the diagnostically-related "sick role" will be replaced by the student's participation in the study and practice of life-related tasks in self-care, work and leisure. Though not unique to occupational therapy, as these tasks are frequently addressed, the educational way in which they are delivered provides an alternate model which encourages student responsibility for skill acquisition. The vital link will be the application of learned material to the natural environment (Bakker & Armstrong, 1976). As Lamb (1976) so eloquently stated, the chronic mental health client will assimilate that

Table 1. Occupational Therapy in Mental Health

	Biomedical Model	Community Mental Health Model	Psychoeducational Model
central focus:	medicine	long-term care	education
environment:	institutions; clinics	community; some institutions	educational settings
therapeutic role:	clinician	clinician or case manager	educator
recipient's role:	dependency	semi-dependency	independent/interdependent
recipient's expectation:	"get well"	"maintain" or improve	"learn"
recipient's name:	patient	client	student
responsibility:	therapist responsible for client	dependent on CMH's philosophy	client responsible for self
control:	therapist directs treatment	mutual responsibility	student selects learning opportunities
referral to service:	can be coercive/ involuntary	mixture	non-coercive/voluntary
service base:	treatment plan	treatment plan	course syllabi

basic skills are learned and not magically bestowed talents or abilities that some have and others do not. Consequently, much of the mystique about "making it" in the world is taken away.

Developing a Psychoeducational Program

In developing a psychoeducational program for persons with chronic mental illness, several suggestions concerning the setting, curriculum and students are necessary. The school-like setting should be characterized as a learning environment preferably outside the typical mental health service environment which encourages dependency and identification with the "sick role," and in which the students are further integrated into the community, such as an adult education program or continuing education unit in a local college or university. By locating the program in an educational setting, the role is one of a student engaged in learning new skills versus a patient hoping someone will be able to rid him or her of the symptoms. The teachers may be multidisciplinary professionals such as occupational therapists, vocational rehabilitation counselors or adult educators, volunteers from the community, program graduates or students in health or education careers who have [the] skills to be educators and tutors. Though a school nurse may be present, planned intervention with severe symptomatology is non-existent except during medical emergencies. Students are expected to have symptomatology controlled sufficiently in order to benefit from the educational program. Thus, it is desirable to be in contact

with the community mental health center and inpatient psychiatric unit should services be needed during a student's medical leave of absence from the educational program. Tuition for the program can be charged and, if a nominal amount is paid by the student, is considered to enhance student motivation. Most programs run in similar duration to other educational units using the semester or quarter format which enhances the student's ability to respond to schedules, facilitates goal-directed behavior and allows testing of behavior generalization at semester or quarter breaks (Spiegler, 1977).

The curriculum is planned by developing educational goals and objectives into logically coherent didactic and experiential learning opportunities with assigned homework for practice in the naturalistic setting, such as the student's current residence. Persons currently teaching in academic environments could serve as excellent resources in preparation of classroom activities and materials. Topics could include: money management, leisure time, job hunting, self care, communication, sex education, nutrition, meal preparation, household safety, transportation, assertiveness training, and stress management, to name a few of the limitless options (Fidler, 1984; Lillie & Armstrong, 1982; Arbesman, Armacost, Hays, Rauschi and Swindle, 1984). Use of videotaping, films, field trips and guest speakers with expertise for the classroom topic would be advantageous. For example, contacting the local dental hygienists group can result in a presentation on dental care or, by contacting the local dairy council, charts on the nutritional value of various foods along with workbooks on nutrition can be obtained. With microcomputers, practice with various information on a wide array of daily living topics is available which also gives students experience with a socially-valued and current technology. Most educational software programs are listed through software directories and educational software distributors. Use of software should supplement, not replace, classroom learning activities. All educational opportunities should provide training in new skills and develop problem-solving strategies for independent living based on the individual needs of the student.

The person with chronic mental illness must be ready to voluntarily identify himself as a learner and not a patient. Key elements to this process include student participation in planning the curriculum, assessment of skill ability and learning need in relation to student goals and attitude of educator, in order to reinforce learner responsibilities instead of the expectations associated with patient-therapist relationships. The student role must be encouraged and begins with an assessment of learning needs in a skill area by a student advisor who provides information concerning appropriate coursework for the student to reach [his or her] goals. Evaluations which may serve as useful tools include: the Kohlman Evaluation of Living Skills (McGourty, 1979); Task Check List (Lillie & Armstrong, 1982); Phillip's Social Skills Criteria Scale (Phillips, 1978); Solving Community Obstacles and Restoring Employment (Kramer, 1984); Basic Living Skills Battery (Skolaski and Broekema, 1975); and Scorable Self Care Evaluation (Clark and Peters, 1984) as each evaluation gives specific but different composites of living skills. Two other sources include general educational tests over specific content domains and the development of community/life skills questionnaires which reflect course objectives or content and community skill needs. To individualize course content, a portion of the assessment should solicit student goals which can be used to develop open topics in each class as well as plan the student's course of study. This cooperative planning process sets a tone of reciprocity between student and teacher, each with [his or her] own prescribed responsibilities. Students should be encouraged to take notes, do homework, collect related handouts and meet timelines while instructors prepare coursework, give feedback to the students concerning their performance and provide student evaluation of overall course success.

Two psychoeducationally-related programs for persons with chronic mental illness will be briefly exemplified:

Case Study #1

In a local community mental health setting, persons seen in a partial-care program were invited to participate in a basic living skills program designed to assist with problems in living. Each potential student was informed about the educational format of the program and assessed using the Basic Living Skills Battery (Skolaski & Broekema, 1975), which was adapted to reflect the community in which the students resided. An interview identified their goals and interest in participation. The program was developed and instructed by two community mental health occupational therapists. The majority of students were not coerced into participation.

Clients selected the content groups they desired based on the skills they wished to acquire and were informed that they must attend and participate in each session. Participation included: listening, practicing skills while in the group, completing homework based on the new information learned and sharing (the following week), their success in completing their homework.

Based on the initial group's cumulative assessment, the occupational therapists began initially with three separate programs on interpersonal communication, self-care, and nutritional meal preparation. Eventually, the programs were expanded to topics on leisure planning, vocational readiness skills, financial management and communication. Program entrance was voluntary.

Example: Though all members had some degree of problem with cleanliness, one particular female will be discussed. During the assessment, she indicated that she washed her hair, took a bath and brushed her teeth once a month. During the interview, she indicated that the day on which all this happened was a very busy one for her. Later, one of the sessions was allotted to dental care. A local hygienist was invited to instruct the course. She demonstrated proper dental brushing and flossing as well as explored healthy snack foods. A highlight of the demonstration was the red-dye tablets each member chewed to demonstrate brushing deficiencies. In addition, each member was given a free toothbrush. The previously mentioned female student agreed to brush her teeth daily and a chart was developed for her to keep track of her homework assignment. At each consecutive session, she reported progress on her contract. A generally successful change was noted by the end of the class sessions which was maintained after the class terminated. In fact, more than this behavior changed due to the cumulative impact of contracts added at the end of each session.

The program was viewed by agency administrators and accreditors as beneficial to not simply maintaining clients in the community but also improving their quality of community life. A major hindrance to this program was that the clients were still seen in the mental health environment (day care program) and it would have been interesting to see their performance in a strictly educational setting. This program is related to usual day care programs but is different due to the expectations for student acquisition of new skills and the teacher-student relationship in contrast to the usual therapist-client one.

Case Study #2

Through contacts with the local community mental health center, the vocational rehabilitation division, and support groups for families of the chronically mentally ill, it is becoming apparent that a vital community service-link is missing. Several persons with chronic mental health problems wanted to be "normalized" within the community and no longer identified with mental health services. It is known that these persons are employable, but hiring is easy compared to retention on the job due to maladaptive secondary behaviors which prevent job survival. Families of the chronically mentally ill desire increased options for their family members which go beyond recreational diversions only. Simultaneously, the free-standing sheltered workshop for persons with chronic mental health problems was moved to the same enclosure as one for the developmentally disabled amidst concerns for economics and promises for new, unique job training which has not been forthcoming over the past two years. This has created frustration among staff and consumers in the community.

In response, three occupational therapists are in the initial stages of developing a psychoeducational program to be housed at the university, instructed by community persons/professionals on given topics, [with] tutors made available through students completing occupational therapy practicums. Initial evaluation of persons with chronic mental illness interested in the curriculum format will decide which course content to develop first. The overall outcome of the program will be job evaluation and placement by providing skill courses in work readiness behaviors. Though an eventual training grant will be applied for to support the complete development of the program, the initial pilot studies are being conducted through the resources of the university (primarily the occupational therapy department and the division of continuing education), the local community mental health center, and, hopefully, the division of vocational education. By housing the program within the university environment, an educational atmosphere will be promoted. The initial challenge at this time is to continue to maintain an educator's viewpoint and avoid slipping into a therapeutic model. Collaboration between the three occupational therapists is helping to keep this in check.

Currently, occupational therapy students in a research methods class are performing a needs assessment of the community to identify services needed by the chronically mentally ill. It is anticipated that this initial evaluation will give direction to the curriculum as well as identify potential registrants. Further, it will provide evaluation objectives for the future to assess outcomes of the program.

Future program expansions include developing learning materials for any student regardless of their physical, psychological or social disability as long as they desire to develop new living skills to increase their productive community involvement. Research efforts are planned to document the impact of the program on participants' quality of community living. Both of these programs, one underway and the other evolving, support potential benefits of the psychoeducational model for service delivery to persons with chronic mental health problems. They offer a community-based alternative which from initial entry into the curriculum anticipates student self-responsibility and investment in learning. The student is seen as the responsible change agent and the instructor a guide to resources and skill development. Of course, the success of this program is directly related to students entering who are motivated to learn and the provision of appropriate coursework to meet their objectives. If the two are present, relevance or meaningfulness to the student will become the prime motivator.

Conclusion

The intent of this article was to review the potential benefits of a psychoeducational program to meet the needs of the chronically mentally ill. Psychoeducation and its relevance was described and exemplified via two brief case studies.

This model has broader benefits since there are numerous individuals who are beyond the capacities of usual rehabilitation programs, particularly if they are coping with a long-term, irreversible disability, such as spinal cord or head injury. Programs such as the ones described above focus on problems in living, not diagnosis. Thus, if the instructor is able to adapt his or her teaching strategies, many persons who have peripheral social status due to their disability could benefit from a psychoeducational program. Occupational therapists are professionally suited to provide services in such a holistic manner.

In a psychoeducational model, [those] with chronic mental illness will benefit as they will be participating in a self-development program whose central organization focuses on normalization and self-direction. Occupational therapists will be able to utilize their teaching expertise in naturalistic settings which support underlying philosophies. The community will benefit from more socially independent and productive members who are less dependent on costly mental health services. Additionally, as noted in the second case study, occupational therapy curricula could offer relevant fieldwork experiences to their students. In these days of cost effectiveness and pending prospective payment for mental health services, the advantages of psychoeducation cannot be understated as a community-based alternative in the health care delivery system and the potential contributions of the occupational therapist in providing leadership to these community living skills programs are exemplified.

References

Arbesman, F., Armacost, P., Hays, C., Rauchi, M., & Swindle, S. (1984). *Occupational therapy protocols in mental health.* Baltimore, MD: Betty Cox Associates.

Bakker, C. B., & Armstrong, H. E. (1976). The adult development program: An educational approach to the delivery of mental health services. *Hospital & Community Psychiatry, 27,* 330-334.

Berkell, D. E. (1982). Psycho-educational and task-analysis models. *Educational Technology, 22,* 28-29.

Clark, E. N., & Peters, M. (1984). *Scorable self care evaluation.* Thorofare, NJ: Slack, Inc.

Falloon, I. R. H., Lindley, P., McDonald, R., & Marks, I. M. (1977). Social skills training of out-patient groups: A controlled study of rehearsal and homework. *British Journal of Psychiatry, 131,* 599-609.

Fidler, G. S. (1984). *Design of rehabilitation services in psychiatric hospital settings.* Laurel, MD: RAMSCO.

Hersen, M., & Bellack, A. S. (1976). Social skills training for chronic psychiatric patients: Rationale, research findings and future directions. *Comprehensive Psychiatry, 17,* 559-580.

Hewett, F. M. (1967). Educational engineering with emotionally disturbed children. *Exceptional Children, 33,* 459-467.

King, L. J. (1978). Occupational therapy research in psychiatry. *American Journal of Occupational Therapy, 32,* 15-18.

Kramer, L. W. (1984). Solving community obstacles and restoring employment. *Occupational Therapy in Mental Health, 4,* 1-135.

Lamb, H. R. (1976). An educational model for teaching skills to long-term patients. *Hospital & Community Psychiatry, 27,* 875-877.

Lillie, M. D., & Armstrong, H. E. (1982). Contributions to the development of psychoeducational approaches to mental health service. *American Journal of Occupational Therapy, 36,* 438-443.

McGourty, L. K. (1979). *Kohlman evaluation of living skills.* Seattle, WA: KELS Research Box 33201.

Phillips, E. L. (1978). *The social skills bases of psychopathology.* New York, NY: Grune & Stratton.

Schulberg, H. C., & Killilea, M. (Eds.) (1982). *The modern practice of community mental health.* San Francisco, CA: Jossey-Bass.

Short, R. H., & Pagliaro, L. A. (1981). A psychoeducational model of counseling. *International Journal for the Advancement of Counseling, 4,* 111-118.

Skolaski, T., & Broekema, M. C. (1975). *The basic living skills battery.* Madison, WI: Dane Mental Health Center.

Spiegler, M. D., & Agigian, H. (1977). *The community training center.* New York City, NY: Brunner-Mazel.

Spiegler, M. D., & Agigian, H. (in Press). *Schools for living.* New York City, NY: Brunner-Mazel.

Stern, R., & Minkoff, K. (1979). Paradoxes in programming for chronic patients in a community clinic. *Hospital & Community Psychiatry, 30,* 613-617.

Chapter 25

Day Activities Programming: Serving the Severely Impaired Chronic Client

Mira Coviensky, MS, OTR/L
Victoria C. Buckley, MS, OTR/L

Every mental health system has a history of "treatment failures": those severely impaired chronic clients who have not responded to traditional forms of psychiatric treatment (Anthony, 1979; Sullivan, 1981; Liberman & Foy, 1983). Despite psychotherapy, family therapy, chemotherapy, partial hospitalization, intensive day treatment, electroconvulsive therapy, insight-oriented groups, task-oriented groups, vocational programs, and whatever else has been tried, these clients remain symptomatic and dysfunctional. They may have made gains, but still cannot function even within traditional sheltered mental health settings in the community.

These are clients whose paranoia may decrease but never disappears, who hear voices daily and cannot ignore them to focus on reality, and whose internal world is so chaotic that the slightest change in their external world upsets whatever modicum of stability they may have achieved. These clients' cognitive-perceptual-motor problems make the simplest task into a major challenge, and seriously restrict their role functioning and performance of daily activities. For the most part, these clients are severely depressed and dissatisfied with their lives; their capacity for pleasure has diminished to the point of nonexistence (as noted also by Gruenberg, 1982). Typically, the problems have been of long-term duration, necessitating multiple, extensive psychiatric hospitalizations.

With deinstitutionalization and the creation of community residential programs and nursing home placements, these clients no longer need to spend their lives in hospitals. There is now an "uninstitutionalized generation" of chronic clients (Pepper, Ryglewicz & Kirshner, 1982) who have spent little time in hospitals yet share similar psychiatric and functional limitations with the deinstitutionalized clients.

Without programming designed specifically for their needs, these clients are unable to use their time in a gratifying way. For them, deinstitutionalization without daily structure only increases their social isolation and emphasizes the impoverishment in their lives. Repeated exacerbations and rehospitalizations, known as the "revolving door syndrome" (Liberman & Foy, 1983), emerge as the pattern for their lives in the community.

For these reasons, in 1982, a long-term adult day activities program was designed to be a partner program to an already existing transitional intensive day treatment program. Program designs are not readily transferable from one setting to another due to culture-specific and internal idiosyncratic factors (Bachrach, 1980, 1982). Fully recognizing this, the program description offered below is intended to highlight certain essential principles generalizable to the treatment of the severely impaired chronic client.

The Day Activities Program

Philosophy and Structure

The major goal of the day activities program is to give meaning to the lives of these clients in hopes of both increasing their satisfaction and decreasing the need for rehospitalization. The emphasis on quality of life inherent in this program reflects a model of health different from the traditional medical model, with the focus on occupation as opposed to cure.

The program provides an environment enabling clients to establish a health-enhancing work/play/rest balance (described by Reilly, 1966). Prior to enrollment in the program, the daily pattern of these clients was largely made up of rest and aimless wandering. Clients identified themselves as patients and as disabled. Through changing the pattern of their daily activities, the program provides the opportunity for them to develop both new occupational identities, such as worker and hobbyist, and new social identities, such as friend and responsible adult. The program day has two major components, work and recreation, within a supportive milieu environment. The milieu is based on three tenets: consistency, concreteness, and normalization.

Consistency and predictability are crucial, given these clients' low tolerance for change. In addition, repetition is important for the clients to internalize norms and routines and to develop skills. Within this consistent, predictable framework is built-in flexibility and respect for individuals' needs. Clients exhibit a wide range of abilities and intellectual functioning, as well as varying mental status, and activities need to be adapted accordingly in order to meet clients on their own level.

The clients in the program have difficulty abstracting, and therefore have difficulty accepting the value of a process without a product. The activities and interventions are centered around tangible, concrete elements. The clients' concreteness is also addressed by staff role modeling, allowing clients to learn new skills through direct practical observation.

Normalization is important throughout the program structure. The norms of the larger community are the norms of behavior at the program, and activities are always designed to reflect cultural relevance and the values of the larger community.

Considering the tenets of consistency, concreteness, and normalization, the balance between work, play, and rest must be actually experienced by the clients in a unified way. For this population, using isolated groups focusing on pre-vocational skills or leisure skills will only result in the learning of isolated skills rather than the generalization to the daily pattern of activities. The actual structure of the program must provide the concrete opportunity for clients to routinely experience the balance of work, play, and rest.

Work Component

Much of the clients' sense of failure is due to their repeated inability to succeed in one arena identified as the proper arena for adult activity: work. These are clients who have failed in pre-vocational programs, sheltered workshops, and transitional employment programs. They are keenly aware of the difference between meaningful productive work and "busywork." For this reason, the main criteria for the work activity is meaningfulness: the work must be considered worth doing in the values of the larger community. This sense of being truly productive may be more incentive than earning money.

There are two categories of work at the program. The first is volunteer work for other non-profit agencies, such as the Red Cross, nursing homes, and the hospice. Typical tasks involve stuffing envelopes for mailing and making holiday decorations for nursing homes. The second is work necessary for the program itself. Examples of tasks include chores, preparing meals, gardening, and building furniture. Due to the wide range of task performance skills, the occupational therapist needs to adapt the tasks to each individual's cognitive, perceptual, motor, and psychosocial needs. Staff participate in the work itself for the purpose of role-modeling.

Due to their concreteness, it is difficult for clients to see the value of work that is not readily tangible. Details such as visibly stacking the stuffed envelopes as they are completed, or having clients involved in actually delivering the products to the nursing home, can add to clients' satisfaction with their productivity.

Since the normal pattern in society is to work first and then play, the work activities always take place in the morning. The consistency of this routine is important in addition to the aspect of following cultural norms.

Recreational Component

Chronic clients have an abundance of free time but cannot make use of the recreational resources in the community. This is due to a variety of reasons: poor task skills, unawareness of social norms, bizarre behaviors which set up rejection, paranoia, depression, inability to experience pleasure, agoraphobia, confusion, disorganization, and fear of failure. In general, the clients have little understanding of how to select or adapt recreational activities to their needs.

As for other adults, recreation should provide a balance to work. It is a chance to explore interests, establish different social contacts, and enjoy relaxed expectations of performance. As in the work component, the main criteria for selecting the activities is meaningfulness. For clients to develop a sense of themselves as responsible adults, their recreations as well as their work must be consistent with normal adult values: cards, board games, trivia games, sports, walks, reading, outings, music. Several concurrent recreational activities are offered so that clients can learn to select those appropriate to their abilities and interests. Staff participate, respect individual interests, and adapt activities accordingly.

Recreation normally provides a chance to meet new people. To expand clients' social network, the recreational component of the program is open to drop-in clients from the rest of the mental health system three times a week. This serves the additional purpose of providing programming to clients unable to make a commitment to the full program. Staff again role-model so that clients can develop and practice appropriate verbal and non-verbal social skills in a non-threatening situation.

Due to their need for concreteness and their pervasive inability to experience pleasure, it is difficult for clients to simply have a good time without a concrete task and a tangible product. It has been helpful to provide concreteness to non-tangible events by such things as using prizes for games and having clients bake cakes and make decorations for parties.

Supportive Milieu Environment

As deviants in their society, these clients seldom feel a sense of belonging. Even in hospitals, they are often the ones unable to tolerate therapy groups and are only too clearly able to see the difference between themselves and the less functionally-impaired patients. The milieu is therefore designed to foster a sense of belonging and security.

To encourage group cohesion, the day begins with a brief community meeting to focus on upcoming events and clients' evening or weekend plans. Lunch break provides an unstructured time for socialization in self-selected groups with staff remaining readily available to facilitate interactions.

To feel a sense of belonging, clients must have some control over their environment and choice over their participation. These choices must be respected. Clients are encouraged to be as active in decision-making and activity planning as they are comfortable with doing. Decision-making needs to be graded to not overwhelm the client, beginning with offering a clear choice between two alternatives within a consistent, predictable framework, and then gradually becoming less directive and more open-ended, making more choices available.

Throughout the program, expectations are structured in ways designed to minimize stress. These clients are hypersensitive to the demands of the environment, often misperceiving external demands due to feeling so much overwhelming internal pressure. What to staff is meant as gentle persuasion may be experienced by the client as a stressful expectation. Therefore, although every attempt is made to adapt activities to the individual, varying levels of participation are acceptable and advisable. For these clients, learning how to match the amount of stimulation and interaction to their own level of tolerance is a skill to encourage.

When clients do exceed their tolerance level and lose control, as does occasionally happen, they are given space, both in a physical and in an emotional sense. There is a lounge always kept free from groups to which clients retreat when overwhelmed. Staff interventions are supportive rather than interpretative. Depending on the situation and the needs of the particular client at that moment, one of several approaches is employed to minimize stress. These approaches include redirection, refocusing, distancing, involvement in activities, and, when appropriate, socialization. These interventions seem the most effective with this population and have the added advantage of being generalizable for clients to use in other settings and situations where trained staff are not available.

General behavior or dress inappropriate to the social norms of the larger community is dealt with as it comes up in context. The issue-oriented groups approach usually used with less severely impaired clients does not work due to the concreteness of this population. This population cannot generalize the skills learned in an isolated group, such as a grooming group, to the natural context. Therefore, a more concrete approach is needed. Bizarre behavior and dress have their natural consequences: rejection by storekeepers, stares on the street, avoidance from other clients. Behaviors are addressed by acknowledging these consequences as they occur and by offering specific concrete solutions to target problem behaviors. Self-care issues and task skills are addressed in the same way: in natural context as they arise.

The program encourages integration into the community to the extent that clients are comfortable. Lunch break is often a time during which clients shop. The location needs to be within walking distance from stores and restaurants for this to occur with minimal stress.

The site must be large enough for clients to find their own comfortable physical distance from each other and from staff. This is particularly important as clients begin to feel cohesion and closeness, an unfamiliar and initially unsettling feeling for most of them. Minimally, the program needs several large group rooms, a large kitchen, a client lounge kept free of groups, an area for gardening, and office space for staff. The setting and decor should be as non-clinical as possible to discourage clients from seeing themselves as patients.

Since the program is based on an occupational model, staff must represent disciplines which believe in the value of doing: occupational therapists, expressive therapists, rehabilitation counselors, and recreation therapists. Although volunteers are useful to augment the staff, a full-time core staff adequate for program needs is crucial to provide the consistency and predictability which clients need. Currently, this program operates with a staff:client ratio of one:four.

Coordination of Treatment

These clients need a multitude of services, of which day activities programming is only one. Services provided outside the program include medication monitoring, individual and family therapy, residential placement, case management, and crisis intervention. These additional services must take place at other sites for the day activities program to serve its purpose. Clients cannot develop identities as workers and adults in the same setting where they are treated as patients.

A well-coordinated system of communication among treatment providers is crucial, particularly to ensure smooth transitions and provide support for changes. Each client is assigned a case coordinator from among the program staff, whose role is to collaborate with the client on their treatment plans, to maintain documentation, and to coordinate with other treatment providers.

Discussion

As has been previously stated, programs are not easily transplanted from one system to another. However, basic treatment principles are generalizable, and similar programs will likely encounter similar challenges.

The effectiveness of this type of programming is difficult to assess and to report to funding sources, although there is some evidence from this program and from others that day programs are in fact helpful in maintaining clients in the community (Polak & Kirby, 1976; Task Panel, 1978). Since it is neither the goal nor the expectation, the efficacy of the program cannot be judged by progressive movement out of the program. For many clients, it will take months for them to feel comfortable even within the program. Research has indicated that programs providing more occupational therapy and nonthreatening milieu environments with lowered expectations are more successful with the chronic population than those expecting progressive movement (Linn, Caffey, Klett, Hogarty, & Lamb, 1979).

Changes seen in clients involve the quality of their lives and life satisfaction. The clients smile more frequently, are more socially appropriate and relaxed, and the more verbal clients can state that they feel happier. Research needs to be done, however, to find ways to quantify such intangibles as life satisfaction with this population in order to see if day activities programming meets its stated goal of improving the quality of life. If so, the issue which can then be explored is whether there is any correlation between life satisfaction and the need for other services, particularly rehospitalization.

Although the program was established to be a long-term placement, this has been difficult for other treatment providers to accept. As clients have developed task skills and stability, there has been pressure to "graduate" them to a "higher-level" program, despite repeated evidence from these clients' pasts that this will only lead to decompensation, and despite clients' strong desires to stay at the day activities program. Resistance to long-term placement seems related both to the values placed in society on achievement and upward mobility and the cure-oriented medical model of the mental health system.

Since long-term programs do not discharge clients, they can only expand. This is a problem both with the site capacity restrictions and with availability and adequacy of funding sources. It is also a problem for the clients. As has been noted, a major characteristic of this population is an inability to tolerate change. Each new admission has been viewed as a major disruption, and each new client has had a difficult period of entering a tightly knit group.

For staff, the clients' low tolerance for change can be frustrating. The consistency and predictability so necessary for these clients can become tedious for a creative, energetic staff.

Implications for Occupational Therapy

Many of the program concepts are based on the theories of occupational behavior (Reilly, 1966, 1969; Black, 1976; Heard, 1977; Kielhofner, Burke, & Igi, 1980); however, within community mental health centers, program proposals are often judged by non-clinical administrators and members of consumer boards and need to be written in lay terms. The proposals for this particular program stressed the fact that occupational therapy was the one crucial discipline for staffing, while presenting program concepts in as non-technical language as possible. These proposals provided a unique opportunity to educate consumers and administrators about occupational therapy.

Due to their unique view of the health-enhancing value of a work/play/rest balance and their ability to translate the theory into practice, occupational therapists are particularly suited to design and direct day activities programs for this population. Assertiveness is necessary to advertise this expertise and initiate programming. Occupational therapists must educate others that concentrating on psyche and symptoms can prove non-productive and frustrating. For the severely impaired chronic client, the focus of treatment on occupation is both more meaningful and more fruitful.

References

Anthony, W. A. (1979). The rehabilitative approach to diagnosis. In L. I. Stein (Ed.), *Community support for the long-term patient: New directions for mental health services*, No. 2 (pp. 25-36). San Francisco: Jossey-Bass Inc.

Bachrach, L. L. (1980). Overview: Model programs for chronic mental patients. *American Journal of Psychiatry, 137*, 1023-1031.

Bachrach, L. L. (1982). Program planning for young adult chronic patients. In B. Pepper & H. Ryglewicz (Eds.). *The young adult chronic patient: New directions for mental health services*, No. 14 (pp. 99-109). San Francisco: Jossey-Bass Inc.

Black, M. M. (1976). The occupational career. *American Journal of Occupational Therapy, 30*, 225-228.

Gruenberg, E. M. (1982). Social behavior in young adults: Keeping crises from becoming chronic. In B. Pepper & H. Ryglewicz (Eds.). *The young adult chronic patient: New directions for mental health services*, No. 14 (pp. 43-50). San Francisco: Jossey-Bass Inc.

Heard, C. (1977). Occupational role acquisition: A perspective on the chronically disabled. *American Journal of Occupational Therapy, 31*, 243-247.

Kielhofner, G., Burke, J. P., & Igi, C. H. (1980). A model of human occupation: Part 4, Assessment and intervention. *American Journal of Occupational Therapy, 34*, 777-788.

Liberman, R. P., & Foy, D. W. (1983). Psychiatric rehabilitation for chronic mental patients. *Psychiatry Annals, 13*, 539-545.

Linn, M. W., Caffey, E. M., Klett, J., Hogarty, G. E., & Lamb, H. R. (1979). Day treatment and psychotropic drugs in the aftercare of schizophrenic patients: A Veterans Administration cooperative study. *Archives of General Psychiatry, 36*, 1055-1066.

Pepper, B., Ryglewicz, H., & Kirshner, M. C. (1982). The uninstitutionalized generation: A new breed of psychiatric patient. In B. Pepper & H. Ryglewicz (Eds.), *The young adult chronic patient: New directions for mental health services*, No. 14 (pp. 3-14). San Francisco: Jossey-Bass Inc.

Polak, P. R. & Kirby, M. W. (1976). A model to replace psychiatric hospitals. *Journal of Nervous and Mental Disease, 162*, 13-22.

Reilly, M. (1966). A psychiatric occupational therapy program as a teaching model. *American Journal of Occupational Therapy, 20*, 61-67.

Reilly, M. (1969). The educational process. *American Journal of Occupational Therapy, 23*, 299-307.

Sullivan, J. P. (1981). Case management. In J. A. Talbot (Ed.), *The chronic mentally ill* (pp. 119-131). New York: Human Sciences Press.

Task Panel reports submitted to the President's Commission on Mental Health: Vol. II, Appendix. (1978). Washington, DC: U.S. Government Printing Office.

Chapter 26

The Occupational Therapist as Case Manager in Community Mental Health

Pat Moeller, MS, OTR/L

Leaders in our profession have long identified the shift in the locus of mental health service delivery from the hospital to the community (Ethridge, 1976), yet the majority of psychiatric occupational therapists continue to work in hospital environments. Factors inhibiting the transition include a lack of understanding of the community mental health delivery system and a lack of confidence that our occupational therapy skills which were acquired in academic and hospital settings, will be relevant in the community. In reality, the occupational therapist's contributions are much needed, especially in communities that are trying to serve residents who are seriously mentally ill.

Community Mental Health Service Delivery System

An overview of the community mental health delivery system helps to delineate the need for occupational therapy.

In most communities, a major agency that is involved in delivering traditional mental health services (e.g., psychiatric, therapy, and day program services) is the community mental health center (CMHC). These agencies were formed in the 1960s as a result of a federal mandate that divided most of the United States into catchment areas, each served by a specific CMHC. Unfortunately, many CMHCs have tended to focus on their more verbal, functional clients, disregarding the more chronically and seriously mentally ill (Pepper & Ryglewicz, 1986). Part of the reason for this orientation is that many CMHCs rely on professionals with social work backgrounds whose therapy skills center on verbal interactions with clients. The non-insight-oriented client who does not particularly benefit from discussing problems constitutes a treatment dilemma for a therapist with this background. Many CMHCs are therefore ill prepared to meet the challenges of deinstitutionalized chronic patients and other clients with serious mental illness who are returning to their communities because of the Omnibus Budget Reconciliation Act of 1987 (Public Law 100-

203). CMHCs have received much criticism for neglecting people with serious mental illness and are now more open to the contributions of other professionals, especially professionals like occupational therapists who can bring more of a psychiatric rehabilitation perspective to programming for the long-term client.

However, the CMHCs constitute only a small part of the services necessary to maintain persons with serious mental illness in the community. Their needs extend beyond the traditional mental health services to a whole range of other services. This is where the role of case manager or case coordinator becomes essential.

Case Management for Persons With Serious Mental Illness

Case management is an organized, coordinated process of assessing clients' needs, developing interagency service plans, linking clients to services, monitoring provision of services, and reevaluating client progress. Case management is merely a variation of the treatment planning process with which all occupational therapists are familiar. Occupational therapists can be especially effective at case management with seriously ill clients because of their skills in assessing clients and linking them to services. People with serious mental illness often need to be linked to three or more services to be maintained adequately in a community setting. Psychiatric occupational therapists know that this is a complex process that involves understanding each client's functional level and ability to use a service, modifying the service for the person, and then actively encouraging him or her to use the service. Occupational therapists experienced in assessing clients and in planning and implementing appropriate treatment methods in the hospital environment can easily transfer these skills to assessing the "matchability" of a client and a potential community service—for example, determining whether a service will be too demanding for the person on the one hand or too demeaning on the other. Even when communities have a limited range of service to offer, the occupational therapist can help existing programs modify their structures to better accommodate a client's needs.

The service needs of the person with serious mental illness fall into the areas of physical health, educational/vocational needs, leisure/social needs, parenting/family, housing, finances, and daily living skills (see Figure 1). Although no mental health professional can be expert in all these areas, I will highlight the many areas where occupational therapists have special knowledge and programming expertise that either directly address clients' needs or enable the occupational therapist to make appropriate linkages to other services.

Figure 1. Community Services for People With Mental Illness.

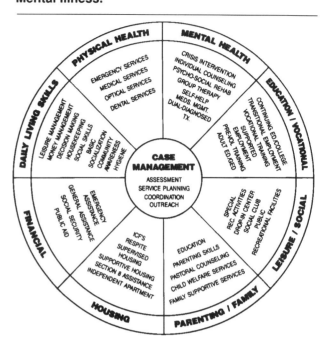

Physical Health

Studies have shown a high rate of medical illness among mentally ill people living in the community (McCarrick, Manderscheid, Bertolucci, Goldman, & Tessler, 1986). This may be due to their lack of awareness of symptoms, confusion over how to pay for services, or lack of understanding of community resources. Occupational therapists' background in physical dysfunction alerts them to symptoms that need attention and helps them link the client promptly to appropriate medical care.

Mental Health

We have already discussed how occupational therapists can help the CMHCs organize programs for people with serious mental illnesses—programs that are based less on insight therapy and more on skills training and socialization activities.

Educational/Vocational Needs

People with serious mental illness need a variety of services in these areas. For example, in the vocational area there is a need for prevocational services, sheltered workshops, supported employment, and transitional employment. The occupational therapist can assess where the client belongs on this continuum and can help establish realistic expectations for progress.

Leisure/Social Needs

In this area, as in the others, communities tend to focus on their more functional clients, making their programs too overwhelming for the more seriously ill. Occupational therapists can suggest less threatening or competitive social and leisure activities.

Parenting/Family

Families are often confused about how to offer support to their relative with mental illness. Some families overdo the caretaking role, fostering unnecessary dependency. Others fail to grasp the severity of the illness and expect unrealistic performance at home, school, or work. Occupational therapists can help families form a more realistic picture of their relative's performance potential and need for support.

Occupational therapists can also assist parents with mental illness to better understand their child's developmental process and to practice good parenting skills.

Housing

Housing for people with mental illness will be a key issue for many communities in the 1990s due to some recent federal legislation. The Fair Housing Amendments Act of 1988 (Public Law 100-430) confronts communities that refuse to allow group homes or other housing for people with disabilities. The Omnibus Budget Reconciliation Act of 1987 cuts federal funding for people with mental illness living in nursing homes and encourages more individualized community placements. Housing for people with mental illness is much more than just finding buildings. Developing appropriate programming is a major concern. Occupational therapists' ability to do functional assessments helps them answer questions regarding the amount of independence clients can handle, their need for supervision and daily living supports, and their ability to learn new skills, get along with roommates, and so on. This knowledge can, in turn, lead to organization of logical program structures for clients functioning at various levels.

Finances

Although occupational therapists usually have no formal training in dealing with complicated public entitlement programs such as Social Security, neither do most other community professionals. This knowledge is gained chiefly through on-the-job experience.

Daily Living Skills

Community work enables occupational therapists to return to a primary area of their expertise: formulating individualized programs for building activities of daily living skills. The hospital environment, with increasingly shortened lengths of stay, no longer allows therapists to do anything more than introduce this area to the patient. In the community, clients' abilities to manage their own money, housekeeping responsibilities, medications, and hygiene become crucial in maintaining community placements.

The Need for Occupational Therapy Services in the Community

Many communities are struggling with the problem of how to adequately serve residents who have serious mental illnesses. Occupational therapists understand how to assess functional levels and implement appropriate programming for this difficult population. We need to move confidently into community positions such as case manager, consultant, and program director. The seriously mentally ill people in our communities clearly need our services.

References

Ethridge, D. A. (1976). The management view of the future of occupational therapy in mental health. *American Journal of Occupational Therapy, 30*, 623-628.

Fair Housing Amendments Act of 1988 (Public Law 100-430), 42 U.S.C. § 3604.

McCarrick, A. K., Manderscheid, R. W., Bertolucci, D. E., Goldman, H., & Tessler, R. C. (1986). Brief report—Chronic medical problems in the chronic mentally ill. *Hospital and Community Psychiatry, 37*, 289-291.

Omnibus Budget Reconciliation Act of 1987 (Public Law 100-203), 42 U.S.C. § 1396.

Pepper, B., & Ryglewicz, H. (1986). Designing/redesigning public policy for the chronically mentally ill: We need a bus! *Tie Lines, 3*(2), 1-4.

Chapter 27

Toronto's Home-Based Mental Health Aftercare Program: An Exciting New Model

Karen Goldenberg, BSc (OT), OT(C)

Forty to fifty percent of all psychiatric patients discharged from a typical inpatient unit will be readmitted within one year (Anthony, Clan, & Vitelo, 1978). The cost of these repeated hospitalizations is high. Unfortunately, the development of adequate aftercare services with psychiatric patients has lagged far behind the impact of deinstitutionalization. In particular, service networks have been slow to develop necessary human links for assuring continuity and coordination of care.

Occupational Therapists Develop Unique Model

Community Occupational Therapy Associates (Comm OT) of Toronto, Canada, has developed a unique model for integrating discharged psychiatric patients into the community. Comm OT is a private, nonprofit health care agency with over 90 full- and part-time therapists providing occupational therapy in metropolitan Toronto, a city of over two million people. Forty percent of the referrals are patients with a primary or secondary psychiatric diagnosis. This represented 1,840 patients in 1985. The program is unique in that it responds to both active rehabilitative and ongoing supportive needs. Active rehabilitation is funded through Provincial Home Care Programs, the agency providing universal health care benefits for Ontarians in the form of short-term, goal-oriented treatment in the community. Traditionally, Provincial Home Care Programs have geared their services to people with physical disorders who rarely request occupational therapy. In 1975, Comm OT and the Metropolitan Toronto Home Care Program began a pilot project at the Clarke Institute of Psychiatry, offering home visiting services to psychiatric patients. This was the first psychiatric facility in Canada to have a formal liaison with a Provincial Home Care Program, and this marked the real beginning of the role for occupational therapy in the home with this population.

The short-term, goal-oriented model was not appropriate for many discharged psychiatric patients. This model permits frequent visits and intensive therapy geared to individual needs, but regression often occurs when treatment is discontinued. The time limitations hinder the achievement of long-term objectives. Thus in 1976, Comm OT applied for and received funding from the Ontario Ministry of Health for a complementary long-term psychiatric program. Comm OT now provides both intensive short-term treatment through Home Care and long-term, less intensive treatment and case management through the Mental Health Aftercare Program (MHAC).

The goal of MHAC is to help psychiatric patients function more actively in the community. Implicit in this is the hope that additional hospitalization and excessive use of outpatient facilities may be significantly reduced. The program links patients with appropriate services and coordinates community agencies and other available resources to improve aftercare as well as providing community-based, traditional occupational therapy interventions.

Psychiatric referrals to Comm OT represent an array of diagnoses, including depression (30%), schizophrenia (18%), Alzheimer's disease (13%), personality disorder (8%), alcoholism (3%), and other (28%). A profile of the population suggests that the typical psychiatric referral to Comm OT is a 40- to 50-year-old depressed woman who is a single homemaker living alone in downtown Toronto. Only 13% of the patients referred are employed full- or part-time.

Referrals come from over 40 different sources, including general and psychiatric hospitals, private physicians, public health nurses, community and social service agencies, nursing homes, homes for the aged, and patients or relatives. Referrals are phoned to the Comm OT office by hospital discharge planners or Home Care personnel in the community. Therapists try to visit within 72 hours of receiving a referral or immediately if necessary. Approximately 65% of the referrals are for patients about to be discharged. Therapists are encouraged to make predischarge visits to develop rapport and to establish continuity between hospital and community. Poorly managed community reentry is a major obstacle to effective aftercare; thus, it is important to establish liaison between hospital and community to achieve effective continuity of care.

Individualized Programs: Key to Success

Following discharge a functional assessment is conducted in the patient's home. When appropriate, other assessments are conducted to establish the need for alternate housing or prevocational readiness. Data from these assessments help to establish client goals, including increasing independence in activities of daily living (e.g., household management, transportation and personal care, increasing medical compliance by assisting with the establishment of drug regimes and appointment compliance, improving family relationships and

child management techniques, developing leisure skills, and reducing social isolation). On the average there are 3.6 presenting problems per patient. To achieve the reduction of social isolation, therapists explore suitable community resources and often escort their patients to social therapeutic programs and other community-based social groups.

Individualized treatment plans result in a variety of visiting patterns. However, the typical psychiatric client receives 10 visits over a period of 52 days through the Home Care Program and 8 visits over a period of 164 days through MHAC. This is a total of 30 hours of service over approximately 7 months. Case management service is offered as ongoing follow-up. The current system enables the transfer of patients in critical health situations from the MHAC back to the Home Care Program. This flexibility prevents repeated hospitalization and facilitates treatment in the least restrictive setting.

The establishment of a case management model and a long-term relationship between patient and therapist significantly increases community tenure. Follow-up for those psychiatric patients discharged from the Comm OT program shows a hospital readmission rate of 12%. Additional data on effectiveness of programs include an early study by Community Resources Consultants of Toronto in 1976, which found, after a two month follow-up, that only 23% of psychiatric clients referred to social therapeutic activities in Toronto continued to attend the program, while 35% of those referred to Comm OT continued to attend. Finally, positive changes in functional status are indicated by client and therapist goal attainment ratings.

A Case Study

The following case study illustrates the treatment approach. Mrs. Brown is a 55-year-old widow with a history of repeated depressive episodes and noncompliance with medication. She also suffers from osteoarthritis. She was referred to Comm OT by a Home Care Program after three months on the psychiatric unit of a general hospital. At the initial visit, Mrs. Brown was sad and tearful. She felt that she had been discharged from the hospital too early and saw little hope for the future. The Comm OT therapist made daily visits for two weeks. Occupational therapy goals were to reduce social isolation, assist with medical compliance, and assess her potential for vocational rehabilitation. A structured and daily schedule, including a medication routine, was established. The patient was referred to a swim program and to a group for widows. She was initially escorted to both programs by the therapist, and she then attended regularly on her own. She became a volunteer in the provincial election campaign and the Cancer Society. As her confidence improved, it became clear that she could return to a job in keeping with her training as a nursing assistant. Mrs. Brown was hired through contacts with therapists to look after a severely disabled woman in the community. Mrs. Brown continued in this position until [the woman] was admitted to a nursing home 1 year later.

Mrs. Brown received 40 visits over a period of 15 months and is now on the MHAC program for monitoring. Although there was a previous history of frequent admissions, she has now been out of the hospital for 22 months. The confidence she gained in her private nursing job has encouraged her to look for another job. After several months of unemployment, she was recently hired to look after another elderly woman in her neighborhood. She continues to swim regularly and to attend the widows group. The therapist maintains informal contact and calls her every 6 to 8 weeks.

This case study illustrates the program's flexibility, which enables frequent visiting during times of crisis to prevent rehospitalization. It also illustrates effective community involvement and the establishment of a drug regimen in the home. In this case, the pattern of frequent hospitalizations was interrupted.

Conclusion

For decades psychiatry has concentrated on verbal and drug therapies. The occupational therapist who uses activities to assist the return of function has been consistently underused. Home care is an essential component to psychiatric aftercare, and yet very few effective home care psychiatric programs have been developed. This highly successful program provides a viable, cost-effective model of aftercare service delivery for psychiatric patients.

Comm OT has continued to provide innovative roles for occupational therapists in the community. Presently, the psychiatric services include the MHAC program, a psychogeriatric program, a boarding home support program, and a social network therapy program for chronic schizophrenics. A formal case management program using a team concept is currently being developed. Comm OT has been on the cutting edge of psychiatric service delivery in metropolitan Toronto for over 10 years and has carved out a prominent role for occupational therapy with psychiatric patients in the community.

Reference

Anthony, W. P., Clan, M. R., & Vitelo, T. (1978). The measurement of rehabilitation outcomes. *Schizophrenia Bulletin, 28.*

Chapter 28

Health Promotion Through Employee Assistance Programs: A Role for Occupational Therapists

Marianne Maynard, PhD, OTR, FAOTA

In the 1970s, a series of articles in the *American Journal of Occupational Therapy* urged therapists to broaden their perspectives and practice to include community health promotion and disease prevention. During this period, health policy agencies also began to place more emphasis on keeping people well through health promotion programs. Occupational therapists, along with other allied health professionals, were encouraged to share their expertise in advocating a healthy life-style through the prevention of disease and disabilities and the maintenance of wellness.

Wiemer and West (1970) found support for the role of the occupational therapist in health promotion and disability prevention in the American Occupational Therapy Association's (AOTA's) definition of occupational therapy as the art and science of directing a person's response to selected activity to promote and maintain health, to prevent disability, to evaluate behavior, and to treat or train patients with physical or psychosocial dysfunction. The authors observed that our practice model was expanding from a hospital-based and treatment-oriented setting to a community-based and health-oriented setting. Walker suggested in 1971 that the emerging model of occupational therapy is concerned with the well community and the maintenance of health and prevention of deficits, disease, and disabilities. She identified areas of practice in home health, maternal and child health, community guidance, and chronic disease care. Wiemer proposed in 1972 that the role of the occupational therapist in preventive and community health should be that of a health advocate and counselor and that, by joining with other health professionals, occupational therapists can promote their special knowledge of the relationship between health and occupation. In the wellness community, therapists can function in all types of settings such as homes, schools, labor union halls, industrial plants, businesses, hospitals, and town halls.

Finn (1972), in her Eleanor Clarke Slagle lecture, traced changes in our professional role in the delivery of health services in the 1960s. She affirmed that, unless we begin to refocus our attention on keeping people well, we will never be able to stem the tide of human suffering in our country. She also urged us to move beyond the role of therapists and become health agents, to progress along the continuum from hospital and clinical services to community and health programs. Occupational therapists can make unique contributions to preventive health care and community programming because they understand the importance of activities in wellness. Grossman (1977) advised us to "be skilled in the techniques of primary prevention: consultation, education, and collaborative efforts to develop community resources, to establish natural support systems, and to use natural caretakers" (p. 351).

The official AOTA position paper on the role of the occupational therapist in the promotion of health and prevention of disabilities (AOTA, 1979) identified a framework to promote health and prevent disease and injury through primary, secondary, and tertiary programs:

> The provision of services for primary prevention most often focuses upon health promotion activities that are designed to help individuals clarify their values about health, to understand the linkages between lifestyle and health and to acquire the knowledge, habits and attitudes needed to promote both physical and mental health. . . . Secondary prevention services that help to prevent or retard the progression of a disorder to more serious or chronic condition normally include early diagnosis, appropriate referral, prompt and effective treatment, as well as health screening, consultation, crisis intervention, and home health care. . . . Tertiary prevention programs encompass the provision of rehabilitative services to assist disabled individuals in attaining their maximum potential for productivity and full participation in community life. (p. 50-51)

Occupational therapists are generally active in all three prevention levels and with most of the risk factors listed. However, their role has only recently become visible. New areas for occupational therapy services in health promotion and wellness activities will continue to emerge. One specific area that is expanding rapidly in business and industry is the employee assistance program (EAP). EAPs address both primary and secondary prevention health issues of employees, and many also incorporate health promotion activities. Occupational therapists can contribute to EAPs by identifying and providing services for workers who are at risk for occupational dysfunction or who have early signs of maladaptive occupational behavior.

Employee Assistance Programs

For some time now companies and institutions as well as local, state, and federal agencies have been using employee assistance programs to handle their employees' personal and job-related problems. The earliest EAP may have been an alcohol rehabilitation program for employees instituted by Macy's department store in 1917. DuPont established the first corporate EAP in the 1940s because of alcoholism among its workers. After World War II, with the increase in drug and alcohol misuse and mental health problems at the workplace, more companies established EAPs. These programs have expanded or have grown from an estimated 50 in 1950 to over 5,000 in 1981 (Sakell, 1985). For example, General Motors' EAP provides services to 44,000 employees at over 130 sites (Galvin, 1983). The list of major corporations, private firms, state agencies, and universities with EAPs continues to grow, with many EAPs expanding their services into areas of health promotion, stress management, and fitness and recreation programs for employees and their families. In general, companies have found it more cost-effective to rehabilitate good workers with problems than to fire them and train new workers (Pelletier, 1984).

Staffing Patterns and Procedures

Depending on the organizational structure and the size of the facility, EAPs may be free-standing units reporting directly to top management or units within employee health or human resource departments. Employee assistance services are usually included as part of the company benefit package. For example, mental and physical health problems may be covered by employees' group health insurance plans.

The staffing pattern also varies in companies, depending on the location in the organizational structure and on the services provided. Most EAPs are staffed by counselors and human services professionals, including mental health and rehabilitation counselors, social workers, and perhaps industrial health nurses and related health personnel. As EAPs expand into health promotion and disease and disability prevention activities, there is a substantial role for occupational therapists to perform as members of the EAP team.

General Operational Procedures

The general purpose of an EAP in industry is to identify, confront, diagnose, treat, and follow up on employees' health problems:

> The eight elements for program support identified by people who work in stress prevention are: (a) a policy statement or performance contract; (b) union support; (c) clearly-defined work performance standards; (d) recognition that performance problems have a variety of causes; (e) a diagnostic and referral agent; (f) comprehensive

treatment resources; (g) insurance coverage that is compatible with the EAP philosophy; and (h) an evaluation program (Gam, Sauser, Evans, & Lair, 1983, p. 62).

Most EAPs' procedures include the following steps: (a) referral of an employee either by supervisor, colleague, family member, or a voluntary referral; (b) screening process, including information gathering; (c) personal interview, assessment of problem/situation; (d) diagnosis of concern, problem, and situation; (e) intervention process, which may include employees' family members or co-workers; (f) intervention in the form of counseling sessions, group support sessions, information and skill building classes, and seminars; (g) continuing follow-up and evaluation of services provided (Sakell, 1985).

If after the initial screening or diagnosis of a problem situation the EAP administrators are unable to handle the employee's problem within their unit, the employee is referred for follow-up to an appropriate community service agency. An important part of most EAPs is the training sessions, which teach supervisors how to identify and refer troubled employees to EAP services. In many cases, the supervisor provides the early guidance and referral that is so important in primary prevention.

The Richmond Employee Assistance Program (REAP), for instance, provides services to 10,000 employees in 16 organizations. Based on request or employees' needs, classes have been offered in assertiveness, communication skills, dealing with depression, financial planning, life planning skills, parenting skills, retirement planning, single parenting, stress management, substance abuse awareness, time management, and two-career family management. REAP also provides support groups for employees and their family members who are concerned about Alzheimer's disease and related disorders, battered women, aging parents, children with special needs, and separation and divorce (Krammer, 1984). Frequent services offered by EAPs are in the areas of retirement planning, stress management, family concerns, financial and legal concerns, and health and fitness. In addition to counseling employees, identifying problems, and finding solutions, the larger EAPs spend a large amount of time organizing and conducting support groups and special seminars and classes for their employees in occupational performance areas where occupational therapists have expertise, such as daily living management and encouraging a balanced work-leisure life-style.

EAPs and Health Promotion

Some corporations include health promotion activities under the EAP, either providing in-house facilities for their activities or cooperating with a local YMCA or YWCA, Heart and Lung Association, or Red Cross to provide their activities. Some corporations provide incentives for employees to stay well, such as memberships in recreational and fitness clubs or discounts on goods and services (Pelletier, 1984).

Most companies disseminate health education information as part of their overall employee health promotion program. The larger companies may focus on stress management and physical fitness programs. Most health promotion programs also provide some type of risk assessment and screening for early detection of coronary, hypertension, and other life-style risk factors.

Health hazard appraisals or health risk profiles are two methods used to determine an employee's probability of becoming ill or dying from a particular cause. The concept of risk implies that there are specific links between habits and disease, such as between smoking and lung cancer or overeating and heart disease. Risk for certain diseases is related to a person's group membership based on heredity, environment, personal history, age, sex, and race. There are three basic types of risk (a) those of potential importance on a probabilistic basis in an otherwise asymptomatic person; (b) those indicating the early manifestation of disease; and (c) those indicative of fully developed disease (Mavis, 1984) [sic].

Employees may volunteer to complete a health risk profile questionnaire or be interviewed for such information. Those employees that evidence a high-risk life-style are especially encouraged to complete a health risk profile. The information is then processed by comparing the person's health data with the national morbidity data base, examining deviation from the average risks for the various causes of death. This process is usually built into the scoring process and interpretation of data with commercially available forms of health risk profiles. The EAP or health promotion counselor will then meet with the employee and family members if this is necessary for interpreting the profile results. The consultation usually focuses on employee habits, helpful resources, and a discussion of a course of action for changing habit patterns. The employee may be encouraged to participate in health promotion classes, exercise programs, or stress management seminars. Periodic follow-ups are made to check progress and provide additional encouragement and resources. High-risk employees are urged to see their personal physicians for monitoring. Health risk assessments have been found to be helpful for promoting a healthy life-style in that they help employees understand the choices involved in risk-taking behaviors in relationship to their life-style. The feedback and interpretation of a profile seems to communicate to the employee a sense of urgency to change risk behavior for a more healthy life-style (Mavis, 1984) [sic].

The Occupational Therapist on the EAP Team

Occupational therapists' knowledge and skills can be used in EAPs, especially in the areas where a recognized void in services exists. Major contributions would be providing employee services in the areas of analysis and enhancement of daily living skills for maintenance of productivity, leisure, and home/family management; assessment and recommendations on adapting the work and home environment to improve health and well-being; task analysis and instruction in work simplification to reduce stress and strain on body parts; and conservation of energy and time for improved job performance. Other areas for occupational therapist services would include the identification and elimination of architectural barriers; instruction in the use of adaptive devices; modification of the work unit for the worker injured or disabled on the job; promotion of a milieu supportive of occupational role performance through interpersonal skill development; and support group process and activities such as health and fitness promotion, stress reduction, and retirement and leisure planning programs.

As EAP team members, occupational therapists would contribute their evaluation skills in functional assessment, self-maintenance, and occupational role performance, as well as their knowledge of adaptive and maladaptive role behaviors. Occupational therapists' experience in program planning, implementation, and evaluation, as well as their experience in collaborating with medical, human services, and education personnel for the purposes of referral, information, and follow-up, could facilitate EAP team efforts in program development and networking.

The Therapist's Approach

Depending on the EAP and organizational structure, the occupational therapist's intervention may include the procedures illustrated in Table 1. These interventions are part of a repertoire of services that may improve the quality of life. Johnson and Kielhofner (1983) suggest that occupational therapy's major contribution to prevention or health maintenance is to enable people to modify their health-threatening life-styles and restore healthy patterns of work and play. The general areas of services of the EAPs either implicitly or explicitly address the occupational behavior perspective as described by Rogers (1983):

> First, there is an emphasis on the *health* of persons in terms of their productive participation in society. Second, health is seen as correlated with *daily experience*, which consists of *work, play, rest,* and *sleep*. Third, daily experiences take place in a complex *physical, temporal,* and *social* environment,

which is a critical factor in shaping behavior. Fourth, occupational dysfunction that may be recognized by symptoms such as boredom, futility, indifference, lack of self-respect, immobility, and disorientation, disrupts daily life. Fifth, daily life may be reorganized through engagement in occupations, such as work, play, crafts, and sports. Sixth, the occupational therapists assist the process of organizing behavior by habit training and socialization of patients to the expectations of the culture. (p. 97-98)

The human development through the occupation model as described by Clark (1979a; 1979b) could also serve as a guiding framework for a therapist working on an EAP team. It can help in identifying the worker's (consumer's) problems, setting goals, facilitating role performance, and enhancing behavioral functioning. Employers are finding not only that an increasing number of workers are developmentally delayed or impaired in basic skills and knowledge such as cognitive, motor, and social performance areas, but also that they are psychologically handicapped in their ability to handle stress and interpersonal relationships. This model recognizes that developmental delays can have a major impact on occupational performance and provides some directions for the therapists to deal with this problem. The basic concepts found in both these models seem to be compatible with the EAP's holistic approach to intervention.

Practice Considerations

Today, consumers have two alternatives for selecting health services: the medically oriented, doctor-centered, hospital-based treatment program or the community-centered, health promotion, disease prevention, and consumer-involved program. Therapists also have choices in considering community practice. Although job opportunities in hospital acute-care programs are on the decline, more opportunities for practice exist in community programs, such as home health agencies, business and industry, public school systems, community mental health programs, day care programs for the elderly, private and group practices, and health maintenance organizations.

However, to take advantage of these opportunities, therapists must be prepared to work not only with pathology but also with health concepts within the normal life continuum of health-wellness and illness-disease. They need an understanding of the impact of personal life-styles, environmental and sociocultural influences, and economic resources on health. In community health programs, occupational therapists must be prepared to intervene anywhere along the health-illness continuum as the need arises, be it in the home, school, agency, or institution. Our focus will be on the maintenance of health and the prevention of disease through life-style management in primary and secondary prevention programs. We will also continue to be active at the illness-disease dysfunctional end of the continuum, providing treatment, reeducation, and skill development in tertiary programs.

Education Considerations

Grossman (1977) suggests the following:

> Students must be introduced to career opportunities other than the clinical model. The concepts and skills of community programming can be an integral part of theory and practice courses. Field placement in the community should emphasize interdisciplinary training for outpatient and outreach services. These experiences are better integrated when assigned after hospital-based placements with clear role models. More importantly, students should be exposed to multiple systems (family, hospital, community) and develop varied interactional patterns. (p. 354)

Academic courses should stress critical thinking and problem solving along with disease prevention, health promotion, and treatment concepts and skills. Programs used in the industrial and business community, such as EAPs, require that the therapists have skills in interviewing, counseling, and group process.

One option for education programs is to provide fieldwork experiences in a community-based program such as an EAP. If there is no occupational therapist to supervise the student, an occupational therapist faculty member, a consultant, or a private practice therapist in the community could work with a staff member at the agency and provide the on-site supervision. Such collaborative ventures would not only promote the profession of occupational therapy, but also open new employment opportunities for therapists in community practice. For example, a 2-month affiliation with an EAP program under the cooperative supervision of a school faculty member and an EAP counselor would enable the students to enhance their skills in program planning, assessment procedures, teaching, group process, job and task analysis, and skill development. My own exploration with EAP directors has convinced me that they would welcome such an arrangement. Those located near universities are already providing field experiences for social work, rehabilitation, and psychology students, and several EAP directors have expressed a willingness to provide training sites for graduate level occupational therapy students.

Another way that occupational therapists can become involved in EAPs is to provide training sessions for

Table 1. Sample Profile of Occupational Therapy EAP Intervention Plan

Intervention Goals	Principles of Behavioral/Situational Change	Techniques Used for Behavioral/Situational Change	Criteria of Success
To obtain information on worker's support networks and significant others that may be helpful in intervention plan.	Assess worker's dysfunction areas, identify occupations and resources beneficial in meeting worker's need.	Additional exploration, information gathering, and identification of resources. Collaboration with significant other in worker's network.	Reeducation in high-risk habits and behavior detrimental to health.
To support optimal health and well-being of workers by promoting a healthy and safe workplace, supportive milieu, and balanced life-style of work, play, and rest.	Design an intervention plan to improve worker's deficits and/or environmental conditions. Facilitate and promote worker's and significant others' involvement and commitment to intervention plan.	Problem solving sessions. Goal setting and action planning.	Resumption of normal occupational roles and function in work, home, and community settings.
To assess worker's behavior and performance in terms of occupational role components (work, leisure, and self-maintenance) and areas of developmental delays (sensory, motor, cognitive, and psychosocial).	Assess worker's occupational role performance, adaptive behaviors, and skills to determine areas of deficit needs and overall capabilities and strengths.	Observation of work unit and situation. Consultation with employee, supervisor, and significant others.	Improved state of health and well-being based on worker's self-report and reports from significant others.
To assess work environment and milieu as to compatibility with worker's needs, skills, job requirements, and work condition.	Assess environmental conditions (home, work, and community) that may be supportive or nonsupportive of worker's performance.	Interview and occupation history. Assessment of worker's role, tasks, and performance.	Acquisition of skills. Improved occupational performance.
To promote, improve, reestablish, or maintain worker's occupational role performance, adaptive behavior, and skills.	Validate and share findings, make recommendations, and follow up results.	Group sessions, educational classes, seminars, skill development or remediation, development, prevention, maintenance.	Engagement in health-promoting life-style behaviors.

employees on a contractual basis. Many EAPs contract with either individuals or other agencies to provide specific classes in areas of employees' needs. Occupational therapists have the knowledge and expertise to conduct such classes, especially those related to lifestyle management and occupational performance. Role delineation tends to be more flexible in EAPs than in the hospital care system. Each staff member works in an area of expertise in addition to sharing tasks that are germane to all human services workers. The social worker may be focusing on the worker's family situation, the rehabilitation counselor on the job climate, and the psychologist on the emotional well-being or psychosocial adjustment of the worker. The occupational therapist can complement these efforts by placing emphasis on the worker's occupational dysfunction in work, play, leisure, and rest, and on the maintenance of a balanced life-style in daily living activities.

Summary

The rapid expansion of EAPs provides a natural area for occupational therapy programming in the well community. If occupational therapists apply their skills and knowledge in the corporate work site, they are able to intervene in the health care continuum earlier than at the acute care stage. Occupational dysfunction can be corrected while the person is still functioning on the job. This approach provides a saving in both time and money for employees, employers, and society.

Occupational therapists are encouraged to take advantage of the opportunities to work as team members in EAPs. Educators can encourage students to consider this job opportunity by promoting fieldwork experiences at EAP facilities and by collaborating with faculty and agency staff for on-site supervision. As EAP team members occupational therapists have the opportunity to inform the public about their services, to promote and maintain health and well-being, to prevent disease and injury, and to correct and improve occupational performance. We provide primary, secondary, and tertiary programs for children with impairments in the public school system. Let us also provide primary and secondary programs for adults in their place of work by assuming a place on the EAP team.

References

American Occupational Therapy Association. (1979). Role of the occupational therapist in the promotion of health and prevention of disabilities [position paper]. *American Journal of Occupational Therapy, 33*(1), 50-51.

Clark, P. N. (1979a). Human development through occupation: A philosophy and conceptual model for practice, Part 2. *American Journal of Occupational Therapy, 33*, 577-585.

Clark, P. N. (1979b). Human development through occupation: Theoretical frameworks in contemporary occupational therapy practice, Part 1. *American Journal of Occupational Therapy, 33*, 505-514.

Finn, G. L. (1972). The occupational therapist in prevention programs. *American Journal of Occupational Therapy, 26*, 59-66.

Galvin, D. (1983). Health promotion, disability management, and rehabilitation in the workplace. *The Interconnector, 6*(2), 1-6.

Gam, J., Sauser, W., Evans, K., & Lair, C. (1983). Implement an employee assistance program. *Journal of Employment Counseling, 20*, 61-69.

Grossman, J. (1977). Preventive health care and community programming. *American Journal of Occupational Therapy, 31*, 351-354.

Johnson, J., & Kielhofner, G. (1983). Occupational therapy in the health care systems of the future. In G. Kielhofner (Ed.), *Health through occupation: Theory and practice in occupational therapy* (pp. 179-195). Philadelphia: F. A. Davis.

Krammer, T. (Ed.). (1984). REAP: The Richmond Employee Assistance Program. *REAP Reader, 1*, 1-4.

Pelletier, K. (1984). *Healthy people in unhealthy places: Stress and fitness at work.* New York: Delacorte Press/Seymour Lawrence.

Rogers, J. (1983). The study of human occupation. In G. Kielhofner (Ed.), *Health through occupation: Theory and practice in occupational therapy* (pp. 93-124). Philadelphia: F. A. Davis.

Sakell, T. (1985, March 21). EAPs develop human assets: Programs help to alleviate costly personnel problems. *Guidepost*, pp. 1, 12.

Walker, L. (1971). Occupational therapy in the well community. *American Journal of Occupational Therapy, 26*, 1-9.

Wiemer, R. B., & West, W. (1970). Occupational therapy in community health care. *American Journal of Occupational Therapy, 24*, 1-6.

Chapter 29

Vocational Integration for the Psychiatrically Disabled

Susan K. Lang, MBA, OTR, ATR
Elizabeth Cara, MA, MFCC, OTR

This chapter was previously published in *Hospital and Community Psychiatry, 40*, 890-892. Copyright © 1989, the American Psychiatric Association. Reprinted by permission.

Interest in the "vocational rehabilitation" of psychiatrically disabled clients has gradually increased since the mid-1960s, when large numbers of people were being discharged into the community as state mental hospital censuses were reduced. At that time, little effort was made to discover how, or if, this population could be successfully integrated into the work world. The California Department of Rehabilitation, like many state departments of rehabilitation, was more familiar with the developmentally and physically disabled and had little experience with the psychiatrically disabled. Until the mid-1980s, "vocational rehabilitation" for the mentally ill was a combination of well-intentioned but often confusing efforts by a variety of practitioners.

Occupational therapists are among the practitioners who have provided vocational services to the psychiatrically disabled and have expertise in working with their vocational integration. "Integration" is perhaps a more accurate term than "rehabilitation" because the latter implies a change mostly in the client. We believe changes in the provider system are also needed. In this column, we will show why traditional occupational therapy approaches to working with the psychiatrically disabled are specifically appropriate to their vocational integration. We will also describe Community Vocational Enterprises, an organization in San Francisco designed to put these principles of vocational integration into practice.

Poor Job Records

The psychiatrically disabled have been the disability group least successful in getting and keeping jobs. They are employed less often and for shorter time periods than members of other disability groups. The data suggest that 15 percent or less of severely psychiatrically disabled persons are competitively employed (1). We believe four general factors are responsible for this lack of success:

Underemployment of all disabled persons. A Harris Survey in 1986 reported a lack of awareness of disabled people as a group and a definite lack of specific policies, programs, and professionals in the disability field for working with employers in the business world (2). In addition, employers reported a lack of qualified disabled applicants and a pervasive inaccurate perception that costs associated with employing the disabled are higher than for employing regular workers.

Inadequate coordination among providers of care and services. The California Department of Rehabilitation, like those in most states, did not serve psychiatrically disabled clients until the 1940s. There was little collaboration between the department and mental health agencies until the last five years. Although it is still difficult for the department to adapt some aspects of programming to serve psychiatric clients, department administrators recently have made real efforts to increase vocational services to this group.

Criteria for funding. Allocation of funds for vocational services, from both public and private sources, has been based primarily on placement of clients in gainful employment. Clients have been trained in sheltered workshops and then placed in jobs. The current trend is to place clients and provide funds for staff support for them on the job. Thus funding criteria are changing in a way that should greatly benefit psychiatric clients.

The nature of serious mental disorder. Fluctuating vocational performance because of varying mental states, unstabilized medications, and difficulty dealing with change is frequently seen in this group. In addition, inadequate support systems and the lingering stigma of mental illness tend to exacerbate the lack of motivation and poor social skills that often characterize these patients.

Factors Predicting Job Success

All of these factors have combined to make vocational integration of the psychiatrically disabled difficult. However, in the past five years, we have learned a great deal, especially about what factors seem to predict a client's ability to succeed on the job. Many of our traditional ideas about what predicts a client's job success have turned out to be wrong. Some of the factors that do not predict job success are reviewed by Stauffer (3). They are traditional psychological test results, demographic data (age, sex, and race), psychiatric diagnosis, and psychiatric symptomatology. In addition, Anthony and Jansen (4) conclude that functioning in a non-vocational area does not predict job performance.

The research reviewed by these authors indicates that four main factors predict a client's future vocational success: assessment in a sheltered setting of work-adjust-

ment skills (4); previous employment history (3); ability to get along with others (4); and enthusiasm, motivation, and healthy self-concept in the role of the worker (4).

Because those factors do predict future job success, we can design programs that do the following:

- Provide a job so that a work history can be developed
- Provide a setting in which social skills can be developed and assessed
- Provide a setting in which self-concept can be improved
- Allow clients, as much as possible, to choose what specific job they would like to do
- Provide a setting that is not time limited
- Provide a setting with a range of jobs, from entry level to more skilled.

Occupational therapists are uniquely skilled to assist clients in each of the above areas. Assessment of social and vocational functioning, promotion of self-confidence and self-determination, a focus on strengths, and a global outlook on personal development are primary roles of psychiatric occupational therapists. Special skills in functional assessment, activity analysis, and gradation of activities to match functional performance make occupational therapists valuable members of the vocational treatment team.

Appropriate Models

Occupational therapists, as one group of practitioners providing vocational services, employ a variety of models of practice. Two seem especially appropriate for promotion of vocational functioning in psychiatric clients. The cognitive disabilities model of Allen (5) employs a cognitive perspective in which therapists use a theoretical description of six cognitive levels to evaluate the quality of observed performance. This perspective allows a very specific assessment of current task behavior and can, by estimating functioning in other settings, assist with vocational counseling and treatment planning.

The second model, the human occupation model of Kielhofner (6), addresses three subsystems of behavior. The first is the volitional subsystem, which is important because clients who are motivated and who see "working" as consistent with their image of themselves generally do better than those who do not. Through helping clients establish organized and well-thought-out patterns of behavior, occupational therapists promote job functioning in keeping with clients' goals and abilities.

Occupational therapists also assess or simulate specific jobs to evaluate actual and needed performance. These activities address the habituation and performance subsystems of the human occupation model. It seems clear that occupational therapists, because of their overall client-centered approach and their specific skills in functional assessment, have a unique place in the vocational integration of the psychiatrically disabled.

In recent years greater attempts have been made to change organizational structures to meet the needs of the psychiatrically disabled client. Much of this effort has been in nonprofit organizations that use an array of work models such as volunteer placements, sheltered work, enclave models, mobile work crews, clubhouse placements, transitional employment, supported employment, and businesses in the community. Although supported employment has been used with the developmentally disabled for ten years, it has been applied more recently to the psychiatrically disabled. This model provides the current focus for many vocational integration programs for the latter group, and results so far indicate that it shows more promise than other models (1).

A San Francisco Program

A new program for clients in the San Francisco community mental health system takes into account what is known about the attitudes of the disabled and of employers as well as what is known about predictors of vocational success. Community Vocational Enterprises (CVE) coordinates vocational programming throughout the San Francisco community mental health system by providing paid work experiences for clients at varying levels of functional performance. The program is compatible with traditional occupational therapy approaches and principles. Among those hired to establish it were two occupational therapists, who helped develop a model for all clients based on the existing structure of the community mental health system, the need to employ clients, and the functional levels of the clients in the system.

CVE has been established as a nonprofit organization, although its staff are employees of an agency with which the city contracts. Even though CVE functions primarily for the purpose of employing clients, the nonprofit structure also creates avenues for funding from philanthropic organizations and from private donations.

CVE serves clients directly by procuring contracts, usually clerical work such as preparation of mailings, that can be completed by clients in their own day treatment programs, under the supervision of occupational therapists and other staff. Although clients work in their own day programs, they are employees of CVE. This aspect was developed specifically for clients for whom gainful employment is unlikely. It serves to increase clients' motivation and helps change their self-perception from patient to worker. In addition, it provides an arena in which occupational therapists can evaluate

functioning and productivity and help clients make future vocational choices.

CVE also procures contracts that can be completed by mobile work crews, usually custodial and maintenance work. These jobs are done in the community, outside the client's treatment program, although staff from various agencies act as liaison personnel, supervisors, and trainers. The crews are organized so that clients can be permanently employed by CVE. They are, however, able to maintain contact with their treatment center, or, if appropriate, move into more independent work in the community.

CVE has also developed contracts through which a group of clients do custodial work in the mental health system's administrative offices. This "enclave" model is similar to the mobile work crews, but workers are less supervised by staff from the treatment agency, which promotes more integration of clients with other employees.

Work in the day treatment centers and on work crews and enclaves takes into account what we know are predictors of success for this population. Clients are developing a work history and are given opportunities to learn how to get along with others in ways that do not increase anxiety or involve major change. CVE plans to pilot-test supported employment for individuals by developing jobs for clients in companies outside the mental health system. This step will also allow occupational therapists to offer their expertise about the psychiatrically disabled to company managers.

Besides its work programs, CVE serves clients indirectly through its outreach, information, and education components. For example, CVE staff train the staff members of various agencies to supervise clients' work. This provides an opportunity to bring together staff with varied backgrounds and philosophies about employment for psychiatric clients. Through outreach and contacts with businesses, CVE also educates businesses about the employability of the psychiatrically disabled and will recruit businesses as employers for clients. Occupational therapists have a special role in working with businesses, by using their knowledge of activity analysis and translating employers' job descriptions into functional requirements.

The programs of Community Vocational Enterprises have made adjustments for factors that usually exclude the psychiatrically disabled. The programs allow for clients' fluctuating performance or lack of motivation by building work into the treatment setting and by offering work experiences with varied levels of involvement. CVE also uses agencies in the system to provide consistent support for clients and the opportunity for clients to practice their ability to get along with others. The programs are offered throughout the San Francisco commu-

---

nity mental health system in a model that seems to have application for other urban areas.

As a group, the psychiatrically disabled have been the last to benefit from vocational services. What we have learned from research, from employers, and from the disabled has led to the development of vocational integration programs that use traditional occupational therapy skills and provide an expanded adjunct to mental health services.

References

1. Anthony WA, Blanch A: Supported employment for persons who are psychiatrically disabled: an historical and conceptual perspective. Psychosocial Rehabilitation Journal 11:5-23, 1987

2. Harris L and Associates, Inc: The ICD Survey of Disabled Americans: Bringing Disabled Americans Into the Mainstream. Study 854009 conducted for the International Center for the Disabled, New York, in cooperation with the National Council on the Handicapped, Washington, DC, 1986

3. Stauffer D: Predicting successful employment in the community for people with a history of chronic mental illness. Occupational Therapy in Mental Health 6(2):31-49, 1986

4. Anthony WA, Jansen MA: Predicting the vocational capacity of the chronically mentally ill. American Psychologist 39:537-544, 1984

5. Allen CK: Occupational therapy: assessment procedures, in Occupational Therapy for Psychiatric Diseases: Measurement and Management of Cognitive Disabilities. Boston, Little, Brown, 1985.

6. Kielhofner GA: A Model of Human Occupation: Theory and Application. Baltimore, Williams & Wilkins, 1985

Chapter 30

Vocational Transition in Acute Care Psychiatry

Gail Zehner Richert, MS, OTR/L

It has been my pleasure for over a year now to work with some very interesting people from diverse employment settings like medicine, government, law enforcement, education, business and industry, communications, the arts, agriculture, and the volunteer sector. All these people have had two things in common: one, that they were employed and two, that they were patients in a psychiatric hospital, often for the first time. Whether they were a manager, nurse, physician, federal, state or county employee, student, factory worker, policeman, disc jockey, musician, welder, or attorney, they all had similar concerns. This paper is about their concerns.

Literature Review

Historical Perspectives

The origins of occupational therapy spring from the care of the mentally ill with humane approaches or moral treatment arising in 18th C. European "work" programs known variously as occupation, activity, industry, or ergotherapy. In our own country, the founders of our profession clearly articulated the importance of work in their early formulations of the focus and purpose of occupational therapy. Dr. Adolph Meyer, professor of psychiatry at Johns Hopkins University, believed in a balance of work, play, rest, and sleep to produce good health and establish balance in the rhythms of life. He felt treatment of the mentally ill must be a blending of work and pleasure that included both recreation and productive activity (Meyer, 1922). Dr. William Rush Dunton, Jr., a psychiatrist for 29 years at The Sheppard and Enoch Pratt Hospital, believed in the use of occupation for the mentally ill as early as 1895. He is credited with the term "occupational therapy" and for writing the basic concepts of the profession (Forbush and Forbush, 1986).

World War I brought an increased number of injured and mentally ill soldiers and civilians injured in industrial accidents. The reconstruction aides served both abroad in France and in the United States. As military personnel received vocational education and rehabilitative servic-

This chapter was previously published in *Occupational Therapy in Mental Health, 10*(4), 43-61. Copyright © 1990, Haworth Press. Reprinted by permission.

es, society recognized the value of these services. This initiated the rehabilitation movement with legislation in 1916 and 1918 for military personnel and in 1920 (P.L. 66-236) for the general public. The post war period saw the rise of general medicine and the growth of hospitals. World War II brought an enormous increase in the demand for rehabilitative services. War emergency training courses for occupational therapists were designed to teach restorative care in military treatment and reduce disability in the acute and chronic phases of illness. Later, in the era of veterans' hospitals, work preparation resumed, but occupational therapists had mostly abandoned interest in work programs to industrial and manual arts "therapists" (Kirkland and Robertson, 1985).

The history of legislative mandates for civilian rehabilitation programs is an interesting one, as it spans the years 1920 up to the present and beyond, or the end of fiscal year 1990 (P.L. 99-506 and Mitchell, Rourk and Schwarz, 1989). Even more interesting is how the involvement of occupational therapy has waxed and waned during this period. As previously indicated, post World War I involvement in work programs was low and continued up to the Vocational Rehabilitation Act of 1943 (P.L. 78-113). This legislation covered occupational therapy services. Two amendments followed in 1954 (P.L. 83-565) and 1965 (P.L. 89-333). This period saw the profession reevaluate its interest in work-related programs with two national institutes in 1955 and 1956. At this time, strong interest was generated in prevocational services. This period also saw the development of the vocational rehabilitation counseling field. Nineteen sixty marked a high point in the development of occupational therapy services using prevocational exploration and training techniques. During the 1960's, indecision about future direction and serious concern about theory dominated the profession, and participation in vocational programs diminished again and essentially disappeared (Kirkland and Robertson, 1985).

The Rehabilitation Act of 1973 (P.L. 93-112) repealed the act of 1943 and restructured the federal program. Amendments followed in 1973, 1974 (P.L. 93-516), and 1978 (P.L. 95-602). Sections 503 and 504 emphasized affirmative action and nondiscrimination in employment services. This was a change in emphasis from vocational to total rehabilitation, including independent living for the severely handicapped who were to be served first with the federal money.

Occupational behavior theory offered a return to occupation or activity as the major modality and the core of practice in 1979. Coincidentally, with the new statement of philosophy, a position paper was prepared and adopted by AOTA in 1980. The language of this paper was more congruent with vocational rehabilitation and coun-

seling literature than with the recently restated focus of occupational therapy practice (Kirkland and Robertson, 1985). Currently, the term vocational integration is being suggested in place of vocational rehabilitation, as it indicates change within the client (Lang and Cara, 1989). This term represents a positive change in focus.

Since its inception, occupational therapy has participated in various ways in vocational education and rehabilitation. Changing legislation, the growth of vocational rehabilitation counseling as a profession, and the restatement of a professional philosophy which emphasized activity or occupation have significantly affected practice. Occupational therapy standards of practice now identify work as part of occupational performance. Work-related issues, then, are an essential component of a holistic perspective in health care delivery.

Theoretical Perspectives

Because vocational behavior is complex, theorists have approached it from different perspectives including trait-and-factor, sociological, psychodynamic, systems, and developmental theories (Creighton, 1985). Developmental theorists see vocational behavior as part of human growth taking place in predictable stages over the individual's life span (Ginsberg et al., 1951, Super, 1957, and Havighurst, 1964). This theoretical perspective is congruent with the occupational therapy section's developmental and cognitive disability frames of reference (Mosey, 1971 and Allen, 1985). These in turn are compatible with object relations or psychodynamic orientations, common in private psychiatric hospitals.

Program Development

Clinical Needs Assessment

The psychiatric unit is a 22-bed short to intermediate term unit in a private psychiatric hospital which in July 1989 had an average length of stay of 25 days, only two days above that of the short-term unit. While community hospitals may experience lengths of stay considerably below this level, the unit is not altogether different from other programs in that its length of stay has dropped significantly and is continuing to plummet steadily. This necessitates almost continuous assessment of patient and program needs. The unit has a strong education orientation, as it is the entry point for the psychiatric residents for their first six months in the hospital. This means that three residents rotate off and on the unit every six months. There are other clinical education programs as well including nursing, occupational therapy, pastoral counseling, and art and dance therapy. There is considerable variety among adult ages and diagnostic categories including schizophrenia and personality, dissociative, and mood disorders, which include bipolar and depressive disorders. At any time, there may be three or more multiple personality disorder patients since one of the attending psychiatrists is a nationally recognized expert in diagnosis and treatment of the disorder. Increased severity in patient symptomatology has been noted particularly with regard to suicidal impulsivity, manic disorganization, and unstable medical conditions including AIDS. Tying all this together and providing the "psychosocial glue" for the unit is a strong therapeutic milieu in which staff and patients engage actively. Hall meetings convene twice daily to encourage and support discussion of relevant individual and group therapeutic issues. There is also a strong multidisciplinary treatment team comprised of psychiatrists, psychiatric residents, nurses, and Rehabilitation Services staff, including occupational therapists, an art therapist, dance therapist, and a therapeutic recreation specialist. While some patients have multiple psychiatric hospitalizations and are chronically ill, many are admitted for the first time and are experiencing additional fear and bewilderment. Many of the patients, whether acutely or chronically ill, are employed and have numerous concerns about their return to work. Two other short to intermediate term units which have similar populations are also included in the referral base. This unanimity of patient concerns in spite of the diversity of their diagnoses and the unit to which they were admitted led to a review of the continuum of vocational services. The result was the Vocational Transition group adapted to an inpatient population (Richert and Merryman, 1987).

Predictors of Successful Work Performance

Many traditional ideas about what predicts job success have not been accurate. Several factors that do not predict success were reviewed by Stauffer (1986) and included demographic data, symptomatology, diagnoses, and psychological test results. Predictors that have been found to be significant are prior employment history (Anthony, Cohen, and Vitalo, 1978, Mantonakis, Jemos, Christodoulou, and Repapi, 1981, and Stauffer, 1986), the ability to get along with others or social skills, and a healthy self-concept in the role of worker (Anthony and Jansen, 1984). Fortunately, this population already has an established and current employment history. Many of the patients in the group are experiencing first or second hospitalizations and are not yet considered to be chronically mentally ill. Their social skills, however, as well as their enthusiasm, motivation, and self-concept are often seriously compromised by their illness.

Standards of Occupational Therapy Practice

Occupational therapists, with skills in functional assessment, purposeful activity, and activity analysis, are poised to provide essential services to psychiatric patients seeking vocational integration. Shortly after admission, each patient is given a functional assessment of occupational performance (work, leisure, and self-care) and performance components (sensorimotor, psychosocial and cognitive) as well as the need for therapeutic adaptation (AOTA, 1983). Particular emphasis is placed on a complete employment history with previous jobs, including length of time held and reason for leaving, feelings, attitudes, and goals related to current employment, length of time since the last day of work, and future education and career objectives. The patient who meets the protocol's criteria for selection is informed of the group and, with his [or her] consent, is referred.

Protocol for the Vocational Transition Group

A protocol is a structured format defining the parameters of direct services and is developed prior to the implementation of any new group. It is a guide for group leaders, patients, potential referral resources, and for occupational therapy interns being oriented to this service. The structure and content of the protocol follows (Richert and Jurkowski, 1988):

Format identifies the group's basic structure such as time, space requirements, and size. While the group meets 50 minutes once a week, with the decreased lengths of stay experienced in most settings, it could meet twice weekly if necessary. With two group facilitators, eight seems to be the maximum number for attending to each member's concerns during the course of the group.

The *definition* includes the basic premise of the group and is identified as providing the opportunity for open discussion about the experiences, attitudes, values, and feelings of patients who are currently on sick leave or leave of absence from paid or volunteer employment or school matriculation. Vocational issues associated with discharge planning are addressed.

The *goals* and expectations for patient behavior are identified both prior to attendance and during the course of the group experience and are as follows:

1. Develop and report on progress toward self-identified goals. During the first or second session, each group member is asked to identify and subsequently report on progress toward goal attainment.

2. Give and receive feedback from peers regarding progress toward identified goals. This goal is essential for successful participation for all members but, at times, can be problematic depend-

ing on the level of symptomatology among the group members. Group facilitators need to adjust their level of active involvement accordingly.

3. Identify issues related to returning to employment after a psychiatric hospitalization. Since prejudice or fear of prejudice is frequently a major concern, patients develop strategies for returning to work that are consistent with their own values.

4. Explore and learn adaptive methods of dealing with conflict on the job.

5. Examine own values and those of others with regard to employment. Patients need to be open to examination of problem areas and the possibility of changing their behavior patterns.

6. Identify and deal with stresses generated by employment. This is a major area of concern for most people who readily identify job stressors.

In order to assure the patient's successful participation in the group, *criteria for patient selection* or referral are identified as follows:

1. Currently involved in either paid or volunteer employment, school matriculation, or a combination of both.

2. Functioning on or above the egocentric-cooperative level of group interaction (Mosey, 1971).

3. Motivated to maintain employed status. Anyone with ambivalence about making a position, job, or career change is also an appropriate referral, as these issues can be expanded and discussed within the group.

4. Possesses an attention span of 50 minutes or more. As the group is this long, patients can most effectively participate if their concentration usually matches that of the group's length.

One of the most exciting aspects of practice is working within a multidisciplinary department, Rehabilitation Services, recently changed from the name Activity Therapy. There are both rewards and challenges dealing with professional boundary issues, and the rewards predominate if the challenges are met honestly and openly. Having identified the need for a vocational counselor as a cofacilitator, boundary issues were identified and articulated prior to the onset of multidisciplinary service delivery. This included examination of unique as well as shared areas of expertise. Aside from professional education and training, there may also be state regulations, licensure, and personal employment experience issues. *Leadership and approach* are as follows:

1. Qualifications specific to an occupational therapist:
   a. Knowledge and ability to evaluate occupational performance and performance components including vocational skills.
   b. Knowledge and ability to analyze, structure, and adapt vocational tasks to suit individual patient skills.
   c. Knowledge and ability to analyze, structure, and adapt group tasks to meet group needs.
   d. General knowledge of each patient's treatment plan. The occupational therapist coordinates other disciplines in the Rehabilitation Services Department, and acts as the treatment team liaison.

2. Qualifications specific to a vocational counselor:
   a. Knowledge and ability to assess vocational interests, skills, and aptitudes as in testing. If patients in the group are contemplating a career change or a position change within their company, a referral can be made for appropriate interest or aptitude testing. This then can be incorporated into the patient's identified long-term goals.
   b. Ability to assist individuals to attain maximum potential in relation to work (knowledge of the principles of vocational rehabilitation).
   c. Knowledge of employment laws and practices.

3. Shared knowledge:
   a. Knowledge of each patient's vocational goal plan and the ability to facilitate goal attainment.
   b. Knowledge of group process.
   c. Ability to assume a facilitative role in the group.
   d. Knowledge of community resources.

In this case, the *modality* of the Vocational Transition group is the discussion content which is introduced by either patients or facilitators. Group members are viewed as competent and responsible individuals who demonstrate appropriate employment behaviors like promptness and participation in group or individual tasks, duties, and assignments. Most of the time, this approach is successful; however, on occasion, when group or individual symptomatology adversely affects group process, the approach needs to be more directive. This generally involves identification, discussion, and resolution of the current problem, including the addition of structured exercises.

The *methodology* of the group used to accomplish the goals is group process and directed discussion in which group members and facilitators function as resources and a support system.

Evaluation consists of weekly verbal reports to the treatment team on individual goal attainment and process issues. Written documentation is completed on a regular basis.

The *content* of the group includes identified patient issues and therapeutic interventions for stress management.

Direct Service Delivery

Identified Patient Issues

It is impossible to discuss individual patient and group issues without understanding values related to vocational readiness (Mitchell, 1985). Patients' personal and social values are fundamental to all their concerns, and they have identified the following as being of most concern to them.

Returning to work is the most immediate and often the biggest work-related issue patients face. The myths surrounding mental illness exert a powerful hold on our society, and no one is more aware of this than the patient planning a return to work. Many questions arise and one is, what do I tell people, which often begins with what do I tell my boss? While patients may be ambivalent, most decide in favor of honesty with their supervisors. For example, a dairy herd tester believed the best way to protect the job she loved was to have her husband call in "sick" for her. After the first group, she decided to call her supervisor herself and tell him she was in a psychiatric hospital. A cable television manager had done the same thing, and, after role playing the conversation, she left the group, called her supervisor and gave the actual story. An elementary school teacher whose principal already knew she was in the hospital, struggled with whether or not to reveal her own recently uncovered history of child abuse and the anticipated need for additional hospitalizations. Her concern was that long-term treatment and the possibility of long absences from her job would impact negatively on her career as an elementary teacher.

Often a representative of a human resources department or an employee assistance program (EAP), rather than the immediate supervisor, may be the patient's contact in a large state or corporate employer. This may be a less intimidating experience for the patient. In general, most employers are sympathetic and supportive. In instances where the patient suspects the opposite, a reminder that discrimination in employment of people with handicapping conditions is forbidden by law helps to assuage patient skepticism and doubt (Commission on Human Relations, 1986).

Other questions such as what and how much do I tell co-workers are closely related to personal privacy. Some patients choose to inform significant peers, while others decide to reveal nothing to anyone. Still others are willing to be candid. Patient values are determined not only by their own circumstances but also by prevailing attitudes in the work place, and most patients have an excellent sense of these attitudes. Factory workers and supervisors are sometimes unwilling to relate their experiences to co-workers unless those experiences involve substance abuse, which seems more readily acceptable. Many health care workers and teachers seem at ease with relating experiences to co-workers, since they are often supportive. One accounting clerk with multiple personality disorder, who had been hospitalized previously and then returned to work, wisely commented that the first and second days were the most difficult as everyone watched her carefully. After that, it was business as usual.

What will people expect of me when I return is another question that arises and often is the basis of the question, what do I expect of myself? Others' expectations are often determined by one's own expectations. The patient who feels capable and confident can assure doubtful co-workers. Conversely, the patient who lacks confidence in his own capabilities can negotiate with supervisors or employers to reduce job pressure by requesting temporary decreases in time, work load, responsibilities, or even position changes or transfers. One worker planned to speak with her supervisor after discharge and before returning to work. Upon her second admission, she explained to an approving group how she had successfully managed to do this, thereby significantly reducing stress in at least one aspect of her life.

The second area of concern is the environmental and social stress of the work place itself. In a recent episode of Weekend Edition on National Public Radio, three national experts on work relations identified current work environments as having changed dramatically within the past few years. These changes included increased working hours, often 60-70 per week; work that is automated, demeaning, and alienating; jobs that are interchangeable with extensive cross-training; disposable part-time workers such as in fast food places; and electronic monitoring of workers with no one person visibly in charge. Today in the workplace, it is not just the frequency of stress that is increasing but the duration as well. Atlanta therapist Geneva Rowe states that stress today is chronic and unremitting, whereas 25 years ago it was only intermittent. There is little chance to bounce back from one crisis before another one occurs (Miller, Springer, Gordon, Murr, Cohn, Drew, and Barrett, 1988).

Patients relate to these issues and others as well. One young depressed factory worker stated his production quota had recently increased from 95 to 100 percent. This unrealistic expectation was enforced by the daily posting of all workers' votes results thereby increasing peer pressure and competition. Sometimes, the availability of drugs and alcohol in the work environment is problematic. A hospital engineer claimed his chemical dependencies got out of control when his shift was changed from evenings to days where there was increased drug availability. Problems can also arise with co-workers outside the workplace. A young carpenter's apprentice found his drinking and drug use out of control after regularly drinking with co-workers after work. This patient quickly pointed out a similar problem to a part-time restaurant employee who was doing the same thing after late night restaurant closings. Both subsequently decided to seek employment in other areas. Social contact with co-workers after hours, while sometimes supportive, can be illusionary as in the case of the depressed factory supervisor who bought many rounds of drinks for his co-workers in an effort to gain their acceptance and prove he was "one of the guys." He discovered in the hospital that he could have friends without buying them drinks.

Supervisors and managers have additional job stresses. One nurse in a large state hospital was frustrated by an employee who slept on the job during the night shift and her own inability to eliminate this behavior. A public health nurse felt frustrated by several poor management decisions. Numerous dilemmas face middle managers such as the senior line operator who felt caught between legitimate worker concerns and the productivity expectations of senior managers. One owner of a wholesale food distributorship felt overwhelmed by the demands of 35 employees who called him 24 hours a day, continually interrupting his family life. He identified the need to set limits but expressed doubt about being able to do so.

A third area is that of lifestyle and how work affects other aspects of daily living. For example, accepting or refusing a promotion as in the case of the senior line operator who felt he could not respect his prospective new boss. Involuntary termination or firing is exceedingly stressful for all concerned, but the timeliness of a planned termination can be difficult as well. One lab technician wanted to leave her job in which she was overworked by an insensitive supervisor, but, with her recent decision to separate from a husband who was a recovering alcoholic, she decided to wait until her living situation had stabilized. A structural draftsman wanted to leave a highly toxic work environment but decided to remain until he could find another job. The depressed physician, burdened by the demands of private practice, began to weigh the benefits of government employment. Sometimes, patients feel they "owe" their employers for benefits provided during sick leave or leaves of absence and subsequently delay termination. Even the type of termination can be problematic as in the case of the depressed corporate employee who, after 20 years of service, vacillated between straight retirement and disability, as each would affect her benefits in a different way.

Career change, with its concomitant monetary and timing problems, presents other lifestyle issues. A nurse who wanted to change her specialty from psychiatry to counseling anticipated a decrease in her salary but later found out that if she remained in the civil service system, this would not occur. The policeman, stressed out after 18 years of foot patrol in Washington, D.C., needed two more years before he was vested in his retirement plan. Fortunately, his supervisors agreed to put him on a desk job for his remaining time. Hospitalization itself can precipitate interest in career change, as patients may begin a reordering of their work-related values. They may decide on a more service oriented career, as did the carpenter's apprentice who decided he wanted to be an emergency medical technician. The laboratory assistant, however, decided she wanted a more creative job and planned to study floral design. Planning for second careers can also begin as in the case of the policeman who after retirement planned to go into business with his brother, and the corporate employee who was considering how she could transfer skills in training and development to another field.

Another aspect of lifestyle is the balance of work and leisure. Working long hours with little or no time for creative and leisure pursuits or with family and friends is an all too common problem. A welder with post traumatic stress disorder following a serious automobile accident was highly resistant to decreasing his 60-70 hour work week. He loved his work, but his marriage and family life were clearly suffering. It was not until a few days prior to discharge that he acknowledged the need to reduce his work hours.

Therapeutic Interventions

The most significant intervention is the *group process* itself and the support that emerges from shared concerns about work-related issues. The unit's focus on patient involvement in the therapeutic milieu provides an excellent model for involvement in other therapeutic groups like Vocational Transition. Another significant intervention is *humor*. The facilitators share a similar sense of humor which is helpful in finding or providing at least one humorous anecdote per session, and thus [they act] as role models for other group members. This also helps to provide a playful context in which patients feel supported and encouraged to risk change if necessary.

Goal planning plays an important part in the group, and, as previously mentioned, group members are expected to identify a goal for themselves, usually during the second session. This gives focus to the discussion as they report their progress toward goal attainment. This regular reporting also encourages collaboration with other group members. For example, the nurse whose long-term goal was to change her specialty area of practice mentioned that she needed to go [to] the civil service office downtown but did not know how to use public transportation. The carpenter's apprentice, himself considering a career change, offered to go with her and show her how to take the bus while he was obtaining his own career information.

Problem solving strategies are excellent for a dysfunctional or depressed group that needs additional structure or stimulation. This six step process can be identified and used as a whole with a patient's individual problem, or individual aspects can be used alone. The six steps are:

1. Identify the problem
2. Brainstorm strategies
3. Identify pros and cons of each strategy
4. Prioritize
5. Select one
6. Evaluate the results

One part-time government secretary used the entire process within the group to make a decision about handling a problem with her supervisor. A county groundskeeper found it helpful in determining whether to start back to work on a part-time or full-time basis after discharge. The structural draftsman utilized the pro and con strategy only, as he had clearly identified the problem in advance; he determined that he would not return to work nor would he resign until he found another position, hopefully prior to discharge. The cable television manager used the brainstorming strategy to look at her current job dissatisfaction. The group members suggested working part-time or looking at options within the company itself, alternatives she had not previously considered.

Patients often have major problems with *assertive communication* and benefit from the process of identifying, practicing, and planning for change. These strategies are particularly useful in dealing with the environmental and social stresses of the job itself. Most patients suffer from decreased self-esteem and often lack confidence in their ability to return to work. Sometimes they find it helpful to return to work part-time while still in the hospital. This can provide a useful transition and opportunity to discuss concerns and issues before returning to work full-time. Rehearsal of desired behaviors can also be helpful as with the cable television manager who rehearsed her request for a leave of absence after discharge; her supervisor subsequently granted her request. Speaking to an authority like a supervisor can be intimidating, but setting limits can be equally difficult. The food distributor set limits on his 24-hour availability to his employees, and the nurse with the sleeping employee on the night shift left the hospital with a specific plan for modifying the employee's behavior.

Values clarification facilitates resolution of concerns about returning to work and lifestyle. Usually the diversity of group opinion and feedback is instrumental in patients' clarifying their own values. Peer opinion is a powerful persuader. If there is little or no diversity of opinion, or there is general support for one approach, this too, can be helpful. The presence of group members who are themselves employers or managers is very useful in presenting alternative perspectives. On one occasion, a radio station owner gave excellent feedback to a patient with a supervisor problem.

The most significant value issue is usually how much, if anything, to tell supervisors and co-workers about problems or about their psychiatric hospitalization. Patients who value honesty are most perplexed when faced with possible negative reactions from co-workers. This problem, however, is less acute for patients who are already employed than for those who are seeking employment, especially if they have long histories of chronic mental illness and short histories of employment. These people are often faced with explaining large gaps in employment history.

Lifestyle issues most frequently present themselves with patients who have work/leisure imbalances. This is a common problem and may be a mask for avoidance of family or social issues. Helping patients clarify their leisure issues through leisure surveys may help them to see where their values and actual leisure practices are in conflict. The self-employed franchise owner was highly resistant to changing his six-day-a-week work schedule. He valued his involvement in physical activity, and as he began to understand that his practices didn't match his values, he agreed to take off Wednesday afternoons for golf when he returned to work.

Closely related to values clarification is the issue of *time management*. Most people who are employed struggle with this issue, particularly if they have additional roles like those of parent, volunteer, spouse, or student. One young depressed mother and wife, after working individually on her time management issues, decided to terminate her job in her husband's company when she realized she was overwhelmed by her multiple roles and responsibilities.

Identifying *community resources* is preliminary to discharge planning which, on a short-term unit, begins on admission. Many patients are unaware of available resources. Aside from supervisors, most employers have human resources departments which can provide information about leaves of absence, insurance and disability benefits, and accrued sick and vacation days. Employee assistance programs are excellent sources of support for patients (Maynard, 1986), and, on occasion, making contact with one prior to discharge can be an identified goal. One state employee, a disability determiner, had been placed on probation for his decreased productivity prior to hospitalization. When he contacted the EAP, they agreed to assist him when he returned. Conferences with supervisors prior to returning to work can be very useful also, and some supervisors express interest in meeting with patients prior to discharge. A corporate patent attorney met with his supervisor and a representative of the human resources department in the hospital in order to plan a transition back to work. Additional referrals to vocational programs for testing or to the Department of Vocational Rehabilitation may be helpful for those patients considering long-term career changes.

Discharge Planning and Health Promotion

As patients near the time of discharge, it is important for them to identify their plans and what they have learned. If the psychoeducation process has been successful, their plans will include the maintenance and support of positive work habits including outpatient therapy, maintenance of a good work/leisure balance, stress management strategies either in the workplace or outside, and identification of appropriate community resources. When a patient is in his last group session prior to discharge, a considerable amount of time is spent on his discharge plan and identifying what he has learned. In this way, he serves as a role model for newer members of the group.

Program Evaluation

Recently, a vocational transition evaluation form was developed as part of quality assurance. The plan is to give this to each patient prior to discharge in order to determine the effectiveness of the group and to obtain suggestions for change or improvement. Results are too preliminary to report.

Summary

Examination of the historical and theoretical perspectives of occupational therapy in vocational programs, the demographics and clinical needs of an inpatient psychiatric unit, the predictors of successful work performance, and the standards of occupational therapy practice led to the development and implementation of a Vocational Transition group for employed patients, including therapeutic interventions, discharge planning, and health promotion. This program is readily adaptable to inpatient psychiatric units where patients are planning to return to work.

References

Allen, C. K. (1985). *Occupational therapy for psychiatric diseases: Measurement and management of cognitive disabilities.* Boston: Little Brown and Co.

American Occupational Therapy Association (1980). The role of occupational therapy in the vocational rehabilitation process, a position paper. Rockville, MD: American Occupational Therapy Association.

American Occupational Therapy Association (1983). Standards of practice for occupational therapy. Rockville, MD: American Occupational Therapy Association .

Anthony, W. A., Cohen, M. R. and Vitalo, R. (1978). The measure of rehabilitation outcome. *Schizophrenia Bulletin, 4*(3), 365-383.

Anthony, W. A. and Jansen, M., (1984). Predicting the vocational capacity of the chronically mentally ill. *American Psychologist, 39*(5), 537-544.

Commission on Human Relations, MD Code Ann. Article 49B-1-28 (1986).

Creighton, C. (1985). Career development theory. In M. Kirkland and S. Robertson (Eds.), *PIVOT: Planning and implementing vocational readiness in occupational therapy* (pp. 29-34). Rockville, MD: American Occupational Therapy Association.

Forbush, B. and Forbush, B. (1986). *Gatehouse: The evolution of The Sheppard and Enoch Pratt Hospital, 1853-1986.* Baltimore: The Sheppard and Enoch Pratt Hospital.

Ginsberg, E., Ginsberg, S. W., Axelrad, S. et al. (1951). *Occupational choice: An approach to a general theory.* New York: Columbia University Press.

Havighurst, R. J. (1964). Youth in exploration and man in emergence. In H. Borow (Ed.), *Man in a world of work.* Boston: Houghton Mifflin Co.

Kirkland, M. and Robertson, S. C. (Eds.) (1985). Planning and implementing vocational readiness in occupational therapy. In M. Kirkland and S. C. Robertson (Eds.), *PIVOT: Planning and implementing vocational readiness in occupational therapy* (pp. 17-26). Rockville, MD: American Occupational Association .

Lang, S. K. and Cara, E. (1989). Occupational therapy update: Vocational integration for the psychiatrically disabled. *Hospital and Community Psychiatry, 40*(9), 890-892.

Mantonakis, J. E., Jemos, G. N., Christodoulou, G. N., Repapi, M. N. (1981). Factors associated with occupational rehabilitation of psychiatric patients. *Bibliotheca Psychiatric, 160,* 110-116.

Maynard, M. (1986). Health promotion through employee assistance programs: A role for occupational therapists. *American Journal of Occupational Therapy, 40*(11), 771 -776.

Meyer, A. (1922). The philosophy of occupational therapy. *Archives of Occupational Therapy, 1,* 1-10 .

Miller, A., Springer, K., Gordon, J., Murr, A., Cohn, B., Drew, L., and Barrett, T. (1988, April 25). Stress on the job. *Newsweek,* (pp. 40-45).

Mitchell, M. (1985). Values. In M. Kirkland and S. Robertson (Eds.), *PIVOT: Planning and implementing vocational readiness in occupational therapy* (pp. 45-49). Rockville, MD: American Occupational Therapy Association.

Mitchell, M., Rourk, J. D. and Schwarz, J. (1989). A team approach to prevocational services. *American Journal of Occupational Therapy, 4*(6), 378-383.

Mosey, A. C. (1971). *Three frames of reference for mental health.* Thorofare, NJ: Charles B. Slack.

National Public Radio (1989, September 3). Weekend Edition, interview.

Rehabilitation Act Amendment of 1974 (Public Law 93-516).

Rehabilitation Act Amendments of 1986 (Public Law 99-506).

Rehabilitation Act of 1973 (Public Law 93-112), 29, U.S.C.

Rehabilitation Comprehensive Services and Developmental Disabilities (Public Law 95-602) (1978).

Richert, G. Z. and Jurkowski, J. (1988). A4/A5 Vocational transition protocol. Unpublished.

Richert, G. Z. and Merryman, M. B. (1987). The vocational continuum: A model for providing vocational services in a partial hospitalization program. *Occupational Therapy in Mental Health, 7*(3), 1-20.

Stauffer, D. (1986). Predicting successful employment in the community for people with a history of chronic mental illness. *Occupational Therapy in Mental Health, 6*(2): 31-49.

Super, D. E. (1957). *The psychology of careers.* New York: Harper and Row.

Vocational Rehabilitation Act of 1920 (Public Law 66-236), 41 U.S.C.

Vocational Rehabilitation Act of 1943 (Public Law 78-113), 57 U.S.C.

Vocational Rehabilitation Amendments of 1954 (Public Law 83-565), 68 U.S.C.

Vocational Rehabilitation Amendments of 1965 (Public Law 89-333), 79 U.S.C.

Chapter 31

Vocational Treatment Model

Frances Palmer, MS, OTR
Donna Gatti, OTR

ABSTRACT: A major component of psychiatric occupational therapy is the restoration of functioning: work, play and self-care. For the adult psychiatric patient working represents a significant life skill challenge. Vocational programs offered by the Rehabilitation Services Department at McLean Hospital are structured to assist patients [to] identify and evaluate work behaviors which either enhance or inhibit successful performance. This paper will present a description of the Clinical Vocational Assessment Program (CVAP) at McLean Hospital, including a list of common referral goals and the Patient Performance Checklist. The remainder of this article will consider several facets of person-environment interactions relevant to the CVAP, with primary emphasis on the Open Door Thrift Shop program. Finally, a clinical case will highlight some of the concepts discussed.

It is difficult to predict the impact of psychiatric illness on a patient's ability to resume previously acquired competencies. To provide assessment in the critical area of work behavior, the McLean Hospital Rehabilitation Services Department offers a multi-faceted work activity: the Clinical Vocational Assessment Program. McLean Hospital is a private, non-profit psychiatric facility with a 328 inpatient capacity and approximately 900 patients registered in 11 separate outpatient clinics. The work activity program is available to both inpatients and outpatients. McLean Hospital is situated on 200 acres in a suburb 11 miles west of Boston, MA. Modeled after the European cottage system, there are 40 buildings, most clustered in the center of the campus. Two of the four work activity environments discussed are located in the Rehabilitation Building: the Food Service Training Program facilities, the Coffee Shop and Restaurant; and the Patient Library with the adjacent Clerical Training area. On campus, but located away from the center of hospital activity is the Greenhouse, and within a ten minute walk from the hospital is the community-based Open Door Thrift Shop.

Food Service Training Program

This program includes the basic coffee shop training component and the advance restaurant segment. The Coffee Shop area and a 24 seat dining room serve as the location for the on-the-job training portion of the program. This fast food facility services the visitors, patients and staff of the McLean community. It is staffed entirely by Rehabilitation management personnel who work in conjunction with the program supervisor to provide supervision and training for the patients. Classrooms, training kitchen, and reference library round out the facilities that complement the program. The on-the-job training segment of the program consists of 90 hours in the Coffee Shop working in one of the three following positions: counter person, grill and fry, salad bar. Participation is gradually scheduled from quiet to busy periods as the patient's ability and confidence increase. The ultimate goal of this phase of the program is to give the patient a basic knowledge and understanding with an entry level degree of proficiency. The Restaurant segment provides the patient an opportunity to learn fundamental vocational and interpersonal skills necessary for entry level employment in the restaurant field or to support continuing in higher levels of education now offered in food service and the culinary arts field. The patients may experience one or all of the three different occupational categories: (1) Host/Hostess, (2) Waiter/Waitress, or (3) Cook.

Library-Clerical Training Program

The Patient Library and adjacent clerical training room are the sites for this jointly supervised program. The Library stocks over 40 monthly periodicals, 3000 fiction and non-fiction books, vocational and career education reference books, and local and national daily newspapers. The area is open and available to patients, staff and visitors and typifies a small community reading room. The clerical area resembles a large office production environment with four secretarial work stations and two computer work stations. Files, shelves, tables, telephones, practice typewriters and other business machines complete the room. Each area has a distinct vocational skill development component; however, many of the task projects cross these boundaries. For example, inventorying new books involves labeling, cataloguing and shelving. These tasks are shared library and clerical efforts. The production of a patient newsletter also in-

volves a broad array of patient endeavors. Article writing, layout design, editing, word-processing, and distribution are some of the singular tasks associated with the project. The program supervisor is able to match the patients' interests and pursuits with demonstrated skill proficiency. New skills can be learned, present skills evaluated, and former skills re-learned. Environmental factors contribute to a patient's program choice and often the subdued atmosphere of the Library contrasts the busy task production in the clerical area. Both clerical and library tasks are largely individual skill efforts; typing or answering the telephone or reshelving books involve only the activity and the individual.

Greenhouse Program

The 60 foot greenhouse is located away from the center of hospital activity and overlooks a meadow and an apple orchard. Its quiet setting is conducive to the individual task efforts associated with horticulture. Specific tasks in the program include soil preparation, propagation of plants, continuous plant care, preparation, planting and care of gardens, and maintenance chores related to the facility. Along with those activities, several projects are organized throughout the year to introduce production oriented experiences. A sample of these projects is seasonal plant sales; supplying the floral arrangements for the evening Restaurant program, or wreath construction and sale during the Christmas season. This aspect of the program requires more cooperation among the patient participants and provides exposure to other vocational skills such as pricing, selling, and marketing. The program supervisor varies the assignment of tasks as well as the composition of group participants. As many as 15 people could be involved in one project or during one daily session 15 participants may be involved in very separate activities. A project may also be solely one individual's effort. Each circumstance is dependent on the patient's interest, rehabilitation treatment objective, and psychosocial tolerance level. The program space both indoors and outdoors permits this high level of flexibility. The variance in patients' functional abilities and behavioral manifestations can also be accommodated. If a patient can tolerate a half hour of attention to the activity then that individual could be assigned the task of watering the decorative plant foliage in a specific building. If a group of patients are addressing work-related production skills then the organization and implementation of a plant sale may be appropriate. A significant benefit to this program is the availability of employment in this field. The labor market is receptive to the temporary or part-time employment requirements of many of our patients.

Open Door Thrift Shop

The Shop program includes a full range of tasks from highly structured, repetitive activities such as inventory sorting, pricing and tagging, and housekeeping assignments, to the less structured multi-step demands of window displays or the pronounced organizational and communicational requirements of cashiering. Task assignments are under the direction of the program supervisor and are specifically geared and modified to meet the individual's needs, with monitoring of psychosocial stimulation via the use of either upstairs or basement work locations. The overall treatment approach assesses not only areas for remediation but recognizes and utilizes the client's existing functional strengths. The basic objectives of the program are twofold: to permit formal and informal evaluation of clients' social, emotional, and basic vocational functioning; and to provide a transitional community setting for the habilitation or rehabilitation of work adjustment skills. General program expectations include a dress code which is appropriate to community retail standards, and the ability to maintain control over behavior disturbing to fellow workers and customers or to recognize impending loss of control and return to the hospital. Also, there is the expectation to arrange appointments that do not conflict with the established work schedule, to make arrangements for travel between the hospital and Thrift Shop, and a general ability to understand directions and maintain a minimum level of verbal communication.

Program Structure

Rehabilitation staff are responsible for referring patients to the Clinical Vocational Assessment Program (CVAP) and directly supervising each program site. The program supervisor plays a complex role. As a therapist, the supervisor observes the patient for a sufficiently protracted period to detect behaviors preventing adjustment to work. The therapist manipulates those conditions of work that will help the patient move toward a more adequate set of work behaviors. The patient is a vital and active part in this rehabilitation process: the patient chooses the specific CVAP placement, negotiates the treatment goals to be addressed, and participates in the evaluation of specific work-related behaviors. By emphasizing the negotiation and self-evaluation procedures designed in the CVAP, the patient is encouraged to own and control the experience. The Patient Performance Checklist focuses the treatment interaction for the program supervisor and patient. This multi-item behavioral protocol is filled out by the patient and supervisor together at regular intervals. There is a 3 part rating scale: needs much improvement; needs some improvement; or, acceptable level of performance. It is around this concrete focus that important information is exchanged and reinforced: patient's goals and sense of progress, level of skill development, as well as attitudinal and emotional adjustment factors. It is the responsibility of both therapist and patient to justify their ratings of each work behavior with specific observations. The items on the evaluation protocol are generic to any job. The patient is encouraged to relate these items to organize and understand their experiences on previous jobs, to assess current performance in the hospital program, and to anticipate the types of demands he (or she) may encounter in his (or her) next vocational step. The following 47 work-related behavioral descriptions comprise the checklist.

Patient Performance Checklist

PRODUCTION AND WORK SKILLS

Concentrates on Tasks	Accuracy in Use of Numbers
Follows Verbal Directions	Completes Tasks in Assigned Time
Follows Written Directions	Paces Own Time
Retains Directions Over Time	Consistent in Task Performance
Accuracy in Written Tasks	Plans Ahead in Task Assignments
Establishes Task Priority	Organizes Two or More Tasks
Able to Shift from Task to Task	Able to Learn New Tasks
Physically Coordinated for Task	Physical Tolerance (standing/sitting)
Can Work in a Noisy Area	Aware of Consumer Needs
Uses Tools/Equipment Properly	Handles the Unexpected

COOPERATION

Discusses Work Problems with Supervisor	Works with Fellow Workers
	Willing to Redo Tasks

Patient Performance Checklist (cont.)

MOTIVATION

When in Doubt, Asks Questions	Checks Own Work
Attempts Tasks Until Correct	Avails Self of Suggestion to Improve
Uses Independent Judgment	Sets Own Work Goals
Eager to Learn	Shares Improvement Ideas

RESPONSIBILITY

Attends Regularly	Arrives Punctually
Notifies Work Area When Absent	Takes Breaks as Scheduled
Maintains Organized Work Area	Directs Others in Tasks
Follows Safety Procedures	Familiar with Environment of Area
Accepts Work Standards	

WORK TRAITS

Separates Personal and Work Issues	Appropriate Dress/Hygiene
At Ease in Work Setting	Use of Verbal Communication
Pride in Work Completed	Uses a Sense of Humor
	Accepts Praise

The referring rehabilitation clinician continues to counsel the patient regarding adjustment and progress in the setting. The focus is kept on eventual transition to other less restrictive vocational opportunities. Since each program site varies in its occupational activity, the total program is unified around specific treatment objectives. The referring clinician specifies goals to be addressed over the course of placement. The 14 common goals for CVAP referral include:

1. Assessment of functional abilities, and social and emotional behaviors in a work setting.
2. Provide identification and discussion of interfering work traits.
3. Establish positive work identity.
4. Improve realistic self-assessment.
5. Increase interpersonal skills, both with co-workers and supervisor.
6. Transitional/preparatory experience.
7. Learn to assume responsibility.
8. Instruction in work skills/behaviors/work adjustment training.
9. Provide patient with successful work experience.
10. Learn to separate personal and work issues.
11. Capitalize on existing functional strengths and maintain self-esteem.
12. Vocational exploration.
13. Provide ongoing feedback regarding capabilities.
14. Patient-stated goal of eventual competitive employment.

Application of Environmental Theory

The environmental themes conceptualized by Roann Barris (1982) provide a useful framework for understanding the clinical impact of the CVAP. Expanding on the model of human occupation, Barris focuses on 3 facets of person-environment transactions: (1) environmental characteristics that influence the volition subsystem and a person's decision to participate in a setting; (2) the influence of a setting's demands on the habituation and performance subsystems, and (3) factors which affect the individual's capacity to perform over an increased range of settings. Among those environmental characteristics which Barris considers influential to a person's desire to participate in a setting is that environment's arousal potential. She defines arousal potential as a composite of variables: psychophysical variables—the quality or intensity of physical stimuli; ecological variables or the meaning that event has to a person; and finally collative variables—properties of the setting, such as ambiguity, novelty, complexity, and incongruity. Barris views the collative variables as most likely to produce exploratory behavior and stresses that the therapist must determine an optimal level of arousal for each client. Too much or too little arousal may impede the urge to explore. Barris also proposes that when a setting's innate value and interest resonate with those of its client, then there is a greater likelihood of satisfying participation and thus the chance for a sense of efficacy in one's environment.

In viewing the 4 CVAP work sites from the characteristic of interests and values, it is clear that the environments provide a broad continuum of experience in these areas. In addition, not only do the settings provide quite different arousal experiences from one another, but within each setting there is varying ability to grade the intensity of such stimuli. At one end of the continuum lies the community-based Thrift Shop setting, which easily surpasses the other settings in terms of variety and intensity of psychophysical, collative, and ecological variables.

The Thrift Shop is a veritable bombardment of the sensory/perceptual apparatus; a person entering the shop is likely to be greeted by a cacophony of background street noises, shop telephone, shop radio, customer and worker voices, plus the visual experience of assorted clothing and housewares occupying every available floor, wall, and shelf space. Predictably, very few of the 80 patients who enter this program each year are neutral about its initial impact. Surprisingly, perhaps, the vast majority form an immediate positive cathexis based largely on the arousal factor. The very variety of the Thrift Shop's psychophysical properties lends itself to all of the collative variables: complexity, novelty, surprise, incongruity, and ambiguity. Where else would one find the unlikely combination of objects, human and non-human, in one cluttered setting. For the many psychiatric patients whose interpersonal skills are shaky at best, the wide array of inanimate objects is often a safer start to relationships outside the hospital. The patient who likes clothing and finds comfort and competence in learning to price and tag, size, arrange garments on racks, and not incidentally set aside a few things for his or her own purchase is one example. The shop's motto "We have something for everyone," is as applicable to its patients' interests as to its customers', from dressing mannequins to truck work, to tinkering with mechanical objects in disrepair. The nature of the store, a recycling of used merchandise, its low prices, and the wide variety of task opportunities suggest a broad base of both interest and value appeal to patients.

Clearly, the Thrift Shop has some potent environmental characteristics, and for at least some referred patients these characteristics are noxious. The potential for too much arousal in this setting is obvious. The hypomanic patient whose volition subsystem may well direct him toward this kind of stimulation, nevertheless will often be unable to perform even previously acquired skills or engage in new learning.

In a sense, the manic patient is an individual whose volition subsystem has hypertrophied; he is filled with a drive toward enactment of his multiple interests and goals combined with an overblown sense of efficacy, while his actual ability to perform, his level of skills lies at best in a state of splintered disarray, and at worst is nonexistent. For these patients the possible harmony between the volition subsystem and the Thrift Shop setting is pathological. Such patients are usually best directed toward a setting with less sensory overload, although an occasional hypomanic patient can make a satisfactory adjustment at the Thrift Shop by having his work space individually tailored. Thus, he might do tasks initially in the confinement of the supervisor's small office, in the back corner of the store removed from heaviest customer traffic, or in the basement location at a table facing the wall.

Another group of patients for whom the Thrift Shop environment is incompatible are those whose values do not include public service work, a belief in the ecology of recycling used merchandise or whose interests in a work subculture include a need for order, formality of dress, and high standards of cleanliness. There is invariably program failure for this group of clients whose values and interests are not well-matched to the Thrift Shop setting, with one curious treatment exception. One hospital unit at McLean which specializes in the treatment of severe obsessive-compulsive disorders, typically hand-washing and bathroom rituals, has routinely insisted that all such patients participate in at least a brief stint at the Thrift Shop. The Thrift Shop environment becomes in effect, part of the behavioral flooding program of this unit whereby the individual is exposed to a massive amount of the feared item, such as dirt, dust, or human contamination. Thus, desensitization is achieved through continual overexposure, not only in the hospital ward setting, but in a community-based, "real-life" environment as well. It is perhaps a dubious distinction for the Thrift Shop that it succeeds in desensitizing individuals to less than sanitary conditions, but [it is] an interesting process to interpret from Barris' concepts.

At the time of interview at the Thrift Shop, the typical "hand-washer" is outraged at being referred and [is] exquisitely uncomfortable in the Shop, clear that the only reason for his or her presence is the absolute coercion of hospital ward staff. Yet by the end of most of these individuals' stays in the program, some resonation has occurred between the patients' volition subsystems and their environment. What happens? Initially the obsessive-compulsive patient is threatened and overwhelmed by the nature and level of arousal at the Thrift Shop. Deprived of the freedom to act defensively, albeit pathologically in the form of his [or her] compulsion, the patient feels frightened and out of control. But no longer able to maintain the same actions, the handwashing for instance, a small break is made in the otherwise fixed vicious cycle for new feedback, and thus for a reorganizing of this new information by the individual. By itself, simply deterring the compulsive behavior is not enough. It is a combination of limiting the opportunity for the pathological action plus providing some successful competition for the individual's energy and attention, in a sense crowding out the obsessive ruminations with a more interesting agenda. Here lies the value of the Thrift Shop by virtue of its powerful arousal potential and the immediate chance to gain some measure of control over the environment through task performance.

To summarize, the compulsion is temporarily halted at the Thrift Shop, allowing the individual time and energy to perceive new information and demands for performance from a stimulating new environment, to organize and process such information and demands, and hopefully, to result in new actions and perceptions. By loosening the harsh constraints of obsessive-compulsive behavior, the individual may well find his urge to explore in the Thrift Shop setting awakened by the sheer variety of stimuli, his interests broadened, his sense of personal causation enhanced by the development of new vocational skills and routines.

In terms of its psychophysical variables, the library-clerical environment in this vocational model lies at the other end of the spectrum from the Thrift Shop. An orderly setting, it has no striking physical stimuli save the occasional multiple clicking of typewriter keys; even that noise level is well-muted by rugs. For the seasoned clerical worker, the setting would hold few impressive collative variables. Certainly for the novice, however the library-clerical environment could represent complexity and novelty. Probably the strongest arousal factor for this program resides in its ecological variables, the meaning of learning or relearning to type, using the computer, or filing. In short, the arousal potential of this environment is much less intense and varied than that of the Thrift Shop but certainly relative to the experience and perception of the entering patient. Unlike the Thrift Shop, the library-clerical program is a highly defined work subculture, with predictable environmental artifacts, task schedules, and work jargon. Given the specificity of its subculture, the match between this environment and the individual's interests and values would be vital. Without it, the person has little hope of program success.

Environmentally, the Coffee Shop and Greenhouse vocation programs lie somewhere between the polarities of Thrift Shop and clerical sites, and share some aspects of each. Like the clerical program, the Food Service Training Program has its circumscribed subculture. Again, the predictable artifacts exist; cash register, counter, grill, ice cream machine, and soda dispenser. Uniforms standardize the dress code and there is a vocabulary for ordering food items. The Coffee Shop and

Restaurant possess considerable arousal potential; sounds, smell, temperature, and color, and a fair degree of complexity and novelty for the inexperienced referral. Both the Thrift Shop and Food Service sites are stimulating environments which can potentially exceed the optimal threshold of arousal for individuals, but are rarely guilty of insufficient arousal.

The Greenhouse program claims some of the order and predictability of the clerical setting, and a moderate degree of certain psychophysical variables, including a warm, moist climate, smells, tactile experiences, and color. The most striking arousal aspects of this setting are its novelty and ecological impact; the process of nurturing—whether plants or people—is hardly a neutral event to most individuals. It is an environment which may be of value and interest to people both avocationally and vocationally and is usually perceived by patients as the least interpersonally competitive program.

In the remainder of Barris' paper on environmental themes, she considers several properties of the interaction with the setting, and an event called the trajectory of increasing occupancy. Press, or environmental demands is one property to consider in an individual's interaction with his environment. Press is defined simply as an expectation for a certain kind of behavior.

> Just as arousal is the match between volition and environment, press is the match between environmental demands for performance and the system's ability to perform. Arousal tells us how likely a person is to attempt a performance; press tells us what the person is required to do and how likely he or she is to succeed. (Barris, p. 640)

The density of people in a setting is another property discussed by Barris with its implications for performance. Research findings around this issue suggest that individual responsibility and satisfaction are inversely correlated with the level of manning. Thus, in so-called undermanned environments, [with] fewer people than necessary to carry out normal group activities, there appear to be more desired opportunities available to each person and subsequently more chance to develop competence over a range of skills.

In relating some of these properties to the work-related programs at McLean, the concept of press is helpful in understanding the common discrepancy between descriptions of ward-based patient behavior and patient behavior in the CVAP placements. Patients may be reported engaging in a variety of pathological behavior on the ward (threatening, aggressive behavior, isolation, apparent hallucinatory activity) and yet nevertheless manage an hour or more of appropriate performance in a hospital work setting. Clearly the work placements may elicit expectations for performance which at least temporarily supercede more maladaptive behavior.

By their sheer physical set-ups, the library-clerical and food service areas connote some very clear expectations for behavior, whether it be the associated tasks of filing books, typing, or running the cash register. While the tasks of the Greenhouse and Thrift Shop may be less immediately clear and somewhat more varied, ranging from solitary to group or structured to creative, nevertheless there are strong task expectations for each of the work placements. This in contrast to the many ward-based environments where the main gathering place is a central foyer comprised primarily of chairs, ashtrays, and patients. That physical environment creates almost no press except one of absolute passivity, and in such a void of both structure and stimulation, it is little wonder that intrapsychic aberrations flourish. Of some interest in this regard is that the hospital-based work programs are sometimes negatively contaminated by their location on hospital grounds, in spite of the contrast of their own discrete settings. Thus, for some patients, the work program is not very "real," its expectations not to be taken seriously, since after all, it is only a hospital program. In essence, it appears that the press of the ward is simply generalized to the work site. Fortunately, with continued contact, most patients are eventually able to perceive the particular press of the work environment and adapt their behavior accordingly, but in a few cases termination has proved therapeutic as a means of ultimate feedback on behavior which fails to conform to the standards of the setting. The wearing of uniforms at the Coffee Shop certainly helps patients discriminate the press of the food service area. And the Thrift Shop, which is located ¾ of a mile from the hospital, almost never suffers the blurring of its press with that of the hospital wards. In fact, the concept of press may explain why many long-term patients are often referred to the Thrift Shop as a means of interrupting the process of institutionalization. While still inpatients, these people can begin to experience community and work demands in a setting outside the hospital, and thereby ease the course of their transition.

One last comment remains in regard to press and the psychiatric patient. There seems to be a temporal component to this concept. That is, patients are often noted to make a satisfactory adjustment to one of the work settings for one or two hours, but after a certain amount of time their ability to meet the previous level of expectations declines. Fatigue may be a simple explanation. Where the physically disabled patient may evidence such fatigue in excessive perspiration or tremor, the ramifications for the psychiatric patient are often the gradual re-emergence of pathological behavior, clearly a cue that the patient's physical and emotional tolerance has been reached, and that the originally optimal level of press is no longer optimal.

In terms of density characteristic, the general experience in the CVAP certainly corroborates Barris' notion that overmanning of an environment tends to restrict participation, while undermanning often encourages individual responsibility and satisfaction. There are, however, some interesting considerations related to overmanning and the functional mix of patients found at each of the work sites. The two work programs with the most multi-faceted press, the Thrift Shop and Greenhouse, have a great variety of task demands ranging from very structured and repetitive to highly creative within each setting. This permits a degree of overmanning that is not counterproductive. The Thrift Shop, for instance, could be effectively run by two full-time people. Yet both the Thrift Shop and Greenhouse tend to be heavily subscribed programs that are able to accommodate a daily census of 20 patients on overlapping schedules as long as the group reflects a diversity of functional levels. When the balance shifts to a majority of either high-functioning or low-functioning individuals, then the overmanning becomes more problematic. In both cases there would be difficulty in meeting the breadth of program needs and selected work would end up being duplicated ("busy work"), plus the supervisory burden increases. With the highly functioning majority there is the need to generate sufficient challenging opportunities; with the lower functioning there is the obvious requirement for more supervision and instruction. Fortunately, since all the work programs are open referral sites, there is rarely the problem of many clients simultaneously existing on one functional plane, if only because they enter at different times and thus have different amounts of experience behind them. For the food service and library-clerical areas with fewer but more structured and defined task expectations, overmanning almost always has negative consequences for the patients regardless of functional mix.

A few words about undermanning. While potentially a more therapeutic state could be created since participants would have greater opportunity to become involved, undermanning backfires in those programs with the public service component. When there is already pressure to get a product out, whether a hamburger or a sales slip, undermanning can create excessive pressure and ultimately impede performance of all but the most high functioning individuals.

The last concept that Barris covers in her consideration of environmental themes is the trajectory of increasing occupancy, or the theory that as people master performance expectations in one setting, they will usually seek new settings in which to both practice their acquired skills and increase their skill repertoire. Similarity between settings facilitates the transfer of behavior, but if they are too alike, if a person's life spheres have been too constricted or unchanging, then the opportunity for new learning and behavior will be limited.

The trajectory of increasing occupancy is very germane to this discussion of vocational rehabilitation with the psychiatric patient. On the one hand there is an effort to make each of the work programs a close simulation of its community counterpart to facilitate eventual transition by the patient; to promote success, however, the task demands made on each patient are carefully titrated, his daily schedule is limited, and community standards are selectively imposed. Thus, expectations for performance vary from patient to patient. It is always a delicate balancing act, and one which sometimes fails. There is the "truncated" trajectory, the patient who leaves when the work expectations, real or imagined, become too overwhelming, or the patient who leaves because he is bored or because the stigma of a hospital work placement is overpowering to him. There is also the "fizzled" trajectory, representing the patient who is never quite ready to leave, who makes a satisfactory adjustment to the safety and security of the work site as long as the hospital umbilicus remains intact.

The case study which follows illustrates some of the theoretical material discussed.

Case Report

Bob is a bright, 29 year old single male who experienced a three year course of intensive psychiatric treatment, both as an inpatient and outpatient. He was hospitalized in a confused, agitated state with active suicidal ideation. The reported precipitating life stress was the added pressure of clinical assignments as a 4th year medical student. His admission diagnosis was mixed affective disorder with a questionable temporal lobe seizure disorder. Since Bob possessed a medical background, the potential neurological explanation for his psychiatric condition became central to his acceptance of the problem. Medication trials and various neurological tests were compatible treatment interventions for this patient and his medically sophisticated family. Although Bob reported a history of learning disability in elementary school, his academic achievements were consistently successful. He maintained an interest in the arts and enjoyed athletics. His social relationships were few, although he maintained one childhood friend and did single out at least one other person in whatever environment he presently found himself. Dating relationships were extremely stressful.

While an inpatient for 2 years, Bob was active in directing his treatment program; his volition subsystem remained largely intact. He participated in the milieu structure, maintained an individualized physical fitness program, was a consistent member of a ceramic group and music relaxation group [and was] involved in a placement in the Food Service Training Program. The initial rehabilitation treatment goal is best stated in Bob's own words: "to learn to work better during periods of personal difficulty." All of the selected treatment environments were compatible with Bob's values and interests, called upon some of his previously learned skills and were sufficiently stimulating. An initial evaluation of his performance capacity revealed interfering behaviors to be (1) an inability to prioritize relevant information, (2) an overly self-critical attitude, (3) dependency on structures provided by school or family, and (4) generalized disorganization in the face of strong emotional stimuli. After a considerable period of time some of his maladaptive performance behaviors diminished; his task pace and accuracy improved, and overall concentration and performance stabilized. Interpersonal interactions continued to suffer from inconsistent behaviors idiosyncratic to his moods. At times he was withdrawn and at other times he was very sensitive and responsive to others. Equally inconsistent was his self-appraisal and his ease in exploring new situations.

Bob was discharged with the belief that only neurological follow-up was necessary. However, this proved insufficient. Within weeks after discharge, Bob quickly began to experience increasing social isolation and cognitive disorganization. Bob then contracted for a rehabilitation outpatient program and re-entered individual psychotherapy. His reasons for participating in the outpatient program continued to highlight the central theme of medication trials but now included other needs such as a supportive environment, social network, and developing a sense of productivity. As an outpatient, he was determined to rehabilitate himself; again the volition subsystem proved to be a prime mover. He rejoined the ceramic group because of his attachment to the group leaders, became a member of two outpatient counseling groups, and started a nine month involvement at the Thrift Shop. Bob quickly developed a proficiency in all of the Thrift Shop tasks. Though the Thrift Shop is an environment very different from Bob's previous work and school experiences, he immediately embraced the store's philosophy of recycling and selling inexpensive items particularly to people in need, and developed an interest in the vast array of merchandise available.

In a sense, the Thrift Shop became Bob's medical laboratory and an internship of a different order. The Shop's limitless variety of objects paired with Bob's imagination and creativity led to a sustained and productive level of arousal. Clearly, all of the environmental variables associated with arousal had an impact on Bob. He set up displays, repaired broken appliances, and was often able to find that special object to match a customer's special request. He helped to outfit a number of patrons looking for a unique Halloween costume. With the discovery of possible rare book acquisitions, Bob called numerous book dealers to appraise the worth of these finds. He composed an advertisement for an upcoming sale and suggested several store improvement ideas. One facet of the press of the Thrift Shop environment is to invite participation on many levels, and for this patient little prompting was needed to identify and fulfill many of the different demands presented. As Bob's sense of competency grew in this work role, he became eligible and applied for the Senior Clerk position at the Thrift Shop. This position is part of a transitional employment opportunity, and as such, requires a 20 hour commitment. He was responsible for knowing all Shop procedures, managing the store independently at times, closing out each evening, making deposits, training the vocational assessment patients, and handling customer requests.

Although a transfer of physical settings was not involved in Bob's movement to the Senior Clerk position, nevertheless the trajectory of increasing occupancy is represented here by all the additional responsibilities of the new position. Unlike the routine CVAP participation, Senior Clerk carries with it the expectation for a global understanding of the Shop program, as well as heavy emphasis on initiative and independent decision-making. Bob attained a high level of skill in the new position, though occasionally exceeded his authority and tended to over identify with staff, becoming too involved in the problems of the patients. His physical energy level tended to wax and wane; one day he might be enormously productive in re-organizing merchandise and on another day take little initiative around the store. Initially, Bob attributed the shifts in energy or any other dysfunction to his "unique and poorly understood" neurological problem. The inconsistencies were recognized and discussed using the Patient Performance Checklist. As Bob grew more confident and competent in his role, he perceived himself as more in control, and less a passive victim of some disease process. Gradually, the disparities in his performance diminished. At termination, Bob reported that the program experience was extremely beneficial because it gave him the opportunity to help others, to learn about himself and his various responses to situations, and to explore options for future employment. More importantly, he perceived himself as a rehabilitated person rather than a marginally functioning, neurologically disabled person. He could translate the sense of accomplishment as a productive store manager to exploring other career fields that were less conflicted and pressured than medical school.

Summary

There are always a number of variables considered when a patient is referred to one of our work-related programs. The most compelling and prognostic factor, however is the patient's desire to participate, [or] the involvement of that person's volition system in choosing a setting. As Barris explains:

> choosing a setting involves resonation between the volition subsystem and the environment. Arousal is a form of resonation between the urge to explore and feel control, and the novelty and complexity of the setting. The possibility of engaging in enjoyable behavior or fulfilling goals reflects resonation between the person's interests and values, and the environment. (Barris, p. 639)

Helping the patient to use his [or her] experiences in the work program to seek further vocational challenges is the task of the supervising clinician. Clarifying with the patient the purpose of his [or her] participation is critical and is reinforced during the evaluation sessions. The multi-item performance checklist focuses attention on those behaviors which either need to be improved or are positive attributes for the patient. This evaluation process helps to make the trajectory of increasing occupancy a cognitively reinforced experience; no longer are a person's past work history, current participation, and future vocational plans simply a series of discontinuous, discrete occurrences. The opportunities, qualities, and activities of each setting can be related to their impact on the patient's performance: identifying strengths and weaknesses, and using this information to establish a realistic vocational plan with the patient. A patient whose sense of efficacy is stimulated by a setting and whose values and interests coincide with the opportunities presented by that environment represents a therapeutic formula for success.

Reference

1. Barris, R.: Environmental Interactions: An Extension of the Model of Occupation. Am J Occup Ther 36: 637-656, 1982.

Chapter 32

Transitional Employment for the Chronically Mentally Ill

Jane L. Dulay, OTR
Mary Steichen, OTR

A concept that is becoming increasingly popular in community based treatment of the chronically mentally ill is that of transitional employment. Many discharged psychiatric patients find the transition from the hospital to the community difficult, particularly in the area of work. They find upon returning to the community that traditional job placements are not open to them. Although former patients often possess the necessary work skills to function on a job, they are unable to secure employment.

There are many factors contributing to the lack of opportunities available to the chronically mentally ill. These include a psychiatric history, a poor work history, a lack of recent job references, the inability to pass a job interview, and a lack of initiative in seeking employment. Transitional employment is a means of removing these barriers and aiding the former psychiatric patient toward becoming a functional member or the work force.

The first transitional employment program, referred to as TEP, was instituted in 1958 at Fountain House, a psychosocial rehabilitation program in New York City (Bean & Beard, 1975). Since that time new programs have been developed in many community based rehabilitation centers throughout the country. A survey conducted by Fountain House in March of 1981, revealed that 89 community mental health centers offer transitional employment, with a total of 935 former psychiatric patients employed in TEP positions (Transitional Employment, 1981).

TEP offers discharged psychiatric patients an opportunity to become employed in the community, rather than in a sheltered work program, which traditionally has been the only type of employment situation available to them. TEP serves as the stepping stone between these sheltered work programs and competitive employment in the community. TEP contracts with businesses for positions within their companies. These positions are usually part-time, entry-level positions. TEP members rotate through these positions, holding a particular position for six months.

TEP offers the employing businesses a potentially never ending supply of labor. The initial screening and interviewing for the positions and on-the-job training for each member assuming a position are provided by TEP staff members. As a major incentive to employers, the TEP staff guarantees the work shift will be covered in the event a member is unable to work on any day that he is scheduled.

Since these positions are reserved for TEP, the members are given an opportunity for employment regardless of their past psychiatric or work history. Many members who lack the confidence and initiative to compete for jobs in the community are given an opportunity to apply for a job that is readily available to them. After members have completed a TEP placement, they possess current work experience and a recent job reference which leaves them better equipped to enter the competitive job market.

The Towne House Creative Living Center, Oakland, California, (hereafter referred to as Towne House) is the only pre-vocational program in the San Francisco Bay Area that offers TEP to adults with a history of chronic mental illness (Hill, 1980). In 1980, the passage of state legislation, Bates Bill AB3052 (allocating state monies for a community residential treatment system), provided the financial impetus for Towne House to expand its center-based, pre-vocational program and develop a TEP program. An occupational therapist was hired to develop and implement a TEP program similar to that of Fountain House, New York.

The Role of the Occupational Therapist in the Development and Implementation of a TEP Program

While designing the new pre-vocational component offering TEP as the major treatment service, the occupational therapist identified 3 key elements essential for a comprehensive rehabilitation program: 1) developing jobs for the chronically mentally ill in the business community, 2) developing criteria for entrance into the TEP program, as well as screening members for employment placement, and 3) providing a therapeutic link between the employment placement and Towne House via an ongoing support group for TEP members.

Job Development

Two important factors were considered for securing jobs in the business community: 1) assessing the special pre-vocational needs of the chronically mentally ill members who came to Towne House and 2) identifying appropriate employment placements which could provide the therapeutic conditions necessary for successful work performance of the TEP employee.

Of the 25 members who entered the TEP program in the first year, 64% were male, 36% were female; 44% had less than a high school education, 28% received only a high school education, and 28% received some college education. In terms of work experience, 44% had 0-5 months of work experience, and 56% had over 5 months of work experience. These figures reflect the results of a pilot study conducted by Howe in 1976 (Howe, Weaver, & Dulay, 1981). Her findings indicated that the pre-vocational program at Towne House appealed to young males with a high school education or less, who had never held a steady job, but valued paid work. All members had more than one psychiatric hospitalization prior to their involvement with Towne House and were receiving some type of financial assistance such as supplemental security income (SSI). 52% lived in supervised situations such as board and care homes, 14% lived with their families, 14% lived in semi-independent situations such as halfway houses and satellite housing, and 19% lived independently in apartments or hotels.

A review of the current job market indicated that the employment positions available and suitable for the Towne House members were the unskilled, entry-level positions that fell into three areas: janitorial, food services, and clerical. Companies which were most receptive to reserving job positions for TEP were those with job openings due to high turnover rates, absenteeism, and undesirable working hours such as weekend shifts, and were supportive of the mental health system.

A task analysis was conducted on each job secured for the program. The following conditions were observed to be important therapeutic indicators for successful work performance of the TEP members. Arrangements were made with the employer to adapt the TEP position to meet as many of the conditions as possible.

Type of activity. Structured, concrete, routine tasks that changed little from day to day gave the TEP employees a sense of competence early in employment.

Variety of techniques. Tasks that could be performed by a variety of methods with a minimum number of tools required to complete the task seemed to eliminate the pressure of the "right and wrong" way to do a task.

Rates of achievement. Tasks that allowed the TEP employee to perform at his [or her] own speed and that emphasized quality rather than quantity, decreased the pressure to work at a predetermined rate.

Space. An open, uncrowded work environment that was stable and relatively free of noise, decreased the possibility of overstimulation and distraction for the TEP employee.

Mental-motor coordination requirements. It has been expressed by TEP employees that sustained heavy physical labor, large gaps of inactivity requiring initiative and judgment to keep busy, or fine motor activities lead to frustration and feelings of inadequacy or exploitation by their supervisors. These feelings have been observed to trigger internal preoccupation and decreased attention span and concentration. Employers have, at times, interpreted this behavior as laziness or a tendency to daydream. Therefore, gross motor and simple cognitive level responsibilities such as sweeping, setting tables or collating papers are preferred and seem to provide the opportunity for concentration and an increase in attention span.

Social interaction. Interpersonal interaction seemed best when limited to one supervisor and two to three co-workers. Little or no public contact helped a TEP employee gradually learn to work and socially interact in an unsheltered, unsupported environment.

The occupational therapist, by adapting the work environment, plays an important role in assisting the chronically mentally ill attain their occupational goals. Johnson states that "occupational therapists have a contribution to make to most persons who, because of personal or environmental or social barriers, are unable to influence their environments in such a way as to enable them to fulfill their personal needs" (Johnson, 1971).

Currently, the TEP employment opportunities include janitorial positions at McDonald's restaurant, kitchen aide positions at a psychogeriatric nursing home, meal handler positions at senior nutrition sites, and clerical positions at a ticket agency.

The TEP job placements range from 2-4 hours a day, 1-5 days a week. The gradation of job responsibilities is according to the number of hours and days per week a TEP employee is physically and psychologically ready to handle.

Gradation of the number of hours in a work shift also serves to minimize a member's fears of termination from social security disability income or supplemental security income. Under existing social security administration regulations, disabled persons are allowed to earn up to $85.00 per month. Any earned income over that limit is divided in half and subtracted from their monthly check. A person is entitled to work 12 months in a given disability period. More than 12 months of employment may result in a review of eligibility by the social security administration (Social Security Amendments, 1979). [Readers are advised to check with the social security administration for current regulations.] The fear of losing disability or supplemental security income is a major work disincentive for the chronically mentally ill.

Screening Process

The occupational therapist agrees, as part of the contract with the employer, to send the most qualified person for the job. A 5 step screening process encourages members to apply for TEP job openings. At the same time, this screening process allows members who have unrealistic employment goals or who need more work

adjustment to eliminate themselves at various stages of the process. Emphasis is on independent decision-making and a realistic appraisal of one's capabilities.

1. *Application.* TEP job openings are announced at the Towne House weekly member-run business meetings, posted on the bulletin board as well as advertised in the center newsletter. Interested members are requested to fill out the employment application required by the company. These employment applications also aid the occupational therapist in assessing a member's ability in reading, writing, and comprehension. At this time, members can join the TEP program. This requires an interview with the occupational therapist where a psychiatric and work history is gathered, and a commitment to attend the weekly support groups.

2. *Field Trip.* All applicants are required to take a field trip to the employment site via public transportation. This opportunity to become familiar with the transportation system, to see the actual work environment, and to meet the prospective supervisor and co-workers can aid a member in independently deciding whether he can meet the job expectations and/or if the job is a safe and meaningful work environment. At this point in the screening process as many as half of the applicants often decide not to continue.

3. *Work supervisor evaluation.* Most members applying for TEP placement are involved in the center-based prevocational program in activities such as recycling, landscaping, janitorial and food services. A recommendation, through the use of an assessment tool developed by the membership at Towne House, is requested from a member's work supervisor. This assessment tool evaluates a member's performance in work areas such as attendance, punctuality, ability to deal with authority, ability to get along with co-workers, ability to do a variety of jobs, and ability to follow directions (Howe, Weaver, & Dulay, 1981). Members who receive a high recommendation from their work supervisor are then selected to take a work sample evaluation.

4. *Work sample evaluation.* The occupational therapist develops a work sample evaluation for each TEP segment. See Figure 1 for an example of a work sample evaluation. Patterned after the Bay Area Functional Performance Evaluation (Bloomer & Williams, 1979), each work sample is divided into three major parts. The main objective is to assess and predict work behavior and vocational potential.

Part I evaluates the member's ability to meet specific company requirements. For example, McDonald's does not permit beards. Is a member with a beard willing to shave it? A member is also evaluated on the ability to locate the company phone number, the use of the telephone, and the ability to remember the days and hours of his work shift.

Figure 1.

NAME: TEP PROGRAM
DATE: Towne House Creative Living Center
RATER: 412 Monte Vista Ave.
                                                      Oakland, CA 94611

                                            CLERICAL WORK SAMPLE EVALUATION

I. COMPANY REQUIREMENTS (if member able to answer YES to all questions proceed to tasks)   YES   NO
    1. Work a 6 hour shift
    2. Work on Saturdays
    3. Use public transportation to San Francisco

II. BASIC WORK SKILLS—I am going to give you a series of tasks to do that are similar to what will be required of you at Ticket Easy. I will first give you the instructions of the task. I would like you to summarize the instructions for me as you understand them and then proceed with the task. Are there any questions?

TELEPHONE USE
You will be working at Ticket Easy, located at 655 Stockton St., San Francisco. You may need to call them if you are unable to make it to work or will be late for work due to an emergency. I would like you to tell me how you would find out the telephone number of Ticket Easy.
Do you understand the instructions?
If YES—would you summarize each step that I've asked you to do.
Go ahead and begin.
Any of the possibilities are correct:
Dial 411 for information _____   Look up in the telephone book _____
Have member do either one and check with the correct number: 421-6407
Why do you think I have asked you to do this task?

TIME
Your shift will be: Saturdays, approximately once a month from 10:00 am to 4:00 pm, with an hour lunch break. I would like you to tell me the days and hours of your work shift and how long of a break you have each day.
Do you understand the instructions?
If YES—would your summarize each step that I've asked you to do.
Go ahead and begin.
Why do you think I have asked you to do this task?

III. WORK TASKS—I will be timing you in the following tasks, so work as quickly, but accurately, as possible.

ATTACHING LABELS
Here are some address labels and ____ envelopes. I would like you to apply the labels onto the center of the front of the envelopes.

Do you understand the instructions?
If YES—would you summarize each step that I've asked you to do.
Go ahead and begin.
Why do you think I've asked you to do this task?

SORTING
Here is a stack of envelopes. I would like you to sort them into piles according to zip codes.
Do you understand the instructions?
If YES—would you summarize each step that I've asked you to do.
Go ahead and begin.
Why do you think I've asked you to do this task?

COUNTING
Here is a stack of cards. I would like you to count out 20. Do this 3 times.
Do you understand the instructions?
If YES—would you summarize each step that I've asked you to do.
Go ahead and begin.
Why do you think I've asked you to do this task?

IV. PROBLEM-SOLVING—I am going to describe several situations and would like you to tell me how you would handle each one.

    1. It is Saturday morning and you have to go to San Francisco this morning to work. How will you go about getting to work?
    2. You are in San Francisco, but you are lost. What would you do?
    3. Your boss is the kind of person who likes to talk to you while you are working. He asks you what kinds of things you like to do. What would you tell him?
    4. Your supervisor tells you you are working too slow. What would you do?
    5. One of your co-workers is giving you a hard time. What would you do?
    6. There is a large mailing to be done. You must complete 2000 mailings in 2 hours. What would you do?

Part II involves evaluation of the member's functional ability to carry out tasks similar to those that will be required on the job. The member's level of function is assessed in the following areas: (a) ability to paraphrase verbal instructions, (b) productive decision making, (c) organization of time and materials, and (d) ability to follow instructions leading to correct task completion.

The work sample concludes with a series of situational questions geared to assess a member's judgment in handling common problems or crises that may arise on the job.

A member who best meets all of the above screening requirements is chosen to be interviewed by the prospective employer. Once approved, a member completes two days of on-the-job training on a volunteer basis, and then is officially hired and placed on the company payroll. The TEP employee is paid the prevailing wages.

5. *On-the-job training.* The fact that the TEP staff will provide on-the-job training at no extra cost to the employer is a major selling point for involving the business community with the chronically mentally ill. Within the past year, TEP members who have successfully completed a placement have begun serving as TEP trainers, assisting the occupational therapist in teaching new TEP employees on-the-job responsibilities. A major reason for promoting this concept is that members related more readily to a peer rather than a staff member while learning a new job.

At the same time that a TEP employee is hired, another TEP member is also hired and trained to serve as a substitute in the event that the TEP employee cannot meet his [or her] work schedule. This provides the opportunity for members to learn reliance upon their peers rather than dependence on staff. The use of substitutes also promotes social networking among TEP members as they must know each other's phone number as well as where they cay be reached during the day. It is the responsibility of the TEP employee to contact the substitute if he [or she] is unable to work a shift.

Once officially hired, a TEP member is asked to sign a contract drawn up by the occupational therapist. This contract clearly states the name of the supervisor, the length of employment, the requirements of the job and TEP program, and the names and phone numbers of [the] substitutes. A TEP placement is a maximum of 5 months. At the end of that time, the screening process is repeated. As part of the TEP program requirements the TEP employee is expected to continue attending the support groups.

TEP Support Groups

Whereas the actual job placement provides the opportunity for members to be engaged in a real work situation, the support groups, which meet three times weekly for 45 minutes, provide the crucial link for members to work on dealing with psychological problems and issues they face as they work to master occupational goals. It has been our experience that the psychotic defenses arising from psychological issues around the meaning of work are primarily responsible for a TEP member's inability to function successfully on the job, rather than an absence of specific work skills.

A model for day treatment and group therapy for chronic schizophrenics developed by Gootnick (1971, 1975) is used as the clinical orientation of the support groups. According to Gootnick the group structure provides a therapeutically safe environment for the schizophrenic to work on personal goals. The intense transference complications generated in individual therapy that intensify conflicts of right-wrong, pleasing-displeasing, submission-defiance, dependence-independence, etc. and immobilize the patient from functioning are greatly diminished in the group experience. Thus, the group experiences in the TEP support groups provide opportunities for social relationships and for the identification with a group of peers who are experiencing similar psychological problems and achieving similar social and occupational goals.

To counteract the passive roles the chronically mentally ill assume in social and verbal exchanges and in making decisions, the emphasis in the TEP groups is on healthy, adult, member-to-member interaction, placing them in active, "doing" roles. The major role of the therapist is in minimizing member-to-staff interactions and acting as an observing ego, intervening only when the group members are unable to work as a group. For example, a common group occurrence that happens when a new member enters the group is that old group members will ignore the new member. One of the ways to address this issue would be for the therapist to ask the group if anyone noticed there was a new member in the group. Using this technique, the responsibility for social exchange is placed on group members to think and ask basic social questions such as, "what is your name, what brings you to join the TEP group, what kind of job are you looking for, etc?" As a result, members are in a position of practicing normal, everyday, social interactions which are critical for learning and integrating new skills or recovering lost skills.

When individual psychological issues surface, again the primary therapeutic feedback comes from the group members themselves. As members are exposed to each other's difficulties and disturbed thought processes as well as healthy resources, there are opportunities for reality testing concerning personal and occupational goals. Distortions that members have about themselves or others are often brought out and clarified, corrected, as well as consensually validated by their peers.

A case in point was a young man, C. R., who was officially hired for a janitorial position. His two days of volunteer on-the-job training proved he was capable of meeting the job requirements and the thoroughness of his work won the praise of the management. However, on the third day of employment, C. R. became increasingly anxious to the point where he was immobilized from walking through the door of his place of employment. He decided to quit his job. C. R. was encouraged to attend the group meeting to talk about this sudden change of attitude.

Members asked him why he did not want to work anymore. Was it because he did not like the work, or that the supervisors were mean to him? After much exploration, C. R. was able to express the notion that if he were to work and be successful, his mother would die. Some group members could empathize with this feeling and thought C. R. was making the right decision to quit his job. Others voiced the opinion that it was a ridiculous idea. If everybody thought that way, no one would be working today. One member shared with C. R. he used to think that if he worked his mother would die, too. However, he had to take the risk, and she has not died yet. After hearing these shared experiences, C. R. was able to recall the time he had a volunteer job a year ago. His mother barred the doorway to prevent him from going to work. He also shared with the group that when he told his mother, who is his payee and controlled his money, that he had gotten a paid job, instead of being pleased she was upset with him for jeopardizing his SSI benefits. These experiences meant to him she did not want him to work, and that his working caused her to become upset and sick. C. R.'s ability to relate these thoughts to the group members demonstrated several significant steps for C. R.: his ability to trust the group to share his problems in reaching his goals; his ability to gain some control over his sense of omnipotence in the destruction of his mother; and the fact that the group did not act ruined like his mother around his wanting to work. As a matter of fact, after they had heard his reasons for quitting, they recommended he should stick with his job.

According to Gootnick (1975) "experiences in groups are responsible for enhancing the healthy part of the ego, that part of the schizophrenic ego involved with reality, so that defenses against the psychotic aspect of the self can be maintained. As a result, the patient's self-esteem is elevated and this leads to the ability to become involved with and relate to reality at a higher level." In TEP, this ability to become involved with and relate to reality at a higher level is demonstrated in several areas: increased care about personal appearance, increased social interaction with peers, moves to more independent living situations, and the ability to successfully complete a TEP job placement.

Performance Evaluation

Two performance evaluations are given by the immediate employment supervisor during a member's 5 month placement. The final written evaluation becomes a current job reference.

For many members who have never held a steady job, completing a 5 month placement is a major developmental achievement. Certificates of completion are awarded publicly at Towne House and photographs of the TEP members at work are displayed. Local newspaper announcements and articles have been helpful in creating a climate in the community that the chronically mentally ill can hold a job and be a productive member of the community.

The Future Role of Occupational Therapists in TEP Programs

It has been documented that occupational therapists have the skills and knowledge base to provide prevocational services to the mentally disabled (American Occupational Therapy Association, 1980). As more occupational therapists become involved in community based programs, new therapeutic modalities need to be explored outside the traditional realm of treatment activities used in hospital based treatment with the mentally ill. TEP can be an effective therapeutic modality in assisting the chronically mentally ill engage in productive, meaningful activity. This form of activity is not only age-stage specific, but also one of the few socially acceptable ways to integrate the chronically mentally ill into the community. Igi (1979) spoke of the need to provide "an arena that enables patients to acquire skills in a low stress environment and to experience a process they can replicate in their daily life to facilitate continued skill building and a sense of competence and mastery." TEP can be that arena as well as a cost-effective way to rehabilitate the chronically ill in the face of shrinking mental health funding. Finally, TEP is one of the rare opportunities open to a segment of the population who, because of their history of mental illness, have been denied the experience of gainful employment which is critical to being part of the mainstream of society.

References

American Occupational Therapy Association, "Position Paper—The Role of Occupational Therapy in the Vocational Rehabilitation Process," *American Journal of Occupational Therapy*, 34:13, December 1980, p. 881-883.

Bean, Bonnie R., Beard, John H., "Placement for Persons with Psychiatric Disability," *Rehabilitation Counseling Bulletin*, June 1975, p. 253-258.

Bloomer, J., Williams, S. *The Bay Area Functional Performance Evaluation*, San Francisco, California, c/o Rehabilitation Therapy Department, Langley-Porter Institute, U. C. S. F., 401 Parnassus Avenue. 1979.

Hill, Helen. *Vocational Rehabilitation Services in the San Francisco Bay Area Mental Health Program*. Albany Press. October 1980.

Howe, Margot, Weaver, Cecile, Dulay, Jane, "The Development of a Work-Oriented Day Center Program," *American Journal of Occupational Therapy*, 35:11, November 1981, p. 711-718.

Gootnick, Irwin, "The Psychiatric Day Center in the Treatment of the Chronic Schizophrenic," *American Journal of Psychiatry*, 128:4, October, 1971.

Gootnick, Irwin, "Transference in Psychotherapy with Schizophrenic Patients," *International Journal of Group Psychotherapy*, 25:4, October, 1975.

Igi, Cynthia Heard, "Apprenticeship. . .Skill Building in the Marginally Disabled," paper presented at the Mental Health Symposium of the Occupational Therapy Association of California, Los Angeles, California, November 1979.

Johnson, Jerry, "Consideration of Work as Therapy in the Rehabilitation Process," *American Journal of Occupational Therapy*, 25:6, June 1971, p. 303-308.

Social Security Amendments to the Social Security Act, 1936, "Section 6714. The Trial Work Period, March 1979, and Section T6400. Revised Earnings Guidelines for Evaluation or Substantial Gainful Activity, April 1979."

Transitional Employment, Survey Memorandum 218, Fountain House, Inc. New York, New York, April 24, 1981.

Chapter 33

Occupational Therapy in Geriatric Mental Health

Susan Trace, OTR
Timothy Howell, MD

Elderly persons with mental illnesses present a complex picture to geropsychiatry teams. Problems such as dementia, depression, and psychotic disorders are often compounded by nonpsychiatric problems. For example, health problems or physical disability, changing or stressed support systems, loss of major life roles, and impaired performance of activities of daily living all may exacerbate the impact of the psychiatric disorder on the older person's life. The occupational therapist, with an eye toward functional skills and limitations and an educational background in physical, psychosocial, and environmental factors, can provide important information and insight to the multidisciplinary team as it strives to provide optimal services for this population.

This article describes the specific contributions of the occupational therapist to the mental health of the aged. On the basis of our clinical experience, we have identified three important outcome areas of occupational therapy intervention: preserving autonomy, enhancing integrity, and increasing personal and community safety.

Older persons with psychiatric disorders are often at risk of losing their independence at many levels, ranging from being deemed unable to choose where to live to being restrained in a geriatric chair. The occupational therapist can assist these persons in maintaining independent living (or in instituting the least restrictive measures necessary) and maximal autonomy.

The engagement or integration of older people within their life context is vital to their well-being and integrity. Detachment and inactivity are often seen among this population. The occupational therapist can contribute to the support system that is often required to enhance the integrity and productivity of aging persons.

Concerns about unsafe behaviors associated with psychiatric impairment are often paramount in the treatment of elderly persons. Measures taken to ensure safety

This chapter was previously published in the *American Journal of Occupational Therapy, 45*, 833-838. Copyright © 1991, The American Occupational Therapy Association, Inc.

may at times oppose the older person's desire for autonomy. While the health care team sorts through the clinical and ethical questions surrounding these issues, the occupational therapist can help to support the older person's autonomy while improving his or her safety.

Barriers to the provision of occupational therapy services to this population include limited resources, inadequate alternatives, an insufficient number of occupational therapists, need for an improved knowledge base in occupational therapy, need for quality assurance methods, and the underutilization of mental health services by the elderly.

Preserving Autonomy

Difficulties in performing instrumental activities of daily living are often experienced by persons with dementia, depression, or other psychiatric problems. These limitations raise a question as to whether a supervised setting may be required for such persons to function adequately. These persons may be capable of living independently but may have one or two limitations in instrumental activities of daily living. A thorough evaluation of their ability to perform such instrumental activities as managing money, keeping house, preparing food, and managing medications along with an evaluation of external available resources (Williams et al., 1991) allows the occupational therapist to assemble information about their abilities and areas of difficulty as well as available informal supports needed.

Often, if a problem and its cause can be identified, a solution may be reached through adaptation or assistance that can postpone or eliminate the need for institutionalization. Once the nature of the problem is determined, various measures can be implemented. Examples of adaptations for the improvement of instrumental activities of daily living abilities are enlarged telephone buttons, compartmentalized daily medication boxes, and checkbooks printed in large type. Other physical adaptations may facilitate the client's mobility or compensate for physical or perceptual difficulties. When more than adaptation is necessary, the therapist can refer the client with limitations in instrumental activities of daily living to services designed to support independent living, such as chore services, meal delivery services, and visiting nurses. These services often deter a move from the home to a nursing home or group home. To ease the caregivers' stress, the therapist may refer the family to respite programs or adult day-care centers, which also may facilitate the person's remaining in the home longer.

If the client wishes to remain in the home and has the requisite skills or resources, the therapist may advocate the client's position to the family, the clinical team, or the legal system by proposing alternatives. In areas where services, living options, and other types of resources are limited or unavailable, the therapist can advocate for these persons by increasing public and government awareness of their problems and needs. Advocacy is a natural role for occupational therapy; our therapeutic tradition has been one of subscribing to the value of independence and respecting the individual's right to choose (see Harvey, 1984, for a description of this role).

Chemical and physical restraints are used more often with the elderly than with any other population (Robbins, Boyko, Lane, Cooper, & Jahnigen, 1987). Restraints are used to control behaviors considered to be dangerous or disruptive (e.g., falls, agitation). Recent legislation limits this practice and challenges the interdisciplinary team to find alternatives to controlling these behaviors (Omnibus Budget Reconciliation Act of 1987 [Public Law 100-203]). The engagement of a person in a meaningful task usually reduces his or her agitation, anxiety, and wandering by channeling energy in a positive direction, thus reducing the need for restraints. Selection and modification of an activity that will be both accepted by an agitated person and successful, however, can be difficult. Activity selection requires consideration of the client's motivation, task simplification, and potential for risk if agitation escalates (e.g., the use of sharp or heavy objects is not wise when working with agitated clients). Engagement in activity can provide not only therapeutic value but also information on the precipitants of agitation, aggressive behavior, or catastrophic reactions. The therapist can share this information with other health care professionals and with caregivers to develop strategies to prevent these behaviors from recurring.

When people are restrained to prevent falls secondary to unsteadiness, poor judgment, or both, they may become physically deconditioned and thus more unsteady. Often, there may be treatable but overlooked reasons for the unsteadiness (e.g., orthostatic hypotension, sedation from psychotropic medications). Because the occupational therapist focuses on maintaining or improving function, he or she may be able to recommend interventions other than restraints. The risk of falling must be weighed carefully against the psychological and physical risks involved in the use of restraints.

Enhancing Integrity

Purposeful activity is essential to one's integrity and well-being throughout the life span (Erikson, Erikson, & Kivinick, 1986; Smith, Kielhofner, & Watts, 1986). Withdrawal or disengagement of one's usual level of activity can be a major consequence of mental illness. Due to performance deficits associated with mental illness (e.g., changes in memory, perception, energy level, or coordination), persons may develop increased expectations of failure, avoid activities, and thus experience a decline in their skills. The occupational therapist can interrupt this cycle by ensuring success or partial success in activities. Clients can thus regain a sense of productivity or even mastery, which in turn increases the likelihood that they will participate in future activities.

The loss of life roles, common in the aged, contributes to the exacerbation of a psychiatric disorder. By interviewing the client or using a role-oriented assessment tool such as the one offered by Oakley (1982), the therapist can gain insight into the current status of valued roles and how role changes have affected the client. This information, together with an idea of the client's current abilities and limitations, allows the therapist to help the client reactivate roles, even through alternative means, if necessary (Levy, 1990). For example, with the move to a sheltered living situation, one may expect to lose the roles of home maintainer, hobbyist (e.g., gardening), and religious participant. Although these roles have been strongly valued and central to a person's identity, they may no longer be assumed because the client believes that he or she can no longer participate in the activity. The therapist can help the client identify the importance of these roles and ways to continue practicing them. In the sheltered facility, the client may be able to do his or her own laundry, have a window-box garden, or be escorted to religious services. With help in identifying the importance of valued life roles and support in continuing them, the client is less likely to lose those roles.

Anhedonia, or lack of pleasure in previously enjoyable activities, is a major symptom of depression and other psychiatric disorders and can disrupt activity patterns that are conducive to good health. Activities with successful outcomes are likely to improve the client's appraisal of his or her own abilities, facilitate a belief in his or her skills, and foster a renewed sense of pleasure from doing. A determination of the presence of anhedonia is diagnostically valuable in the identification of depression and in the differentiation of depression from dementia. Persons with depression may have the component skills needed to complete a task but may show little enjoyment initially. Conversely, persons with dementia will generally enjoy a task until their skills fail them and they are unable to continue. They then may provide a spurious excuse (i.e., "My hands are sore" or "I have other things to do") to avoid a sense of failure.

Group activities are efficacious in working with this population, not only because of the inherent therapeutic benefits of group process, but also because the therapist's use of time is maximized. Due to the clients'

decreased initiation of and involvement in activities, the enlistment of their participation in a group activity becomes problematic without skilled and patient intervention. Persons with psychiatric impairments living in nonspecialized (e.g., nursing homes, retirement centers) or minimally staffed settings may never engage in the groups available. Group leaders, therefore, must understand the dynamics behind a person's reluctance or refusal to participate as well as provide the time and support necessary to help the person over the hurdle of first attempting to participate. This process can be time consuming, especially with clients with dementia. Zgola (1987) described the difficulty that patients with dementia have in initiating activities as well as ways in which to facilitate engagement. She interpreted a client's refusal as being a "response to the stress resulting from an inability to conceptualize what is expected, a difficulty in initiating, and the fear of failure" (p. 70). Clear directions, concrete cues, and specific first-step instructions are some of the techniques that Zgola employed to get beyond a client's reluctance to engage in the group.

In selecting activities for clients with performance anxiety or deficits, the therapist may find it helpful to build on the clients' existing skills and special interests as well as to use familiar tasks rather than tasks requiring new learning. Compensating for mistakes rather than drawing attention to them is usually more therapeutically valuable in working with persons with depression or dementia. For example, by pointing out to a woman with dementia that she is redrying dishes that she has already dried, the therapist is augmenting the client's inability to remember. Conversely, by putting the dried dishes away, redirecting the client to the wet dishes, and acknowledging the client's contributions, the therapist will be more helpful in improving the client's feelings of self-worth and integrity.

In group activities, a playful and safe arena together with positive regard for the aged client provides an encouraging foundation for exploratory behavior and helps to minimize interpersonal failures. The therapist facilitates a therapeutic psychosocial environment by modeling playful behaviors, providing an atmosphere of acceptance, and minimizing the consequences of failure. We have found the Directive Group Therapy Model (Kaplan, 1988) to be most useful in maximizing performance and facilitating group process in lower-skill-level groups.

Increasing Safety

Elderly patients with cognitive impairment who no longer retain skills adequate to cope with the perils of everyday life may engage in a variety of unsafe behaviors (Howell & Watts, 1990). Risky behaviors, such as reckless or inattentive driving, unsafe use of heating devices, and careless smoking, may jeopardize both the client and the community as a whole. Other examples of risky behaviors include the mismanagement of medications, neglect of nutritional and health concerns, and consumption of spoiled food. Memory loss, inability to recognize or appreciate the consequences of actions, and lack of insight concerning physical or mental impairments may contribute to such behaviors. Restrictive decisions (e.g., selling the car, hospitalization) are often made by the family, medical team, or legal system and compromise the client's personal liberty. The risk of an activity and its consequences must be carefully weighed against other factors, such as whether the benefits of protection are worth the loss of autonomy (Watts, Cassel, & Howell, 1989). The discovery or development of measures that will improve safety with the use of the least restrictive means will yield workable solutions in such situations. The insights that the therapist lends to this search can help ensure that the goals of safety and autonomy are optimally balanced.

Functional assessment is of critical importance and is a key contribution of the occupational therapist in the assessment of safety issues. By using assessment tools and observing task performance, the therapist obtains information about the client's ability to maintain safe behavior and the likelihood of a risky situation recurring. For example, watching the client perform the simple task of making a cup of instant coffee allows the therapist to observe the client's judgment, memory, ability to understand the implications of abstract concepts (i.e., heat), coordination, and praxis. Does the client remember to attend to the pot without cues? Does he or she handle and pour hot materials safely? Does he or she turn off the stove when finished? Through observation, the reasons for an unsafe behavior like hazardous cooking can often be identified. For example, unsafe use of the stove may be due to problems with memory, awareness, judgment, or vision. Once the reason is ascertained, the therapist can recommend specific environmental adaptations or treatment to decrease the recurrence of the unsafe situation.

In the home or institutional setting, the occupational therapist can suggest critical environmental adaptations that may decrease the older person's risk of harm to self or others. For example, the therapist can mark stairs and remove or tape down throw rugs to compensate for the client's perceptual difficulties and to prevent falls, thus preserving mobility and saving costly medical bills. Adaptations to a stove unit also may improve safety. Marked dials for improved visibility or automatic shut-off features to compensate for forgetfulness are examples of such adaptations. Visible cues such as labels or pictures on

doors or drawers may assist persons with memory or orientation deficits. The removal of items that could be misused by a person with cognitive impairment (e.g., poisons, sharp objects, weapons, heating devices) may also decrease the risk of harm. (See Skolaski-Pellitteri, 1983, 1984, for more information on this topic.)

Medication management can be important for the maintenance of safety and well-being. Elderly persons are prone to misuse both prescription and over-the-counter medications (Carruthers, 1986). They commonly have multiple medical conditions, each of which requires medication, thereby adding to the complexity of medication management. Additionally, because elderly persons are often more sensitive to medications than are younger people, there is less margin for error in the avoidance of side effects. The occupational therapist can assess the skills needed for the independent administration of medication, including the client's memory, orientation to time, fine motor dexterity, vision, and understanding of possible side effects. This assessment may indicate the need for a supervised trial of self-medication. Adaptations such as pillboxes holding premeasured amounts, easy-opening containers, large print, and color-coded labels may facilitate the client's independence in this task. Simplification (e.g., having the physician adjust times or dosages) may also improve the potential for correct medication use.

Another related role of the occupational therapist is to monitor functional performance as psychotropic medications are titrated (Allen, 1985). With the narrowed margin of effectiveness of such medications in the elderly, close monitoring can prevent improper medication or overmedication. Medication may have adverse effects on mobility, attentiveness, continence, communication, and cognition. These effects may be associated with akathisia, confusion, incontinence, sedation, and even delirium. The occupational therapy session provides a more natural environment in which to observe a person for a longer period than that usually provided in a brief visit with the physician.

Barriers to Optimal Service Provision

One cannot discuss occupational therapy in geriatric mental health without also addressing barriers to optimal outcomes of intervention. In the health and social service systems, as well as within the profession, there is often a lack of sufficient resources to best meet the client's needs.

Although the range of care alternatives for the elderly client has grown considerably in recent years, for most clients options for services are inadequate in several ways. There continue to be, especially in rural areas, limited sheltered housing options, too few respite or day-care programs, and unavailable or sparse independent living services. There are often waiting lists of 6 months to a year or even longer for services. Because psychiatric admissions are often related to clients' level of stress and the burdens placed on support networks, services need to be available on discharge to decrease the risk of readmission.

The shortened hospital stays resulting from efforts to reduce costs make time a limited resource as well. Elderly persons usually require a longer assessment period due to a slower response time, possible communication difficulties, and the often complex nature of their combined medical and psychiatric problems. These factors emphasize the necessity of an immediate focus on discharge planning, better coordination of inpatient and outpatient services, and maximization of patient contact hours. Gibson (1990) suggested structuring more frequent presentations of core activities, making documentation more efficient by moving from a narrative style to checklist formats, and minimizing "unnecessary, redundant or poorly focused activities" (p. 268).

Much debate exists concerning the expense and allocation of the nation's health care resources. Resources for the elderly for housing, health care, and home services are limited and in danger of becoming more so. Discharge plans are often hampered by the lack of options, and creative or compromised solutions are often required. These solutions may not be in the elderly person's best interest or even the most cost-effective. For example, an elderly person with a schizophrenic disorder may be able to return to an independent living situation but may need regular and predictable opportunities for socialization and assistance. If these opportunities are unavailable or inconsistent (e.g., a facility may experience a high staff turnover due to underpaid workers), the person may require rehospitalization.

An additional barrier to optimal service provision lies in the population itself. Many elderly persons do not seek treatment for mental health problems (Kale, Ouslander, & Abrass, 1984), and, if they do seek treatment, it is often from their primary physician and for medications only. Such clients usually do not seek mental health services until a crisis occurs. If we can eliminate the stigma associated with mental health problems, more elderly persons may be willing to seek help.

The second set of barriers lies within the profession. The personnel shortage makes recruitment in this practice area difficult. Of the personnel available, few therapists specialize in mental health or gerontology, and even fewer in both. In fact, the total number of therapists in mental health and geriatrics combined is less than the number in either pediatrics or physical disabilities (Ezersky, Havazelet, Scott, & Zettler, 1989).

One reason that the geropsychiatric arena draws few therapists may be related to the idea of making a difference. Hasselkus and Dickie (1990) identified this theme as being of primary importance for therapists in achieving job satisfaction. Elderly patients are often seen as hopeless or not worth the effort. Those therapists who work with the elderly have come to realize that even limited interventions, although producing small functional gains, nonetheless can have a great impact on the person's well-being. An additional 20° of motion in the shoulder may allow an elderly person to dress independently. Similarly, a boost in self-confidence may enable the client to visit the senior center or prepare a meal.

Lack of visibility and understanding of occupational therapy services is too common among physicians and other support staff. Many geriatric evaluation teams have no occupational therapist on staff. Increased visibility of occupational therapy services within the referral setting and the education of team members concerning occupational therapy's role may help to remedy the situation.

The literature on occupational therapy in geriatric psychiatry is also limited. Comparatively few research projects within the profession have dealt with this domain. Because the population is aging and the number of persons with dementia and other psychiatric disorders is increasing, a better definition, understanding, and identification of occupational therapy contributions in this area is warranted.

Quality assurance, which is necessary for the maintenance of standards of care and reimbursement, is another challenging area in geriatric psychiatry. Conditions that are progressively degenerative (e.g., dementia) make it difficult for the therapist to set goals that reflect improvement. Even maintenance goals are ultimately impossible given the certainty of decline. With treatment, decline in abilities may be slowed, but there is currently no way to predict or measure this. Many useful and relevant treatment goals involving quality of life are difficult to measure (e.g., greater self-esteem, enhanced safety).

Conclusion

Geropsychiatry holds many challenges for the occupational therapist. Although it affords the therapist an opportunity to make an important contribution to the overall quality of elderly persons' lives, it presents obstacles. With the occupational therapist's training in creating innovative adaptive solutions, the possibility of meeting these challenges is enhanced. By expanding the knowledge base through research and disseminating that knowledge through the literature and educational curricula, we can help to improve the standard of practice. These efforts will also increase the visibility of the geropsychiatric specialty area within the profession. Higher visibility is of primary importance in continued efforts by the profession to recruit therapists in geriatric mental health.

The need for standardized, validated assessments for elderly persons with psychiatric problems will continue. Measures of abstract concepts (e.g., quality of life) are needed for quality assurance. Advocacy and education of the public and government to increase awareness of the growing needs of elderly persons with mental illness and their families will continue to be important issues for both the practicing therapist and the profession as a whole.

References

Allen, C. (1985). *Occupational therapy for psychiatric diseases: Measurement and management of cognitive disabilities.* Boston: Little, Brown.

Carruthers, S. G. (1986). Principles of drug treatment in the aged. In I. Rossman (Ed.), *Clinical geriatrics* (pp. 114-124). Philadelphia: Lippincott.

Erikson, E. H., Erikson, J. M., & Kivinick, H. Q. (1986). *Vital involvement in old age.* New York: Norton.

Ezersky, S., Havazelet, L., Scott, A. H., & Zettler, C. L. B. (1989). Specialty choice in occupational therapy. *American Journal of Occupational Therapy, 43,* 227-233.

Gibson, D. (1990). The challenge of adaptation: Shaping service delivery to meet changing needs. *Hospital and Community Psychiatry, 41*(23), 267-269.

Harvey, L. (1984). Advocacy and the aged: A case for the therapist-advocate. *Physical and Occupational Therapy in Geriatrics, 3*(2), 5-15.

Hasselkus, B., & Dickie, V. (1990). Themes of meaning: Occupational therapists' perspectives on practice. *Occupational Therapy Journal of Research, 10,* 195-205.

Howell, T., & Watts, D. (1990). Behavioral complications of dementia: A clinical approach for the general internist. *Journal of General Internal Medicine, 5,* 431-436.

Kale, R., Ouslander, J., & Abrass, I. (1984). *Essentials of clinical geriatrics.* New York: McGraw-Hill.

Kaplan, K. (1988). *Directive group therapy: Innovative mental health treatment.* Thorofare, NJ: Slack.

Levy, L. (1990). Activity, social role retention and the multiply disabled aged: Strategies for intervention. *Occupational Therapy in Mental Health, 10,* 1-30.

Oakley, F. (1982). *The Model of Human Occupation in psychiatry.* Unpublished master's research project, Virginia Commonwealth University, Richmond.

Omnibus Budget Reconciliation Act of 1987 (Public Law 100-203). Title IV, Subtitle C, Nursing Home Reform.

Robbins, L. J., Boyko, E., Lane, J., Cooper, D., & Jahnigen D. W. (1987). Binding the elderly: A prospective study of the use of mechanical restraints in an acute care hospital. *Journal of the American Geriatric Society, 35,* 290-296.

Skolaski-Pellitteri, T. (1983). Environmental adaptations which compensate for dementia. *Physical and Occupational Therapy in Geriatrics, 3,* 25-32.

Skolaski-Pellitteri, T. (1984). Environmental intervention for the demented person. *Physical and Occupational Therapy in Geriatrics, 3,* 55-59.

Smith, N. R., Kielhofner, G., & Watts, J. H. (1986). The relationships between volition, activity pattern, and life satisfaction in the elderly. *American Journal of Occupational Therapy, 40,* 278-283.

Watts, D., Cassel, C., & Howell, T. (1989). Dangerous behavior in a demented patient: Preserving autonomy in a patient with diminished competence. *Journal of the American Geriatric Society, 37,* 658-662.

Williams, J., Drinka, T., Greenberg, J., Farrell-Holtan, J., Euhardy, R., & Schram, M. (1991). Development and testing of the Assessment of Living Skills and Resources (ALSAR) in elderly community dwelling veterans. *Gerontologist, 31,* 84-91.

Zgola, J. (1987). *Doing things.* Baltimore: Johns Hopkins University Press.

Chapter 34

An Expanded Community Role for Occupational Therapy: Preventing Depression

Alisa Ofsevit Eilenberg, MS, OTR

This chapter was previously published in *Physical and Occupational Therapy in Geriatrics, 5*(1), 47-57. Copyright © 1986, Haworth Press. Reprinted by permission.

Depression is a formidable illness currently threatening the well-being of countless community elderly. Their social isolation, the physical changes of aging and a societal focus on youth and the roles and skills of the young cause this group to be particularly vulnerable to depression. Therapeutic approaches employed by occupational therapists can be effectively applied to promote mental health and prevent depression in the community elderly.

After several years of working with institutionalized elderly psychiatric patients, many of whom had been admitted for depression, the author's focus turned to prevention stimulated by a course taken in the advanced Occupational Therapy Program at Columbia University. As part of a related practicum at a senior center, the author designed and implemented a time-limited program to foster independence and prevent depression, as well as to observe the multidisciplinary efforts being made toward this end on an experimental basis. This preparation helped in the planning of the theoretical and practical aspects of the "Wellness Program" now carried out at the Mamaroneck Senior Center in Westchester.

Frames of Reference

The "Wellness Program" is based on several frames of reference that form a comprehensive approach to preventing depression and promoting the health of the community elderly. The first frame of reference is developmental. Erikson, as cited in Belkin, described the chief challenge of old age as a struggle of "ego identity versus despair." Successful resolution of this life stage involves a sense of peace and acceptance of life's accomplishments and failures, an overall sense that one's life has been worthwhile. He suggests that depression results if this perspective is not attained (1980). Peck, as cited in Weiner, elaborates on Erikson's view by listing more specific tasks of old age, including adaptation to work and family role changes by the establishment of varied, valued activities. He stresses the importance of transcending physical and cognitive limitations and discomforts while enjoying social interaction. A further task is the focusing on making some contribution to the welfare of future generations rather than the preoccupation with death that so often accompanies depression (1978). The Wellness Program seeks to help members attain these goals and overcome the limitations of aging as each individual finds him or herself at a different point of development.

A sensory-integrative frame of reference focuses on the human need for adequate, varied and meaningful stimulation. Ideally, this input is then processed by the brain and permits daily adaptive behavior. Sensory integration is typically compromised in the elderly. Sensory systems such as sight, hearing, taste and smell are commonly diminished. The sense of joint movement and position in space may be impaired because of arthritic changes and reduced nerve conduction. The consequences of these changes are frequently slowed and cautious movement and decreased overall activity.

Socialization, a most important type of sensory and mental stimulation, is also compromised in the aged. This is due to death and relocation of friends [and] relatives (particularly spouses), and the scarcity of extended family systems in this society.

The author's previous research into the sensory-integrative needs of the elderly indicates that disuse of existing sensory-motor abilities only accelerates the deterioration of these systems. The inactivity and withdrawal that can accompany these losses puts the elderly at great risk of depression. Numerous studies of sensory deprivation demonstrate that inadequate stimulation and/or processing of information have devastating physical, cognitive and emotional effects, including vulnerability to disease, confusion, decreased motor skills, irritability and general withdrawal (Ofsevit, 1980).

Given the importance of sensory-integrative function, it is crucial that these needs be addressed in any program designed to prevent depression in the elderly. In the Wellness Program, a dance and movement part of each session is an important tool in meeting sensory-integrative needs of members.

A learning model is another useful frame of reference in the design of the Wellness Program. There is an assumption that given the motivation new skills can be learned and changes made in a lifestyle late in life. Mosey (1971) states that learning takes place as a consequence of positive reinforcement. In the Wellness Group, the reinforcement includes peer and leadership support for constructive changes, as well as the innate satisfaction that comes from mastery of one's environment. The forming of individualized goals, which, when met, increase members' sense of their autonomy, is a valuable approach to preventing the sense of helplessness that so often accompanies depression. The group problem-solving approach is a useful means to this end.

An additional frame of reference is the systems approach. This approach is useful in understanding the structure of any organization: staffing patterns, membership composition, goals, mandates, [and] constraints of the institution. It was helpful in initially determining how occupational therapy skills could be applied toward furthering the existing goals of the senior center through the implementation of a new program and in maintaining open lines of communication for the ongoing success of the program.

Program Setting

The Mamaroneck Senior Center has a membership of approximately two hundred from the Westchester area. It provides hot lunches Monday through Friday, daily activities, special events, and referrals for members in need of community services. Mamaroneck Human Resources is particularly involved in this regard. Staffing includes a chief administrator, site manager, a secretary, assistants, kitchen workers, as well as volunteers and consultants who conduct activity programs. The senior center is supported by federal funds which are scheduled to be gradually phased out, as well as by the town of Mamaroneck. Local community organizations frequently contribute toward special needs or events at the center.

The senior center aims to meet the social and recreational needs of its membership. There is also an awareness of the increasing frailty of members and the difficulties faced by them in terms of remaining well and independent in the community. The administrators were thus receptive to the idea of a Wellness Program which would have the aim of promoting health in this group at risk for physical deterioration, social isolation, and depression.

In introducing the Wellness Program at the center the author described the role of occupational therapists in different settings and with varied age groups. Life tasks change with the aging process. Older adults have tremendous adjustments to make to role changes, as children leave home, retirement arrives, and a spouse dies. The many physical changes that occur with aging often begin to interfere with the performance of daily activities. The purpose of the Wellness Program was to help older people make the fullest possible use of their abilities and to stay well and able to live in the community as long as possible.

An open discussion and written survey were provided to determine the unique health concerns of this population. Large and small group meetings were held as well as two consecutive sessions with individuals. Physical concerns expressed included arthritis, managing household tasks, improving posture, coping with pain, and getting adequate exercise. Psychosocial subjects of concern included living alone, using time more fully, and meeting new friends.

Following the written survey, members were invited to sign up for the Wellness Group. Potential participants were encouraged to give the group a try. The group was to be conducted in time-limited phases, after which members were free to continue or to leave. Individuals were pleased to know that the program would be geared to their needs, [and] that no one would be pressured to participate beyond what was comfortable for them. Staff was helpful in identifying individuals who could benefit from the program. The response was enthusiastic. So many members signed up that a waiting list had to be started.

Methodology

The Wellness Group's objectives were influenced by the expressed needs of the population. This approach fostered the objectives of helping participants to discover and make use of their strengths, express their health needs and thus to realize the impact they can have on shaping their lives and environment. Another objective is for group members to form a supportive network of friendships at the senior center. A further objective is for members to gain and share knowledge about preserving physical abilities and compensating for deficits as these relate to activities of daily living. Yet another objective is for participants to understand a balanced, fulfilling use of time for them personally.

The group has a maximum enrollment of fifteen members per eight-week phase; each phase covers a specific topic. Every group begins with a one-hour discussion, using a group problem-solving approach. A half-hour of movement follows, including posture, breathing and warmup exercises along with selected ballroom, folk and free style expressive dance. The author meets with individuals during the final half hour. At the end of each eight-week phase, members are asked to assess the program via discussion and written survey.

The senior center's site manager helps publicize the group through the monthly calendar, weekly announcements and an attitude of enthusiastic support. Senior center staff set up the group's meeting area in advance. Periodic meetings are held with the site manager and the chief administrator to discuss the outcome of the group, and any difficulties or questions that arise.

The Wellness Group meets in the one long, large, often crowded room that comprises the temporary accommodations for the senior center during its renovation. A corner of the room is set up with a record player and a circle of chairs. Tables are pushed away to allow for needed space. The membership is asked to assist the group by keeping their voices lower than usual, since a high noise level interferes with discussion.

Sample Sessions

Physical discomforts and increasing dependency that stem from arthritic conditions so common in the elderly can produce feelings of depression. The first series of sessions was devoted to arthritis and learning joint protection concepts, since this was the main priority indicated in the initial survey. Topics covered included resources for relieving and coping with pain, safety and management issues around the home, posture and body mechanics, and resources for coping with arthritis.

The theme of one particular session was finding a balance between rest and activity. The group was asked how they determined whether a household or other task was too much for them to handle. One woman described the enormous task of cleaning her fish tank. She had made it more manageable by emptying it out cup by cup. It was still exhausting and she felt that the only solution was to give up having the fish. Although this solution would be acceptable if the fish were no longer important to her, it was suggested that an alternative might be found if an effort were made to creatively solve the problem. That led to the topic of when, whom and how to ask for help. Possible resources, such as family and friends, were mentioned. The group discussed the advantages of calling upon them, the "price paid" for doing so or for not doing so. The importance of the timing of a request was discussed, along with consideration of the resource person's mood and obligations.

The tone of voice and attitude of the person making the request were explored. Participants pointed out that a demanding or hurried tone could make others less willing to help. It was also noted that firm self-advocacy was at times needed in case of hazards, such as when one member's window would not close during a harsh winter.

Mamaroneck Human Resources was mentioned as an additional resource. Members had heard that high school students and retirees were available for assistance with heavy tasks such as household repairs and that senior center staff might know more about specifics.

The group concluded with posture, breathing, and warmup exercises. There was dancing in pairs and as a group to oldtime jazz. All were encouraged to take part within their individual limitations and capacities. The mood of the group was lighthearted and cheerful. There was much enthusiastic participation.

The second phase of the Wellness Program dealt with developmental social concerns that can be handled constructively or make the elderly more vulnerable to depression. In this sample session, the group discussed the benefits and drawbacks of living alone. One member said that she thought it was fine for younger people to live alone, but that she would not want to do so at this time of life. Another woman had managed to live alone with no difficulty for many years. After her marriage late in life, however, when her husband was hospitalized, she found it a shock and nerve-wracking to suddenly be alone again.

One participant is usually withdrawn, in pain and has memory problems. He complained that it was terrible to live alone. When the group suggested he consider taking in a "boarder," he was emphatic that such a step would impinge on his freedom and independence. He didn't want to answer to anyone or be dictated by their needs. The group laughed in response to his description of some of the benefits of living alone.

A member whose husband lives in an institutional setting expressed her contentment with the flexibility of living alone. No one tells her when to go to sleep or get up, and she feels able to find all the company she needs outside of her home. Her one concern was security. She had worked to improve the building's security by fighting to get a front entrance lock, and so was no longer afraid of break-ins.

The group discussed security problems and measures to be taken, including getting a free security appraisal by the police.

Another member of the group had never married. Living alone was never a problem until recently, when she began to feel the need to have "someone around." We discussed the fact that needs often change over time. The group discussed housing alternatives and the fact that many older people are trying group living situations and taking in roommates.

The movement session following the discussion included warmups, dancing in pairs to square dance music, and free-style expressive dance.

Other topics covered in this phase were members' work and family backgrounds, current living situations, relocating, and making friends later in life.

Additional Group Topics

The extensive leisure time that older people are often faced with after retirement can be a source of new enjoyment or it can be a source of burdensome loneliness. A fulfilling use of time is quite important in preventing depression. It is vital in meeting sensory-integrative needs for variety and meaningful stimulation. A twelve-week phase of the program was devoted to the developmental task of exploring options to enhance or improve the use of time.

This particular session focused on adult education. The group was asked whether it was harder to learn earlier or later in life. One woman said she was concerned that she would not retain as much information now as she could when she was younger. Others had the

same concern. We talked about ways to compensate for slight memory losses that affect many older people. One method mentioned was to have the instructor review material to reinforce learning. Other approaches discussed were practicing skills at home, reviewing with a classmate, and taking notes. It was pointed out that some types of courses such as film or music appreciation do not rely heavily on memory. It was noted that another aspect of successful learning later in life is one's attitude. If older students take a realistic and tolerant view of their abilities, they may enjoy the experience of learning without constantly comparing themselves to other learners.

Transportation as an issue that can help or interfere with taking classes was discussed. Accessibility and cost of transportation were considered. We discussed car pools, taxi pools, buses, and the possibility of exploring town funding to help older people attend classes.

The group concluded with exercise and dance to international folk music. Increased participation of members who had been reluctant to take part earlier was noted.

Additional topics covered during this phase were volunteer and work options, museums, theater and concert attendance, and other recreational options.

Obstacles Encountered

Several factors have interfered with the group. One has been the physical setting of the Wellness Program. Leading a small group within a single, large and busy room has caused frequent distractions and interruptions. It poses a particular challenge to participants who are hearing impaired or distractible. This difficulty should be resolved with the completed renovation of the original senior center which will include small meeting rooms.

Another problem has been the varied demands on participants' schedules. In the community, events such as holiday preparation or even clothing sales can reduce attendance. Weather and illness inevitably interfere as well. Although flexibility is needed, participants should be reminded that attendance is a commitment and that each member is an important and valuable part of the group. The site manager has been most helpful in reinforcing the importance of attendance and in locating members who fail to attend.

Funding has severely limited the time that can be devoted to the Wellness Program. A more extensive program could reach more people, allow for more teaching and reinforcement of the kinds of adaptive skills mentioned earlier, and permit leadership in time-consuming projects that would benefit a large portion of the senior center membership.

Assessment of the Program

After the first eight-week phase of the group, a written survey was provided to assess the effectiveness of the group. Eleven of the thirteen regular members completed the survey. The following quotations are some representative responses to the questions, "How did the group benefit you, if at all?" and "Has the group influenced your lifestyle in any way?"

1. "I realized not to feel bad when I can't do ordinary things but to accept it and work around it. There always is a way." "I exercise more often."

2. "It helped to talk about the problem and bring it out in the open." "I realized I've got to get a little more exercise."

3. "It was a time to participate in the different exercises and to get to know the other people." "Made more friends, made me aware of how to help myself in many tasks, and to know where to look for help should I ever need it."

When asked how the group might be improved, participants who responded in the earlier survey expressed complete contentment with the structure of the group, praising the leadership as being motivating and enthusiastic. Only in the most recent survey were members at all critical. There were requests for a larger group, for craft instruction, and for more time to be devoted to movement. This suggests that over time, group members have become more secure and autonomous in terms of voicing their needs.

The group and leader have made various observations about members during the course of the sessions. The group spontaneously told one member who had been initially lethargic that she looked more awake and happy. Another participant reported feeling much more energetic after practicing some of the exercises at home. In time, this same group member took on greater responsibility within the senior center and demonstrated considerable creative abilities in that setting for the first time. Another participant who had always considered herself "just a listener" found that to her satisfaction, she was eventually able to express her own opinions. Two members began volunteer jobs in the course of the sessions, and one decided to take driving lessons in order to take fuller advantage of leisure options.

These changes occurred over weeks and months. The size and supportive nature of the group, as well as the structure, which is carefully tailored to address the needs of a specific group of older adults, has greatly helped members to make the most of their abilities and promote their health on many levels. Those who entered the group withdrawn and isolated clearly benefited from the program at least for short periods of time. Members who came with greater personal strengths have made fuller use of their resources and inspired their peers in the process.

Implications for Occupational Therapy Practice

There is a vast and increasing population of community elderly in need of preventive services. Some are obviously depressed, while many experience low levels of depression which are not dramatic, but nevertheless take a heavy toll in terms of socialization, disuse of existing living skills and physical abilities. Their potential contribution to their own welfare, to their families and communities is being lost.

Occupational therapists have the potential skill for organizing preventive programs. Our holistic training provides a perspective on the developmental needs of each age group. Our schooling in the basic sciences gives us a grasp of the physical changes and sensory-integrative needs of old age. We are creative teachers equipped to assess individual needs, teach living skills, and motivate clients in the face of many obstacles.

Occupational therapy educational programs need to focus more on prevention and the burgeoning needs of the elderly. Training must include an understanding of and practical experience in community organizations to help therapists feel secure in noninstitutional settings.

At the highest levels of the professional association, occupational therapists must take an active role in paving the way for community practice. Most community organizations that serve the elderly either are unfamiliar with occupational therapy or associate any kind of therapy with hospitals and the ill. The scarcity of funds for new programs within community organizations makes it equally difficult if not impossible for occupational therapists to support themselves doing preventive work in the community.

As a professional body, occupational therapists need to lobby government officials and endeavor to educate the public about the at-risk community elderly and how our services might be used to keep older people independent and well in the community as long as possible.

Occupational therapy can and should assume a substantial role in preventive services for the elderly. Prevention programs address a relatively neglected area: keeping older people healthy. The possibility of preventing unnecessary use of more costly care needs to be carefully explored through research. The author's experience indicates that much of the isolation, despair, boredom, and physical deterioration that face the community elderly can be reduced and to some extent reversed by preventive occupational therapy programs.

References

Belkin, Gary S., *An Introduction to Counseling*. (Dubuque, Iowa: Wm. C. Brown Company, 1980), pp. 262-263, 270, 280-281.

Mosey, Anne Cronin, *Three Frames of Reference for Mental Health*. 3rd ed. (Thorofare, New Jersey: Charles B. Slack, 1971), p. 109.

Ofsevit, Alisa, "The Effect of a Sensory Integration Movement Group on Life Satisfaction for the Frail Elderly" (unpublished Occupational Therapy Master's Thesis, Columbia University, 1980).

Weiner, Marcella Bakur, Brok, Albert J., and Snadowsky, Alvin M. *Working with the Aged—Practical Approaches in the Institution and Community*. (Englewood Cliffs, New Jersey: Prentice-Hall, Inc., 1978), pp. 27-29.

Bibliography

Burnside, Irene: *Working with the Elderly—Group Process and Techniques*. 2nd ed. Monterey, California: Wadsworth, Inc., 1984.

Butler, Robert and Lewis, Myrna: *Aging in Mental Health: Positive Psychosocial Approaches*. 3rd ed. St. Louis: C. V. Mosby Co., 1977.

Caplow-Lindner, Erna, Harpaz, Leah, and Samberg, Sonya: *Therapeutic Dance Movement—Expressive Activities for Older Adults*. New York: Human Sciences Press, 1979.

Chapter 35

Program Planning in Geriatric Psychiatry: A Model for Psychosocial Rehabilitation

Danielle N. Butin, OTR, MPH
Colleen Heaney, BS, MA

This chapter was previously published in *Physical and Occupational Therapy in Geriatrics*, 9(3-4), 153-170. Copyright © 1990, Haworth Press. Reprinted by permission.

Psychosocial rehabilitation in geriatric psychiatry is based on the premise that success in self-care, leisure and work is crucial to mental well-being. The objective of program planning is to comprehensively assess function and to promote optimal performance in areas of cognition, interpersonal skills, self-care, leisure, work, and utilization of community resources. Maintaining levels of activity involvement with adaptability and flexibility is an essential component of late life satisfaction. The geriatric activity program at the New York Hospital is a comprehensive rehabilitation model that positively impacts on patients' well-being.

The Westchester Division of the New York Hospital-Cornell Medical Center is a university based non-profit voluntary psychiatric facility. The 322 bed inpatient clinical service has a separate division of geriatric services, with three units totaling 66 beds.

Separate departments of medicine, nursing, social work, psychology, and therapeutic activities comprise the multi-disciplinary team. Three of the five therapeutic activity professionals who treat geriatric patients are represented on each unit, and serve as case managers for their patients. The arbitrary age for admission to the geriatric service is 55 with potential range from 55-98 years old. The average length of stay is five weeks. Though a wide variety of neurological and psychiatric disorders are represented, the majority of patients are admitted for diagnosis and treatment of an affective disorder or an organic mood disturbance. Diagnosis, prognosis, chronological age and expected discharge environment often do not influence placement on any particular unit because bed availability is an over-riding concern. Those persons with affective disorders, dementia, or long term chronic psychiatric illness may live on the same unit.

The wide variation in developmental and chronological age for this heterogenous group, and the brief length of stay presented a significant challenge to activity program planning and treatment. Equally challenging for activity rehabilitation is that a medical model of treatment prevails, and in the past, psycho-social rehabilitation had been minimized or disregarded. Elderly patients, family members and many professional staff readily abdicated all clinical decisions to professionals, and symptom relief was seen as the ultimate answer. Prior to aggressive efforts to restructure activity rehabilitation, geriatric patients were treated biologically, received individual and family therapy, and participated in a largely diversional activity program. The patients generally were discharged free of major psychiatric symptomatology and were given a suggested aftercare plan. However, maladaptive behavior patterns and skill dysfunction that can accompany mental illness or result from loss of esteem and confidence was manifest throughout the hospitalization and evident at discharge. Patients were often at risk for non-compliance in following discharge recommendations, were unsuccessful in adapting to their discharge environment, and were risks for recidivism.

Over the past five years, the authors have worked extensively to develop a program that would more definitively address psychosocial aspects of rehabilitation and challenge patients, families and staff to acknowledge the importance of it. The complexion of professional staff in the Geriatrics Therapeutic Activity Division include a gerontological counselor, an occupational therapist, two recreational therapists, and a creative arts therapist. A liaison vocational counselor is also available for those persons who have work as a priority goal. Through collaborative efforts of these professionals, a framework for treatment has been established that uses counseling techniques to promote purposeful involvement in activity. Activity rehabilitation has gradually, but consistently become integrated into treatment in the geriatric division, and is currently recognized as tantamount to recovering from mental illness.

Frame of Reference

Although the disengagement theory suggests that older people naturally become more self-involved and less interested in others or external events, clinical observations and scientific studies dispute this view of universal disengagement (Neugarten [sic], 1965, Havighurst, 1968). Disengagement theorists claim that this reaction is a response to inner needs and not a response to socio-cultural pressure (Cummings [sic], 1961). A universal disengagement process is an overgeneralization, and lacks the consideration and integration of an individual's lifestyle as a predictor of successful aging (Neugarten, 1965). In fact, social involvements and commitments are the factors most strongly associated with well-being during the natural adjustment to old age. Greater life satisfaction has been found amongst seniors who are active in both community activities and family roles. Since life satisfaction is more closely related to

levels of activity than inactivity, older adults who maintain greater amounts of activity report high levels of gratification and contentment (Havighurst, 1961). Activity theory stresses the need for older adults to maintain active involvement and to augment and replace activities to assure continued satisfaction and mental well-being (Pikunas, 1969). Older adults age favorably if they remain active, cope with major life losses, and find meaningful replacement activities for those relinquished. Generally, older adults have the same psycho-social needs as middle aged adults, with the exception of biological and health related changes (Havighurst, 1961).

As older people age, however, activity levels may decrease with restrictive opportunities for interpersonal pursuits. Life satisfaction tends to be greater when physical and mental health states are sound (Maddox, 1965). People limited in activities of daily living, access to community services and vocational opportunities are least likely to report feeling satisfied and fulfilled (Smith, 1972). Psychogeriatric patients are frequently faced with the dual burden of coping with a major psychiatric disorder, while attempting to adapt to physical changes and limitations. Skills in carrying out activities of daily living, working or volunteering at a relatively satisfying job, enjoying avocational and creative pursuits, and relating interpersonally are frequently impaired amongst psychiatric patients (Mosey, 1970).

The overall goal of psychiatric rehabilitation is to promote patient satisfaction and provide learning opportunities for the skills necessary to accomplish tasks of everyday living (Fidler, 1984). The necessary components for a meaningful activity program for older adults with psychiatric illness are sensory stimulation and reality orientation for the cognitively impaired or severely regressed; remotivation for patients who are socially withdrawn and alienated from their surroundings but capable of coherent interactions and able to perform graded simple tasks; complex and challenging activities for those whose social and functional skills are relatively intact; [and] transitional activities or volunteer work to meet the needs of those returning home with community responsibilities (Weiner, 1978).

Following initial assessments of their needs, capabilities, and wishes for rehabilitation, patients are referred for individual or group treatment. This process encourages skill development and incremental progress toward attainment of individualized activity goals that are vital to the well being of the elderly patient.

Assessments

Comprehensive assessments are the cornerstone of psychosocial treatment in the geriatric division. These assessments help determine assets and liabilities in cognition, interpersonal skills, task performance, physical ability, leisure and social involvement and utilization of community resources. The assessments guide treatment, maximize individualized interventions and promote programming that is responsive to the expressed interests of each patient.

The rehabilitation process is initiated (within a few days of admission), when the Therapeutic Activities Representative meets with the patient and engages him/her in a planning dialogue. The Rehabilitation Activity Assessment helps determine the patient's overall goals in self-care, work, and leisure and elicits participation in identifying and prioritizing skills and behaviors needed to attain their goals. Patients who have the cognitive skills to participate meaningfully in this process value this tool as it promotes participation in a rehabilitation plan that is self-generated. This model gives patients the opportunity to identify goals, determine needed skills, select methods for skill acquisition and augment or modify their goals in relationship to their ongoing performance.

Sometimes the patients are seriously cognitively impaired, or too psychiatrically ill to realistically determine their goals and needs. In these cases, the Therapeutic Activity Representative provides assistance in referring to groups and recommending discharge plans that are consistent with their needs for support.

Consistent application of this initial dialogue with geriatric patients has generated some common rehabilitation goals and skills needed to achieve the goals. Individual and group treatment that reflects the patient's priority needs in self-care, work or leisure and focuses on their level of functioning have been conceptualized with regard to the patient's expressed interest for rehabilitation.

Self-care treatment generally focuses on skills needed for the patient to manage in [his or her] living environment following discharge. Treatment in the leisure category addresses the skills needed for the patient to spend free time qualitatively. Treatment in the work category focuses on skills needed to resume paid employment or acquire a volunteer job. Some common examples of overall rehabilitation goals and required skills in these areas are as follows.

Self-Care Rehabilitation Goals

1. I will go to a nursing home when I am discharged from the hospital.
2. I want to move to my daughter's house when I leave the hospital.
3. I want to return home to my apartment when I am discharged from the hospital.

Skills:

- identifying self-care strengths and weaknesses
- improving attention to hygiene
- following schedule
- improving nutritional awareness
- managing money
- accepting help from a home health aide
- managing transportation
- cooking and meal planning
- expressing opinions
- tolerating others
- improving confidence
- expressing satisfaction
- following routine
- researching residences

Leisure Rehabilitation Goals

1. I want to participate in the activity program at the nursing home when I am discharged.
2. I want to find people to play bridge with in my location when I leave the hospital.
3. I want to join a senior center when I leave the hospital.

Skills:

- clarifying current and past leisure interests
- enriching or renewing leisure interests
- improving skill in a leisure activity
- finding community leisure options
- increasing confidence and independence in using community resources
- initiating leisure involvements
- initiating contacts with peers

Work Rehabilitation Goals

1. I want to be productive in my nursing home environment.
2. I want to find a volunteer job in the community when I leave the hospital.
3. I want to find paid employment in the community when I leave the hospital.

Skills:

- clarifying work/volunteer history and aspirations
- identifying concerns regarding retirement
- improving awareness of post-retirement options
- accepting supervision in the work setting
- increasing willingness to accept challenge and responsibility in work setting
- working cooperatively with others
- organizing tasks
- increasing productivity in tasks
- exploring community services
- interviewing for job
- identifying work related skills

The described assessment and planning dialogue almost always signals a need for additional assessments to supplement, validate or help patients measure the congruence between their goals, assets and liabilities.

The SHORT-CARE (Comprehensive Assessment and Referral Evaluation) (Gurland, 1984) is often used to gather additional functional information. The SHORT-CARE discourages reliance on typical symptoms only for resolution of psychiatric illness. It encourages a probing look at the etiology of specific areas of psychosocial dysfunction. This standardized, multidimensional semi-structured interview provides clinicians with scales for depression, dementia, and disability. The SHORT-CARE assists therapists in becoming more cognizant of each patient's individual needs for rehabilitation and aftercare.

Patients are also assessed with the Activities Health Assessment. This tool provides both therapists and patients with information about time management, involvement in meaningful activities, and discharge planning.

Finally, patients are constantly assessed and observed while participating in functional activities. They have opportunities to critique their own performance while receiving feedback about the specific skills needed to attain their overall rehabilitation goal.

Program Description

The primary objective of activity rehabilitation in geriatrics is to help each patient identify [his or her] specific goals and needed skills in self-care, leisure and work. Because the therapeutic activity professionals recognize the broad range of dysfunction, there is commitment to meeting individual needs. The program and the therapists are highly flexible while maintaining a core structure that provides stability. This is accomplished by offering groups that closely parallel the expected plans for the individual's discharge environment. It is also accomplished by expecting the therapist to individualize treatment within the context of the group. For example, in a verbal group, one patient may be working on expressing opinions, while another patient might be working on the acquisition of listening skills because they are dominant interrupters. A moderately demented patient might cook in a group with patients preparing for discharge because they have maintained a skill in that one area.

Groups are generally organized with regard for the patient's functional status and need for different amounts of support. This assures successful involvements while challenging the patient to continually use skills that have been neglected.

After assessments are completed, findings are collected and analyzed. The patients are then referred to groups that can provide them with skill acquisition that they, or the therapist, have determined as essential for success in their discharge environment. Patients are given large print schedules with a detailed description of groups. The schedules have a space for the therapist and patient to list the specific skills requiring attention within the context of each group. Since each group has a clearly defined protocol, therapists are aware of the specific guidelines and objectives for that group. As an example, the Leisure Planning Protocol is described in Table 1.

Table 1. Leisure Planning Protocol

Days: M-W-F   **Time:** 1:30 - 2:45 pm

Problems
1. Patient unable to identify leisure interests.

2. Patient unable to independently plan or participate in meaningful activities.

3. Patient is unaware of leisure resources or how to access these services in the community.

Short Term Goals
1. Patient will identify one or two interests within the group.
2. Patient will cooperatively plan and participate in one community activity per week with peers on the unit.
3. Patient will call two or three community resources per week to heighten awareness of available programs.

Long Term Goals
1. Patient will commit to two-three community based activities based on identified interests.

2. Patient will initiate suggestions and plans for weekly community outing.

3. Patient will develop a resource file of meaningful activites in the community prior to discharge.

Interventions
1. *Identifying Leisure Interests*
Leader provides leisure interest finders and value surveys to encourage identification and exploration of interests.
2. *Planning*
Leader encourages group to cooperatively identify and plan one community activity. Patients utilize resource file to make arrangements and calls.
3. *Implementation*
Leader accompanies group on the community trip. Patients secure names on mailing lists and independently seek out information for their involvement.

Each program cluster (self-care, work and leisure) has groups that respond to the requirement for maximum, moderate or minimum levels of support. As patients improve or plateau they are encouraged to participate in increasingly challenging activities. Examples of the program are provided to illustrate how assessment findings are applied to the level of support needed in group treatment.

Group Structure Offering Maximum Support

Patient Population

This population is quite regressed due to depression, chronic schizophrenia, or dementia, and is moderately to severely cognitively impaired. They are alert, but frequently disoriented. If their level of function remains the same throughout hospitalization, these patients are usually discharged to an institutional facility, or return home with significant home care, and a structured day program.

Self-Care

Assistance and encouragement is needed in all activities of daily living, and patients are unable to follow simple 1-2 step directions. Decisions do not show good judgement and supervision is required to maintain safety. These are patients who have a limited investment in how they look, how they spend their time, and often deny, minimize or overlook difficulties.

Self-Care Skills:
- Following simple directions while grooming
- Eating independently
- Dressing with minimal cuing and encouragement
- Finding room on the unit
- Using notes to compensate for memory problems

Leisure

Activity participation is limited. They cannot generate interests or skills, and require constant encouragement and stimulation to remain engaged in purposeful activity. They minimally communicate with each other, and are withdrawn and isolative.

Leisure Skills:
- Attempting an adapted version of an activity from the past
- Tolerating the presence of others
- Initiating and completing a task within one group setting

Work

Patients are unable to work productively in organizing tasks to completion. They are easily frustrated and have no tolerance for stress. Difficulties sequencing logical steps in an organized manner are noted.

Work Skills:
- Asking for clarification or assistance
- Maintaining participation in task activities for 15 minute periods
- Sequencing simple steps in a logical order
- Following simple directions

Activity groups organized for this population illustrate ways to engage the seriously regressed geriatric population. The severely regressed begin each day with sensory stimulation and exercise. Old familiar show tunes lead even the most regressed patient through pleasurable movements. Balloon volleyball ends this daily session with increased alertness and heightened sensitivity to the environment.

Simple repetitive tasks are provided to encourage basic responsibility for one's immediate environment. Examples of volunteer jobs on the unit include folding laundry, ringing meal bell, dusting tables, and changing tablecloths. Jobs are listed weekly on the unit bulletin board, with the patient's name, and cuing is provided consistently by the inter-disciplinary team.

Many strategies of an adaptive function model are incorporated in the remotivation group. Modalities utilized to increase socialization, and sensitivity to the immediate environment are memory games, elder trivia, reminiscent slide shows, pet therapy, nature outings, murals, improvisation, and simple baking.

For the more regressed, individual work includes sensory stimulation, and in some cases holding stuffed animals has been therapeutic.

Group Structure Offering Moderate Support

Patient Population

This population represents those older adults with partial symptom resolution following biological, milieu, activity and counseling therapies. As patients improve, they need new challenges. Although they are alert and oriented, they may be mildly cognitively impaired, and still depressed. If their condition remains stable, they are usually discharged to a senior residence, or home with senior day treatment. Moderate support is required because the therapist must organize components of their projects, while encouraging greater self-reliance amongst group members. The leader encourages interaction, and promotes opportunities for group feedback, but must continue to be the facilitator.

Self-Care

Although needing help with problem solving, most can perform activities of daily living with minimal assistance. They are able to recognize areas of difficulty and may begin to ask for help and feedback.

Self-Care Skills:

- Following activity schedule independently
- Participating in meal planning and preparation
- Making bed
- Cleaning bedroom
- Organizing datebook with telephone numbers and appointments

Leisure

Interest and motivation for leisure involvements is inconsistent. They initiate activities within structured settings, but not outside of group opportunities. These are people who have difficulty asking peers to join them for a casual activity or conversation. They are dependent on a group leader for initiating interaction, and rarely generate involvement independently.

Leisure Skills:

- Setting up supplies needed for a group activity
- Attending all scheduled activities
- Identifying interests to pursue upon discharge

Work

Patients derive genuine pleasure from involvement in work-related projects, or commitments that improve the lives of others. They continue to rely on [the] group leader for directions and instructions to follow-through on tasks appropriately.

Work Skills:

- Identifying ways to remain committed to meaningful work-related activity
- Improving investment in quality of work
- Increasing confidence in familiar tasks

Patients in this phase of treatment are expected to be familiar with unit and activity routines. They often begin their day with discussion of current events, and are encouraged to bring at least one or more topics of interest to the group. This intervention provides them with a non-threatening way to participate in discussions.

Often patients demonstrate increased independence by participating in a cooking group. By making snacks for their unit, and initiating luncheons for peers, family members, staff or guests, they begin to regain confidence in a wide range of skills. A leisure skills group provides an opportunity to get acquainted with peers who share similar interests. Group leaders facilitate opportunities for patients who value bridge, Scrabble™, shuffleboard, [etc.] to know one another and make commitments. This is important for those who will return to a center, because they will be expected to initiate and join social activities.

Finally, exposure to volunteer activity is popular at this phase of treatment. Community service projects help patients move outside themselves and offer something to others. This group has frequently made and contributed toys to homeless children, participated in clerical tasks needed for fund raising events, maintained bulletin boards, designed advertisement flyers and contributed information to the patients' newsletter. The leader usually needs to provide tasks, direction and encouragement.

Group Structure Offering Minimum Support

Patient Population

This group is approaching discharge and has resolved a major depressive disorder. After a major depression has been treated with medication, maladaptive behaviors are often apparent. Patients continue to struggle with dependency; helplessness; anger over losses; and poor coping mechanisms. They can use insight oriented experiences to understand maladaptive patterns and initiate and practice alternate coping mechanisms. This population generally returns home with a clearly defined plan to pursue for community involvement. The therapist encourages increased leadership and opportunities for problem solving by operationalizing decisions made within the group, and helping members to see the carryover process. Although they are cognitively intact and usually physically healthy, they frequently have lifelong difficulties with adaptation, making and keeping friends, and interacting meaningfully in the community. They need careful individualized programs to help compensate for life-long problems reaching out for help.

Self-Care

Any limitations in activities of daily living are minimized because of fears of dependency. They struggle with issues of interdependence, and lack the ability to comfortably ask for help. Familiar tasks, like cooking or balancing a checkbook, are resisted because of anxiety or lack of familiarity with the task (following the death of a spouse). Some self-care tasks may be difficult due to dependency and anxiety.

Self-Care Skills:

- Planning and ordering food for meals
- Arranging transportation for passes
- Practicing asking for help
- Identifying strengths in self-care

Leisure

Although motivated and interested in meaningful activities, they need encouragement and support to participate in new or challenging activities. They are quite anxious about engaging in community outings and returning home.

Leisure Skills:
- Identifying activities to pursue upon discharge
- Participating in a few community outings per week
- Planning and arranging details for community based activities
- Asking peers to participate in unstructured activities
- Initiating meaningful activities during unstructured time

Work

They are motivated to translate interests into community service or employment. These skills are practiced while hospitalized and only assistance with major decisions is needed.

Work Skills:
- Identifying specific volunteer/paid employment interests
- Practicing skills needed for expected job
- Exploring community options for work
- Arranging details and interviews
- Identifying strengths and deficits

This population is approaching discharge to the community following treatment for a major depression. Generally, they have reacquired essential concrete skills, but maladaptive behaviors may resurface or continue to be apparent as the patient faces discharge without the intense support [he or she] had during hospitalization. Struggles with dependency, anger over losses, fears of incompetence and interpersonal problems are highlighted as expectations for more challenging functioning are indicated. Essential in this phase of treatment are opportunities to verbally express concerns and get support, but shift emphasis away from the activity therapist and toward themselves and others. Counseling groups that focus on increased autonomy, choice, and responsibility are introduced along with more challenging activities. These interventions help patients to identify concerns, explore coping strategies and practice activities designed to rekindle feelings of competence and worthwhileness.

The Leisure Planning Group is a three part group that helps older adults identify interests, community events, and plan a weekly community outing. An extensive file of community resources is available. Group participants are expected to make appropriate calls and arrangements.

Goals Group uses activity and cognitive therapy models to empower and assist in re-gaining some control and mastery of life tasks. The action oriented verbal-task group stresses exploration of coping and problem solving skills, emphasizes collaborative involvement and encourages goal directed activity that alters the person's role from that of subordinate to peer group member responsible to themselves and others. Homework is given and participants are encouraged to practice specific strategies to optimize their independence in preparation for discharge.

To practice better communicating strategies with their grandchildren, an intergenerational meal group was established in collaboration with hospitalized adolescents. An older adult patient was matched with an adolescent to foster and learn appropriate interactive strategies to carryover at home. The dyads inter-changed responsibilities for meal planning, and each dyad assumed responsibility for the preparation of specific components of the meal. Older patients used past meal planning skills, while practicing appropriate interactive styles necessary for healthy relationships at home.

For those patients who have work as a priority goal, Vocational Services provides them with opportunities for volunteer jobs throughout the hospital. The placement is viewed as a vital reality testing tool. Examples of volunteer jobs used by hospitalized older adults have included a plant operations director volunteering in the hospital maintenance department, a retired secretary volunteering as a research librarian, and a knitting teacher volunteering as an instructor with older and younger long term patients.

Conclusion

The geriatric psycho-social rehabilitation program has become well regarded and integrated into the fabric of comprehensive, multi-disciplinary treatment.

Initial and ongoing assessment assure that the patient is continually being evaluated so that [his or her] treatment is specific and relevant to changing needs. Well designed groups and flexible group leaders guarantee a structure that is perceived as stable, while being responsive to the unique needs of each patient.

The Geriatric Therapeutic Activities staff's distinct contribution in clinical rounds has impacted upon all disciplines planning for treatment, family therapy and discharge. The patients report valuing the program because it gives them the varied opportunities and support they need to meet the challenges of growing older with dignity and purpose.

References

Cumming, E., Henry, W. (1961). *Growing old: the process of disengagement.* New York: Basic Books.

Fidler, G. S. (1984). *Design of rehabilitation services in psychiatric hospital settings.* Laurel, MD: RAMSCO Publishing.

Gurland, B., Golden, R. G., Teresi, J. A., Challop, J. (1984). The SHORT-CARE: An efficient instrument for the assessment of depression, dementia and disability. *Journal of Gerontology,* Vol. 39, No. 2, pp. 166-169.

Havighurst, R. J. (1961). Successful aging. *Gerontologist,* Vol. 1, pp. 8-13.

Havighurst, R. J., Neugarten, B. L., Tobin, S. S. (1968). Disengagement and patterns of aging. In B. L. Neugarten (Ed.) *Middle age and Aging,* Illinois: University of Chicago Press, pp. 161-172.

Maddox, G. L. (1965). Fact and artifact: evidence bearing on the disengagement theory from the Duke Geriatrics Project. *Human Development,* Vol. 8, pp. 117-130.

Mosey, A. C. (1970). *Three frames of reference for mental health.* New Jersey: Charles B. Slack, Inc.

Pikunas, J. (1969). *Human development: an emergent science.* New York: McGraw Hill.

Smith, J. J., Lipman, A. (1972). Constraint and life satisfaction. *Journal of Gerontology,* pp. 77-82.

Weiner, M. B., Brok, A. J., Snadowsky, A. M. (1978). *Working with the aged.* New Jersey: Prentice-Hall, Inc.

Chapter 36

Occupational Therapy Approaches to Treatment of Dementia Patients

Karen Crane Macdonald, MS, OTR/L

The dementias are now recognized as prevalent disorders which affect multiple areas of physical and psychosocial functioning. Statistics which identify Alzheimer's disease as the fourth leading cause of death (Clark, 1984), and as the primary diagnosis of at least one half of institutionalized long term care patients (U. S. Dept. of Health and Human Services, 1984) have provided the impetus for health professionals to more closely examine these diseases.

In the past five years, an explosion of literature has been published which examines possible etiologies of Alzheimer's disease, discusses diagnostic procedures, describes current research, and explores support strategies for caregivers (which include family and staff members). There is less literature which responds to the frequent question, "Isn't there something we can DO for Mrs. Smith?" This question implies that beyond the provision of basic care and assurance of safety, the dementia victim has additional needs which relate to the quality of life. The occupational therapist is a professional who can assess, plan, and provide intervention for these important needs.

Within this paper, the generic term dementia will be used to represent the variety of diagnostic labels which include Alzheimer's disease, multi-infarct dementia, primary degenerative dementia, organic brain syndrome, and cerebral atrophy. The author realizes that the etiologies for these various types of dementia are dissimilar, but is focusing upon the similar sequelae of these diseases which result in decreased functional abilities.

Role of the Occupational Therapist

Dementia victims present symptoms of decreased skill in the cognitive, motor, sensory integrative, social, and psychological areas of functioning. These areas of dysfunction affect occupational performance in self care, work, and leisure (Mosey, 1981, and Hurff, 1984). All of these areas of dysfunction are within occupational therapy's traditional domain. Because of the progressive nature of dementia, the occupational therapy process emphasizes maintenance and preventive intervention, with lesser emphasis upon restorative treatment.

The occupational therapist may be involved in intervention in a variety of settings where dementia victims may be patients or clients. These settings include long term care facilities, convalescent facilities, general hospitals, adult day care programs, senior centers, and home care.

This paper will present clinical information related to the role of the occupational therapist in working with dementia victims. Following [a] brief reference to assessment, three areas for intervention will be discussed: activities, environment, and communication. These three areas are important considerations in all aspects of care of the dementia victim, and will be discussed here in reference to occupational therapy treatment.

Assessment

The occupational therapist may utilize standardized and non-standardized tools to assess a patient's functional status. Evaluations may be performed on an individual patient, or on a group of patients (for example, to determine level of social skills). The reader is referred to Kane and Kane, *Assessing the Elderly*, for a full description of assessment techniques. In general, the occupational therapist must be aware of sensory impairments, especially visual and auditory, which may compound confusion. Observation of these deficits, when demonstrated by performance in occupational therapy, should be referred to other appropriate sources for examination.

Activities

Following an assessment which determines the type(s) and degree of functional impairment, the occupational therapist selects, analyzes, and applies purposeful activities as primary treatment modalities. The patient's interests should be considered as an integral aspect of the treatment planning.

Activity analysis is an essential prerequisite which serves to determine the appropriateness of selected activities. General considerations in planning group activities for dementia victims include selection of tasks which are structured, concrete and short term in nature, offer the opportunity for positive reinforcement, are adaptable for grading the level of difficulty, and promote interpersonal contact. Additional factors to consider include the activity's demand in terms of energy, frustration tolerance, neatness, creativity, and also therapist preparation.

Other elements of the activity analysis include attention to sensory components, and the desire to offer stimulation, yet avoid bombardment which may increase the patient's confusion or agitation. Although a patient's level of functioning may be low, the therapist seeks to avoid activities which are infantile in appearance, or which foster regression. For most patients, the best tasks

are those which are repetitive in nature, do not have multiple steps, and are conducive to both verbal and demonstrated instructions.

Concrete end products are especially meaningful, and serve as evidence to family and staff members of existing abilities, remaining skills, and strengths. The therapist must maintain flexibility and creativity when planning and implementing activities, because apraxia and limited attention span often influence the patient's task performance.

Depending upon the therapeutic setting and the overall patient population, individual and/or group therapy may be indicated. The emphasis here is upon the "ideal" group of four to eight patients, all of whom are functioning at a similar level of ability.

A number of verbal and activity group approaches have enjoyed varied popularity in the last decade. These include reality orientation (Taulbee and Folsom, 1968 [*sic*]), resocialization and remotivation (Burnside, 1976), validation therapy (Feil, 1982), movement therapy (Sandel, 1978), reminiscing, music therapy (Batcheller, 1972 and Bright, 1972), art therapy, exercise, and activity groups. The author has used the majority of these approaches, and generally finds an eclectic approach with goal oriented purposeful activities to be most effective.

Depending on the level of functional ability of the group members, activities are selected to enhance particular occupational performance components. In determining patient level of functioning, Reisberg (Reisberg, 1984) defines seven specific categories of cognitive ability and dysfunction. Categories one and two describe normal cognitive functioning or minimal impairment. Categories three and four have clinical manifestations such as difficulty with abstract concepts, decreased understanding, denial, forgetfulness, and avoidance of unfamiliar situations or tasks. Categories five and six are manifested by decreased judgement, awareness and planning, increased disorientation and memory loss, and difficulty with self care. Category seven patients have minimal speech, motor skills, or awareness.

The author has grouped Reisberg's categories to identify three levels of activity groups for occupational therapy intervention. The groups address the needs of patients falling within categories three through seven, inclusive. The categories or levels will be described separately with category three/four the highest level of functioning, and category seven the lowest.

Category Three/Four

Motor

Exercises: Incorporate imitation of postures and identification of body parts to reinforce existing skills, touching other members, and choices of props such as: theraband, dowel or towel, scarves, hula hoops, parachute with ball, long plastic (garden type) link chain. Creative movement with music and imagery are also popular and successful methods to encourage full active range of motion.

Table tasks: Discrimination games or puzzles which identify: size, shape, color, number, textures, two versus three dimensions, directionality and laterality. Sorting tasks and peg board type activities are also tolerated well.

Games: Ring toss, bean bag, adapted bingo, pokeno, basketball, bowling, and horse races are recreational activities which promote a host of physical and emotional responses (Hamill, 1980). Other recreational/leisure pursuits may include gardening, baking, dancing, sing-alongs, puppetry, and pet visitation.

Arts and Crafts: Painting, collage, clay, printing, yarn projects (wrapping and braiding), mosaics, woodworking, weaving, stuffing and sewing, cutting paper for projects, and leather work.

Verbal

Current events, modified trivia-like memory games, complex reality orientation concepts, poetry writing, reminiscing, group story telling, and focused discussion.

Activities of Daily Living/Self Care

Discussion, demonstration, and practice with simulated or actual devices and utensils. May focus on separate areas of meal preparation, grooming, home management, or dressing. Emphasis is upon temporal adaptation and approaches for labelling, sequencing, and/or adapting self care devices and techniques.

Category Five/Six

Motor

Gross (exercises) and fine (table task) activities are graded for simplicity from category three/four, requiring a lesser degree of decision making and problem solving.

Verbal

Reality orientation with more extensive visual aids, word games, expression of feelings, story telling, poetry reading, and resocialization.

Sensory

Stimulation through activities, props, and related discussion of visual, auditory, and olfactory senses.

Category Seven

The emphasis is upon prevention of total regression. Some passive involvement in verbal or activity groups may be possible along with the activities below.

Sensory

Tactile: Nylon netting balls, vibrator, lotion, touch, hugging.

Visual: Ball, lights, colors, movement.

Auditory: Noisemakers, handclapping, music.

Gustatory: Ice water, cookies.

Olfactory: Coffee, clove, cinnamon, potpourri, perfume.

Vestibular: Slow rocking movements.

Kinesthetic: Passing weighted objects.

For categories three through seven, Ross suggests five stages for structuring an individual group session (1981):

1. Opening and orientation: an alerting activity which welcomes members.
2. Movement activities: elicit bodily response.
3. Perceptual motor activity: facilitate integration of senses.
4. Cognitive stimulation: verbal activity for "cool down" period.
5. Resolution and termination: close session with review, refreshments, and positive reinforcement.

Overall approaches to groupwork with dementia patients would also include consideration of stages of group development and group process issues.

Environment

There are a myriad of elements in the dementia patient's nonhuman environment and physical surroundings that the occupational therapist must assess. The non-human environment is defined as factors which influence behavior such as time of day, sensory stimulation, and objects in the surrounding environment. These factors are discussed separately from physical surroundings, which refer more to architectural and safety considerations.

A. The Non-Human Environment

For the patient with dementia, every incoming stimulus may result in an unpredictable effect, depending on a variety of influences which may not be readily observable by the untrained person. Three elements of the non-human environment, time, sensory stimulation, and objects will be discussed briefly.

Time

Dementia victims are influenced by circadian rhythms, as are all people. Alertness levels tend to be higher in the mid-morning, followed by a slow, drowsy period following lunch, and increased energy and activity in the late afternoon. The entire period preceding dinner until bedtime is an unpredictable period in which "sundowning phenomena" may exist. This is characterized by increased wandering, agitation, and calling out. In facilities where change of shift occurs, there may also be a time-influenced period of confusion and agitation.

Because dementia victims are generally confused about time, multiple cues are necessary to reinforce accurate interpretation of the time of day. To encourage awareness of time, and to capitalize upon patient cycles of alertness, the occupational therapist may be involved in selecting visual time cues and activity schedules for the patients. Time cues include large print clocks and calendars, printed and accessible activity schedules, and attention to the patient's watch bearing the correct time. When windows are available, opened curtains may demonstrate light or dark for the patient who has confusion related to reversal of day and night.

Repeated reference to time issues during activity and verbal groups are helpful to alleviate anxiety about time. In day care centers, "going home anxiety" is often demonstrated by repeated questions about time. In this situation, a planned transitional activity helps to prevent anxiety which quickly escalates if not dealt with appropriately.

Sensory stimulation

The occupational therapist helps to identify and maintain a balance between prevention of sensory deprivation and prevention of sensory bombardment. Generally, the occupational therapist may act as a patient advocate in interpreting reactions to sensory stimuli. Some possible influences upon patient behavior are described below.

Visual: Bright colors and frenzied motion may excite a patient. Objects utilized in activities of self care tasks should be readily identified, with special consideration to figure ground difficulties (Powell, 1983).

Tactile: Surfaces and objects should be safe in nature. Certain textures may be perceived as irritating, for example, a patient who refuses to wear a terry cloth robe. Physical contact, through gentle touch, hand holding, and hugging, is especially beneficial for the isolated or withdrawn individual.

Auditory: Patients may have difficulty with auditory figure ground, and become increasingly confused and disoriented when attempting to discriminate between a variety of volumes and noises such as voices, buzzers, alarms, telephones, and cleaning machines. The occupational therapist may act as an observer for monitoring the levels of preventable noise. The occupational therapist may also act with other team members to explore auditory or visual hallucinations. One patient, for example, who "suffered from hallucinations" of hearing voices in the walls was actually reacting to her roommate's intercom system.

Gustatory: The occupational therapist may serve as a role model to nurse aides by assisting with meals and engaging in food related conversation with the patient. The food may be identified and described (especially if chopped or pureed), with reminders of the name of the meal and time. The occupational therapist may also work with dietary and nursing staff to identify foods that consistently evoke negative or positive responses.

Olfactory: Certain pleasing or noxious odors may elicit responses. The occupational therapist may work with the patient to eliminate odors which evoke negative reactions, for example, a particular brand of shampoo or soap.

Objects

Objects in the environment often have symbolic value for patients which the occupational therapist may explore with the patient and family members. Certain objects (a favorite sweater) may be comforting, whole other objects (a commode) may elicit distress. The therapist may assist in determining the cause of the distress, and can assist in attempts to alleviate the distress.

B. The Physical Environment

The physical environment is also evaluated and modified to assure safety and ease in functioning. The dementia patient may easily "get lost" in his or her own environment (Powell, 1983). When relocating to a different room, unit, or facility, the patient demonstrates increased confusion and disorientation which the occupational therapist may identify and work through with the patient (Rabins & Mace, 1981). General considerations for the assessment of the physical environment are listed below.

Overall environment: Color, light, sounds, safety, privacy, constancy, carpeting, mirrors (may confuse), temperature, clutter and swallowable objects, clocks, and areas designated solely for activity (versus dining area).

Patient's room: Homelike, familiar objects, accessible furniture, items and pictures labelled, lighting, radio or television functioning, rugs on floor, no objects resembling toilets (garbage receptacles), calendar, large print name sign on door, roommate compatibility.

Bathroom: Accessible towels and toilet paper, familiar looking faucets (non-modern), absence of razors and poisonous sprays and liquids, rubber mat in tub, handrails if needed.

Kitchen: Labels on cabinets, sharp items removed, stove knobs removed if patient is no longer capable of cooking, cleaning substances are locked away.

Living room or solarium: Comfortable, soil resistant chair upholstery, round or curved edged tables, electrical cords are fastened down or concealed.

Hallway: Avoidance of glare, lack of confusing patterned designs on floor, wandering area available, entrance and exits may be locked and/or disguised to prevent unsupervised exit.

The occupational therapist is particularly sensitive to the importance of the environment upon the dementia patient's functioning. It is important to communicate these influences to primary caregivers on an ongoing basis. The environment should also be reassessed as the patient's levels of functioning change over time.

Communication

When working with dementia patients, the occupational therapist uses a variety of consciously selected communication techniques. The therapist must be aware of the patients' and also her own characteristic modalities of communication. These include both verbal and non-verbal (tactile, visual, tone, volume, and proximity) messages. It is especially important to anticipate how the patient perceives messages. For example, a patient may perceive certain types of touch as seductive, irritating, or pleasant.

General approaches for communication with dementia victims include speaking slowly and clearly and using direct statements. If a patient does not understand, the therapist should repeat the message before rephrasing, as this may only confuse the person. The therapist should face the patient, and speak directly to him or her, not over the heads of others. The therapist should be prepared to spend time in speaking with the dementia patient, who is often aphasic and has great difficulty expressing a thought or need. It is recommended that questions that start with "Wh", such as why, what, where, when, and who be avoided, as the cognitively impaired may have difficulty processing the answer and become frustrated (Gugel, 1984). It is helpful to use closed ended questions with the more impaired dementia patient. It is also wise to avoid demanding or ordering a patient, rather the command should be phrased as a request. Whenever possible, the use of demonstration of a desired response is preferable to simply telling the patient what is expected of him.

Patients with dementia demonstrate a variety of behaviors which may be extremely trying for all caregivers. These behaviors include repetitiveness, withdrawal, sexual expressiveness, monopolizing, agitation, and attention seeking. Although each behavior requires unique approaches, responses which are generally effective include kind firmness, positive regard for the patient as a person, and redirection. Redirection is the most frequently utilized approach, where the therapist diverts the patient's attention from one behavior, and focuses upon another topic or object. In using this approach, the therapist must assess what need the patient is trying to express, and respond with an alternate suggestion related to the underlying need.

The occupational therapist may take an active role in serving as an advocate and interpreter for a patient. Aphasia and poor impulse or emotional controls may cause a dementia patient to say things that are highly offensive to family, staff, or peers. The therapist should reinforce the idea that the patient is not responsible for these undesirable behaviors, and cannot necessarily control [his or her] speech or actions.

The foregoing material reflects techniques of direct intervention offered by the occupational therapist. In the application of these techniques and approaches, the therapist often works cooperatively with nurses, aides, social workers, recreation staff, music therapists, physical therapists, dieticians, speech pathologists, and family members in collaboration with physicians and psychiatrists.

Summary

This paper presented practical, clinical issues related to intervention with dementia patients. The scope of the paper did not permit full attention to occupational therapy assessment techniques or evaluation of treatment programs. The occupational therapist may offer valuable intervention in a variety of settings, while serving in differing capacities, including consultation and education. Considering the devastating impact dementia has upon victims and their families, the occupational therapist has an important role in the provision of services which contribute to the patient's continued quality of life.

References

Batcheller, J., & Monsour, S. (1972). *Music in recreation and leisure.* Dubuque, Iowa: Wm. Brown Co. Pub.

Bright, R. (1972). *Music in geriatric care.* Australia: Angus and Robertson Musicgraphics.

Burnside, I. M. (1976). *Nursing and the aged.* New York: McGraw-Hill.

Clark, M. et al. (1984, December). A slow death of the mind. *Newsweek*, pp. 56-62.

Feil, N. (1982). *Validation—the Feil method: How to help the disoriented old-old.* Cleveland, OH: Feil Productions.

Gugel, R. (1984, June). *Communication with dementia patients.* Workshop presented for Aging in America, Sturbridge, Mass.

Hamill, C. M. & Oliver, R. C. (1980). *Therapeutic activities for the handicapped elderly.* Rockville, MD: Aspen.

Hurff, J. M. (1984). Visualization: a decision-making tool for assessment and treatment planning. *Occup. Therapy in Health Care.* 1(2) 6.

Kane, R. A. & Kane, R. L. (1981). *Assessing the elderly: A practical guide to measurement.* Lexington, MA: Lexington Books.

Mosey, A. C. (1981). *Occupational therapy: configuration of a profession.* New York: Raven Press.

Powell, L. S. & Courtice, K. (1983). *Alzheimer's disease: a guide for families.* Reading, MA: Addison-Wesley Pub.

Rabins, P. & Mace, N. L. (1981). *The 36 hour day.* Baltimore, MD: Johns Hopkins Press.

Reisberg, B. (1984). Stages of cognitive decline. *Am. J. of Nursing,* Feb, 225-228.

Ross, M. & Burdick, D. (1981). Sensory integration: *A training manual for therapists and teachers for regressed, psychiatric, and geriatric patient groups.* Thorofare, NJ: Slack Co.

Sandel, S. L. (1978). Reminiscence in movement therapy with the aged. *Art Psychotherapy, 5,* 217-221.

Taulbee, L. & Folsom, J. (1966). Reality orientation for geriatric patients. *Hospital and Community Psychiatry, 17,* 133-135.

U. S. Dept. of Health and Human Services. (1984). *Progress report on Alzheimer's disease* (DHHS Publication No. 84-2500). Wash, DC: U. S. Government Printing Office.

Section IV

Humanistic Approaches in Mental Health: The Patient Perspective

Introduction

Occupational therapy is a caring profession. Caring is firmly rooted in our historical heritage (Schwartz, 1992), our professional philosophy, and our art of practice (Gilfoyle, 1980; Mosey, 1986). Occupational therapists care by helping people maximize their capabilities, adapt to their losses, and engage in satisfying, productive activities—utilizing their assets and minimizing their limitations (Devereux, 1984; Mosey, 1986). This helping requires a collaborative process between the patient and the therapist. Occupational therapists engage *with* patients, facilitating the patient's ability to do for him- or herself; we do not do things *to* patients (Devereux, 1984; Gilfoyle, 1980). We believe each individual has the capacity to change and grow if given the chance. Our caring, therapeutic relationships are based on a strong foundation of empathy, warmth, respect, and unconditional positive regard for the client. Honesty, trust, hope, and patience are also fundamental to our relationships with patients (Brammer, 1985; Mosey, 1986; Rogers, 1961).

To sustain these relationships, the therapist needs to be self-aware and to maintain competence because therapeutic relationships are not static; rather, they are dynamic, ever-changing growth experiences for both patients and therapist (Brammer, 1985; Hutchins & Cole, 1986; Schulman, 1984). At times these experiences may be confusing, tiring, or overwhelming, but the benefits are worth the effort (Schulman, 1984). These benefits include improved functioning and increased ability to cope with life for the client (Rogers, 1961) and enhanced professional skills and strengthened self-image for the therapist (Brammer, 1985). We often gain as much (or even more) from the process of caring and helping than the client does (Brammer, 1985).

However, for therapists to be able to reap the benefits of this enriching experience, we must actively and continually work on our helping skills. Certification establishes competence in a field of knowledge, but competence must be permeated with caring to have any relevant meaning or lasting effect (King, 1980). The chapters in this section clearly describe the vital role caring, empathetic, helping relationships play in facilitating therapeutic change within patients. Although we cannot truly know the patient's experience, it is hoped that reviewing patient perspectives on therapy will increase awareness, understanding, and empathy for clients, thereby enhancing the readers' helping skills.

Chapter 37, by Turner, provides a strong contrast between helping and non-helping relationships. Turner reflects on her personal experiences as a hospitalized psychiatric patient, which ranged from disastrous, dehumanizing, and hopeless to successful, respectful, and life-affirming. Turner clearly identifies characteristics from both ends of the helping continuum. Her vivid descriptions provide readers with a renewed appreciation of the value of respect, kindness, and collaboration in therapeutic relationships and of the need for well-designed, goal-directed treatment programs.

The patient-therapist relationship is further explored in chapter 38 by Peloquin, who describes the therapeutic relationship in occupational therapy as an "evolving blend of competence and caring." Peloquin examines this relationship from both the viewpoint of the therapist and the perspective of the patient. Professional literature and non-fiction patient accounts are reviewed to identify characteristics of helping relationships. Based on an analysis of this literature, Peloquin presents three types of patient-therapist relationships, with the most therapeutic providing a balance between caring and competence.

The need for a balance between caring and competence in therapeutic relationships is strongly presented in chapter 39 by Leete, who chronicles her 20-year battle with schizophrenia. Leete's personal account describes the characteristics of helping relationships and therapeutic programs that enabled her to maintain hope, accept her illness, and pursue a fulfilling and productive life. Her descriptions of beneficial approaches are highly relevant to occupational therapy practice. Patient education; structured, goal-directed activities; support groups; community residences; vocational training; stress management; and social and independent living skills training are all advocated by Leete as vital for gaining control over one's illness and life. As occupational therapists skilled in these areas, we can work in collaboration with clients to develop their ability to cope with their illnesses and to attain a satisfying quality of life.

Hatfield continues this exploration of coping and adaptation to schizophrenia in chapter 40, which reviews a number of narratives written by patients about their illnesses. Based on these personal accounts, Hatfield identifies four internal sources of stress for persons with schizophrenia. She provides poignant, realistic, first-hand examples for each stressor and identifies coping strategies used by patients in dealing with these stressors. This presentation is highly relevant to occupational therapy, as the identified stressors can have significant functional impact on a person's task, social, and occupational performances. The patients' expressed need for structure and predictability in the external environment is also relevant to the occupational therapist who wants to assist clients in adapting to their illness in a functional manner.

The final chapter in this section presents a research study that is also pertinent to occupational therapists who want to increase their understanding of the patient's perspective of his or her illness. The authors found that individuals with schizophrenia are aware of early warning signs that their illness may be exacerbating, and that almost all of the patients take action to manage these increasing symptoms. The most frequent symptom-management actions employed by this study's sample group were activity-based. Adding new activities, focusing on existing activities, and getting busy were identified adaptive strategies that are relevant to occupational therapy practice in mental health.

The need for occupational therapists to utilize their professional skills to structure the environment, adapt activities, teach functional skills, and provide support in a competent, caring, and collaborative manner with psychiatric clients is strongly validated by the chapters in this section. We have a great deal to offer our clients, and we can be enriched by what they give to us. I hope these readings will facilitate the development of in-creased understanding, empathy, and respect for the patient experience and a renewed commitment to developing therapeutic helping relationships.

In closing, I would like to remind readers that being therapeutic does not equal being perfect. Therapists are human, and all of our therapeutic relationships or interventions will not always be ideal. Sharing our humanity is what is vital to a helping relationship. Perfection is not the goal; mutual growth is. The quote below from Schulman reflects on the benefits of maintaining humanity in a therapeutic relationship. Questions for further consideration follow to facilitate the introspection and self-analysis skills that are essential to developing and maintaining caring, therapeutic relationships.

> Each of us brings our own personal style, artistry, background, feelings, values, beliefs, and so on, to our professional practice. Rather than denying or suppressing these, we need to learn more about ourselves in the context of our practice, and learn to use ourself in pursuit of our professional functions. We will make many mistakes along the way, saying things we will later regret, having to apologize to clients, learning from these mistakes, correcting them, and then making more sophisticated mistakes. In other words, we will be real people carrying out difficult jobs as best we can, rather than paragons of virtue who present an image of perfection.
>
> As we demonstrate to our clients our humanness, vulnerability, willingness to risk, spontaneity, honesty, and our lack of defensiveness (or defensiveness for which we later apologize), we will be modeling the very behaviors we hope to see in our clients. Thus, when workers or students ask me: "Should I be professional or should I be myself?", I reply that the dualism implied in the question does not exist. They must be themselves if they are going to be professional. Fortunately, we have the whole of our professional lives to learn how to effect the synthesis. (Schulman, 1984, p. 15)

Questions to Consider

1. What are my needs to be helpful? What motivates me to engage in therapeutic relationships? How do I benefit from this process?
2. What are my helping strengths? What can I uniquely offer a client?
3. What are my values and beliefs? My sociocultural background? How do these influence my ability to help others?
4. What are my helping limitations? Are there clients or topics that make me feel uncomfortable or vulnerable? How do I handle these feelings therapeutically?
5. Do I look for strengths and assets in clients, as well as for their problems and limitations? How

do I relate assessments to my clients?

6. What are the characteristics of helping relationships and therapeutic programs? How do I design my occupational therapy interventions to maximize these therapeutic characteristics? How can I facilitate patient collaboration with goal setting and treatment implementation?

7. What are the potential functional effects of the four stressors identified by Hatfield on a patient's task, social, and occupational skills?

8. How can occupational therapy assist patients in coping and adapting to their illnesses and pursuing satisfying, productive lives? What do patients seem to value and need most? How can I join with a patient to meet these needs?

References

Brammer, L. M. (1985). *The helping relationship: Process and skills* (3rd ed.). Englewood Cliffs, NJ: Prentice Hall.

Devereux, E. B. (1984). Occupational therapy's challenge: The caring relationship. *American Journal of Occupational Therapy, 38*, 791-798.

Gilfoyle, E. (1980). Caring: A philosophy of practice. *American Journal of Occupational Therapy, 34*, 517-521.

Hutchins, D. E., & Cole, C. G. (1986). *Helping relationships and strategies*. Pacific Grove, CA: Brooks/Cole.

King, L. J. (1980). Creative caring. *American Journal of Occupational Therapy, 34*, 522-528.

Mosey, A. C. (1986). *Psychosocial components of occupational therapy*. New York: Raven Press.

Rogers, C. R. (1961). *On becoming a person*. Boston: Houghton Mifflin.

Schulman, L. (1984). *The skills of helping individuals and groups* (2nd ed.). Itasca, IL: Peacock.

Schwartz, K. B. (1992). Occupational therapy and education: A shared vision. *American Journal of Occupational Therapy, 46*, 12-18.

Chapter 37

The Healing Power of Respect—A Personal Journey

Irene M. Turner

This chapter was previously published in *Occupational Therapy in Mental Health*, *9*(1), 17-22. Copyright © 1989, Haworth Press. Reprinted by permission.

It was unnecessary; it was unfeeling; it was humiliating; it invaded my privacy; it made me feel very embarrassed; I felt like slightly less than a child; and there was nothing I could do about it.

I was being admitted to a locked unit of a long-term psychiatric clinic. My belongings were searched, then locked away, and I was stripped and dressed in bed clothes—those horrible green hospital-issued "smock things" that tie in the back with two ill-spaced and sometimes nonexistent ties. Thus clad and dehumanized I was sent to "mingle with the other patients." At that point, they wanted to talk to me about as much as I wanted to speak to them, which was not at all, and at the very first opportunity I retreated to my small room. At least I could hide my face in the privacy of my own space. But not for long! Soon my appointed therapist appeared to talk to me, give me a physical examination, and have me draw some pictures for her. A relationship began which should have helped me during the following months, but on the contrary, it made me feel even worse about myself. How could I believe, at that time, that I was worth anything if my therapist insisted on calling me Mrs. Turner even though I told her it was important for me to be Irene? She did not speak to me in the hall unless I spoke first, and then it was always a formal "Hello, Mrs. Turner." During our therapy sessions, she constantly wrote notes and did not look at me; after ten months of biweekly meetings she *almost* acknowledged my personhood by giving me a formal handshake and wishing me well as I was leaving the hospital.

Some positive relationships helped during the time I spent there. I interacted well with fellow patients, and I discovered that some staff members genuinely cared about their work and wanted to help me just because I was me. Two members of my treatment team, one my primary nurse and the other a mental health worker, were very supportive. They helped by listening to me, often by giving firm reprimands when I became self-destructive, sometimes by just sitting and holding my hand for a short time. The mental health worker forced me to try to concentrate by playing card games or Scrabble with me. The nurse picked out some knitting yarn and a pattern for me and helped me knit a sweater—often watching close-by for several hours as I struggled to concentrate. Two senior staff members who played oboes for a hobby allowed me to play piano with them, and this helped keep me in touch with reality and gave me the opportunity to do something I enjoyed. We three gave several brief recitals for patients and staff. These relationships were especially meaningful to me, in part because many of the activities which were supposed to be of help to me were not fulfilling my needs.

Some of the activity therapies I felt to be insulting. I was insulted partly because of my own perfectionism and rigidity, I am sure, but nonetheless my feelings were real and based on some real shortcomings. Activities such as art therapy and leisure crafts were pitifully lacking in supplies. Searching through the sparse, somewhat chaotic supply of art or craft materials added greatly to my sense of confusion and lack of focus and direction. Often after I found the supplies I wanted I was not able to complete a project because of inadequate time. Storage for unfinished work was not available. Dance therapy did give opportunity for some exercise, but it also made my self-esteem spiral downward. The skips, leaps, hops, and runs were done with a partner or in sequence, like follow the leader, while others watched. I always felt clumsy and uncoordinated, and I hated to attend. Music therapy met none of my needs. Song sheets were distributed so that we could make singing selections, but I was not familiar with many of the songs, and I felt frustrated. I realize that I was reacting negatively because of my musical training, but not having musical notes to accompany the words was disconcerting. I was not able to express my feelings through music as I had once been able to do. I experienced each session as a much too casual, inadequately planned, sing-along. The most meaningful activity at that time consisted of two separate but short sessions in creative writing—something I had never tried before. These sessions were taught by volunteers and when they left, I felt strangely abandoned because they had cared about what they were doing, they had come prepared, and they had tried to help me discover something about myself through use of the written word. Both leaders had treated me with respect and never made me feel like "just a mental case." At the time, I felt keenly the difference between being treated with respect and being merely "treated."

I know that I am an unusually sensitive person and suffer from low self-esteem, but my unhappiness did not come entirely from within. The thread binding together so many of my experiences in that hospital was lack of respect. I received the message that it was all right to offer me activities in ill-equipped, cluttered areas. After all, "I was too mentally ill to notice." I began to care less about myself, to take less care of myself, and to take little pride in what I did. It was likely that I would be unable to finish a project because of time limitation, and any feedback would be extremely minimal. My sense of accomplishment, or even a desire for accomplishment,

dwindled. When some activity therapy staff gave the impression that it was not important for them to prepare for groups, I began to feel less important as a person. At one point, I tried to stop going to these activities, but I was made to feel like a naughty, rebellious child for suggesting such a thing. At that time, I had an unhealthy need to please people at any cost. I returned to the groups, participated in them, and felt increasingly more depressed. Not wanting anyone to know how truly ugly and unworthy I felt, I tried to bury my feelings.

During ten months of hospitalization I had taken several different types of antidepressants. None of them seemed to work very well, however, and my doctor decided that I should take nothing. I had the feeling that I never stayed on one medication long enough to test its effectiveness. No one discussed the meds with me, so I never knew what to expect, and I believed that no one cared enough about me to explain how the meds should work, why I took them, and why I was taken off them. I thought the doctors did not want me to get well.

My self-esteem continued to deteriorate. I felt that I was a "mental patient" who was making no contribution to family or friends. I felt incapable of doing anything well, and the staff gave me the impression that they really did not care about helping me. I felt hopeless, and I had little faith in the treatment I was receiving. Although I felt less like living than before I entered the hospital, I began to prepare for discharge. I tried not to mention suicide, and I talked positively about returning to work because I did not want the staff to know my true feelings about my job. In reality, I hated it and dreaded going back to my office. I feared facing my coworkers almost to the extent of feeling paralyzed. After remaining in that long-term hospital for almost a year, I was discharged having fear, inadequacy, helplessness, and hopelessness as my constant companions. There was [no] follow-up support, aftercare, or suggestions made about any support groups in the community. There had been no discharge planning group of any kind in the hospital. I just left.

The return to work was, in many ways, worse than I had imagined. Although my friends tried to treat me naturally, they could not, and acquaintances treated me with such condescension that I retreated from everyone. One younger employee, for example, offered to show me the way to the cafeteria, in spite of the fact that he knew I had worked in the building for over five years. I was utterly miserable. I received very little support from friends at work and, with the exception of my therapist whom I saw once a week, no support from the psychiatric community.

The transition from hospital to work was more difficult because of some confusion about my job assignment when I returned to the office. For four weeks, I sat at a perfectly clear desk and did nothing but answer a few phone calls. There was no opportunity for me to show my peers or my immediate supervisor that I was capable of functioning in the workplace. When I tried to describe my feelings about having no real work to friends, they merely laughed and said they would like to have "my kind of problem." I sat, did nothing, and felt progressively worse about myself. I, too, began to believe I was crazy and unable to do minimal tasks. By the time someone in authority intervened and began to prepare a new job assignment, I had already determined that I would not go back to that office with its empty desk and no work. I just wanted to die.

One of the activities I still found meaningful was playing the organ regularly for worship services at a small church. Some members of that congregation, and most especially my minister, were supportive and very concerned about me. Their watchfulness over me intensified as they identified increasing depression in me. I felt more hopeless than ever, so I planned to kill myself by taking an overdose of pills with vodka. However, my minister had been making frequent telephone calls to check on me, and he and another friend managed to enter my home when I did not answer the phone and prevented me from taking the entire supply. They took me to the psychiatric wing of a general hospital. I remember very little about that admission process except for a vague memory of thinking it very strange that my friends were with me as a nurse was trying to get me to answer some simple questions, while I wanted only to go back to sleep. Later, when I became fully awake, I was dismayed to discover that I was in the maximum security section.

During the five weeks I stayed there, my contact with life outside that ward was very restricted. My meals were served in a small sitting area next to the nurses' station. I was encouraged to watch television for very short periods each day, but I could not tolerate the shallowness and stupidity of most programming, so often I just stared into space when other patients wanted to watch a program. I could not go to the craft area to work on projects, nor participate in any groups held away from the restricted area. At one point, I had asked if someone could bring a small craft project to the sitting area for me, but there was no one to supervise one-to-one, so I was not allowed to do anything with my hands. The head nurse had suggested that I read some books, and when I protested that the sitting area was too noisy, she permitted me to read in my room during certain hours (it was considered safe because my closet was locked and all toilet articles, even my toothbrush, were kept at the nurses' station). I knew I could not concentrate enough to read, but I seized the opportunity to go to my room. I held a book in my hand for hours and when a nurse checked on me—every fifteen minutes or more often—

I tried to remember to turn a page. I was allowed to have only one visitor—my minister—because others upset me too much. He could not come often, but when he did come I was greatly helped and comforted.

I felt like a prisoner. I was awakened each morning at a certain time, my meals were served at a certain time, I went to bed at a certain time. And in between those certain times I sat in a plastic covered chair in full view of the staff person assigned to me. I was extremely depressed.

Since I had not been able to respond to treatment in the length of time it was possible to stay at that hospital, my doctor decided to transfer me to a different long-term hospital. The memory of my earlier experiences was very fresh, so I was prepared for the worst.

My first impression as my minister, two other friends, and I drove into the hospital grounds was one of spacious serenity. In spite of my resistance, I had a brief glimpse of the security this place could offer me. A bit later my friends and I were shown into a quiet room to await my new therapist. The quietness and the spaciousness were surprises because they were so different from the noisy cluttered hallway I expected since that was my earlier experience. It seemed to matter to the staff of this hospital that my admission be as easy as possible. I appreciated those moments with my friends because even though my thoughts were in turmoil I knew they cared about me. I was so afraid that I was to spend the next few months among people who did not care. The only thing I knew about this new place was that I was to have a woman as a therapist. During that short waiting period I speculated about what she would be like.

My speculations did not prepare me for the doctor who was assigned to me. My spirits took a nosedive when she entered the room. She was beautiful! I saw a woman so impeccably dressed that I was sure she must be uncomfortable. She seemed aloof, stiff, and stone-like. When she began to speak I was completely convinced that she could never help me. How could she help me if I could not understand her Italian accent? After a short interview, she took me to the unit where I was to live. I received the first hint of how wrong my first impressions were during my first hour there. I had appreciated the fact that she took me to the unit and did not send me with some other stranger. Then she did an amazing thing. The mental health worker who was searching my luggage for sharp or other dangerous objects was going to remove a picture of my daughter because it was in a glass frame. When I started to cry, my doctor said I could keep the photograph. It was such a small but tremendous statement, affirming my personhood—my ability to think and feel and react like any normal mother. I am convinced that it was at that moment that I took my first tentative step toward helping this extraordinary woman help me. A relationship which has profoundly affected my life had begun.

When my doctor left me—with my daughter's picture—I felt very alone. But I was relieved to discover that from the first I could wear my own clothes. And in spite of the fact that I was restricted to the sitting room, I did not feel so isolated. The other patients respected my need to adjust to the unit, and thus did not intrude, but offered their friendship and willingness to help. For the moment, the gesture was as significant as doing something specific. The staff members were friendly and tried to make it easier for me to relax.

That evening I was introduced to the first of many, many "hall meetings" and observed how milieu therapy works. We twenty patients plus the staff on duty met for approximately an hour and discussed a variety of things, including housekeeping issues (keep the coffee area cleaner), reminders of activities for the weekend (a dance, of all things!) and also "agenda items." These agenda items turned out to be issues concerning people, and my heart sank when I heard my name put on that agenda. My fear was exaggerated, however. My peers merely wanted to welcome me and give me the opportunity to speak if I wanted to do so. Beyond introducing myself, I had nothing to say and was not pushed to say more at that time. As I listened to the rest of the discussion, I learned that the patients really cared about each other and shared their feelings of support, concern, encouragement, disappointment, anger. When I heard the feedback from those patients, I felt more of a sense of belonging than I had experienced in quite some time. It was ever so small, but coupled with kindness from my doctor, I was beginning to feel something other than a desire to die.

My first several weeks in the hospital were very difficult. I was not restricted to the sitting room the entire time, but I was restricted to the unit since I was still extremely depressed and suicidal. Nevertheless, I felt "bound in," and I believed that I was receiving my just punishment because I was such an evil, unworthy person. I did not want to talk to the other patients, nor did I want to share my true feelings with the staff. I thought that if I simply remained quiet, everyone would assume that I was feeling better, and this would result in early discharge. The staff members were very patient with me. I resented their intrusions and their restrictions, but, at the same time, I dimly recognized their actions as evidence of caring and support. Someone sat with me when I could concentrate on a project, such as an embroidery sampler, which I enjoyed although I was not allowed to keep the needle or scissors. I began to feel less like a prisoner because I was given some freedom and because the staff seemed to respect me and care about my getting well. One mental health worker, in particular, was thought-

ful enough to take me for brief walks outside in the fresh air. I appreciated visiting the vegetable and flower gardens and feeding the rabbits near the greenhouse.

The occupational therapist made some suggestions about things I could do while I remained on hall restriction. She brought some small projects which were simple, and I appreciated just being able to have something to do with my hands. I remember coloring with magic markers and feeling good about the lovely designs which took form. Even as I did these things, I felt support from people who were beginning to be important to me—my doctor often stopped by to make comments, my occupational therapist complimented me, and other patients appreciated my giving them a colorful card. The sense of connections with others was a good feeling.

At the appropriate time, the occupational therapist introduced me to an activity program which was to enhance tremendously the benefits I was gaining from psychotherapy. At first I was most skeptical, because on paper it looked a great deal like the program to which I had been exposed previously. However, a larger variety of activities was offered at this hospital, and I wanted to attend those which the occupational therapist and I had decided would be meaningful. Having input into the final choice of activities was important for my self-esteem, because it implied that what I thought and did as an individual mattered. Thought and concern were given to my selections, and I received the message that I would not be haphazardly assigned to an activity and then "baby-sat" for the time I spent there.

"Referred groups" consisted of ongoing activities to which I was referred for specific treatment objectives, and I was expected to attend them regularly. From that group I helped to choose dance therapy, leathercraft, ceramics, and art therapy. "Skill development groups" consisted of self-selected activities which rotated on a monthly basis, and were designed primarily for leisure. From this group I selected activities such as knitting, creative writing, and nature hikes. "Open activities" involved supervised activities such as swimming, crafts, and beachball volleyball, which were available to all patients. All of these activities were good for me, but some were more significant than others.

I remember being told while I was making a leather notebook that I was too intense: I needed to accept the fact that my design would be good enough and I could accept it even if it were not perfect. I had early learned that to be acceptable I had to please, and in order to please I had to be as nearly perfect as possible. I was always my own strictest judge, and when I did not meet my own standards, my self-esteem plummeted. Because of those feelings, the group leader continued to encourage me to relax and take pride in what I was doing—even with the flaws. Finishing that notebook reminded me that "good" is all right, too, and if that is so with a leather notebook, it could be so for other things in life.

My dance therapist and fellow patients in dance therapy helped me to lose some of my feelings of inadequacy and low self-confidence. The origin of some of these feelings centered on the belief that my musical talent had disappeared. One day my dance therapist sat on the floor and encouraged me to feel the rhythm of the music with my body by moving in any way I felt comfortable. She held my hands and rubbed them in an attempt to make me aware of their importance and their strength. I shall remember the moment for years to come because she respected me and tried to help me rediscover and accept my best qualities.

Perhaps the most important activity for me at the time was art therapy. Initially, I protested being referred to that group because I am not an artist! I could not imagine how I could benefit from drawing pictures of which I would be ashamed. I soon discovered that being artistic was not a prerequisite to reaping benefits from art therapy. One extremely important thing, especially in the beginning, was the fact that there were enough art materials with which to experiment. I was not forced to draw. I could choose to do so, but I could also select other options. As my art therapist guided me in learning to express some of my deepest feelings, I found expression through the use of watercolors, acrylic paints (a special favorite of mine), finger paints, collages, and modeling clay.

When the art therapist introduced me to scribble art, something special happened. My skepticism again came to the fore when she suggested that I loosen up my arms by swinging them around and that I shake my hands to completely relax them. However, by that time I had developed some trust in her and had gained a small understanding of the real value of art therapy. Although it was not difficult to close my eyes and make scribble lines on a piece of construction paper, I believed I would never be able to see images or forms. To my amazement, the lines, angles, squiggles, and circles began to take shape. From the very depths of my feelings pictures formed on the paper with such clarity that it often frightened me. Those scribbles were very valuable to my progress. Often during the following weeks I took the scribbles with me to psychotherapy sessions, since there were times I had been able to express feelings in those scribbles which I had never been able to verbalize. It was helpful to put the pictures on the floor, admit that they meant something to me, and begin to explore their meaning with my doctor. At times I felt that a major breakthrough had been made as a result of discussing the scribbles.

On several different occasions, I had discussed with the occupational therapist my desire to enter a referred group in interpersonal skills. She discouraged my participation in it at that time because she felt that I was not ready for the kind of confrontation which took place there. I had a great deal of difficulty accepting her statement and thought that she disliked me. I began to misinterpret other things the occupational therapist said and did. I allowed myself to be hurt and felt that I had done something wrong. Feelings of rejection were evoked when I could not understand the reason she referred another patient to Interpersonal Skills ahead of me.

Later, when I was ready, I was referred to the interpersonal skills group which was honest, confrontive, supportive, and caring. I learned to communicate more effectively by observing myself and others as we talked together, as we listened to each other, as we gave nonverbal messages by body language, expressions, or eye contact and tried to understand the complex and often incongruous relationship to the verbal ones we shared. As the weeks passed, I was grateful for the fact that my enrollment in that group had been delayed until I was able to hear the feedback given to me without being devastated by it. Again I was reminded that people genuinely cared about me and had my best interest in mind when decisions about my schedule were made.

During the long months of hospitalization I was a member of the patient organization, Patient Activities Committee (PAC), which planned evening and weekend activities for fellow patients. Our responsibilities entailed selecting, organizing, providing leadership during the activity, and evaluating these events. Involvement in PAC helped me to remember that there was a community outside the hospital and that I would be discharged to that community when I was ready. Working with fellow patients to help make our plans become reality gave me the opportunity to improve my interpersonal skills in a supportive environment.

For a long time, I served PAC as secretary to its executive body, thus enabling me to use my secretarial skills, and I felt a real sense of accomplishment when I had completed the weekly typing assignments. On the other hand, it gave me little opportunity to work closely with other patients, so I approached the PAC Coordinator to ask about filling the vacant leadership position of co-chairman. She said she did not think it was wise because I still needed to learn some important things about relating to others in a task oriented situation.

At first it was difficult for me to accept those comments, and it was hard not to feel a sense of personal rejection. However, the important thing about that conversation and the resulting decision to remain as secretary was that at no time was I treated without respect. On the contrary, this respect given to me was, I feel, the basis for my developing a sense of trust which resulted in my ability to listen and try to change. I knew I needed help, and I trusted the Coordinator enough to believe that she could help.

She did! I learned many things from her, but two things are noteworthy. She repeatedly reminded us that while we as patients experienced ourselves as different from nonpatients, the so-called "normals," this was more a function of our feelings of isolation rather than reality. She frequently quoted from Harry Stack Sullivan, "We are all more simply human than otherwise." Recognizing that fact helped me have a sense of connectedness to the outside world. Secondly, she helped all of us examine those of our behaviors which tended to separate us from others and rejoiced with us as we made progress in correcting those behaviors. What a marvelous asset to my psychotherapy that woman was.

I was receiving psychotherapy, and many of the problems which had brought me to the hospital were being addressed in my activities. However, I also began to realize that there was care and concern for me as a total person and not just as a mental patient. Therefore, it did not surprise me to learn that there was a hospital chaplain, and I appreciated the fact that religious services were provided regularly for patients. During the early weeks of my hospitalization, I had not felt comfortable enough with my own feelings about the church to attend those services, but my doctors suggested that I do so. My academic training had been in organ and church music, and my professional involvement with the church was of long standing. Once again being a part of a communal worship service met many of my deepest spiritual needs. After I had attended a few services, my doctor further suggested that I make an appointment to speak with the chaplain. I did so, but I had such anxiety, fear, skepticism, and doubt about the usefulness of such a meeting that I almost canceled the appointment. I am so grateful that I did not do so, because the chaplain also became a special "significant other" in my life. My sessions with him were very important. Some of my fear of men, especially ministers, began to disappear, and my self-esteem grew with his acceptance of me. I often took my "scribbles" from art therapy to discuss with him. Together we explored the pictures' meaning, and the insight I gained helped me understand the origin of many of my fears. He gave me a sense of security and stability, and he often gave me very direct advice. He told me once, "When you feel like harming yourself, pick up a pencil or pastel chalk to use rather than a knife or a razor." It worked!

There was hope for me, because I was beginning to believe there was hope. That tiny grain of hope needed nurturing, and I was gratefully amazed as I moved closer and closer to a discharge date that I received support from many staff members.

A vocational counselor, who helped me plan how to re-enter the work force, administered some vocational tests and discussed their findings with me. We discussed the job market, updated my resume, and addressed the questions of revealing my psychiatric hospitalization or changing occupations. In preparation for work, I was given a work therapy assignment in the hospital. Work expectations were discussed, and my performance was evaluated. Vocational counseling and work therapy did not take away all the fear of returning to work, but it helped prepare me. My work therapy assignment was one which used the secretarial skills I planned to use when I left the hospital. Being regular in attendance, and being on time, both to start work and to end work, were goals I was expected to meet.

The transition to work outside the hospital began before I was discharged. Fortunately I was able to obtain a part-time job in a small law office which suited my needs and interests. Although I enjoyed the job, even though it was stressful at times, I was grateful that I could return to the hospital after my work day and talk about what had happened. Receiving valuable feedback helped my transition from the hospital.

The discharge planning group in which I participated was helpful in a special way. During my stay in the hospital I had been focused inward. The practical side of living had not concerned me for many months. In this group, we focused on living arrangements, budgets, meal planning, entertainment, dealing with family and friends, [and] handling free time. The occupational therapist who led the group made valuable specific suggestions to each patient about groups or activities in the community. She gave me the name and schedule of a community chorus which I joined in order to use my musical talents as well as to make some social contacts. I remember reflecting during the discharge planning group that I would not be "just leaving" this hospital as I had left the other hospital months earlier.

Leaving and saying "goodbye" were things that were very difficult for me because they provoked feelings of abandonment. I was encouraged, along with every other patient who left, to set aside specific times for saying farewell to the patients on my hall, to individual staff members, and to members of activity groups which I attended. The process of actually saying goodbye did take some planning and coordinating of schedules, but the help I received was worth the effort. I discovered that it was all right to say goodbye. It did not mean that I was being abandoned or that I was being rejected because I was not perfect enough to please everyone. Nor did it mean that there was no one to care about me any more.

This part of my discharge process was both sad and happy. I would miss a group of good friends, but I would take with me many lessons learned from them: lessons about caring, for others and for myself; lessons about acceptance, of others and myself; lessons about honesty, with others and myself; lessons about listening without feeling personally attacked.

Discharge planning is one important thing. The actual discharge is enormously different! I was petrified. Even though I knew my plans were well made I had gigantic doubts about my ability to implement them. Many of my worst fears from my past reappeared to haunt me. I could not trust my own feelings, but fortunately I trusted the hospital staff and they had faith in me. Their attitude often gave me the courage I needed.

My tenure as an inpatient ended on a beautiful day in May 1987. Going through the locked door of the hall which had been my home for so many months created an extraordinary mixture of emotions. I was happy, but a bit sad; I was eager, but a little uncertain; I was confident, but somewhat insecure; I was prepared, but I also had doubts; I felt alone, but I knew I still had the support of the hospital staff to help during the transition period. That support continued to be very important to me. I was extremely fortunate to be able to work as a volunteer in the Activity Therapy Department of the hospital after my discharge. The work consisted of secretarial duties similar to those I had as a paid employee outside the hospital, but the difference in the two jobs was significant. In the hospital, I had feedback and support from several sources but especially from my supervisor who had known me during the long months of my hospitalization.

During the hours when I was doing my volunteer job, my supervisor did not discuss therapy issues but only issues related to my work habits. I learned so much about the way I functioned in a work related environment. For the most part, my work skills were solid, but I needed honest feedback and suggestions about the way I worked with people—my supervisor, my peers, people I might need to supervise. Because of my volunteer job I became better prepared for independently working outside the hospital.

My relationship with the hospital chaplain continued to be most important. He gave me honest, straightforward and caring feedback and encouraged me to explore how I felt and to verbalize feelings clearly. He also encouraged me to use my musical training by playing the organ for worship services for the patients. I believe that in this way I made a small contribution to the life of the hospital.

During that transition period, I was never without the encouragement, the support, the feedback, the care, and the listening ear of my doctor. Often it was her concern for me and my love for her that made it possible for me to try to get through a day. There were times when I would tell myself, "Hang in there until you see your doctor because you know she cares."

Not long ago, my doctor had the flu, and she called to cancel our appointment. After a brief moment of panic, I discovered that I was more concerned about her health than my own fear that she would not come back soon. I knew that she would return when she recovered. The panic of a lost child abandoned by her mother was not there. I believe that was a significant realization since it meant that I was moving slowly toward becoming the kind of adult my doctor always said I could be. My relationship with her will not stop for a while. My love for her will never end, but perhaps it will not be such a dependent love.

One of the statements that my doctor used a great deal was, "You must learn to look at the half-full glass. The half-empty glass that you always saw is not good for you."

I believe that, in a sense, I have done that in describing my recent hospitalizations. There were regressions, conflicts, disappointments, fears, aloneness, but they all dimmed as I thought about all the help I received after the disastrous experience I had during my first long-term stay. When I was admitted to my second long-term hospital my experience was different. I believe this was because the underlying attitude that governed all aspects of hospital life was respect. It was this most important quality which made me begin to feel better about myself and want to do something to help myself. I made use of every aspect of hospital life that was available to me. And now, I have, with some confidence, grasped my half-full "glass of life." I can now affirm that it is indeed half-full and not half-empty. Furthermore, it can become even fuller as I continue my journey, one step at a time.

Chapter 38

The Patient-Therapist Relationship in Occupational Therapy: Understanding Visions and Images

Suzanne M. Peloquin, MA, OTR

This chapter was originally published in the *American Journal of Occupational Therapy, 44*, 13-21. Copyright © 1990, The American Occupational Therapy Association, Inc.

The stories patients tell about their experiences with occupational therapists often tell more about their views than [do] structured responses to surveys. The following fictional story tells much about one patient-therapist relationship:

> Brunhilde, the misplaced Viking Lady, comes tapping on my door every afternoon in an effort to intimidate me into going to Occupational Therapy. She marches around the seventh floor telling all the patients that their doctor has "ordered" Occupational Therapy and they must come IMMEDIATELY. She herds them out in the hall and they mill around until she lines them up in two columns and goosesteps them out the door. (Rebeta-Burditt, 1977, p. 114)

A fuller reading of the story reveals that this patient, Cassie, accurately perceives expressions of concern from other health care professionals. Her satirical barbs target those whose demands for control and order threaten her autonomy. Because Brunhilde seems uncaring, the image of the occupational therapist in this story is disturbing.

Clinically, patients derive images of their therapists from their interactions with them. Image forming as a process includes an exchange: The therapist brings to each exchange some understanding, or vision, of what a therapeutic relationship (and perhaps what a "good patient") should be, and the patient brings needs, memories of past experiences, and expectations of how a helpful caregiver should behave. The exchange of needs, visions, and expectations helps to shape the image that each person will hold of the other. In the above story, Cassie is frustrated by an occupational therapist who does not demonstrate the kind of personal concern that she wants and expects. She sees a paternalistic therapist, an intimidating Viking Lady. The novel does not reveal the vision of the therapeutic relationship that the therapist brought to this exchange. One can only wonder what happened beyond the patient's unmet expectations to yield such a negative image.

The therapeutic relationship promoted in occupational therapy has been an evolving blend of competence and caring. Therapists have interacted with patients in a variety of ways, depending in part on their interpretation of the occupational therapy vision. It follows that images of occupational therapists in patients' stories have also varied. This [chapter] will examine the patient-therapist relationship envisioned by therapists and experienced by patients. Thoughtful consideration of both views—the visions therapists have of the relationship and the images patients hold of their therapists—can remind practitioners that concern about the patient as a person remains essential to effective practice.

The Patient-Therapist Relationship: In Search of the Occupational Therapy Vision

Perhaps no source better illustrates the evolution of the profession's understanding of the patient-therapist relationship than *Willard and Spackman's Occupational Therapy*. From the first edition (Willard & Spackman, 1947) to the sixth edition (Hopkins & Smith, 1983), this text has presented contributions from therapists working in a variety of practice arenas. *Willard and Spackman* has been a primary tool in the education of occupational therapy students and has often served as a therapist's first introduction to the vision of the therapeutic relationship.

The therapeutic relationship, however, has been treated in a fragmented way in this basic text. Between 1947 and 1983, no chapter has specifically addressed the therapeutic relationship. No references are made in either the table of contents or the index to concepts such as *rapport* or *relationship*, or to key relational words such as *empathy* or *trust*. The 1947 edition has brief sections entitled "Approach to the Patient," "Personality Qualifications," "Normal Atmosphere," and "The Attitude of the Therapist." The 1983 edition has pertinent sections called "The Therapist," "Observation," "Humanistic Approaches," and "Psychological Considerations." A discussion of patient-therapist communication as it affects the evaluation process is listed in the index under the heading Communication, and a discrete section entitled "Therapeutic Relationship" is in the chapter on functional restoration. It seems significant, however, that within a definitive text on occupational therapy, one can find the profession's vision of the therapeutic relationship only after a chapter-by-chapter search.

If each treatment chapter addressed relational considerations for the patient population in question, one could argue that the concept of the therapeutic relationship is so basic that it permeates the text. But this is clearly not the case. Most of the material articulates the assumptions, theories, and methodologies essential to the application of occupation. Although this emphasis is essential in an occupational therapy text, the minimal acknowledgment that occupational therapy occurs within the context of the patient-therapist relationship suggests the curiously marginal status of this fact. Because fragments of information about the therapeutic relationship are scattered throughout several chapters, the reader cannot gain a clear understanding of the vision from this one source. The fragmented manner in which the patient-therapist relationship is covered compromises its significance and clarity.

The Evolving Vision: From Competence to Care

The vision articulated in *Willard and Spackman's Occupational Therapy* has changed over the years, largely through changes in emphasis. Earlier contributors advocated skill-oriented and professional (impersonal) patient-therapist relationships; the emphasis was on competence. Later contributors focused on the essentially personal character of the patient-therapist relationship, with the emphasis on care.

For example, in the 1947 edition of *Willard and Spackman*, Wade characterized the development of the therapeutic relationship in treating the mentally ill in a rather impersonal way:

> The development of a good psychiatric approach does not occur spontaneously, nor is it a natural gift but, like many other accomplishments, it is acquired through diligent effort, study and experience. (p. 83)

Wade viewed a good patient-therapist relationship as an achievement attained by a skilled therapist who could "command respect, admiration, hope and confidence" (p. 83). She identified "courage, patience, tolerance and friendliness" as innate personal characteristics that could be directed toward the achievement of a good approach (p. 83). Wade additionally characterized the successful therapist as one who had mastered two specific skills that supported patient equilibrium. First was the ability to make a "tactful approach," one in which "adjustment is always made to the patient by the worker" (p. 84). Wade explained the rationale for this guarded approach: "These patients are hypersensitive to implications expressed in words, by tone of voice, mannerism or facial expression" (p. 84). Second, the therapist needed "complete self-control in order to prevent untimely expression of a spontaneous emotional reaction" (p. 84). Self-control and personal adjustment seemed critical to patient equilibrium; spontaneity and personal expression were suspect.

Other skills entailed reaching out to the patient, but always within the context of professional objectivity. The therapist had to identify with the patient, but at the same time maintain an objective attitude: "The technic [sic] of doing this is similar to that used by the adult in correlating his thoughts with those of a child" (Wade, 1947, p. 84). The therapeutic goal was primary; caring expressions were a means to that end. The therapist needed to be a good listener, for example, because "it is frequently necessary to play this role" (Wade, 1947, p. 84). The patient-therapist relationship was to be kept "within normal limits" and "restricted to matters of impersonal interest" (Wade 1947, p. 85). The bottom line during interactions with the mentally ill was that one remain "impersonal in relationships" (Wade, 1947, p. 84).

This emphasis on competence was not restricted to practice in mental health. Fay and March (1947) discussed the development of the therapeutic relationship in both general and special hospitals:

> Skill in making the professional approach to each patient for occupational therapy may come more easily to some than to others, but it comes with experience in correlating the patient's history with the character as revealed by his face to one who is interested in enlisting the patient's cooperation. (pp. 124-125)

The relationship had to be professional. Toward that end, Fay and March enumerated several guidelines for a suitable approach. The following guidelines are representative of the list's precision and direction:

Do's

3. Stand or sit where you can be seen easily.
4. Be encouraging and hopeful and foster a desire in the patient to get well.
5. Be understandingly sympathetic.
6. Be friendly and sincere.
7. Be courteous, not flippant or bold.
11. Be patient and resourceful.
12. Be impersonally personal.

Dont's

3. Don't show alarm, horror or sorrow.
5. Don't be physically objectionable by body odor, the use of strong perfume or by having the clothes permeated with cigarette smoke.
7. Don't argue. Be a good listener.
8. Don't talk of depressing or distressing subjects.
9. Don't make promises that cannot be kept.
10. Don't hit or jar the bed.
12. Don't show racial, religious or political prejudices. (pp. 125-126)

The predominant vision of the patient-therapist relationship in this 1947 edition reflected a self-conscious striving for precise skills that could professionalize the patient-therapist relationship. Personal, warm traits were seen as tools requiring guidance, monitoring, and objectification. Perhaps the closest any contributor in the 1947 edition came to the idea of personal investment and care in relationships with patients was Gleave in her chapter on pediatric services:

> The occupational therapist should be an understanding, friendly and cheerful person. . . . Ability to talk *with* children rather than *to* or *at* them is an asset. Every effort should be made to bring out the child's ideas, to get him to express himself freely and naturally. In all contacts with the patient, the therapist should strive to keep the tone of her voice pleasant and well modulated. She must make the child feel that she is his friend while holding his respect and maintaining discipline when problems arise. (p. 148)

Gleave alone alluded to the concept of friendship in the therapeutic relationship. Her emphasis on a caring expression seemed acceptable in 1947 within the context of working with children, for whom, perhaps, the need to project a professional image seemed less crucial.

By the 1983 edition of *Willard and Spackman's Occupational Therapy*, however, the term *therapeutic relationship* had taken root, and the therapist's caring attitude had assumed greater significance than personality traits or interactional skills. As if in recognition of prior emphasis on competence and professionalism, Hopkins and Tiffany (1983) cited a new image: Purtilo's characterization of "the personal-professional self" (p. 95). Purtilo (1978), a physical therapist, proposed a synthesis of personal and professional characteristics to facilitate the therapeutic relationship. She tried to minimize conflicts for therapists struggling with personal-professional tension in relationships with patients. This brief portion of Purtilo's (1978) characterization reveals her vision:

> [The personal-professional self] incorporates actions that communicate caring into the patient health professional interactions; he recognizes efficiency as a trait which can express caring when it does not impose rigid limits on the interaction.
>
> He is interested in the patient as a person with values, needs, and beliefs, but does not encourage a relationship that will lead to over-dependence (detrimental dependence). (p. 148)

This more balanced view of the therapeutic relationship communicated a sense of helping. Hopkins and Tiffany (1983) believed that patients need to feel that they can be helped and argued that "the therapist in a treatment setting is, by definition, a helper" (p. 94). The helping process required personal trust—a trust built on confidence in and respect for the patient:

> Without the establishment of trust between the client and therapist, it is unlikely that a truly collaborative effort will be possible. . . . The therapist's own self-confidence, the therapist's ability to be honest and open in the relationship, and the extent to which the therapist is able to communicate "unconditional positive regard" and empathy for the client will affect the client's ability to invest trust in the relationship. (pp. 94-95)

Tiffany (1983) underscored her view of the therapist's role: "Occupational therapy is attuned to the principle of facilitating the client's own personal search for purpose, meaning, and self-actualization" (p. 291). Open communication between the therapist and patient seemed critical to understanding the patient's purpose and personal values. Smith and Tiffany (1983) elaborated: "The communication process...lays a foundation for rapport and trust. The client needs to feel that communications have been heard and understood by someone who has not only some empathy but also some knowledge and skill" (pp. 144-145). A personal relationship was critical to this new vision. It was the *relationship* that might well "determine the success or failure of the treatment plan" (Hopkins & Tiffany, 1983, p. 94), and within that relationship, "activities are used as facilitators for transactions between people" (Hopkins & Tiffany, p. 95). This singular distinction ought never be forgotten; occupational therapy's vision of "being with" is essentially a vision of "doing with."

This later vision of the therapeutic relationship, with its emphasis on care, on the importance of each person, and on helping, transcended the awkward and self-conscious vision of earlier years. Both visions grounded themselves in competence and caring, and both highlighted competencies and styles of caring thought (in their respective eras) to be important and effective. A young profession, striving to be recognized as scientific, might emphasize competence. A more secure profession, leery of the objectification inherent in scientific practice, might more readily emphasize care.

When one pieces together the ideas of 1947 and 1983 regarding the therapeutic relationship, the ensuing vision lends itself to much individual interpretation. One therapist may feel that earlier directives to be "impersonally personal" should yield to more recent appeals for warmth; another may favor a relationship marked by more traditional objectivity and distance. If therapists demonstrate competence and caring in different ways in contemporary practice, this is consistent with their having been exposed to a fragmented and evolving vision of the patient-therapist relationship over the years.

From Therapist's Vision to Patient's Image

Stories about occupational therapists tell much about their relationships with patients. In this next section, I will attempt to explore stories from the 1940s through the 1980s that develop the therapeutic relationship, citing the stories wherever possible. Although in a previous article (Peloquin, 1989) I emphasized that fiction can contribute powerfully to therapists' understanding of their functions, I here draw primarily from nonfiction so that the stories will ring truer to those who might dismiss fictional accounts as fantasy.

A Pioneer: Ora Ruggles

One biography in particular presents a therapist with a clear vision of what she believes the therapeutic relationship should be. *The Healing Heart* (Carlova & Ruggles, 1946) portrays a competent and caring reconstruction aide and pioneer, Ora Ruggles. Ruggles's bold and humane vision contrasts markedly with that of her 1940s

contemporaries; it reflects a patient-therapist relationship more characteristic of the vision of the 1980s. Her drive to relate to patients is clear: "It is not enough to give a patient something to do with his hands. You must reach for the heart as well as the hands. It's the heart that really does the healing" (p. 69). Healing permeates the story. As Ruggles helps wounded soldiers at Fort McPherson, she says, "I have more to offer than pity. I'm here to help these men" (p. 12). Others say of her, "She [has] an intense desire to help every one, to give freely and fully of her strength, her skills, her compassion and courage" (p. 63). She realizes that a significant part of helping means caring for each patient, and she acknowledges the cost:

> She and the other therapists had to fight to keep from becoming emotionally weakened by their atmosphere. If they turned hard, as many of the nurses did in self defense, they would lose the sensitivity and enthusiasm so necessary to their work. If they allowed themselves to be touched too deeply by the tragedy around them, they would become mentally disturbed—as, in fact, several young therapists did. (p. 77)

Ruggles maintains her sensitivity, as Major Benson acknowledges:

> The work that Miss Ruggles has accomplished here is little short of a miracle. . . . The camp has been transformed into a model of its kind. The men's morale has risen. Patients who had quite literally resigned themselves to death are more alive than ever. . . . (p. 130)

Ruggles describes an early insight into caring as she reflects about a particular patient:

> He hadn't done very well when I first started with him, but he's doing fine now. I asked myself why, and the answer suddenly came to me—the patient had improved because I had. I had become truly concerned about him. I wanted him to gel well and I made him know I wanted him to get well. (p. 69)

Ruggles listens intently and understands her patients' values and goals. She responds by structuring activity options to meet the expressed needs of patients. She believes in the patient as primary healer. The story overflows with examples of Ruggles's responsiveness. One poignant example is her successful work with an angry and unruly patient who cannot tolerate sedentary crafts:

> "No, baskets aren't for you, Kilgore, and we both know it. I want you to make some spurs I've designed."
>
> His interest was immediately aroused. "Say, that sounds good. I used to be a cowboy you know. . . .'"
>
> From the moment Kilgore went to work in the blacksmith shop, he never got into a fight. His gambling ceased entirely and he drank only moderately. After his discharge from the Army, he started an iron work plant which grew into one of the largest in the Southwest. (p. 91)

Ruggles describes her aim: "Most people have resources and reserves they don't even know about. My job, as I see it, is to bring out those resources and reserves. . . ." A captain responds, "Tell that to a man with no legs" (p. 52). Ruggles's rejoinder endorses the therapeutic caring specific to occupational therapy:

> "Oh, these aren't things you tell," Ora hastily explained. "These are things you do. The man with no legs would probably feel useless and unwanted. . .my problem is to get him to produce with his own hands something useful, beautiful or satisfying. . . . By personally making something useful, he feels useful—and wanted. He belongs." (p. 52)

Ruggles acknowledges personal gain from helping others: "I don't see what's missing, I see what's there. I see real manhood. I see great courage. I see tremendous strength. I see true spirit. That's what gives me courage, strength, and spirit. I gain as much or more as the men I try to help" (p. 76). Her sense of the mutuality in helping, her caring, and her competence enables her to help others.

One passage in *The Healing Heart* creates a lasting image. Paul, Ruggles's fiancé, tells her, "You're an artist in the greatest medium of all. You're an artist in people" (p. 92). She reflects that "it was indeed true that there was artistry in her work as a healer. She dealt with the soul, the heart and the spirit rather than paints and palette" (p. 92). The image the reader takes from this story is one of a therapist personally committed to each patient. This image is congruent with a vision of a personal relationship that balances competence in technique with caring in a relationship. Ruggles is a professional therapist; she is also a friend.

The Occupational Therapist as Technician, Parent, and Covenanter

Not all images of occupational therapists convey Ruggles's balance of competence and caring. Other stories present occupational therapists who seem bossy or preoccupied with crafts. One wonders how to characterize these images, how to begin to name them, in order to better understand and evaluate them. I have found it particularly helpful to turn to the writings of another person who thinks about professional relationships in terms of images.

May (1983) finds images helpful, both in clarifying functions and in establishing standards. He argues that "the image tells a kind of compressed story" (p. 17). An image is storylike in that it describes not only the basic character (in this case the physician), but also the person with whom the basic character interacts. If one thinks of a physician as a priest, for example, the priestly image suggests a relationship in which the physician is powerful and inspires awe in the patient. May (1983) discusses various images that he feels characterize physicians: Three of the images—the technician, the parent, and the covenanter—seem relevant to this discussion of occupational therapy because they emerge from stories about occupational therapists. Technical occupational therapists are chiefly concerned with technique and technical issues, parental occupational therapists perceive and relate to their patients as dependents or children, and covenanting occupational therapists see their patients as bonded partners in the pursuit of therapeutic goals. Each of these images mirrors a markedly different understanding and manifestation of competence and caring.

The occupational therapist as technician. The therapist who functions as a technician commits to excellence in technical performance (May, 1983). Competence in technique preempts relationships; the therapist refines technical skills above all else. Although this image may seem cold, the basic impetus is humanitarian, because to the technical therapist only superior technical performance, efficiency, and use of correct procedure serve the patient's best interests. The occupational therapist whose primary focus is on methodology, percentage of function, or the task at hand is perceived by the patient as a technician.

In *No Laughing Matter* (Heller & Vogel, 1986), Heller describes his ordeal with Guillain-Barré syndrome and his experience with an occupational therapist who, though pleasant and humane, "possibly will be surprised or contrite to find out now of the very considerable anguish I experienced so often in my sessions with her or one of her co-workers" (p. 166). Methodology and gain are clearly important to this therapist:

> But in occupational therapy, as soon as I could sand a block of wood (with a need to rest both arms, it was written, after seven repetitions), a change was made to a coarser grade of sandpaper, increasing the amount of force required, and it was just as punishing and demoralizing for me to have to execute them as it had been in the beginning. (pp. 166-167)

Heller's overall impression is that "what they intended was to keep me always at a standstill" (p. 166). His personal need seems clear: to experience and then to savor a sense of gain. The therapist, oblivious to this need, implements a strategy to improve a condition. Treatment goals become the therapist's and clearly do not emanate from a collaborative relationship in which Heller's personal need has meaning.

Seabrook (1935) tells of his stay in a private mental institution for the treatment of his alcoholism. Although Seabrook's experience of occupational therapy is generally positive, he, too, views the occupational therapist as a technician. He describes one therapist/superintendent as "conscientious and probably having a kind heart, but nobody like[s] him" (p. 62). The superintendent values technique over relationship. Any personal or collaborative function that can be associated with occupational therapy rests with Paschal, Seabrook's psychiatrist. Paschal mediates with the occupational therapist for different crafts and a more individualized approach to Seabrook. The occupational therapist provides competence; the psychiatrist provides care.

Another patient's story, this one in verse, portrays a predominantly technical occupational therapist. The opening lines introduce both the therapist and the elderly patient: "Preserve me from the occupational therapist, God. She means well, but I'm too busy to make baskets" (McClay, 1977, p. 106). The young therapist supports activity for its own sake. She makes no attempt to hear the patient or to discuss meaningful occupations; the patient-therapist exchanges merely parody the relationship:

> Oh, here she comes, the therapist, with
> scissors and paste.
> Would I like to try decoupage?
> "No," I say, "I haven't got time."
> "Nonsense," she says, "You're going to
> live a long, long time."
> That's not what I mean,
> I mean that all my life I've been
> doing things
> for people, with people. I have to
> catch up
> on my thinking and feeling. . . . (p. 107)

The concept of therapy as something that uses purposeful and meaningful activity to promote healing is predicated on some mutual understanding of personal meaning and interest. This therapist matches technique to patient type; she uses age, diagnosis, and disability to determine the choice of activity without regard for the patient's meaning and need. Activities chosen because protocol and the provider consider them meaningful may be reasonable forms of occupation, but they are questionable forms of occupational therapy.

The occupational therapist as parent. The image of parent is clearly a more personal one than that of detached technician. The parental image, typically associated with the provision of order and nurture, can be positive or negative depending on the manner in which order and nurture are provided (May, 1983). An excess of either order or nurture can compromise the relationship; helpers become paternalistic while patients become rebellious or dependent. The best parental figure, although excelling in knowledge and skill, bridges the power/knowledge gap through caring self-expenditure and compassion (May, 1983). I believe that he or she projects the positive image of a supportive parent who guards against

exercising imbalance in the provision of order and nurture. The occupational therapist who threatens the patient's autonomy, rigidly and unilaterally enforces rules, or preempts the patient's decisions and fosters overdependence, however, conveys a negative parental image. Conversely, the therapist who supports the patient while trying to meet his or her need for order and nurture conveys a positive parental image.

The story of Brunhilde cited earlier illustrates the overauthoritative parent figure who wields power for the patient's own good (as defined by the therapist). Rule-bound Brunhilde eschews adult autonomy; caring, for her, is parenting gone awry. By contrast, Hanlan (1979) praises the parental occupational therapists who treated her husband:

> I was...impressed with the equanimity of occupational and physical therapists as they worked all day with severely handicapped people, some with terminal illnesses. . . . If helping personnel—social workers, physician, or whoever—conceived of their function with the terminally ill as helping with discrete, day-to-day problems, I believe they would have less trouble just "hanging in there," which is really the most essential ingredient. (p. 28)

The steadfastness of therapists who help patients with simple daily activities evokes a positive parental image.

The following fictional story about an activities therapist named Meg illustrates the parental therapist's vigilance against overnurture and overorder. Meg comes up with the idea of having patients in a private psychiatric hospital design and make living room drapes as a therapeutic activity. She benignly manipulates the patients into regarding the idea as their own, and they are enthusiastic about "their" project. The psychiatrist later commends her for her skillful handling of the situation. [Meg] acknowledges that it was "handling" and questions the appropriateness of her conduct. Her psychiatrist friend answers:

> I don't think you did any—violence to their being; the idea was in them or you couldn't have wooed it out. And dealing with patients always takes some handling, the question is only is it for their benefit or yours. (Gibson, 1979, p. 51)

The psychiatrist's rationalization for this benignly paternalistic intervention is typical: The intervention is justifiable if it is for the patient's own good.

The occupational therapist as covenanter. May's (1983) image of the occupational therapist as covenanter illustrates a relationship equivalent to friendship. A friend (as covenanter) acknowledges an element of gift in human relationships. For one who covenants with another, a sense of reciprocity characterizes the giving and receiving. The professional steeped in the spirit of covenant regards his professional skills as gifts to be shared with a community of others. Services rendered occur within the context of a trusted relationship, and both parties receive as well as give. Although reciprocity characterizes the relationship within a covenanted bond, the stronger partner uses strengths and skills to nourish and build up the weaker (May, 1983). Above all, the friend, as covenanted person, professes commitment to the patient, based on personal respect. Within the context of this friendship, the therapist collaborates and cooperates with the patient's self-actualization. Petersen (1976) describes a way of collaborating in self-actualization that includes activity. It could well represent an occupational therapist who is a friend:

> There is a shouting spirit deep inside me:
> Take clay, it cries,
> Take pen and ink,
> Take flour and water,
> Take a scrub brush,
> Take a yellow crayon
> Take another's hand
> And with all these
> Say you,
> Say loving.

Certainly the image of Ora Ruggles from *The Healing Heart* is that of a friend. Other patients' stories also portray occupational therapists as friends: Benziger (1969) tells of her hospitalization for depression, remembering the occupational therapist as her "new friend" (p. 48). She notes her first impression of the therapist:

> A few days later the first person I had met there who made any real sense came into my room. She was the occupational therapist—a term I've always hated. She was kind, interested, enthusiastic, full of ideas, and intelligent. (p. 47)

The occupational therapist trusts Benziger, follows through on promises made, and supports a desire to get well. Crafts serve as catalysts for their interactions about life. The following exchange shows how the occupational therapist is responsive to Benziger and respects her strengths:

> "You know, you go at your work too hard, too fast, too desperately—and too frenetically."
> "I guess I do, but that's the way I feel. Time stands still for me now, it is endless, and yet if I have something to do, I get the sense that there will not be time enough to finish it, or that someone will stop me. . . ."
> She said, "You are an intelligent person, and you will help yourself to get well quickly."
> "You know," I answered, "you're the first person who has mentioned intelligence versus non intelligence, instead of sanity. You make me feel like a human being. . . ." I was grateful. I should not forget her. (p. 49)

A third image of occupational therapist as friend appears in Donaldson's (1976) autobiographical account of his unwanted and unwarranted 15-year confinement in mental institutions. That Donaldson could, under the circumstances, perceive any staff as friendly comes as a surprise. Nonetheless, Donaldson considers the occupational therapy worker, Baldylocks, a friend:

> While I waited, I found OT fun. Young, overweight Baldylocks had about five of us. He was a zealous worker in his church, and did not swear, drink, or smoke. He translated his religion to his work by showing compassion and understanding to all of us. He let me spend afternoons learning the touch system of typing. . . . Baldylocks started taking the OT men and a half dozen from upstairs for a two-hour walk on the grounds each Wednesday. Under the umbrella of all this warmth, I began watching the news on TV again. (pp. 245-246)

In occupational therapy, Donaldson exercises, cooks, and learns lathe work—all fulfilling activities selected in a spirit of collaboration and cooperation. Donaldson sees clearly this occupational therapy worker's commitment to caring, trust, and respect.

Patients' stories, then, suggest that occupational therapists can project an image of technician, parent, or friend, because therapists understand the therapeutic relationship in different ways. Images from patients' stories mirror the manner in which various patients experienced demonstrations of therapists' competence and caring.

Variable Emphases on Competence and Caring

Patients' positive images of occupational therapists reflect both competence and caring. Negative images reflect either a failure to commit personally to care or competence or caring gone awry. May's images are helpful both in characterizing occupational therapists and in understanding various interpretations of the occupational therapy vision of relationship. Each of May's three images—technician, parent, and friend—emphasizes competence and caring in a slightly different way. For the technical therapist, competence in performance is the primary expression of caring. Personal investment in the patient stimulates the pursuit of excellence in technique. The positive parental therapist, on the other hand, demonstrates caring, but the caring is powerful; the therapist must guard against falling into handling or managing the patient. Unlike the technician, for whom competence is assumed to be caring, a parental therapist's care presumes competence. The parental caregiver determines how care should be given. Although many patients value care, they challenge the assumption that the caregiver always knows best. The therapist-as-friend image works to resolve the caring-competence struggle found in parental and technical images by assigning equal value to both care and competence. A therapist who would be a friend to the patient commits to competence and caring because the patient is a person who deserves both.

Although there will always be individual patients who want therapists to function as technicians or parents, many patients and occupational therapists call for a different image, one that equalizes competence and caring and that generates images of occupational therapists as friends. Public distress over impersonal care has resulted in a series of measures to acknowledge patients' rights: quality assurance requirements, the Patient's Bill of Rights, informed consent legislation, and the regulation of experimentation on human beings. These measures create a systematic defense against a powerful and technologically advanced medical system that tends to depersonalize the individual patient. The health care system demands scientific and technical competence; the legal system demands the acknowledgment of individual rights. Practitioners must be competent to function in the health care system without creating a service that is devoid of caring. Commitment to caring about a person cannot be legislated; it can, however, be part of a profession's vision.

Hodgins (1969) powerfully describes his post-stroke experiences in his article, "Whatever Became of the Healing Art?" He mourns the loss of the family physician who "was a friend to his patients, one function among many others which most of today's practitioners have completely given up" (p. 838). He values occupational therapists who "have so much more a satisfactory grasp on the real needs of the stroke patient" (p. 841). Hodgins wonders about the patient in today's health care system:

> From whom, then, is he to draw the courage without which he will not truly recover? Not from a silent practitioner; not from a stuffy practitioner; not from a practitioner, whether doctor, therapist, or nurse, who is aloof. He will draw courage as he perceives human understanding underlying the professional techniques of those into whose care he has been given. (p. 841)

In 1980, several therapists addressed the concept of caring at the 60th Annual Conference of the American Occupational Therapy Association. Together their remarks echoed those of Hodgins; they endorsed a vision of the therapeutic relationship that approximates that of pioneer Ora Ruggles, that of the therapist as friend. At the heart of this vision is the belief that the patient-therapist relationship is integral to practice. Baum (1980) writes, "We are nothing more than a bystander in the life of [the patient] until a relationship is formed' (p. 514). Competence and caring remain key elements in the vision, but both are effective only insofar as they reflect

sensitive commitment to a patient who is first of all a person. Activity selection and treatment goals must have personal meaning for the patient; meaningful choice is essential because it fosters personal control. Baum (1980) clarifies the process: "Occupational therapy harnesses will and gives the individual control through activity. That is human, that is care" (p. 515). Technical skills work only within the context of a relationship: "Skills promote movement and flexibility within our therapeutic relationships. . . . Skills in caring provide us with the ability to modify the technique according to another person's needs" (Gilfoyle, 1980, p. 520). King (1980) identifies the commitment to caring that must permeate competence: "Occupational therapy is one of the 'helping' professions, with the assumption that help is the outgrowth of caring" (p. 522). Competence must be rooted in caring for a person.

Caring also needs to be rooted in commitment to the patient as a person. Gilfoyle (1980) writes:

> The caring therapist directly knows a client as a unique individual, as someone in his or her own right, not as an average, a generality, or a number on the Gaussian curve. . . . Implicit knowledge is the art of "being with the person"; it is something you feel. (p. 520)

The person is experienced and respected as an "other" with strengths and capabilities; "the 'caring' is not the taking-care-of the person, but helping the person learn to take care of himself/herself" (Gilfoyle, 1980, p. 519). The same principle can be stated in another way: "Through our professional relationships we reach out and with empathy show that we care hoping that from this caring. . . . the person will find his or her own strength" (Baum, 1980, p. 515).

Yerxa (1980) regards deliberations on caring as calibrations of the profession's success. She says. "Our practice in the future should be evaluated not only on the basis of measurable scientific outcomes, but also by what it contributes to individual human dignity, a sense of mastery and self-respect" (p. 534). She identifies the challenge of the future as that of preserving and embracing a climate of caring "in the face of a society increasingly dominated by technique and objectivism" (p. 532). This type of caring resembles a friendship in which "patient and therapist enter into a partnership, and in which patients have the authority to determine their own needs" (p. 532).

Conclusion

The vision of the therapeutic relationship in occupational therapy has, despite its evolving emphasis and sometimes fragmentary form, encompassed two essential features: competence and caring. Images that patients have held of occupational therapists have varied, partly because of the ways in which therapists have understood and acted on their understanding of how to balance competence and caring during their interactions with patients. Negative images of occupational therapists found in patients' stories suggest that therapists who present themselves primarily as technicians or parents are more apt to disappoint the patient.

A health care system that depersonalizes patients challenges occupational therapists to assess the vision of the therapeutic relationship that has inspired their practice. Recommitment to regarding the patient as a vital partner—as a friend—can lead to exchanges marked by mutuality, caring, and competence. Commitment to a balance of technical competence and personal caring, for the sake of a friend, can shape a healing image.

Acknowledgments

I thank Sally Gadow, PhD, and Anne Hudson Jones, PhD, of the Institute for the Medical Humanities, University of Texas Medical Branch at Galveston, for their encouragement and suggestions. I also thank Paula Levine, School of Allied Health Sciences, University of Texas Medical Branch, for her editorial suggestions.

References

Baum, C. (1980). Occupational therapists put care in the health system. *American Journal of Occupational Therapy, 34,* 505-516.

Benziger, B. (1969). *The prison of my mind.* New York: Walker.

Carlova, J., & Ruggles, O. (1946). *The healing heart.* New York: Messner.

Donaldson, K. (1976). *Insanity inside out.* New York: Crown.

Fay, E. V., & March, I. (1947). Occupational therapy in general and special hospitals. In H. S. Willard & C. S. Spackman (Eds.), *Principles of occupational therapy* (pp. 118-137). Philadelphia: J. B. Lippincott.

Gibson, W. (1979). *The cobweb.* New York: Atheneum Press.

Gilfoyle, E. (1980). Caring: A philosophy of practice. *American Journal of Occupational Therapy, 34,* 517-521.

Gleave, G. M. (1947). Occupational therapy in children's hospitals and pediatric services. In H. S. Willard & C. S. Spackman (Eds.), *Principles of occupational therapy* (pp. 141-174). Philadelphia: J. B. Lippincott.

Hanlan, M. (1979, November). *Living with a dying husband.* Pennsylvania Gazette, pp. 25-28.

Heller, J., & Vogel, S. (1986). *No laughing matter.* New York: Avon.

Hodgins, E. (1969). Whatever became of the healing art? *Annals of the New York Academy of Sciences, 164,* 838-846.

Hopkins, H. L., & Smith, H. D. (Eds.). (1983). *Willard and Spackman's occupational therapy* (6th ed.). Philadelphia: J. B. Lippincott.

Hopkins, H. L., & Tiffany, E. G. (1983). Occupational therapy—A problem-solving process. In H. L. Hopkins & H. D. Smith (Eds.), *Willard and Spackman's occupational therapy* (6th ed., pp. 89-100). Philadelphia: J. B. Lippincott.

King, L. J. (1980). Creative caring. *American Journal of Occupational Therapy, 34,* 522-528.

May, W. (1983). *The physician's covenant: Images of the healer in medical ethics.* Philadelphia: Westminster Press.

McClay, E. (1977). *Green winter: Celebrations of old age.* New York: Reader's Digest Press.

Peloquin, S. M. (1989). Sustaining the art of occupational therapy. *American Journal of Occupational Therapy, 43,* 219-226.

Petersen, J. (1976). *A book of yes.* Illinois: Argus Communications.

Purtilo, R. (1978). *Health professional/patient interaction.* Philadelphia: W. B. Saunders.

Rebeta-Burditt, J. (1977). *The cracker factory.* New York: Bantam.

Seabrook, W. (1935). *Asylum.* New York: Harcourt, Brace.

Smith, H. D., & Tiffany, E. G. (1983). Assessment and evaluation—An overview. In H. L. Hopkins & H. D. Smith (Eds.), *Willard and Spackman's occupational therapy* (6th ed., pp. 143-148). Philadelphia: J. B. Lippincott.

Tiffany, E. G. (1983). Psychiatry and mental health. In H. L. Hopkins & H. D. Smith (Eds.), *Willard and Spackman's occupational therapy* (6th ed., pp. 267-329). Philadelphia: J. B. Lippincott.

Wade, B. D. (1947). Occupational therapy for patients with mental disease. In H. S. Willard & C. S. Spackman (Eds.), *Principles of occupational therapy* (pp. 81-117). Philadelphia: J. B. Lippincott.

Willard, H. S., & Spackman, C. S. (Eds.). (1947). *Principles of occupational therapy.* Philadelphia: J. B. Lippincott.

Yerxa, E. J. (1980). Occupational therapy's role in creating a future climate of caring. *American Journal of Occupational Therapy, 34,* 529-534.

Chapter 39

The Treatment of Schizophrenia: A Patient's Perspective

Esso Leete

It has been 20 years since I first became mentally ill. As I approach 40, I find myself still struggling with the same symptoms, still crippled by the same fears and paranoia. I am haunted by an evasive picture of what my life could have been, whom I might have become, what I might have accomplished. My schizophrenia is a sad realization, a painful reality, that I live with every day. I wonder what, if anything, I could have done differently either to avoid developing schizophrenia or to lessen its severity.

After years of turmoil and lack of direction, in 1982 I made a conscious decision to put my experiences with mental illness, both positive and negative, to constructive use, educating others about mental illness and its treatment. This effort has become my mission in life, my passion. Knowing that something beneficial may eventually come from the horror of my mental illness is my consolation. My search for answers to the many questions I had about my affliction has helped me to clarify my thoughts about the needs of individuals with schizophrenia. These thoughts, which are based on my experiences, are presented here.

The Onset of Illness

Let me tell you a little about my history. I probably inherited a predisposition to mental illness; my uncle was diagnosed as having "dementia praecox," an earlier term for schizophrenia. In my senior year of high school, I began to experience personality changes. I did not realize the significance of the changes at the time, and I think others denied them, but looking back I can see that they were the earliest signs of illness. I became increasingly withdrawn and sullen. I felt alienated and lonely and hated everyone. I felt as if there were a huge gap between me and the rest of the world; everybody seemed so distant from me. I watched dispassionately as my two younger sisters matured, dated, shopped, and shaped their lives while I seemed stuck in a totally different dimension.

I reluctantly went off to college, feeling alone and totally unprepared for life away from home. I was isolative and had no close friends. As time went on, I spoke to virtually no one. Increasingly during classes I found myself drawing pictures of Van Gogh and writing poetry. I forgot to eat and began sleeping in my clothes. Performing even the most routine activities, such as taking a shower, rarely even occurred to me.

The First Break

Toward the end of my first semester, I had my first psychotic episode. I did not understand what was happening and was extremely frightened. The experience left me exhausted and confused, and I began hearing voices for the first time. Reality as others knew it had given way to the multiple realities with which I would now live.

I was admitted to a psychiatric hospital, diagnosed as having schizophrenia, treated with medications, and released after a few months. Over the next two years I was hospitalized in psychiatric facilities five times, the longest hospitalization lasting a year. During my late teens and early 20s, when my age demanded that I date and develop social skills, my illness required that I spend my adolescence on psychiatric wards. To this day I mourn the loss of those years.

When I was first hospitalized, I was young, passive, extremely dependent, and naive. I did not understand what was happening, and I was not sufficiently in touch with the world to care. I was so regressed that I hardly spoke and stayed in bed as much as possible, eagerly seizing my voices as companions. I believed I was living on Venus and, according to hospital charts, I stood on chairs and tables speaking in an incomprehensible language (presumably "Venusian").

My identity began to fragment and seemed to blend with my environment. Rather than just enjoying the wind, for instance, I thought I had merged with it. I had to stare at the sun to appreciate its warmth. Yet gradually I was able to see myself as separate from those things. As I neared discharge, I began to feel some stirring of belief in myself. It was not until much later that I made a conscious effort to develop a sense of control, realizing that I had the power to decide what form my life would take and who I would be.

After spending nearly two years in a series of hospitals, I began weekly outpatient therapy and medication management at the local psychiatric hospital at which I had received inpatient care. I attended a local college part-time and was married to my first husband at the end of my first semester. We moved to another state, where I continued on medication and received both individual and group psychotherapy.

My condition improved, and a few years later I discontinued outpatient therapy and requested that my medication be gradually tapered off. Throughout most of this time I was employed, first in a series of fast-food restaurants and later as a secretary at a college. For the next ten years, I did not require hospitalization. During that time, I was divorced from my first husband and married a community mental health center psychiatrist. Although I experienced some acute flare-ups of symptomatology during that period, I had no recurrence of persistent, disabling symptoms.

Exacerbations

When more serious symptoms returned about ten years later, I denied their existence. The more people alluded to my illness, treated me negatively, and recommended I become reinvolved in therapy, the more resistant and angry I became. I had decided that I was not ill, that I did not need the medications, and that I did not wish to be involved in psychiatric treatment. I just did not want to be sick any more, an understandable desire, and I was convinced that if I got rid of the evidence of illness I would be magically cured. It didn't work.

Instead, having discontinued medications years earlier and now withdrawing from other forms of support, I experienced more symptoms. It is my belief that the actions I took were self-destructive responses to my despondency about being mentally ill. I was aided in my downhill plunge, however, by several of the psychiatric institutions at which I was treated.

Dubious Treatment

One private psychiatric hospital in Denver was particularly destructive. I was banned from group therapy sessions, my food was monitored, my time was regulated, and my roommates were removed from my room and thus from my negative influence.

Toward the end of my hospitalization, I was placed in seclusion and restraints every day. I was forbidden to cross a red line painted on the floor, much less leave the unit. Not surprisingly, I did not improve, as such power struggles and automatic limit setting are rarely therapeutic. The more I was ostracized and punished, the angrier I became and the more I rebelled. Slowly, however, my desperation turned to resignation and hopelessness.

To make matters worse, even my psychiatrist would not speak to me. Although he dutifully came to see me about twice a week, he stopped talking to me after the first couple of sessions, regardless of what I said, what I asked, or what I did. One day I had to actually sit on my hands to prevent myself from jumping up and strangling him out of frustration. Not only was his "silent treatment" not helpful, but it contributed substantially to my feelings of despair. Fortunately, with the help of my friends on the unit and daily one-to-one sessions with various staff, particularly two nurses who had compassion and professional integrity, I survived.

After five months on the unit, any therapeutic alliance that had been established was long gone. One day I announced that I would soon be escaping on the locked elevator and calmly began to collect my belongings. The staff seemed skeptical and utterly unconcerned. Within about an hour, I had successfully eloped from the unit, determined to commit suicide.

What I found on the outside, however, dissuaded me. To my real amazement, I found that people did not threaten me, did not yell at me, did not order me around, did not ignore me, and did not treat me alternately like a child or like a criminal. They were actually friendly, and for the first time in a long time I felt pleasure and power. Having felt these feelings, I fantasized that I might hold on to them and find the strength to run my own life. After two days of deliberation and real soul-searching, I decided to check out of my motel room and return to the hospital on my own, vowing to leave there cured.

The Turning Point

Upon my return to the hospital I was met with silent anger. I sensed that staff were disappointed to see me again and that they had secretly wished they would no longer have to deal with me. Naively I had expected that our relationship would be better after I returned voluntarily. I assumed staff would see the evident change in my attitude and resume my treatment with the same optimism and energy I felt.

Instead, virtually all communication between staff and me ceased, and I continued to be banned from group therapy, occupational therapy, and recreational therapy. Naturally I was again restricted to the unit. Once again I experienced daily episodes of seclusion and restraint, which were precipitated by the anger and frustration I felt toward my private psychiatrist for his refusal to talk to me during our sessions.

The situation deteriorated after the staff discovered while reading my journal that I was in possession of a gun (which I had bought while contemplating suicide). I had brought the gun with me onto the unit to defend myself against the possibility of tube feeding, with which the staff had threatened me before I left the unit. I thought the sight of a gun would force them to abandon their attempt at tube feeding. I had not wanted to hurt anyone, and I kept the gun unloaded and brought no bullets with me to the hospital.

Because of my "dangerous and inappropriate behavior," I was immediately placed in seclusion for two days.

At the end of the two days, I learned that the head of the hospital, acting with staff input, had ordered that I remain in seclusion at least until the next visit from my doctor, who did not see me every day. I was distraught. During the two days I had spent in quiet seclusion, I had heard an increasing number of voices, and I was terrified they would seize this opportunity to close in on me. I did not know how I would survive even another five minutes in this room, let alone until I met with my doctor.

I was released from seclusion on the next day, after I saw my doctor and agreed to do everything he wished. He had threatened to send me to a maximum security unit of a state hospital for an indefinite period of time. About a week later, the hospital "released" me into the streets (actually I was kicked out), even though my psychiatrist had implied that I would need intensive ongoing treatment in a locked setting.

After spending two days in a cheap hotel, I decided to investigate Community Care Corporation, a private psychiatric residential halfway house that one of the nurses at the hospital had told me about. I sought and gained admission to the program.

The residential program was very different from the hospital. It was structured and supervised, yet I did not feel imprisoned and at the mercy of an arbitrary staff. Unfortunately I had incorporated some of the negative messages about myself that I had learned at the hospital and had come to believe I was incapable of living successfully on the outside. At Community Care, however, I sensed that the treatment team genuinely cared about me, and therefore I did not feel an ongoing need to test limits, as I had at the hospital.

Unlike the hospital staff, the residential treatment team did not assume authoritarian, confrontative postures that result inevitably in power struggles. Instead, they encouraged and even demanded my input in treatment. They considered me a partner in my own treatment rather than a less knowledgeable inferior. The mutual fear experienced by myself and the staff at the hospital was replaced by mutual acceptance at Community Care. Medication was used in the residential program as an aid in the recovery process. In the hospital it was too often used to sedate patients into submission.

There were other differences as well. In the residential program, I was able to practice social skills in the safety of a community of peers and to learn skills by watching others practice. Psychiatric hospitals had only engendered or exacerbated feelings of dependency and low self-esteem. After several hospitalizations, I had begun to feel hopeless about the future and about my having any part in the world.

The regimentation of the hospital was missing at Community Care. The residential program expected me to take control of my life and led me to believe that I could. Staff attitudes were extremely important in building my confidence. In addition to recognizing and honestly addressing my weaknesses and problem areas, staff also pointed out my strengths and helped me make the most of them by teaching me specific problem-solving techniques and daily living skills.

Each week a staff member and I independently rated my progress in specific areas. The staff did not approach my treatment with a biased view of what I could accomplish, as I felt hospital personnel had done. Staff at this facility believed in my potential, and I began to develop confidence in myself. Gradually I became aware that I was my greatest asset.

There were other benefits to the program, too. I felt that I was part of a family, which motivated me to improve my social skills and interpersonal relationships, a crucial step in the path to recovery. Group therapy showed me that other members of the program had similar symptoms and strengthened my connection to them. I also learned to do reality testing with staff and group members. The encouragement and immediate feedback I received were invaluable.

As a result of my developing confidence in myself and realistic trust in others, I was able to grow. The prejudice I had encountered was supplanted by an emerging understanding of me as a person, and pity became respect. The flexibility of the program to meet my individual needs enabled me to work forward, with the knowledge that a predictable, consistent, and caring support system was available for me should I need it.

I was now ready to take control of my life. My estranged second husband and I moved into an apartment together, and I threw myself into the task of finding employment. With encouragement from Community Care and my husband, I was successful. None of these steps were accomplished easily, but the pieces of my periodically disrupted life were coming back together.

Reflections

So that I may continue to progress, I have looked closely at what has helped me and what has not, and I have tried to understand why my condition has improved. I have come to the following conclusions.

Community-Based Treatment

Hospitals have their place in the treatment and stabilization of acute psychiatric problems. However, it is my opinion that long-term gains in functioning are made most readily and most successfully through treatment in the community. Although some community facilities are better than others, a good community support program can provide vital services for its clients, perhaps the most important of which are a familiar structured environment and close interpersonal relationships.

Living in the community allows individuals with a psychiatric illness to gain understanding and acceptance from members of a treatment program. Peers, family, and friends can also provide recognition of and respect for clients' individuality and special needs.

A community support program can help residents develop a predictable daily schedule to offset their chaotic inner existence and thus make life easier. Any number of structured activities could satisfy this need, but I have found work—a paying job—to be the most helpful. My job gives me something to look forward to every day, a skill to learn and improve, and an earned income. It is my motivation for getting up each morning, not always an easy task for psychiatric patients. My hours at work are passed therapeutically as well as productively, for through steady employment I have learned to value myself and trust in my ability to overcome my disease.

Education and Support

Education about mental illness is crucial for everyone, but particularly for patients. I resent the fact that I was not given information about my illness and the methods used to treat it, some of which I feel were harmful. For example, alternating electroshock with insulin coma therapy in 1966 only served to virtually eradicate my memories while probably adversely affecting my ability to learn new information as well. Doing so without my consent or even my awareness was criminal.

Patients and family members are entitled to education about mental illness, including its symptoms, course, and treatment; more important, perhaps, they also need to know that the disease can be managed and that there is reason to hope that the patient will live a satisfying and productive life.

Peer-run support groups can be extremely valuable to clients by offering support, friendship, hope for the future, and peer-group modeling. We as consumers of psychiatric services should meet socially with others who have had similar experiences to exchange information about coping skills and to take responsibility for ourselves. We must meet with others like ourselves to see firsthand what we have accomplished and what we can achieve.

Support groups and educational groups can help patients and their friends and family members to accept and deal with mental illness. Community mental health centers should be required to hold classes on a regular basis for both families and consumers in which various major mental illnesses can be openly discussed and information about mental illnesses shared by both professionals and clients. In fact, these classes are already taking place. Each week at the Mental Health Center of Boulder County both consumers and family members pack a room to hear the facts about mental illnesses, hoping to gain a better understanding of these perplexing and frustrating diseases.

Medications

I believe there is also a place for medications in the treatment of major mental illnesses. Unfortunately the side effects of antipsychotic medications can often be more disabling than the illnesses themselves, and I have even experienced side effects from the pills I took to control the side effects of antipsychotic drugs. For years I fought against taking medications before I found one that worked while causing a minimum of side effects. Now I would resist discontinuing it. I now know how terrible I feel when I do not take my medication, and I realize how much better I am able to function with it.

Before I reached this important realization, I was caught in a vicious circle. When I was off the medication I couldn't remember how much better I had felt on it, and when I was taking the medication I felt so good that I was convinced I did not need it. Finally, however, I was able to make the connection between taking the medication and feeling better and to realize how very helpful the medication is to me.

I am not advocating that everyone with a mental illness take medication or that we now have medications that will work for everyone, but the use of medication is an option worth exploring by anyone with a mental illness. Letting a doctor "adjust" your brain chemistry may be frightening, and drug therapy is certainly an art when competently done. However, if psychopharmacotherapy is to be successful, the patient cannot be a passive observer; arriving at the proper type and dosage of medication requires a true partnership between doctor and patient.

Dealing with Relapse

Relapses are inevitable. Although they can be triggered by a number of different mechanisms and may have a biochemical or neurophysiological basis, their effects can often be mediated by a strong, positive relationship with one's family or other significant individuals. Above all else, it is important to deal intelligently with relapses when they occur and make the effort to begin again. Those of us with mental illnesses must try to learn what we can from the unfortunate experience of relapse and remember what helped us to recover and what did not. In that way the next relapse may be softened.

Being Realistic

Like those with other chronic illnesses, I know to expect good and bad times and to make the most of the good. I take my life very seriously and do as much as I can when I am feeling well, because I know that there will be bad times when I am likely to lose some of the ground I have gained. Professionals and family members must help the ill person set realistic goals. I would entreat them not to be devastated by our illnesses and transmit this hopeless attitude to us. I would urge them never to lose hope, for we will not strive if we believe the effort is futile.

Strategies for Preventing Relapse

I find that my vulnerability to stress and anxiety decreases the more I feel in control of my life. My coping strategies largely consist of four steps: recognizing when I am feeling stressed; identifying the stressor; remembering from past experience what action helped in the same situation or a similar one; and taking that action.

Generally speaking, I have also learned to have a more positive outlook. I accept myself and my shortcomings (although I try to minimize them), and I have also become more accepting of others, realizing that we cannot all be alike. I attempt to keep in touch with my feelings and to attend immediately to difficulties, including symptoms. For example, rather than letting my paranoia grow, I will take action to satisfy the paranoid feelings. If I feel uncomfortable in a public place because I am convinced someone is after me, I will make it a point to sit facing the door. Having done so, I am able to forget the paranoid feeling and go on about my life rather than letting the paranoia control me.

Because new experiences and environments create enormous pressures, I need the security of a predictable environment. I also know I must go slow when confronted with anything new, avoiding stressful situations if necessary. I have learned my particular limitations and my own sources of stress, and I mentally prepare myself to cope with situations that test my limits or cause stress by anticipating the problems that might occur.

I now know that at times I may need to spend some time alone, and I take "time out." But not too much. I also try to recognize my personal warning signs of relapse (though not always successfully). To successfully avert or diminish relapses, I have been forced to be persistent and to consistently utilize these coping behaviors.

My illness is a sobering reality, yet I am not as vulnerable to it as I once was because of my regular use of coping strategies as well as my new philosophy about my life. I have come to understand that life may be more difficult for me than it is for others and that I must preside over it more attentively for this reason. Yet every individual, regardless of whether he or she has a mental illness, must develop skills in general coping, interpersonal relations, and management of work and leisure time. It is these skills that will allow us to lead successful and happy lives.

Conclusions

There is no magic answer that will eliminate the tragedy of mental illnesses, but we need not be at their mercy. Appropriate treatment can help those of us with a mental illness to understand our disease and to learn to function in spite of it. After multiple hospitalizations, I found that any gains I had made were consolidated in community treatment, where mentally ill individuals are treated as people with strengths and weaknesses instead of mental patients who can never improve. Those with mental illnesses must try not to be disheartened, admittedly a difficult task, for having some hope is crucial.

Despite my lack of formal credentials, I have become somewhat of an expert about my psychosis; having lived with it these many years, I feel I have a personal understanding of it that could not be learned from books. I have tried to use this knowledge to live the best life my disease will allow. We consumers of psychiatric services have much to contribute in the effort to educate the public about mental illness and eradicate its stigma.

More important, however, those of us who are afflicted with a mental illness must work to understand our disabilities so we can conquer them. We must study our illness, appraise our lives, identify our strengths and weaknesses, and build on our assets while minimizing our vulnerabilities. Only then will we realize and fully use our potential and begin to overcome the stigma, discrimination, and rejection we have experienced, Only then will we reclaim our dignity and our autonomy. To achieve these goals we must change the perception of who we are and who we can become, first for ourselves and then for the public.

Although it takes time, those of us with a mental illness can overcome the disease by compensating for our handicaps. I did not choose to be ill, but I can choose to deal with schizophrenia and learn to live with it. I know I must confront my disorder with courage and struggle with my symptoms persistently, never viewing relapse as a permanent defeat and always acknowledging remission as a hard-earned victory.

Chapter 40

Patients' Accounts of Stress and Coping in Schizophrenia

Agnes B. Hatfield, PhD

The concepts "stress" and "coping" are often used by clinicians to explain the behaviors of people with schizophrenia and to develop strategies for working with patients and their families (1-6). The general assumption of these clinicians is that people with schizophrenia have a special vulnerability, probably of biological origin, to internal and external stress (7).

Anderson (8) used the term "core psychological deficit" to explain this vulnerability, which she felt could be exacerbated in the home, work place, or treatment setting. Anderson and colleagues (1), who elected to focus on the family as a potential source of stress, developed and tested a method of psychoeducational treatment that reduced patients' rate of relapse. The treatment involved training families in new ways of communicating and relating that, along with optimum uses of medication, reduced the stresses that led to decompensation. Kopeiken [sic] and others (5), who also considered life events as precipitants of patients' decompensation, directed their efforts toward helping families identify, prevent, and cope with situations that were stressful to the patient.

These studies focused on stressors that are external to the patient. Patients' accounts of their experiences, however, reveal that many sources of stress are internal to the person. There is a growing interest among researchers and clinicians in learning more about the personal side of mental illness to better understand patient behaviors and to establish better rapport with patients (9-13). As Carpenter (9) pointed out, "It is in the subjective and inner world of volition, perception, cognition, and affect that schizophrenia is manifest" (p. 534). The challenge is to find a valid way to learn about this inner world of schizophrenia.

A potentially valuable, but little consulted, source of information about the personal side of mental illness is patients' accounts that have appeared in numerous small publications, consumer newsletters, and small collections of personal stories, as well as in professional journals and, occasionally, in published books. Although several such accounts were published in the 1960s and 1970s (14-17), more recent materials also offer valuable insights.

The purposes of this study were to learn from first-person accounts how the inner experiences of people with schizophrenia become sources of stress for them and how patients strive to cope with these stressors. First-person accounts from a wide range of sources were selected with the assumption that they supply valid and useful data for understanding and helping people with schizophrenia. The research was also guided by Estroff's suggestion (18), based on studies of patients in their natural environments in the community, that patients' perceptions, beliefs, feelings, experiences, and behaviors are the most important units of analysis. Stress theory (19-23), which is briefly explained below, served as a general framework for interpretation of patients' statements.

Stress Theory

Stress occurs when a person's resources are inadequate to meet the demands of the environment. This definition may be interpreted to include both the inner and outer environment. Stress is a painful state of disequilibrium accompanied by feelings of great tension, high anxiety, and fatigue. When individuals are stressed, they struggle to find ways of coping that will reduce their great discomfort.

This paper is not concerned with ordinary levels of stress but rather with stress severe enough to tax an individual's capacity to cope with or adapt to it. Wrubel and associates (24) have identified some characteristics of situations that are likely to produce overwhelming levels of stress. Such situations may be unique in the individual's experience, and the individual may not be prepared to deal with them. On the other hand, stress is also produced by events that occur frequently or that have a long duration. Such situations lead to fatigue and burnout. Also stressful are situations that affect all aspects of one's existence or that are highly ambiguous. Patient accounts indicate that the experience of schizophrenia commonly has these characteristics.

Some theoreticians assume that all human beings have an innate drive toward competence (25-27). In this view, human beings are always striving to survive physically and psychologically. They either attempt to adapt to their environment or change it. Patient accounts usually reveal an active process of coping and adapting in spite of the tremendous difficulties that schizophrenia presents.

Sources of Stress in Schizophrenia

Sources of stress identified in patients' accounts of mental illness include altered perceptions, cognitive confusion, attentional deficit, and impaired identity.

Altered Perceptions

Alteration of senses may involve either enhancement or blunting of perceptions, but enhancement or in-creased acuteness is probably most common. Visual stimuli appear sharper and brighter, and auditory stimuli seem louder. In addition, these sensations appear to change unpredictably. Since everything that we know about the world must come through our senses, people with schizophrenia experience a grossly distorted reality. They suffer high levels of stress and anxiety as they struggle to negotiate between the world as others know it and the world of their inner reality.

Sculptor and writer Mary McGrath (28) provided this account of her experience:

"I know all of the negatives. Schizophrenia is painful, and it is craziness when I hear voices, when I believe that people are following me, wanting to snatch my very soul. I am frightened too when every whisper, every laugh is about me; when newspapers suddenly contain curses, four-letter words shouting at me; when sparkles of light are demon eyes. Schizophrenia is frightening when I can't hold onto thoughts." (p. 38)

McGrath says her illness is a " journey of fear" that is "often paralyzing" and "mostly painful." Still she is hopeful because new research may help ease the burden of the illness and because of the help and caring of mental health professionals. She expresses the difficulty of living between two worlds, as does Nona Borgeson (29):

"Where weighing the odds of probability ends, schizophrenia begins, and paranoia runs rampant. The schizophrenic doesn't think; he/she knows, false knowledge though it be, and his/her world becomes one of polarities—black or white, love or hate, ecstasy or suicidal inclinations, mortal fear or indestructibility." (p. 7)

It is instructive to review patients' descriptions of their inner world in light of what Antonovsky (30) says about human health or the state of well-being. He suggests that a sense of coherence, an "enduring though dynamic feeling of confidence that one's internal and external environments are predictable and that things will work out as well as can be expected," is crucial to well-being (p. 123). The lack of coherence and predictability that plagues the lives of men and women with schizophrenia, who have a "terrific sense of unreality" and who often feel like they are "waking up in a strange room" (17), is certainly striking.

Cognitive Confusion

Patients in Freedman's study (15) of perceptual and cognitive disturbances in schizophrenia described themselves as "confused," "hazy," "bewildered," and "disoriented" (15). They reported that they suffered thought blocking and sometimes felt their minds going blank, and that they were unable to maintain cognitive control over their ideas. Torrey (13) reported the following example:

"My thoughts get all jumbled up. I start thinking or talking about something, but I never get there. Instead I wander off in the wrong direction and get caught up with all sorts of different things that may be connected with the things I want to say but in a way I can't explain. People listening to me get more lost than I do." (p. 18)

Freedman (15) found a variety of disturbances in memory, language, and speech in the 50 autobiographical accounts she studied. Patients reported experiencing a lag between hearing a word, recalling its meaning, and formulating an answer. Speech required great concentration and conscious effort. Freedman provides the following example from a patient:

"Sometimes when people speak to me, my head is overloaded. It's too much to hold at once. It goes out as quick as it goes in. It makes you forget what you just heard because you can't get hearing it long enough. It's just words in the air unless you can figure it out from their faces." (p. 338)

The patient accounts reported by Freedman revealed that the sense of time was often distorted during acute stages of illness. Some patients said they lost all sense of time and with it, all notions of logic, order, and sequence:

"My time sense was disturbed. This was the result of intense cerebral activity in which inner experiences took place at greatly increased speed, so that much more than usual happened per minute of external time. The result was to give an effect of slow motion. The speeding up of my inner experiences provided in this way an apparent slowing down of the external world." (p. 338)

Attentional Deficit

The difficulties of meeting the ordinary demands of the environment due to cognitive confusion are compounded by problems of attention and concentration. More than half of the sample in Freedman's study specifically noted such problems and reported that their minds wandered a good deal. One patient said, "It is not that he [the patient] cannot keep to the point, but there are so many points and all equally and insistently insignificant" (p. 336).

Anscombe (31) suggested that attentional deficit is central to the problem of coping with schizophrenia. The patient often has the sensation of being captured by a stimulus rather than being able to choose what to attend. Objects seem to jump out of the environment and command attention. Patients have a sense of lack of volition and are unable to shift their attention flexibly.

McGhie and Chapman (32) provided this account:

"If I am reading I may suddenly get bogged down at a word. It may be any word, even a simple word that I know well.

When this happens I can't get past it. It is as if I am being hypnotized by it. It's as if I am seeing the word for the first time and in a different way from anyone else. It's not so much that I am absorbed in it, it's more like it is absorbing me." (p. 109)

Finding themselves riveted to a particular stimulus, people with schizophrenia conclude that what they are attracted to has unusual significance (31). David Zelt (33), telling his story in third person, describes his fascination with colors, each of which came to have its own significance:

"Ordinarily unimportant information from external reality took on new dimensions for him. For example, colors powerfully influenced him. At any given moment wherever David went, colors were used to express judgements about his spirituality. People used the colors of their clothes or cars to express positive or negative views of him. Green meant that David was like Christ; white stood for spiritual purity; orange indicated he was attuned to the cosmos." (p. 530)

The patient experiences enormous difficulties in achieving levels of competence adequate to meet ordinary environmental demands. Since the source of these difficulties is invisible, the world generally does not understand the patient's problems and expects more than the patient can produce. As a result, the patient often feels inadequate, anxious, and discouraged.

Impaired Identity

Alterations in the sense of self are common in schizophrenia. McGrath (28) describes her strange feelings: "If I want to reach out to touch me, I feel nothing but slippery coldness, yet I sense it is me." Later she says, "My existence seems undefined—mere image that I keep reaching for, but never can touch" (p. 638). Normally individuals have a clear sense of where their bodies end and the rest of the world begins. Without this capacity, orienting oneself in the world is extremely difficult.

With treatment, the more acute phases of mental illness tend to abate and more energy is available to attend to the external world. But Harris and Bergman (34) observed that getting better can be a mixed blessing for many clients. They are caught between the familiar patient role and the nonpatient role, which is not clearly defined. They are frightened about the future but cannot return to the past. These men and women have the awesome task of learning to accept that life is irrevocably different, and because of this difference, new meaning in life and a new way of living must be found.

Godschalx (35) studied the personal perspective of patients with schizophrenia and found that many of them struggle with issues of identity. They had great difficulty deciding how to characterize what was wrong with them. They stated variously that they had "a nervous breakdown," "spells," "anxiety," or "mental problems." Godschalx found no relationship between acknowledgment of a mental illness and either happiness or level of functioning.

Coping Strategies

The many creative ways that patients use to cope with these distressing symptoms are truly remarkable. Esso Leete (36) has stated that, contrary to popular thinking that people with schizophrenia are withdrawn and passive, they are actively fighting "internal terrors and external realities" to keep their emotional balance and social composure in a world they cannot always translate.

People with schizophrenia may appear rigid and unable to change directions without difficulty. This inflexibility is one way of maintaining stability when the ground keeps shifting beneath them. Structure and predictability in the external world help compensate for the unpredictability of the inner world. Daily routines give pattern and a sense of order to life. By knowing what to expect, the person with schizophrenia can prepare [him- or herself] and thus exert a degree of control over events. Stress and anxiety lessen when events lose their sense of arbitrariness and an appearance of consistency emerges.

Stephen Weiner (37) likened his condition to that of Sisyphus, who was condemned to roll a rock up a hill only to have it slide down again: "So strategy becomes a necessity—learn to anticipate. No caffeine before a predictably stressful situation. . . . A conscious effort to combat the automatic ideas of reference. . . . Remind myself that coincidences do appear" (p. 9).

Jeannette Keil (38) found that she could learn to control her words and actions even if she was unable to control her racing thoughts. She worked diligently to keep her life in balance, and she pressured herself to appear appropriate. Jerry Pearson (39) said he used relationships with people to stay centered in reality: "When I am alone for too long, my thinking and emotions can produce a semihallucinatory state. As long as I know that I have access to other people, I think I will be all right. Living in isolation would be the worst thing that could happen to me" (p. 2). Cara Lawerance (40) found that "having too much time is like living one's life in a cave. . . . One of the first things we should do to help recovery is to schedule our days" (p. 2).

Godschalx (35) found that her subjects were anxious about the terrors of hallucinations, the sense of being different, possible loss of control, and the likelihood of being victimized. The patients tried to deal with these insecurities by monitoring internal tensions, structuring

their thinking, and taking psychotropic medication. Esso Leete (41) found it important to recognize her own warning signs of potential relapse, including decreased sleep, trouble with concentration, forgetfulness, increased paranoia, more frequent voices, irritability, and being overwhelmed by her environment.

A number of men and women with mental illnesses find an acceptable role in life by helping others. Cathy King (42) found her identity in a "fellowship of others of her own kind." In a patient self-help organization, she experienced for the first time what it means to be a part of a group. Esso Leete (41), after a long struggle with schizophrenia, is now a full-time employee at a hospital to which she was once committed. She started the Denver Social Support Group to help others cope with their mental illnesses.

Patients related many philosophical ways that they came to terms with their dilemma. Stephen Weiner (37) dealt with the unfairness of having mental illness by accepting the fact that life is not fair, although it is unfair in different ways to different people. He has chosen to accept his condition "without completely giving in to it" (p. 10).

But in accepting his condition he eschews bravado as a means of coping. "Bravado is an almost inevitable reaction to pain and humiliation," he has written. "It is easier to pretend to oneself that the pain and humiliation never existed" (43). But this tactic is a form of denial of the "almost-heroic reality that the strength to endure and overcome had to arise as a strategic reaction to an unchosen, unforeseen misfortune" (p. 6).

Zan Boches (44) has suggested that life puts various limitations on people. However, freedom to make choices always exists within these limitations. For him, life was worthwhile in spite of the limitations imposed by a serious illness. Barbara Pilvin (45) came to terms with the way mental illness compromised her goals. She stated that her illness "made me understand that there are no guarantees in life, that the outcome of my plans may be beyond my control" (p. 23).

Conclusions

Clinicians now generally recognize environmental stress as a factor in aggravating the symptoms of schizophrenia. They less often acknowledge the role that internal stressors may play in creating anxiety and suffering. To more accurately explain and interpret patient behavior and to respond empathetically to patients, clinicians must learn much more about the inner world of schizophrenia. A rich source for learning about this experience is the body of widely available first-person accounts of patients.

References

1. Anderson CM, Reiss DJ, Hogarty GE: Schizophrenia and the Family. New York, Guilford, 1986

2. Beels CC, McFarlane WR: Family treatments of schizophrenia: background and state of the art. Hospital and Community Psychiatry 33:541-550, 1982

3. Bernheim K, Lehman A: Working With Families of the Mentally Ill. New York, Norton, 1985

4. Clarkin JF, Glick ID: Recent developments in family therapy: a review. Hospital and Community Psychiatry 33:550-556, 1982

5. Kopeikin HS, Marshall V, Goldstein MJ: Stages and impact of crisis-oriented family therapy in the aftercare of acute schizophrenia, in Family Therapy in Schizophrenia. Edited by McFarlane WR. New York, Guilford, 1983

6. Leff J, Vaughn C: Expressed Emotion in Families. New York, Guilford, 1985

7. Zubin J, Spring G: Vulnerability: a new view of schizophrenia, Journal of Abnormal Psychology 86:103-126, 1977

8. Anderson CM: A psychoeducational program for families of patients with schizophrenia, in Family Therapy in Schizophrenia. Edited by McFarlane WR. New York, Guilford, 1983

9. Carpenter WT: Thoughts on the treatment of schizophrenia. Schizophrenia Bulletin 12:527-539, 1986

10. Minkoff WM, Stern R: Paradoxes faced by residents being trained in the psychosocial treatment of people with chronic schizophrenia. Hospital and Community Psychiatry 36:859-864, 1985

11. Reiser M: Are psychiatric educators "losing the mind"? American Journal of Psychiatry 145:148-153,1988

12. Strauss JS: Discussion: what does rehabilitation accomplish? Schizophrenia Bulletin 12:720-723, 1986

13. Torrey EF: Surviving Schizophrenia: A Family Perspective. New York, Harper & Row, 1983

14. Alverez WC: Minds That Came Back. New York, Lippincott,1961

15. Freedman MA: Subjective experiences of perceptual and cognitive disturbances in schizophrenia. Archives of General Psychiatry 30:333-340, 1974

16. Kaplan B: The Inner World of Mental Illness. New York, Harper & Row, 1964

17. Landis D, Mettler FA: Varieties of Psychopathological Experiences. New York, Holt, Rinehart, Winston, 1964

18. Estroff S: Making It Crazy. Berkeley, University of California Press, 1981

19. Coehlo GV, Hamburg DA, Adams JE (eds): Coping and Adaptation. New York, Basic Books, 1974

20. Figley CR, McCubbin HI (eds): Coping With Catastrophe. New York, Brunner/Mazel, 1983

21. Hansell H: The Person-in-Distress: On the Biosocial Dynamics of Adaptation. New York, Human Sciences, 1976

22. Monat A, Lazarus R: Stress and Coping. New York, Columbia University Press, 1977

23. Parad H (ed): Crisis Intervention: Selected Readings. New York, Family Services Association of America, 1965

24. Wrubel J, Benner F, Lazarus R: Social competence from the perspective of stress and coping, in Social Competence. Edited by Wine JD, Smye MD. New York, Guilford, 1981

25. White RW: Strategies of adaptation, in Human Adaptation: Coping With Life Crisis. Edited by Moos RH. Lexington, Mass, Heath, 1976

26. Mechanic D: Social structure and adaptation: some neglected dimensions, in Coping and Adaptation. Edited by Coelho GV, Hamburg DA, Adams JE. New York, Basic Books, 1974

27. Adler P: An analysis of the concept of competence in individual and social systems. Community Mental Health Journal 18:34-39, 1982

28. McGrath ME: First person accounts: where did I go? Schizophrenia Bulletin 10:638-640, 1984

29. Borgeson N: Schizophrenia from the inside, in A New Day: Voices From Across the Land. Edited by Shetler H, Straw P. Arlington, Va, National Alliance for the Mentally Ill, undated

30. Antonovsky A: Health, Stress, and Coping. San Francisco, Jossey-Bass, 1979

31. Anscombe R: The disorder of consciousness in schizophrenia. Schizophrenia Bulletin 13:241-260, 1987

32. McGhie A, Chapman J: Disorders of attention and perception in early schizophrenia. British Journal of Medical Psychology 34:103-116, 1961

33. Zelt D: First person account: The messiah quest. Schizophrenia Bulletin 7:527-531, 1981

34. Harris M, Bergman H: The young adult chronic patient: affective responses to treatment. New Directions in Mental Health Services, no. 21:29-35,1984

35. Godschalx SM: Experiences and coping strategies of people with schizophrenia. Unpublished doctoral dissertation, College of Nursing, University of Utah, 1986

36. Leete E: Mental illness: an insider's view, in A New Day: Voices From Across the Land. Edited by Shetler H, Straw P. Arlington, Va, National Alliance for the Mentally Ill, undated

37. Weiner S: Exhaustion and fairness, in A New Day: Voices From Across the Land. Edited by Shetler H, Straw P. Arlington, Va, National Alliance for the Mentally Ill, undated

38. Keil J: Overcoming the Recurring Nightmare of Schizophrenia. San Diego, K & A, 1984

39. Pearson J: Need for friendship. Alliance for the Mentally Ill of Tucson and Southern Arizona Newsletter 5(1):5, 1988

40. Lawerance C: Having too much time, too little to do. Alliance for the Mentally Ill of Tucson and Southern Arizona Newsletter 5(1):5, 1988

41. Leete E: A patient's perspective on schizophrenia. New Directions for Mental Health Services, no. 34:81-90, 1987

42. King C: Dissolving the barriers: reflections on coming out of the closet. Hang Tough (newsletter of the Marin Network of Mental Health Clients) 2(2):8-9,1987

43. Weiner S: Bravado and the mental health clients' self-help movement. Hang Tough (newsletter of the Marin Network of Mental Health Clients) 2(2):4-5,1987

44. Boches Z: "Freedom" means knowing you have a choice, in Schizophrenia: The Experiences of Patients and Families. Arlington, Va, National Alliance for the Mentally Ill,1989, pp 40-42

45. Pilvin B: And wisdom to know the difference, in A New Day: Voices From Across the Land. Edited by Shetler H, Straw P. Arlington, Va, National Alliance for the Mentally Ill, undated

Chapter 41

Patient Self-Regulation and Functioning in Schizophrenia

Edna K. Hamera, RN, PhD

Kathryn A. Peterson, RN, MS

Sandra M. Handley, RN, PhD

Ardyce A. Plumlee, RN, MN

Elaine Frank-Ragan, RN, MSN

This chapter was previously published in *Hospital and Community Psychiatry*, *42*, 630-631. Copyright © 1991, the American Psychiatric Association. Reprinted by permission.

Although clinicians have often been skeptical that individuals with schizophrenia can identify symptoms of their disease process, research findings dispute such skepticism. Patients appear to be aware of early indicators of exacerbation of their illness. Findings from retrospective investigations show that many patients identify nonpsychotic indicators as early warning signs and symptoms (1, 2). Examples are tenseness and nervousness or symptoms of dysphoria, such as trouble sleeping.

Prospective studies have sought to determine if early indicators predict relapse (3-6). In most of these studies, early indicators were measured by clinicians' ratings, although Birchwood and colleagues (6) used ratings by patients and significant others. The findings from these studies suggest that although patients may experience early indicators, the presence of the indicators does not always predict relapse. Thus early indicators appear to be sensitive but not specific to relapse. However, definitions and measures of relapse differ among investigators, so the findings are tentative.

These prospective studies assume that although patients may identify early indicators of exacerbation of illness, clinicians still need to intervene to prevent relapse. Our previous findings (2) suggested that patients did not react passively to early indicators but took actions in response to them. Our work is based on a self-regulation model adapted from a model of illness representation (7) and control theory (8). The model posits that individuals monitor symptoms that signal exacerbation of their illness and take actions to manage their illness.

Using our model and the findings from Docherty and associates (9), which showed that patients experience a progression from nonpsychotic to psychotic symptoms before relapse, we hypothesized that patients who identified symptoms of depression and anxiety as early indicators would function at a higher level than patients who identified psychotic symptoms. In addition, we explored the relationship between the type of actions patients took in response to indicators and their level of functioning.

Methods

Study participants were selected from among patients enrolled in Community Support Services (CSS) of Johnson County Mental Health Center in Merriam, Kansas. A convenience sample of 51 subjects who had received a DSM-III diagnosis of schizophrenia at least two years previously were interviewed between December 1987 and May 1988. Patients with secondary diagnoses of substance abuse, mental retardation, or organicity were excluded.

Two-thirds of the patients in the sample were male, and 90 percent were Caucasian. Their mean age was 33.5 years, and they had a mean of 12.6 years of education. Thirty-five percent were employed either full time or part time, and 71 percent resided in unsupervised living situations. The majority of subjects (63 percent) had a diagnosis of a paranoid subtype of schizophrenia, all were on antipsychotic medications, and all were being closely monitored by a case manager. In addition, some attended group activities at CSS.

The interviews were conducted using the Self-Regulation Interview for Schizophrenia adapted from our previous work (2). In the open-ended interview, administered by two of the investigators, subjects were asked if they knew when they were becoming ill; if they said yes, they were asked how they knew. From the list of indicators reported, subjects were asked to select one that they particularly noticed. This primary indicator was then coded into one of three categories—anxiety, depression, or psychosis—based on the stages of decompensation described by Docherty and associates (9).

In the interview, subjects were also asked what they did, if anything, when they experienced their primary indicator. The actions reported were coded two ways. First, they were grouped by whether or not they involved contacting health care professionals or taking prescribed medications (medical versus nonmedical actions). Second, the actions were grouped into self-defeating behaviors (use of drugs or alcohol or acting out) and other actions.

Interrater reliability for the responses to the self-regulation interview, assessed independently by two of the investigators, ranged from 89 to 100 percent. Likewise, intercoder reliability for primary indicators and action categories ranged from 96 to 100 percent.

Within a week of the interview, the subjects' case managers rated their level of functioning using the Global Assessment Scale (GAS) (10). The relationship between the type of indicator (anxiety, depression, or psychosis) and the GAS was examined using an analysis of variance with Duncan's post hoc test. T tests were used to determine if level of functioning differed among subjects who took different kinds of actions to regulate their primary indicator.

Results

All 51 subjects identified illness indicators. Forty-one percent of the subjects' primary indicators were categorized as anxiety, 28 percent as depression, and 31 percent as psychosis.

Forty-nine of the 51 subjects reported taking more than one action to regulate their primary indicator; the mean number of actions was 3.1. The most frequent action was to add new activities or focus on existing ones; for example, "get busy" or "concentrate on usual activities." Other frequently reported actions were cognitive strategies such as self-talk and behaviors such as resting or withdrawing. Of the total number of actions (N=132), only 20 were medical actions; that is, taking prescribed medication or contacting health care professionals. Fifteen self-defeating actions, involving behaviors such as using drugs or alcohol or acting out, were reported.

Subjects were asked if the primary indicator of exacerbation of their illness got better, stayed the same, or got worse in response to their most frequent action. Most subjects (N=36) reported that the primary indicator of illness improved as a result of the action. Ten subjects stated the action had no effect, and three said it made the indicator worse.

Subjects with psychotic indicators had significantly lower GAS scores (a mean of 51.17, with a range of 30 to 70) than subjects reporting indicators involving anxiety or depression (F=5.67, df=2,50, p=.01). Subjects taking medical actions did not have higher levels of functioning as indicated by GAS scores than subjects taking nonmedical actions. Likewise, subjects who regulated the indicators of illness with actions that were not self-defeating were not rated as functioning better than subjects who reported regulating behaviors that were self-defeating.

Discussion

The study was undertaken to evaluate the relationship between symptom self-regulation and level of functioning in patients with schizophrenia. Patients who identified non-psychotic indicators of exacerbation of illness functioned at a higher level than patients who identified psychotic indicators. The GAS, which measures level of functioning, includes symptomatology as an index of functioning but also includes job performance and relationships with family members and other people as well as use of leisure time.

The types of actions taken to regulate primary indicators were not related to level of functioning. It may be that actions are not encouraged by health care professionals, so patients have not systematically assessed what they can do to manage primary indicators of illness. Research on specific actions for specific symptom groups is needed.

The relationship between type of indicator and level of functioning found in this study may be supported in other samples and settings with different demographic and treatment characteristics. However, in our previous work (2), the majority of nonhospitalized patients from mental health centers serving lower socioeconomic populations reported monitoring indicator symptoms and taking actions in response to indicators; implicit self-regulatory processes were present.

The findings suggest that individuals with schizophrenia could be taught to monitor early nonpsychotic indicators more effectively, which may improve their functioning and prevent hospitalization. A prospective study is needed to determine if enhancing existing self-regulatory processes is beneficial.

Acknowledgment

This study was funded by research grant SRG 5R2INRO1507-02 from the National Center for Nursing Research of the National Institutes of Health. Roma Lee Taunton, RN, PhD, was principal investigator and Kathryn Peterson, RN, MS, was project director. The authors thank Leslie Young, MSW, and the case managers at the community support program of Johnson County Mental Health Center for their assistance in data collection and Ronald L. Martin, MD, for comments on previous drafts.

References

1. Herz M, Melville C: Relapse in schizophrenia. American Journal of Psychiatry 137:801-905,1980

2. McCandless-Glimcher L, McKnight S, Hamera E, et al: Use of symptoms by schizophrenics to monitor and regulate their illness. Hospital and Community Psychiatry 37:929-933, 1986

3. Heinrichs DW, Carpenter WT: Prospective study of prodromal symptoms in schizophrenic relapse. American Journal of Psychiatry 142:371-373, 1985

4. Marder SR, Mintz J, Van Patten T, et al: Prodromal symptoms as predictors of schizophrenic relapse, in Predictors of Relapse in Schizophrenia. Edited by Lieberman JA, Kane JM. Washington, DC, American Psychiatric Press, 1986

5. Subotnik KL, Nuechterlein E: Prodromal signs and symptoms of schizophrenia. Journal of Abnormal Psychology 97:405-412, 1988

6. Birchwood M, Smith J, Macmillan F, et al: Predicting relapse in schizophrenia: the development and implementation of an early sign monitoring system using patients and families as observers: a preliminary investigation. Psychological Medicine 19:649-656, 1989

7. Leventhal H, Norenz D, Strauss A: Self-regulation and the mechanism for symptom appraisal, in Psychological Epidemiology. Edited by Mechanic D. New York, Neale Watson Academic Press, 1982

8. Carver C, Scheier M: Control theory: a useful conceptual framework for personality, social, clinical, and health psychology. Psychology Bulletin 92:111-135, 1982

9. Docherty J, Van Kammen D, Siris S, et al: Stages of onset of schizophrenic psychosis. American Journal of Psychiatry 135:420-426,1978

10. Endicott HJ, Spitzer R, Fleiss J, et al: The Global Assessment Scale: a procedure for measuring overall severity of psychiatric disturbance. Archives of General Psychiatry 137:766-771, 1976

Section V

Family Interaction and Social Supports: Promoting Adaptive Behaviors

Introduction

There are more than 30 million people in the United States who have physical and/or mental disabilities that are severe enough to limit their ability to perform daily activities. However, only 5% of all disabled Americans reside in institutions; the remaining 95% live in the community, residing alone or living with their family, friends, and/or professional attendants (Krauss & Stoppard, 1989). The number of Americans with significant disabilities who reside in the community is expected to increase as a result of the continuing deinstitutionalization movement and the prospective payment system (Carpentier, Lesage, Goulet, Lalonde, & Renaud, 1992). In addition, the consumer advocacy movement and the implementation of the Americans with Disabilities Act (ADA) will result in an increased demand for community integration for all persons with disabilities (AOTA, 1991; Javernick, 1991).

However, residing in one's community does not automatically ensure successful adaptation to disability or full integration into the life of the community. Persons with disabilities are often discharged into the community with inadequate skills for community living and with limited resources for adaptation (Carpentier et al., 1992). Economic barriers, limited accessibility, and social stigma may all contribute to increased social isolation and decreased adaptive functioning (Christiansen, 1991). The very nature of a disability and the presence of performance component deficits may also contribute to increased stress and a diminished ability to cope with the demands of one's living environment (Burton, 1990; Christiansen, 1991). The families of persons with disabilities are also challenged by changes in the families' lifestyles, role expectations, and daily tasks (Mosey, 1986; Versluys, 1980). Underlying all of these challenges to the adaptive abilities of the individual and the family are the emotional responses to the illness itself. Shock, anger, grief, and denial may be expressed as the individual and family struggle to accept and adjust to the realities of the disability (Burton, 1990; Christiansen, 1991; Mosey, 1986).

Successful adjustment to community living and effective adaptation to disability have been strongly linked to the provision of a supportive social network. Self-help groups, stress management, psychoeducation, and social skills training have all been found to improve significantly the patient's prognosis and to enhance the quality of life for both the person with the disability and for his or her family (Ascher-Svanum & Krause, 1991; Burton, 1990; Christiansen, 1991; Liberman, 1988; Mosey, 1986; Pedretti, 1990). Therefore, it is vital for occupational therapists to become adept at evaluating clients' and their families' social support needs and at providing appropriate intervention and prevention strategies to enable clients and their families to cope with the daily stresses of physical and/or psychosocial disability. It is insufficient for the occupational therapist to teach functional skills without considering the social context of these skills (Javernick, 1991; Johnson, 1986).

The chapters in this section provide an overview of the collaborative processes needed to build social support networks with clients and their families. A number of social support programs for community treatment centers and for institutional, residential settings are described. These programs have successfully assisted clients and their families in functionally adapting to the challenges of living with disabilities.

In chapter 42, Bernheim outlines eight generic principles for developing a comprehensive, collaborative approach for involving families in the care of persons with chronic mental illness. She provides clear, practice-oriented examples to substantiate each principle. She also gives constructive ideas to empower families to become part of the collaborative treatment process and to be advocates for improved quality of care. Although Bernheim's presentation focuses on the families of the chronic mentally ill, readers will find her principles applicable to families of persons with many types of chronic disabilities. These principles provide essential guidelines for the occupational therapist working with families, and their application is vital for development of effective family intervention programs.

Bernheim expands upon these collaborative principles in chapter 43, in which she describes a support program whose aim is to develop close working relationships between the families of persons with chronic mental illness and the staff of a community residence where these patients live. She identifies the elements of an effective family support program and provides descriptive examples of methods utilized to engage families and to maintain positive collaborative relationships. Bernheim also addresses staff concerns regarding working with families and provides constructive suggestions for dealing with these issues. Bernheim again focuses on the families of persons with chronic mental illness, but readers will find her family support program description highly relevant to most residential settings in which positive professional and family collaboration is desired (i.e., nursing homes, developmental centers).

In chapter 44, the authors also emphasize a collaborative approach among patients, families, and the interdisciplinary treatment team; however, their focus is on the acute care, inpatient psychiatric unit. They describe a short-term psychoeducational program that utilizes a holistic team approach to meet the needs of patients and their families. Psychiatrists, nurses, occupational therapists, social workers, and an administrator all work together to educate patients and their families about the nature of mental illness and to develop the skills and resources needed for effective coping. The chapter identifies the separate components of the psychoeducational program and describes the roles and responsibilities of each professional member within the program. Of particular interest to readers will be the description of the Life Skills Curriculum provided by the occupational therapy department. The utilization of individual, family, and group methods and the empathetic individuation of treatment provide patients and their families with invaluable support to develop the functional skills essential for community living.

The issue of developing functional skills for community living takes on a special meaning in chapter 45.

Parenting involves a number of vital skills that may be lacking in persons with mental illnesses. Waldo, Roath, Levine, and Freedman present a program that aims to teach parenting skills to mothers with schizophrenia. They describe the program's admission criteria, staffing pattern, treatment activities, and intervention outcomes. Their presentation is highly relevant to occupational therapists, who can combine their knowledge of infant and child development with their skills in activity analysis, synthesis, and group process to provide relevant intervention to parents with disabilities. The success of a structured approach in teaching parenting skills is well documented by this chapter's authors. Positive concurrent results of this educational approach for group members were the development of a strong social support network and the prevention of rehospitalizations.

The value of developing strong supportive networks is further explored in chapter 46, by McConchie. This chapter outlines the process utilized to develop a support group for persons with physical and psychosocial disabilities. The questions posed by the author in developing this program provide relevant guidelines for the development of support groups in a diversity of treatment settings. The goals, format, and structure of the program are described. Issues regarding co-leadership and logistical concerns are realistically discussed. The description of the positive effect of the support group on members' personal growth and community advocacy efforts validates the relevance of support groups for persons with physical and/or psychosocial disabilities.

In chapter 47 Mueller and Suto present stress management principles and techniques that are also applicable to a variety of patient populations and a diversity of treatment settings. Evaluation methods, intervention techniques, and group procedures utilized in their stress management program are discussed. A psychoeducational approach is used to increase members' knowledge of stress and to acquire effective coping skills.

The therapeutic value of acquiring situational coping skills is expanded upon in chapter 48, by Courtney and Escobedo. The authors describe an extensive, long-term stress management treatment program that begins on the inpatient psychiatric unit and continues after discharge as an outpatient, community-based treatment program. Patient referral criteria, evaluation methods, intervention techniques, and a comprehensive case example are clearly described. The authors' strong emphasis on continuity of care assists the client in developing the support network and coping skills needed for community living.

The development of a supportive social network provides the basis for chapter 49. In her presentation, Woodside describes a community day treatment program for persons with chronic mental illness that developed into a "surrogate extended family" for its members. Patient population characteristics, program philosophy, and the developmental process of the program are presented. Mutual trust, respect, dignity, and friendship are emphasized throughout the presentation.

The final chapter in this section addresses the special needs of families coping with Alzheimer's disease. The authors, Teusink and Mahler, present a five-stage reaction process that a family goes through in response to the diagnosis and course of Alzheimer's disease. Behavioral examples and relevant suggestions to assist family members during each reaction stage are described. While the authors emphasize issues unique to Alzheimer's disease, readers will find their empathetic discussion of family concerns relevant to many devastating illnesses. Education and support are emphasized throughout their discussion as vital for adjustment to the disease process.

The resources of education and support have provided the foundation for this section on promoting adaptive behaviors in the family and in social systems. I hope readers will utilize the information presented in this section to evaluate clients' (and their families') social support resources and needs and to model their interventions in the collaborative manner presented by each chapter's authors. Questions for further consideration are provided below to stimulate thought about these issues. In addition, a number of resources and references for family and social support are provided at the end of this text to assist readers in their evaluation, intervention, and referral process. Patient self-help groups and professional organizations (e.g., Alzheimer's Disease and Related Disorders Association, Alliance for the Mentally Ill) have a wealth of knowledge and experience to share; readers are urged to contact relevant organizations for further information about available services.

Questions to Consider

1. What are the major concerns and potential reactions a family may have when a family member has a physical and/or psychosocial disability? What are the unique issues a family must deal with if the disabled family member is a parent? A child? A spouse? A sibling?

2. How may the social stigma associated with a number of illnesses (e.g., AIDS, schizophrenia, Alzheimer's disease) affect the patient's and family's adjustment to an illness? How may individual personal reactions to disability affect the adjustment process?

3. How can occupational therapists build collabo-

rative relationships with clients and their families? What are relevant occupational therapy intervention goals and methods for building family and social supports?

4. What are the essential situational coping skills for community living? How can an occupational therapist facilitate the development of adaptive coping skills in patients and their families?

5. How are maladaptive signs of stress exhibited in patients' and families' behaviors? How can stress management techniques be integrated into an occupational therapy program?

6. What are the potential concerns of families who have a member of their family in a residential, institutional treatment setting? What steps can be taken by staff to maintain positive family involvement in institutional settings?

7. What are the unique social support needs of the chronic mentally ill? How can occupational therapists structure a treatment program that maintains a balance between goal-directed treatment and the provision of social support?

8. What resources do patients and/or their families need to maximize adaptive adjustment to disability? What are the social support options available to patients and their families? How can occupational therapists network with these resources to facilitate their use?

References

American Occupational Therapy Association. (1991, December 5). Occupational Therapy and the Americans with Disabilities Act. *OT Week*, pp. II, III.

Ascher-Svanum, H., & Krause, A. (1991). *Psychoeducational groups for patients with schizophrenia: A guide for practitioners*. Rockville, MD: Aspen Publishers.

Burton, G. (1990). Psychosocial aspects and adjustment during various phases of neurological disability. In D. A. Umphred (Ed.), *Neurological rehabilitation* (2nd ed.) (pp. 163-180). St Louis: Mosby.

Carpentier, N., Lesage, A., Goulet, J., Lalonde, P., & Renaud, M. (1992). Burden of care of families not living with young schizophrenic relatives. *Hospital and Community Psychiatry, 43*, 38-43.

Christiansen, C. (1991). Performance deficits as sources of stress: Coping theory and occupational therapy. In C. Christiansen & C. Baum (Eds.), *Occupational therapy: Overcoming human performance deficits* (pp. 69-96). Thorofare, NJ: Slack.

Javernick, J. (1991, November 28). Moving toward therapist/consumer partnerships. *OT Week*, p. 15.

Johnson, J. (1986). *Wellness: A context for living*. Thorofare, NJ: Slack.

Krauss, L. E., & Stoppard, S. (Eds.). (1989). *Chartbook on disability in the United States*. Washington, DC: National Institute on Disability and Rehabilitation Research.

Liberman, R. P. (Ed.). (1988). *Psychiatric rehabilitation of chronic mental patients*. Washington, DC: American Psychiatric Press.

Mosey, A. C. (1986). *Psychosocial components of occupational therapy*. New York· Raven Press.

Pedretti, L. W. (1990). Psychosocial aspects of physical dysfunction. In L. W. Pedretti & B. Zoltan (Eds.), *Occupational therapy: Practice skills for physical dysfunction* (pp. 18-39). St Louis: Mosby.

Versluys, H. P. (1980). The remediation of role disorders through focused group work. *American Journal of Occupational Therapy, 34*, 609-614.

Chapter 42

Principles of Professional and Family Collaboration

Kayla F. Bernheim, PhD

The past decade has witnessed a tremendous resurgence of interest in working with families of chronically mentally ill persons. This interest has been spurred by several factors, including deinstitutionalization; documentation of the enormous emotional, financial, and interpersonal impact of an individual's serious mental illness on family life (1-3); and the demonstrated effectiveness of psychoeducational interventions in reducing relapse and recidivism rates of some (mostly schizophrenic) patients (4-6). Widespread critical reevaluation of theories about the family's role in the etiology of major psychiatric disorders has resulted in the suggestion that the conceptual framework of "coping and adaptation" should replace that of "family pathogenesis" as the basis for clinicians' approach to families (7).

While, on the whole, the professional community is moving toward greater empathy for and cooperation with patients' relatives, there are still pitfalls ahead. Consider, for example, the frequently exhibited "we-do-that" syndrome. When asked whether an agency works with patients' relatives, the director answers, "Of course, we do that! We provide six sessions of psychoeducation." Are family members invited to treatment planning sessions? "Well, no." Do you have a family advisory committee? "No." A mechanism for relatives to communicate grievances? "No." Do your psychiatrists regularly check with relatives before changing patients' medications? "I don't know." Have staff members been trained to understand family burden and family coping? "Not formally, no."

Genuine collaboration with families is widely advocated in principle, but elusive in practice. Each of the following eight generic principles is a necessary component of a comprehensive approach to family involvement in the care of chronic mentally ill patients.

Principle 1: View relatives who desire to participate as empowered members of the caregiving network. The experiences of relatives and, indeed, of consumers themselves have long been discounted and are only now being taken seriously by mental health professionals. However, family members may have expertise in identifying behavioral signs of impending decompensation, specifying situations that are likely to prove stressful to their ill relative, remembering which medications have been most or least helpful, and describing the likely impact of various behavioral and social interventions.

Family members have knowledge that may be otherwise inaccessible to clinicians about who the patient is as a person and what his [or her] temperamental style, needs, aspirations, values, and interests are. A coherent history of the patient's illness and treatment can rarely be obtained from a stack of discharge summaries. Rather than begin treatment de novo at each decompensation, good care requires continuity that can be immeasurably enhanced by adding families' expertise to that of clinicians.

Principle I also implies mutual decision making. Here again, both patients and families have, until recently, been disenfranchised. Assuming that the patient consents, both formal and informal strategies for involving relatives in planning can be used. While some relatives may wish to be present at formal treatment planning sessions, others may prefer meeting with a single staff member before or after such sessions. Some may wish to be involved only at points of transition or trouble, while others may prefer regular contact.

A prerequisite for implementation of principle I is mutual respect. Insofar as clinicians' thinking about families is still framed in pejorative language that includes such concepts as dysfunctional family systems, overprotective mothers, double binds, communication deviance, sabotage, denial, infantilizing, and high expressed-emotion family, we will be unable to engage in genuine collaboration.

Principle 2: Provide adequate orientation. The mental health system, which is often complex, arcane, and jargon filled, presents a formidable barrier to [a family's] successful adaptation to the mental illness of a relative. Family members are likely to interact with multiple providers from many different agencies simultaneously. Inadequate orientation often causes or contributes to friction between staff, patient, and family members.

Each agency or service provider has the obligation to help the patient and family understand its own particular functions, roles, and rules. They should be explained both face to face and in writing (for reference at a later time). After orientation, family members should understand how the agency fits into the overall rehabilitation plan, should know the names and roles of each of the relevant staff members, and should be aware of the conditions under which the patient would be terminated or transferred from the agency's care. In addition, relatives should recognize ways they can be involved in the patient's rehabilitation plan and should be able to identify the mechanisms available for ongoing information exchange between staff and family.

Principle 3: Provide multiple channels for communication. Both formal and informal mechanisms for exchanging information are desirable. Such mechanisms include regular phone calls inviting relatives to treatment or rehabilitation planning sessions, a newsletter, a family grievance procedure, a family advisory group, and social gatherings for patients, relatives, and staff.

Principle 4: Aim services toward reducing family burden. Psychoeducational programs described in the literature have generally been based on the theoretical construct of "expressed emotion" as a presumed causal factor in psychotic relapse. This construct has come under significant criticism (8).

Within the alternative framework of coping and adaptation, it is common sense to provide services designed to reduce family burden. Doing so would be expected to decrease the level of stress and tension within the family, to the benefit of all members. Such services include a combination of emotional support, information, education, advice, skills training, crisis intervention, respite care, and case management. In addition, family members' sense of isolation could be decreased by bringing them together with others in a similar situation through referral to local Alliance for the Mentally Ill support and advocacy groups.

Principle 5: Develop individualized service plans. Numerous intra- and interfamilial differences contribute to the need for an individualized approach to families. Cultural background, educational level, density of social networks, preference for group versus individual services, previous experience with mental illness, and each relative's own typical responses to hardship and grief are just a few of the variables that must be considered in designing services (9). Patients' parents are likely to require different services than patients' siblings or children.

Clearly, a variety of services must be provided in each locality. However, agencies within a given region can cooperate to provide a range of services rather than duplicating services within each agency. The service plan for each family should be developed in the context of an initial consultation phase in which relatives and staff can make a joint assessment of the family's needs and wishes (10).

Principle 6: Respond flexibly to changing needs over time. Just as treatment plans are reviewed regularly, plans for family involvement should also be updated. This activity requires mechanisms for obtaining feedback about the family's perceptions and wishes. With respect to individual cases, informal mechanisms can be used. They include regularly reviewing relatives' goals and objectives and asking participants at the end of an hour's consultation or a psychoeducational session whether the time seemed well spent. Other, more formal consumer satisfaction measures, such as surveys and questionnaires, can also be used.

Principle 7: Involve family representatives in systemic planning and oversight. Family advocacy constitutes a healthy redirection of [the] relatives' wish to be useful and provides the professional community with a rich source of energy and insight. Only from consumers and their families can clinicians learn how the system meets, or fails to meet, the subjective needs of those it is meant to serve.

Mental health professionals who are also consumers or relatives of consumers can be particularly valuable in bridging the gap between principles of autonomy and consumerism and those of professional care and treatment. Efforts to recruit and train these professionals should be a priority. Systemic family involvement, like individual family involvement, should be reevaluated regularly and modified as needed.

Principle 8: Make an ongoing commitment to staff training, consultation, and support. Collaboration with families of patients is a relatively new concept. Many staff have been trained in models of family pathogenesis that are antithetical to these new ways of working. Their professional identities and skills are tied to those models. They may feel threatened, frightened, and angry about families' newfound assertiveness and [be] unable or unwilling to develop a working alliance with patients' relatives.

Collaboration raises some new issues for staff, including concerns about how confidentiality principles should be interpreted, particularly when relatives function as caregivers. Other issues include shifting of priorities to accommodate family work when time and money are limited and management of loyalty conflicts when families are active participants in treatment.

Clearly, staff who feel inadequately skilled and anxious cannot be instructed successfully to work with families. Staff will initially require sensitization to the needs of families, updates on new theoretical models, and skills training, followed by regular supervision and case consultation in responding to families' needs. The period of transition to greater cooperation with families can be expected to last a year or more. Procedures for orienting new staff should be revised to include a module on family-professional collaboration as it is enacted in the particular agency or system the new staff are entering.

Conclusions

Family-professional collaboration is currently in vogue. Clinicians are struggling to bring down old barriers to collaboration and experimenting with new ways of relating to patients' relatives. To prevent a return to business as usual when initial enthusiasm has passed and to avert hesitation at the threshold of real partnership, a thoughtful systemic approach to change is needed. It is hoped that the principles offered here will encourage such an approach.

References

1. Hatfield AB: Psychological costs of schizophrenia to the family. Social Work 23:355-359, 1978

2. Lefley HP: Aging parents as caregivers of mentally ill adult children: an emerging social problem. Hospital and Community Psychiatry 38:1083-1089, 1987

3. Francell CG, Conn VS, Gray DP: Families' perceptions of burden of care for chronic mentally ill relatives. Hospital and Community Psychiatry 39:1298-1300, 1988

4. Leff J, Kuipers L, Berkowitz R, et al: A controlled trial of social intervention in the families of schizophrenic patients. British Journal of Psychiatry 141:121-134, 1982

5. Falloon IRH, Boyd JL, McGill CW, et al: Family management in the prevention of morbidity of schizophrenia: clinical outcome of a two-year longitudinal study. Archives of General Psychiatry 42:887-896, 1985

6. Anderson CM, Reiss DJ, Hogarty GE: Schizophrenia and the Family. New York, Guilford, 1988

7. Hatfield AB, Lefley HP: Families of the Mentally Ill: Coping and Adaptation. New York, Guilford, 1987

8. Kanter J, Lamb HR, Loeper C: Expressed emotion in families: a critical review. Hospital and Community Psychiatry 38:374-380, 1987

9. Terkelsen KG: The meaning of mental illness to the family, in Families of the Mentally Ill: Coping and Adaptation. Edited by Hatfield AB, Lefley HP. New York, Guilford, 1987

10. Wynne LC, Bernheim KF, Wynne AR: Key issues for training in family therapy with the long-term seriously mentally ill and their families. Presented at the National Forum for Educating Mental Health Professionals to Work With the Long-Term Seriously Mentally Ill and Their Families, Chevy Chase, Md, Sept. 18, 1988

Chapter 43

Promoting Family Involvement in Community Residences for Chronic Mentally Ill Persons

Kayla F. Bernheim, PhD

During the past decade, several factors have combined to highlight the importance of mental health professionals supporting, educating, and collaborating with families of chronic mentally ill patients. First, families have been more outspoken about their experiences in caring for ill relatives (1,2). They have clearly expressed their views of professional services (2,3) and of what they want from service providers (4,5).

Second, a model that focuses on family coping rather than on family pathology and that supports families as partners in rehabilitation is now available (6). Third, family-based interventions have been shown to reduce relapse and recidivism (7-9). As a result of these developments, many agencies, representing a variety of inpatient and outpatient settings, have established programs of family support or education.

Families of chronic mentally ill patients and the staff of community residences where patients live have much in common and potentially much to offer each other in managing the day-to-day problems in living posed by chronic mental illness. However, they have historically had little contact. In this report, we describe an attempt to develop closer working relationships between families of chronic patients and staff of a community residence, with particular emphasis on managing staff anxieties about increased involvement of families in patients' rehabilitation.

Program Description

East House Corporation, based in Rochester, New York, serves both seriously mentally ill patients and recovering alcoholics. Its mental health program, which will be the focus of this report, includes a quarterway house with 18 beds, four supervised group homes with a total of 54 beds, and scatter-site apartments that provide a total of 46 beds with various levels of supervision. Some of the agency's residential components had informally involved patients' families in various ways for several years. However, since the fall of 1987, the agency has trained staff and developed a multifaceted, formal family support program. The program is currently in place within the mental health component and is being developed within the alcoholism component.

The elements of the family support program include orientation, family consultation, group activities, and ongoing communication with families.

Orientation

Relatives appear to find careful orientation to the agency's services, policies, rules, and procedures very valuable. When a prospective resident is initially interviewed, the intake worker explores the person's family situation and identifies the family members who constitute the immediate support network. The agency's philosophy about including families in the rehabilitation effort is explained to the prospective resident. This discussion provides the opportunity to work through any resistance the patient may have about staff working with relatives.

In our experience, the overwhelming majority of residents and families respond positively, often enthusiastically, to staff's attempts to involve family members. Situations in which prospective residents are initially completely unwilling to allow family involvement are handled on a case-by-case basis and are generally resolved through negotiation and compromise.

Before admission, family members are offered a tour of the house and are oriented to the agency's intention to involve and support relatives. After the resident's acceptance for admission, relatives are invited to meet with staff to share information. An initial plan for family involvement and services is developed and placed in the resident's record. If the family is unable or unwilling to attend a meeting, staff contact the family by telephone to discuss the plan. Program staff adopt a welcoming attitude that relatives and staff can capitalize on later if either chooses. An orientation packet containing East House materials and information about community resources is provided to relatives during this initial phase.

Individual Family Consultation

Since the needs of each family and resident are unique, individualized plans for contact are made whenever possible. For some families, an occasional phone call may be all that is required, while for others, weekly telephone contacts that follow patients' home visits may be instituted. Other families may prefer face-to-face meetings to coordinate approaches to various problems.

Flexibility is the cornerstone of individual family consultation. As needs change, so do the frequency and format of contacts. For example, transitions, particularly those in which residents move to a more independent living situation, are as difficult for relatives as for residents. Program staff increase contact with family members as they work through their concerns about the move and become oriented to the prospective setting.

Group activities

Family members participate in organizing support groups, educational seminars, and social events. Some of these events are agencywide, and others are limited to individual residences. The educational and social activities include residents as well as relatives and staff.

Communication Channels

The agency's annual report, agencywide newsletter, orientation brochures, and bimonthly newsletter for families are available to residents and family members.

To ensure ongoing feedback from family members, all interested relatives are invited to join an advisory group that meets with administrative staff four times a year. This group has participated in the development of a survey of family attitudes, has suggested topics for educational offerings, and has reviewed anticipated changes in agency policies and services. The group is open to families of prospective residents and past residents as well as families of current residents. In addition, about one-quarter of the members of the agency's board of directors have experienced mental illness, alcoholism, or substance abuse in their family.

Training Issues

Staff members were understandably skeptical about the agency's plans to develop family services. Most had been heavily influenced in their previous training by theories that implicate the family in pathogenesis. Staff members' implicit orientation had been that the therapeutic community is a benign substitute for a dysfunctional family of origin. The majority had little, if any, experience interacting with residents' relatives.

Training has focused on helping staff develop empathy for relatives. Issues such as family burden, stages of adaptation, responses to stigma, variability in coping styles, cultural background, availability of other supports, and attitudes toward mental illness have been addressed. Listening to family members tell their own stories has been an essential element in this sensitization process.

Staff were particularly concerned about confidentiality issues. A problem-solving, case-specific approach to issues of confidentiality is needed in family support programs that rely in part on sharing of information among staff, patients, and family members. New staff members, particularly those who had come from agencies or institutions with rigid confidentiality policies, needed to learn to approach each situation that required a judgment about confidentiality thoughtfully and creatively.

During their orientation, new staff receive four hours

of training about working with families. This training includes but is not limited to the confidentiality issue. Even experienced staff needed both formal training and informal support and consultation to develop a more flexible approach to this complex, anxiety-producing area.

Staff were also fearful about conducting family therapy. They were uncertain about their skills and felt that if they opened the door to family work, they would be unable to set limits appropriate to their role. In addition, they wondered if they would find themselves overwhelmed by a double caseload when they tried to respond to the needs of family members as well as to residents' needs. They were also concerned that if they developed empathy for relatives, they would be unable to fulfill their role as advocate for residents.

To address these concerns, the agency promoted an atmosphere of experimentation within which staff could feel comfortable trying out new behaviors, working through their feelings with colleagues and supervisors, and gradually developing greater ability to identify the needs they could reasonably expect to fill. A recent 50-item survey of attitudes about families and family services completed by all program staff indicated that staff have overwhelmingly favorable attitudes toward family work and have found the positive response of both residents and relatives surprising and gratifying.

Family members' responses to a 43-item survey on satisfaction with services provide an indication of the success of staff training. The survey was conducted by mail in late 1988. Eighty-three surveys were returned for an overall return rate of 63 percent (79 percent of families whose relatives were served by the agency's mental health component and 18 percent of families whose relatives were served by the alcoholism component in which family services had not yet been extensively developed). Eighty-five percent of respondents felt that staff were doing a good job with families, and 78 percent felt staff were adequately trained to work with families.

Discussion

Rather than hiring specialty staff to work with families, East House chose to integrate family work into the jobs of all counseling staff. Clearly, this approach requires extensive staff training and preparation. However, as has been argued elsewhere (10), we feel this approach results in a higher level of satisfaction for residents, relatives, and staff.

It can be argued that family support and education should be provided by community mental health center staff rather than by community residence staff. However, our experience shows that brief family psychoeducation, which is frequently provided by mental health centers, is no substitute for ongoing, open communication that facilitates rehabilitation planning and reduces family members' anxiety. Furthermore, even if community mental health centers consistently were to support families' involvement in rehabilitation, communication between community residence staff and families, who share both interest and experience in the management of day-to-day problems in living with chronic mentally ill people, would still be important. All agencies that serve this population should reach out to families, each from their own unique perspective. The content of the contacts is less important than establishing a process of collaboration in which families who wish to be engaged as partners in rehabilitation have the opportunity to do so.

To summarize, keys to family support at an agency or institutional level include an attitude of welcome and cooperation, individualization of services, and multiple mechanisms for communication. Flexibility in planning, continuous evaluation and change to meet consumers' needs, and ongoing commitment to staff training, consultation, and support are also necessary. Ideally, these elements should be available in all settings in which the chronic mentally ill are served.

Acknowledgment

The author thanks Jim Sorrentino for his helpful suggestions for revision of this paper.

References

1. Doll W: Family coping with the mentally ill: an unanticipated problem of deinstitutionalization. Hospital and Community Psychiatry 27:183-185, 1976

2. Hatfield AB: Psychological costs of schizophrenia to the family. Social Work 23:355-359, 1978

3. Holden DF, Lewine RRJ: How families evaluate mental health professionals, resources, and the effects of illness. Schizophrenia Bulletin 8:628-633,1982

4. Hatfield AB: Help-seeking behavior in families of schizophrenics. American Journal of Community Psychology 7:563-569, 1979

5. Yess JP: What families of the mentally ill want. Community Support Service Journal 2:1-3, 1981

6. Hatfield AB, Lefley HP: Families of the Mentally Ill: Coping and Adaptation. New York, Guilford, 1986

7. Anderson CM, Reiss DJ, Hogarty GE: Schizophrenia and the Family. New York, Guilford, 1986

8. Goldstein MJ, Kopeikin HS: Short- and long-term effects of combining drug and family therapy, in New Developments in Interventions With Families of Schizophrenics. Edited by Goldstein MJ. San Francisco, Jossey-Bass, 1981

9. Leff J, Kuipers L, Berkowitz R, et al: A controlled trial of social intervention in the families of schizophrenic patients. British Journal of Psychiatry 141:121-134, 1982

10. Bernheim KF, Switalski T: The Buffalo family support project: promoting institutional change to meet families' needs. Hospital and Community Psychiatry 39:663-665, 1988

Chapter 44

An Interdisciplinary Psychoeducation Program for Schizophrenic Patients and Their Families in an Acute Care Setting

Linda Greenberg, MS, CSW

Susan B. Fine, MA, OTR

Cynthia Cohen, MSPH

Kenneth Larson, RN, MPA

Arlene Michaelson-Baily, MS, OTR

Phyllis Rubinton, MLS

Ira D. Glick, MD

This chapter was previously published in *Hospital and Community Psychiatry*, 39, 277-282. Copyright © 1988, the American Psychiatric Association. Reprinted by permission.

Clinical efforts to provide "state of the art" treatment of schizophrenia in acute settings are influenced by several factors, including biomedical advances, the patient's special vulnerabilities, family relationships, and staff expertise. The limited availability of community-based resources and constraints on reimbursement and length of hospital stay, as well as high relapse and rehospitalization rates, further confound the picture.

Medication, structure, a protective environment, and family intervention are considered important components of treatment of acute schizophrenic episodes (1, 2), but there are few substantive data and little agreement about the specific elements that make up an effective brief-treatment "package" during acute episodes of the illness (3, 4).

The crisis intervention and symptom reduction models that currently prevail in the treatment of schizophrenia do not adequately address primary deficit symptoms, social adjustment, and community tenure. Mobilization for discharge is often perfunctory and influenced by factors external to the differential needs of the schizophrenic patients. Patients frequently return to the community poorly prepared to deal with environmental stressors.

The time is long overdue for reordering and clarifying the goals and content of the time-limited inpatient phase of schizophrenia treatment. This paper describes a psychoeducational treatment program at the Payne Whitney Psychiatric Clinic in New York that we believe is responsive to the needs of acutely ill schizophrenic patients and their families as well as to the constraints imposed by the larger health care system. The paper delineates the program's goals and techniques and describes the multidisciplinary staff's role in achieving the program's objectives. A rationale is provided for implementing the program in other acute care facilities with comparable populations and lengths of stay.

Psychoeducation: A Model

While education has been a component of the treatment repertoires of many mental health disciplines (5-11), it has often taken a backseat to psychodynamic, interpersonal, and biological methods. During the past decade, however, psychoeducation has gained considerable visibility as an important treatment for schizophrenia.

The psychoeducational model is a systematic, goal-directed, psychosocial technique that uses a collaborative approach in which clinicians, patients, and their families learn from each other. The goals of the process are to impart information and to enhance understanding of the illness, needed treatment resources, and supportive services; to increase daily living skills and adaptive capacities; to acknowledge patients' and families' capacities and their right to know about the illness; and to create a more productive alliance between patients, families, and mental health professionals (12, 13).

The rationale and efficacy of these efforts in long-term institutional and community-based settings have been well documented in the past decade by the pioneers of the psychoeducation movement (14-21). A few clinicians within acute care settings have also reported their efforts to provide psychoeducation to patients or families (2, 22-25). However, to the best of our knowledge, there have been no reports of a comprehensive interdisciplinary treatment program designed to meet the needs of schizophrenic patients and their families during brief hospitalizations.

Program Setting

The setting for the psychoeducation program is the 104-bed inpatient service at the Payne Whitney Psychiatric Clinic of the New York Hospital—Cornell Medical Center. The inpatient service is made up of five units, each staffed by an interdisciplinary team of mental health professionals, trainees, and support personnel.

While inpatient programs, such as the psychoeducation program, are developed and initiated at all levels, guidelines for clinical practice are formulated by the director of inpatient services, as well as by unit and discipline chiefs. Administrative staff support policy and programs.

The distribution of leadership and the ongoing collaboration among the disciplines involved in the psychoeducation program have served to diminish staff burnout and sustain the staff's interest and expertise throughout the four years in which the program has operated. In addition, inservice training and supervision of staff are considered necessary to update practice, introduce educational techniques to new personnel, overcome existing biases, and enhance efficacy.

Although numerous questions about schizophrenia remain unanswered, the psychoeducation team adheres to the stress-vulnerability view of schizophrenia (26). According to this position, symptoms are exacerbated when "…biological vulnerability increases, stressful life events overwhelm the individual's coping resources, [and] the individual's social supports diminish" (27).

The clinic's patients and their families are representative of the socioeconomic and educational mix of our urban setting. Patients range in age from 18 to 65 and include some experiencing their first episode of schizophrenia as well as those with more chronic conditions.

The 30-day average length of stay at the clinic requires rapid diagnostic assessment, treatment, and discharge planning. The majority of discharge referrals are made to outside agencies and practitioners. Continuity of care and utilization of community-based resources, therefore, are influenced by many factors arising after the patient has left our facility.

Program Description and Objectives

The program consists of several components, each administered by one or more members of various mental health disciplines. Separate components are conducted by psychiatrists, nurses, occupational therapists, and social workers; a program administrator participates in family workshops. Each component has been designed to meet the distinct needs of patients and family members. However, all components work toward enhancing participants' cognitive and interpersonal strengths and adaptive capacities and decreasing their feelings of guilt and hopelessness.

The program's objectives are fostered by

- Providing participants with an overview of current information about schizophrenia, which emphasizes the relationship between a "biological vulnerability of unknown origin" (20) and a susceptibility to stress and overstimulation.
- Teaching participants about symptoms and the effects of medication to encourage compliance and prepare patients and family for early warning signs of relapse and side effects of medication.
- Increasing participants' awareness of environmental stress and its relationship to relapse.
- Creating a working alliance between the patients, their families, and staff to diminish resentment and blame, identify and implement short-term goals, and establish a foundation for ongoing treatment during the fluctuating course of the disease.
- Identifying individual strengths of the patients and the families and teaching them strategies for managing activities of daily living, positive and negative symptoms, and other distressing behaviors.
- Providing the patients [with] opportunities for practice, repetition, and reinforcement of adaptive skills to encourage their generalization and durability after discharge.
- Encouraging networking among families to lessen isolation and stigma.

- Supporting realistic hope by informing the patients and their families of the most current research information.
- Establishing contacts for the patients and their families with mental health professionals who support these goals in the community.

These services are thought to complement rather than replace medication and other needed treatment; therefore, the patients have an opportunity to benefit from the additive effects of combined biopsychosocial therapies.

Referrals to each of the program's components are coordinated through each unit's chief psychiatrist and multidisciplinary team. This forum deals with such issues as when and how to inform the patient and the family of the diagnosis, their readiness for information and involvement in the program, and their responses to the educational content and techniques. All patients and families are assessed for their need for psychoeducation, and if they are admitted to the program, for their level of progress.

Psychoeducation is not suitable for some individuals, but most patients on the inpatient service are treated in one or more psychoeducational components. Monitoring and maintaining the balance between individual capacities and program content and techniques are particularly high priorities; it is this balance that facilitates the application of psychoeducation to an acute population.

Components of the Program

The Psychiatrist as Coordinator

The psychiatrist has a dual role that involves coordinating and consulting with the unit-based team and directly introducing psychoeducation into the patient's treatment package. The psychiatrist's use of educational techniques during individual sessions with patients represents an expansion of the psychiatrist's traditional armamentarium.

To the degree that the patient's acute symptoms and cognitive difficulties allow, the psychiatrist spends at least two sessions reviewing the patient's symptoms and diagnosis in a simple and empathic manner. Whenever possible, these sessions precede the psychiatrist's discussions with the family. This information, as well as material about the patient's treatment and prognosis, is repeated and expanded on throughout the hospitalization until the patient manifests changes in behavior and compliance indicating he [or she] has adequately comprehended the material.

Depending on the sophistication of the patient and the family and the nature of the patient's recovery process, the psychiatrist may discuss the patient's vulnerability to stress and problems in information processing, offer information about medications and their side effects, introduce the subject of etiology, and present schizophrenia as a fluctuating but chronic illness that can be managed.

Within this model, the relationship between the patient and the psychiatrist becomes more collaborative, as the patient is encouraged to actively contribute his [or her] experience with symptoms and medication to the treatment process. If the patient is too cognitively impaired throughout the hospitalization, the collaborative exchange described above occurs only with his [or her] family.

Nursing Education Sessions

All of the nurses on the inpatient service teach patients about schizophrenia and its treatment. They also recommend strategies for minimizing stress based on their daily observations and information obtained from admission assessments. The nurses use a specific teaching assessment instrument developed for schizophrenia that outlines instructional techniques and incorporates questions about the patients' understanding of the illness and its treatment. Mental health workers reinforce information provided by the nurses and encourage more positive behaviors under the direction of the head nurse.

The nurses present information in individual sessions as soon as the patient's diagnosis and treatment plans have been established and the patient appears able to understand the material. Teaching is not initiated for patients who appear overwhelmed or extremely fearful or who need to deny the illness until staff establish a stronger alliance with them and they become more accessible. The patients may be given reading material before they attend a teaching session if it appears that they would be less threatened by a written introduction. Modifications in the patients' diagnoses or treatment plans may require additional educational contacts.

The nurses also provide informal instruction about the patients' day-to-day experiences and expectations as a way of augmenting more formal contacts and providing the patients with greater understanding of their illnesses and a better opportunity to actively participate in the management of their treatment.

Life Skills Curriculum

The Life Skills Curriculum, offered by members of the occupational therapy staff, addresses basic aspects of community adjustment through the use of formal instruction and task-oriented techniques. The principal objective of the curriculum is to maximize the patient's potential to function in the community, a goal as relevant for the patient hospitalized for 30 days as it is for one with a lengthier institutional tenure (28).

The curriculum is offered during five weekly classes and in a flexible number of one-on-one tutorials, a format that aims to be both manageable for the patient and relevant to his [or her] needs. The lessons address such issues as personal goal setting, stress management, social skills, self-care, time management, home management, leisure-time planning, and use of community resources.

All of the curriculum's modules emphasize problem-solving and communication skills that can be generalized to a variety of life situations and establish an expectation that problems can be solved. Patients identify their problems, strengths, learning needs, and progress through self-assessments completed before and after they take the course.

The curriculum uses group discussions, lectures by staff and patients, role playing, simulated tasks, video and audio tapes, computerized and paper and pencil exercises, reading assignments, and other resources to facilitate individual and group goals. Patients have opportunities to practice skills through "homework" assignments, which they complete on the inpatient units, in the program's mental health library, while attending other clinic-based rehabilitation programs, or during visits to the community.

While formal data on the outcomes of the curriculum are not available, patient self-assessments, an important element of the psychoeducational process, indicate that they have gained a sense of satisfaction from mastering basic elements of independent living and from playing an active part in improving their own functioning.

Family Sessions

Because schizophrenic patients are discharged in increasing numbers to the care of family members (29), a social worker leads family sessions, with a psychiatric resident present during the early meetings to offer psychiatric diagnoses. The sessions are geared toward helping the family develop cognitive and behavioral skills with which to deal with both the acute and the ongoing manifestations of the patient's illness.

Four to ten family sessions take place during the course of the patient's hospitalization. The first meetings focus on establishing an alliance between the family members and the clinicians (15). These early contacts, which do not include the patient, provide an opportunity for the family to express anger, frustration, guilt, and anxiety about the patient, about the mental health system, and about the future. The clinicians focus on current issues rather than on lengthy family histories, which tend to reinforce the family's feelings of blame and guilt (17).

Once the diagnosis of schizophrenia has been discussed, the social worker meets alone with the family to help them process information about the patient's diagnosis, treatment, and discharge planning. These sessions address the family's ongoing concerns about the future, strategies for coping with the patient's bizarre behaviors, the relationship between stress and symptoms, the patient's continued compliance with effective treatments, and the importance of a predictable, nonintrusive home environment that supports the patient's assets and a gradual increase in his [or her] responsibilities (22).

Giving information and advice in a timely fashion and using forthright and empathic responses to the family's questions are characteristic of this problem-solving and collaborative technique. The family members are encouraged to offer their ideas about management strategies, for they are viewed as experts in their own right. Siblings and children of the patient are encouraged to attend family sessions or to meet separately with the therapists. Patients are generally included in the sessions after they have discussed their diagnosis with their psychiatrist or their nurse.

The contacts with the staff provide families with support in dealing with the stigma of having a schizophrenic family member and the burden of assuming a caretaking role. Family members of all ages often need permission to fulfill personal needs that have long been ignored.

Because continued support in the community is so critical to the family, the social worker actively cultivates and makes referrals to clinicians who use a family-focused treatment model. Unfortunately such referrals are not always feasible, as more traditional interventions for families of schizophrenic patients sometimes prevail.

Mental Health Library

As the psychoeducational program developed, it became apparent that patients and their families had a need for suitable literature about schizophrenia, other mental illnesses, human development, and daily living skills. The Phyllis Rubinton Mental Health Resource Library (30), paid for through private funds, began as a joint venture of the clinic's psychiatric library and occupational therapy department.

Occupational therapy staff oversee the collection and disseminate information about the library, as well as current ideas and developments in patient and family education, to other staff through formal presentations, distribution of materials, and a bimonthly mailing of selected articles suitable for patients and families.

Patient access to the library is monitored by an occupational therapist. The therapist guides patients to resources relevant to their interests, stress tolerance, and cognitive abilities; deals with their immediate emotional reactions to materials; leads a discussion group that provides support and reinforces intellectual mastery of the material; and communicates with staff about the patients' selections and responses. The multidisciplinary team, in turn, uses the readings in individual and family sessions to facilitate treatment goals.

Patients with good functional histories seem the most motivated to use the library. Selections focusing on symptoms and medication, vignettes about people who have adapted to their illness, and guidance in managing time are of particular interest. Families are drawn to literature dealing with diagnosis, prognosis, the natural course of the disease, treatment approaches used by leading experts, and ways of coping with specific stressors.

Family Workshop

A workshop taught by a team of professionals provides another arena for helping the families to understand and manage the patients' illness. The workshop is modeled on the Survival Skills Workshop on Schizophrenia at the University of Pittsburgh (18), but has been modified to meet the intramural and family needs that arise within a short-term setting.

The three- to six-hour workshop takes place on Sundays or in the evenings in order to maximize attendance. An interdisciplinary team consisting of a psychiatrist, a social worker, an occupational therapist, and an administrator present a historical perspective on schizophrenia and review symptoms, somatic treatments, rehabilitation, and family coping strategies. The administrator provides an overview of methods for dealing with the mental health delivery system, reviewing such topics as obtaining insurance for the chronic mentally ill, negotiating bureaucracies, expediting referrals to agencies, and registering complaints within the institution, as well as information about the rights of the mentally ill.

The more didactic components of the workshop are balanced by informal discussions, in which team members work to clarify information, answer questions within the limits of available knowledge, and stimulate problem solving by the families. The staff collaborate in a cohesive but open and nondogmatic manner to provide the families with needed respect and empathy as well as clarification and guidance.

Coordination and referrals to the workshops are managed by a social worker. Referrals may be made any time after the patient has been on the unit for a week until a week after his (or her) discharge, provided there are at least two other families available to participate; the maximum number of families that can attend a workshop is six. Children under 12, family members who are actively psychotic, and the patients themselves are not included in workshops.

A controlled study indicated that six months after completing the workshops, participants demonstrated a statistically significant increase in knowledge about schizophrenia and a trend toward improved attitudes about the patients.

Conclusions

Limiting the objectives of brief hospitalization to symptom reduction and crisis intervention in the face of limited aftercare services may undermine the tenuous gains patients have made by the time of their discharge and contribute to the high human and economic costs of schizophrenia. On the other hand, a brief, focused, interdisciplinary psychoeducational program, designed to respond to the strengths and special vulnerabilities of schizophrenic patients and their families, can provide a foundation for posthospital adjustment and longer-term management of this disorder.

This treatment model involves the active participation of both patients and families in a range of structured, gradually more complex learning experiences that emphasize the here-and-now, stimulate cognitive and social-interpersonal capacities, and offer information and guidelines that contribute to greater understanding of the illness and its ramifications. When introduced in a timely, individualized, and empathic manner, this model promotes greater responsiveness among patients and their families to other important biological and psychological treatment approaches during both the inpatient and the aftercare phases of treatment.

Controlled research studies will more accurately evaluate the impact of this effort, but the need for new models for brief inpatient treatment of schizophrenia is already clear—sufficiently clear, at least, to stimulate other practitioners to address the problem.

Acknowledgment

We dedicate this article to the late Phyllis Rubinton, MLS, in recognition of her innovative ideas and dedication to psychoeducation.

References

1. Drake RE, Sederer LI: Inpatient psychosocial treatment of chronic schizophrenia: negative effects and current guidelines. Hospital and Community Psychiatry 37:897-901, 1986

2. Glick ID, Clarkin JF, Spencer JH, et al: Inpatient family intervention: a controlled evaluation of practice: preliminary results of the six-months follow-up. Archives of General Psychiatry 42:882-886, 1985

3. Collins JF, Ellsworth RB, Casey NA, et al: Treatment characteristics of effective psychiatric programs. Hospital and Community Psychiatry 35:601-605, 1984

4. Maves PA, Schulz JW: Inpatient group treatment on short-term acute care units. Hospital and Community Psychiatry 36:69-73, 1985

5. Heinrichs DW: Recent developments in the psychosocial treatment of chronic psychotic illnesses, in The Chronic Mental Patient. Edited by Talbott JA. Orlando, Fla, Grune & Stratton, 1984

6. Narrow BW: Patient Teaching in Nursing Practice. New York, Wiley, 1984

7. Falvol DR: Effective Patient Education. Rockville, Md, Aspen, 1985

8. Haas LD: Practical Occupational Therapy, 2nd ed. Milwaukee, Bruce, 1946

9. Goldstein AP, Gershaw NJ, Sprafkin RP: Structured learning therapy. American Journal of Occupational Therapy 33:635-639, 1979

10. Hollis F: Casework: A Psychosocial Therapy. New York, Random House, 1964

11. Crow MS: Preventive intervention through parent group education. Social Casework 48:161-165, 1967

12. Anderson CM: Family intervention with severely disturbed inpatients. Archives of General Psychiatry 34:697-702, 1977

13. Hatfield A: What families want of psychotherapists, in Family Therapy in Schizophrenia. Edited by McFarlane WR. New York, Guilford, 1983

14. Paul GL, Lentz RJ: Psychosocial Treatment of Chronic Mental Patients. Cambridge, Mass, Harvard University Press, 1977

15. Lamb HR: An educational model for teaching living skills to long-term patients. Hospital and Community Psychiatry 27:875-877, 1976

16. Liberman RP, Massel HK, Mosk MD, et al: Social skills training for chronic mental patients. Hospital and Community Psychiatry 36:396-403, 1985

17. Anderson CM: A psychoeducational program for families of patients with schizophrenia, in Family Therapy in Schizophrenia. Edited by McFarlane WR. New York, Guilford, 1983

18. Anderson CM, Reiss, DJ, Hogarty, GE: Schizophrenia and the Family. New York, Guilford, 1986

19. Falloon, IRH, Boyd, JL, McGill CW, et al: Family management in the prevention of exacerbations of schizophrenia: a controlled study. New England Journal of Medicine 306:1437-1440, 1982

20. Snyder, KD, Liberman, RP: Family assessment and intervention with schizophrenics at risk for relapse. New Directions for Mental Health Services, no 12:49-60, 1981

21. Leff J, Kuipers L, Berkowitz R, et al: A controlled trial of social intervention in the families of schizophrenic patients. British Journal of Psychiatry 141:121-134, 1982

22. Anderson CM, Reiss DJ: Family treatment of patients with chronic schizophrenia: the inpatient phase, in The Psychiatric Hospital and the Family. Edited by Harbin HT. Jamaica, NY, SP Medica & Scientific Books, 1982

23. Thomes LD, Bajema SL: The life skills development program: a history overview and update. Occupational Therapy in Mental Health 3:35-48, 1983

24. Ogren K: A living skills program in an acute psychiatric setting. Mental Health Special Interest Section Newsletter (American Occupational Therapy Association) 6:1-2, 1983

25. Fine SB, Schwimmer P: The effects of occupational therapy on independent living skills. Mental Health Special Interest Section Newsletter (American Occupational Therapy Association) 9:1-3, 1986

26. Zubin J: Chronic schizophrenia from the standpoint of vulnerability, in Perspectives in Schizophrenia Research. Edited by Baxter C, Melnechuk T. New York, Raven, 1980

27. Falloon IRH, Liberman RP: Interactions between drug and psychosocial therapy in schizophrenia. Schizophrenia Bulletin 9:543-552, 1983

28. Fine SB: Psychiatric treatment and rehabilitation: what's in a name? Psychiatric Hospital 11(Fall):8-13, 1980

29. Goldman HH: Mental illness and family burden: a public health perspective. Hospital and Community Psychiatry 33:557-560, 1982

30. Michaelson A, Nitzberg L, Rubinton P: Mental health resources library: a consumer guide to the literature. Psychiatric Hospital 15:133-139, 1984

Chapter 45

A Model Program to Teach Parenting Skills to Schizophrenic Mothers

Merilyne C. Waldo, MA
Margaret Roath, MSW
Winifred Levine, RN, MA
Robert Freedman, MD

Because of the emphasis on community treatment of schizophrenia and the fact that the illness often does not appear until the late 20s, an increasing number of schizophrenic women are marrying and having children (1-2). Less than 20 percent of these children become schizophrenic themselves (3), and a surprising number become superachievers (4). Thus early intervention may be particularly valuable for them. However, most mental health facilities are not able to provide targeted assistance in mothering to schizophrenic women. Only a few such programs have been developed (5-7), and most reports have not included enough information about their clinical functioning to allow others to benefit from their experience.

This paper describes our work at the Denver Mothers' and Children's Project, which was established in 1982 to address the special needs of schizophrenic mothers and their preschool children.

Program Description

The goals of the Mothers' and Children's Project are to teach mothering skills to schizophrenic mothers, to monitor the developmental progress of their children and provide early intervention when needed, and to develop a model for the establishment of similar programs.

Because the program is designed to supplement other mental health care, women entering the program must be registered patients with a mental health clinic or a private psychiatrist. They must meet the diagnostic criteria for schizophrenia and must have a preschool child with whom they have a significant, ongoing relationship. Although most of the children live at home, mothers whose children are in temporary foster care are also accepted.

Mothers are referred to the program from public social service agencies, domestic courts, mental health clinics, and maternity wards. A mother is visited at home by the program director (MCW), who reviews her diagnosis and assesses her level of functioning. This visit offers us a realistic view of the home environment and any special difficulties a mother may face with living space or family problems.

The staff consist of a psychologist who works ten hours a week with the program; a child development specialist and a social worker who each work four hours a week; five volunteers, experienced and successful mothers recruited by word of mouth; two research trainees; and one paid domestic assistant who provides lunches for the weekly meetings.

Currently the program is functioning at full capacity, with ten mothers and their 12 preschool children. The mothers may remain in the program as long as they feel it is helpful to them. The focus of the program is a two-and-a-half hour meeting held once a week in a community church. The mothers attend the meeting with their preschool children. Transportation is provided to ensure that when the mothers are more symptomatic, they need not make a special effort to attend.

The meeting begins at 10 a.m. and lasts until 12:30 p.m.; mothers and children spend the first 45 minutes in small groups led by a volunteer supervised by a child specialist. The groups focus on developmental education, directed play, and role modeling. Nearly all the children show language delays; the mothers often do not talk to the children because they do not appear to understand. This problem is addressed by modeling good language behavior and also by having the mothers spend short periods of time talking to their children about what they are doing. In addition, the mothers often do not know what their child should be doing developmentally and thus do not encourage age-appropriate activities. Specific tasks that the children should be doing are highlighted, and the mothers are urged to encourage the children to undertake them.

The small groups give mothers the opportunity to discuss problems with staff and peers and to observe other mother-child interactions. Each week one mother and her child meet with the child specialist to discuss individual issues.

Juice and crackers are provided at the end of this period to facilitate a smooth transition to the next period. The children spend the rest of the morning in a therapeutic nursery while the mothers meet in a separate group.

The mother's therapy group, led by a social worker and a volunteer, provides a forum to discuss parenting. Group direction is determined by the mothers. A number of recurring themes have evolved: What does it mean to be schizophrenic? How does being schizophrenic complicate child care and family life? How does one resolve feelings of ambivalence and conflict about men, social

services, and medication? Didactic sessions address specific areas of concern such as discipline, toilet training, and birth control.

The meeting ends with lunch, which gives staff additional opportunities to model appropriate mothering behavior and instruct the mothers in good nutrition. Staff can also help the mothers with any feeding and eating problems their children may be having. After the mothers and children leave, staff meet for an hour to discuss clinical issues.

The mothers have come to rely on each other outside the program. Our experience has been similar to that reported by Liberman and associates (8) in that many of the women in the group have formed the first real friendships they have ever had. They often help each other during crises and will offer to babysit, provide transportation, or teach each other various skills.

Two problems have required us to define the limitations of the program. The first is attempts by the courts to use the program in evaluations for custody cases, and the second is the need for treatment of schizophrenia itself. In the first case, we refuse admission to any mother when it can be determined that the reason for referral is to establish her inability to parent. At the same time, mothers who decide that they are not able to provide a nurturing environment for their child are supported in their decision. In the second case, we refer problems back to the treating service, offering our observations and suggestions when requested. We educate mothers to become aware of early signs of increased symptomatology and advocate early and aggressive intervention.

Characteristics of Program Participants

As of May 1986, a total of 52 women had been referred to the program, of whom 21 were refused admission. The most common reasons for refusal were that the diagnosis of schizophrenia was not confirmed, the woman's children were permanently separated from her, there were no preschool children in the family, or the primary reason for referral was persistent and life-threatening child abuse or the court's attempt to establish the woman's inability to parent.

The 31 women who participated in the program ranged in age from 19 to 45, with a mean of 26.7 years. Three of the women attended only once. Two of these mothers realized that they were not capable of providing adequate care for their children and relinquished custody within 24 hours after attending the program. The third mother was only minimally ill and was referred to another parenting program.

Three women attended only irregularly for periods

ranging from two weeks to three months, and the remaining 25 women attended regularly for at least six months. These 25 women had a total of 48 children, ranging in age from birth to 27 years, and each had at least one preschool child. Twenty-six of the children were living with their mothers, seven had been permanently placed with relatives, three were adults living on their own, and two had been previously placed in adoptive homes. Ten children were in protective custody when the mothers entered the program. After the mothers had attended for six months, six of the children were returned to their mothers, two were placed in adoptive homes, and two remained in protective custody.

Discussion

The effectiveness of our program in helping schizophrenic women and their children depends on several factors, including the mothers' participation, the volunteer staff's continuing involvement, and the program's success in meeting specific goals. Most women who are accepted into the program attend faithfully each week and enjoy the group. Mothers who have left the program continue to drop in during difficult periods and may call long distance to get advice from the group. The children talk about the group during the week and show obvious pleasure in arriving each week.

Since we rely heavily on our volunteer staff, it is also necessary to provide a setting that can attract and keep qualified people. This goal is enhanced by offering an hour-long staff meeting each week, where our volunteer staff's experience is supplemented by a discussion of ongoing issues with the professional staff. Since few established guidelines exist to teach mothering skills to schizophrenic women, the experience of the volunteer mothers is a primary source of information. Most of our volunteers have been with the program for more than three years.

The program has been successful in improving parenting. The number of children in temporary foster care has dropped significantly. Social workers and therapists surveyed by the authors noted that interactions between mothers and their children were significantly improved, and 83 percent of the mothers were judged to have shown significant improvement in their treatment compliance, contributing to a nearly total elimination of rehospitalizations.

In 1987, the program costs for each participant were approximately $1,200, including transportation, lunches, special outings and parties, and staff salaries.

Overall, the program has had considerable success in teaching mothering skills to schizophrenic women. The volunteer staff of experienced mothers represents a community resource that can be used effectively in parent education.

Acknowledgements

The authors thank Cynthia Kendrick for her contributions to the project. They also thank the volunteer staff—Sally Lonegren, Diane Olsen, Lynn Hurst, Anne Fairbairn, Pamela Owen, and Anne Frieze—without whom the program could not continue.

References

1. Seeman MV: Gender and the onset of schizophrenia: neurohumoral influences. Psychiatric Journal of the University of Ottawa 6:136-138, 1981

2. Bland RC: Demographic aspects of functional psychoses in Canada. Acta Psychiatrica Scandinavica 55:369-380, 1977

3. Kety SS: Genetic and biochemical aspects of schizophrenia, in The Harvard Guide to Modern Psychiatry. Edited by AM Nicholi. Cambridge, Harvard University Press, 1978

4. Kauffman C, Grunebaum H, Cohler B, et al: Superkids: competent children of psychotic mothers. American Journal of Psychiatry 136:1398-1402, 1979

5. Waldo MC, Roath M, Freedman R: Schizophrenia and parenting. Presented at the American Psychiatric Association annual meeting, Washington, DC, May 10-16, 1986

6. Grunebaum H, Cohler B, Kauffman C, et al: Children of depressed and schizophrenic mothers. Child Psychiatry and Human Development 8:219-228, 1978

7. Goodman SH: Children of emotionally disturbed mothers: problems and alternatives. Children Today, March-April 1984, pp 6-9

8. Liberman RP, Wallace CJ, Vaughn CE, et al: Social and family factors in the course of schizophrenia: towards an interpersonal problem-solving therapy for schizophrenics and their families, in The Psychotherapy of Schizophrenia. Edited by Strauss JS, Bowers M, Downey TW, et al. New York, Plenum, 1980

Chapter 46

Establishing Support and Advocacy Groups

Susan Delaney McConchie, OTR

Establishing community-based support groups can be a new challenge for occupational therapists. Do you have a yen to explore new directions or to develop new roles for yourself? You have the skills and the background to be of tremendous help to persons in your community, agency, or hospital. Your local newspaper will list support groups or self-help groups that are already operating. Reviewing these listings may give you the impetus to start a group to help meet an identified need in your practice or program.

Several years ago I joined the staff of a community mental health agency. As I continued to work there, I realized that many of our clients had problems that went beyond their stated diagnoses. With the administration's approval, I developed a simple questionnaire to circulate to the staff. The results did confirm my observations: A total of 75 patients, or 8% of the outpatient caseload, carried a secondary diagnosis of such disorders as cerebrovascular accident, cerebral palsy, multiple sclerosis, heart conditions, and so on. Some of the major reasons these clients had been referred to the mental health clinic were such problems as marital conflicts, depression, and feelings of isolation. They were having problems adjusting to the physical aspects of their disabilities, and problems dealing with agencies and service providers; these needs had not been addressed. Armed with these findings, I approached the agency director and persuaded him that we could better address the dual needs of these people by establishing a support group designed specifically for them. This was agreed upon, and a very rewarding chapter in my occupational therapy career began. What follows is an outline of the process we used to develop our group, a description of the group, and a partial discussion of subsequent issues and developments.

Getting Started

Work or Volunteer Project?

The first thing to decide is the context of the project: Do you want to establish a group as part of your regular work load or as a volunteer project within your community? In terms of productivity, payment for services, and so on, you will have to weigh the pros and cons of each option carefully—including agency policies and politics. My own opinion is that it is better to undertake the project as a staff member, because you will have more resources available to you and the group in that context. The task then becomes one of providing education and training skills to the consumers involved, thus enabling them to take over the running of the group themselves. The leaders can then become consultants, which is a less time-consuming role.

Identification of Community Needs

What are some of the needs you have identified in your work setting that are not being met by your existing program? List them first, and then brainstorm with co-workers for additional needs they have identified. You may have some community requests to consider as well: As local community members became aware of our programs, requests came in to the agency for assistance in developing a variety of other groups, such as one for family members of persons with chronic mental illness, one for persons with eating disorders, and another for pregnant teenagers.

Time and Coleadership Issues

If you have decided to have a coleader, identify someone who shares your ideas and enthusiasms and is willing to assume new roles. Having a similar theoretical orientation is also important, and it is helpful to have a coleader with background in the content area you have chosen to stress—perhaps someone who works in a different agency or setting.

Coleadership takes time, and it is important to be sure that your administrator or supervisor understands this. Coleadership does not mean that the group can be twice as large. Time is needed for preparation and for postgroup processing. You will have to decide how much time you can realistically devote to this new project, because—as you will see when you begin—you are not leading a traditional occupational therapy treatment group. In the initial planning stages, 3 hours per week may be needed for planning, phone contacts, group meetings, and processing; later, 2 hours should be sufficient. It is, however, easier to schedule more time initially than to create it later on!

Establishing the Format

Early decisions might include the size of the group, how transportation will be arranged, the meeting location, and whether or not to have a coleader. Other considerations are the age range of participants and how long the group will run (will it be ongoing or time limited?).

Another variable is group content. What type of group format do you envision? Will your group be strictly educational, with films and lectures, or do you envision a self-help model in which the group members determine the agenda? Do you want to provide a purely supportive group environment, or do you want to teach members advocacy skills? To a large degree, answering these questions determines the leaders' roles. For the remainder of this article, it is assumed that you have decided to combine aspects of both support and self-help groups and that your ultimate goal is to see this group maintain itself in the community. Eventually, your role would be that of some kind of informal consultant.

Other Considerations

Additional questions to consider before starting a group might include these: What will your referral process be? How will you screen interested people for membership? How will in-group emergencies be handled? What about general communication with referring staff? Will the agency charge a fee, or will contributions be voluntary? Will refreshments be made available? Consulting the literature on various support and self-help systems may help you decide these questions: you may also want to attend local meetings of other groups and talk with group members.

As with any kind of program, record keeping is extremely important. Because ours was a new venture, keeping detailed notes proved very helpful when we decided to expand the program into new areas. Records were also kept of any critical issues that needed to be passed on to clients' primary therapists (clients agreed to allow them access to this information). Attendance records were also maintained.

Support Group for Persons With Physical Handicaps: Description of Pilot Group

A description of this group is presented to help illustrate client and staff development and growth as this agency-based support group changed to a community-based self-help and advocacy organization.

The data generated from the aforementioned questionnaire proved quite helpful in establishing our group. Appropriate clients were identified within the agency. An outpatient therapist with three such clients in his caseload expressed interest in coleading the group. He was selected as coleader, and we began our planning by discussing the kinds of needs his clients presented. The questionnaire also helped us identify other clients and their primary therapists for further referrals.

Goals and Plans

We set specific goals for the new group, including (a) facilitating a support network among the members, (b) using the group as a forum for sharing information and resources, and (c) teaching clients to become their own advocates. Transportation was determined to be the client's responsibility, although suggestions to meet this need would be available. Because the clients would retain their primary therapists, case management issues would be directed to the original therapist.

All initial members of the group had come to the agency with symptoms of depression, and in one case suicidal ideation was an issue. We suspected that the members' depressions might increase as members shared the stresses of their disabilities, so we decided to teach group members early on how to use the agency's existing emergency services and similar emergency services in the community at large.

We then interviewed prospective members, explaining the purposes of the group. This allowed us to evaluate the clients' communication skills informally, identify their primary issues, determine the main reasons they were interested in joining the group, and verify other agency contacts or connections they might already have.

Group Members

We were cautious at first, so our original group consisted of only six members (three other potential members were placed on a waiting list). Though the following thumbnail sketches are limited at best, I think they will help the reader begin to understand the group's makeup. The extraordinary variety of backgrounds in the group should be noted.

Sue was a 35-year-old widow with two pre-teenage children. She had severe multiple sclerosis and had recently begun using a wheelchair. Derek, in his early 30s, had juvenile diabetes. Blind since 19 years of age, he had recently gone through a divorce and was learning to live by himself. Greg, Derek's friend, was 55 years old and nearly blind. He was quite depressed over his increasing dependence and near isolation (he lived on a farm in a rural community). Mary, 35 years of age, had severe scoliosis as well as other physical problems. She was severely depressed and at times suicidal. Carla, a 17-year-old high school student, had moderate cerebral palsy and evidence of learning disabilities and speech impairments. She frequently threatened to act out her feelings as a means of coping with her depression. Finally, there was Bill, 35, who had sustained a severe head injury in his work as a farmer. Bill was phobic and had many residual difficulties from his injury.

The First Meeting

The group's first meeting was scheduled, and all members were in attendance. We began by asking them to share something about themselves, especially about their disabilities and needs. As coleaders, we also shared briefly about ourselves and more specifically about our interest in this group and why we felt the group could be useful. We were amazed at the outpouring of feelings that took place; clients said that it was the first time that anyone had shown interest in their disabilities. They talked about events that had been crushing to them, and about what it meant to them to be labeled. They also shared feelings of loneliness, fear, and severe isolation. All were experiencing family problems (including, in many cases, marital problems) that seemed directly related to their physical conditions. They also evidenced an astonishing lack of knowledge about their various disabilities and their resulting difficulties. They suffered from fragmentation of services, and had little idea of how to access needed benefits and services, such as transportation or social security income. Access to buildings was very limited at that time. Financial problems were evident, and members had great fears for the futures of their children. The list of unsolved issues went on and on.

The group bonded early on, and little by little started to create an additional network outside of the agency. Group members made telephone calls to one another between meetings. The leaders noted the expressions of anger in the group and supported self-advocacy efforts as they emerged. After a few months of meetings, it became clear to all of us that we needed a concrete way to focus members' feelings of outrage over a general lack of services and accommodations for people with physical disabilities. As coleaders we supported the clients' idea of writing a letter about their issues to the agency director and board. We were somewhat worried about our job security as a result, and spent some time reassessing our position and its consequences. Although we remained somewhat anxious about the agency's response, we came to the conclusion that actions needed to follow ideals. The letter was written by the group and typed by an agency secretary.

This turned out to be a critical turning point for our group and for us as coleaders. We had been the leaders, they the clients, but now that distinction was blurred to some extent. We had become activists.

In response to the letter, the agency director came to a group meeting and listened to the group's complaints. Together we came up with a plan to remedy the most essential issues. Accessible, if not glamorous, bathroom facilities were provided, as were parking lot signs, a buzzer system to open the door near the ramp, and another railing on the stairway. Group members worked with agency staff members to get these tasks completed outside of group time, while we as coleaders spent extra time on the telephone with our rather nervous consumers, supporting them, helping them decide what to say to staff involved in the renovations, and so on. We soon found that we had in effect two groups, one needing ongoing support at meetings and the other wanting to take our time to address issues in the community. This latter group wanted to get other persons with disabilities involved in advocacy.

The Next Stage

At about this time, a flyer about a leadership skills training program appeared on our agency bulletin board. We took advantage of this program and helped three of our group members enroll. They came back to group sessions full of ideas and ready to establish another group in the community to tackle additional issues. We saw that establishing this type of community group would empower these clients and could provide a mechanism where advocacy and self-help would be the norm rather than just a new service within the agency. We spent several of the next support group sessions planning the community group, deciding on a name, coming up with topics of general interest, and compiling a speaker list. We discussed when and where this new group would meet, how to secure a meeting place, and the need for publicity to reach others who could profit from such a group. We provided transportation to meetings with staff persons from other agencies, and provided guidance and suggestions on additional topics as they were raised.

The original group of six clients formed the core of the new group, Handicaps for Handicaps, that began to meet on a monthly basis in the local Salvation Army gym. For the members, choosing a name for this new group seemed to be part of the needed process of freeing themselves for this next stage of development. These early members became the officers of the new advocacy group; my coleader and I served as consultants. The initial support group continued within the agency.

As time went on, referrals began coming from other agencies to both groups. My coleader and I continued to meet regularly and learned to divide issues between the groups. We discovered that we had created a type of aftercare group that we could recommend to clients when they had "graduated" from the agency support group. The support group continues to meet at the agency today and continues to provide long-term support for clients. The community group, which later changed its name to The Coalition of the Handicapped, became a true advocacy group. Among this group's accomplishments were marked parking spaces for disabled people, ramps and curb cuts in downtown areas, and increased awareness of and adherence to federal, state, and local codes for all new public construction. It was instrumental in improving transportation networks for disabled people in our area. Social events and an informal telephone network sponsored by this group helped members feel less isolated.

The Coalition of the Handicapped served as a rallying point and as a forum for client-agency interaction. Representatives from a variety of health-related agencies were frequent observers, speakers, or guests at monthly meetings; interagency collaboration grew as a result of the group's efforts. Community consciousness was raised as well, because the group refused to have its concerns overlooked or ignored. Group members also became active members of their communities, and attended such local meetings as city council meetings.

In addition to The Coalition of the Handicapped, the original agency-based support group served as a stepping-off point for several other community-based self-help groups, including two groups for parents of students with special needs and an educational and support group for people with diabetes and their families. Staff training models were developed to help agency and community caregivers more fully understand the dual diagnoses represented by clients with both emotional problems and physical disabilities. Eventually, a presentation was made at a regional mental health conference about this program.

Summary

I've tried to share the beginnings of one effort in advocacy. I believe that the role of occupational therapy in the development of such systems is a natural extension of community practice. I hope that this article provides food for thought and gives you the impetus to review the needs of your own system.

I would like to thank Richard Stayton, MSW, who served as coleader of the pilot group described in this article, and Carolyn Crane Nicholson, MEd. Both are employed at Monadnock Family Services in Keene, New Hampshire.

Chapter 47

Starting a Stress Management Programme

Sharon Mueller, RN
Melinda Suto, OT

Within the last few years, stress management has become the subject of numerous lectures and workshops. They are sponsored by educational institutions, health care agencies and the business community. What precisely is meant by the phrase "stress management" as it relates to (mental) health care services? For our purposes, we have defined stress management as the "coping behaviors that are learned to reduce the effects of over-stress resulting from the environment, the social and cultural milieu, and specific life events." The purpose of this paper is to convey general knowledge of stress and how it affects people, and to explore individuals' stresses and find effective ways to cope with them.

Although most people could benefit from learning skills with which to cope with life stresses, there exists a high-risk population that we will focus on in this paper. Specifically, these people are: patients (and their families) with a psychiatric disorder, patients who are chronically ill (e.g., diabetes, rheumatoid arthritis), the elderly and the physically handicapped.

People chosen for this group had a variety of psychiatric diagnoses (except those currently psychotic or suicidal), but it was more useful to judge their degree of maladaptive coping behavior than to rely solely on medical diagnoses. Referrals were accepted from the local Community Care Teams, and for people currently in the Day Programme. Those clients who attended the Day Programme and the stress management group had increased opportunities to practice their new skills within a supportive setting and receive feedback on their attempts.

In developing this program, material was used from books by Hans Selye[2,3] and Friedman & Rosenman[1], and prevailing theories on subjects such as nutrition, yoga, balancing exercise, work and play, etc. The treatment program used an educational model and allowed for group discussion. This format encouraged group support, problem-solving and a sharing of personal experiences. During the two and one half hour, once-weekly meetings, homework was discussed, new information presented, and the final half hour involved application of relaxation techniques (i.e., yoga, progressive relaxation, etc.). A handout covering the day's material was also available to participants during this five-week period. Specific outlines for each stress management session are summarized below, followed by a detailed discussion of selected topics.

Session one dealt with the aims of the group, confidentiality, and participants' responsibility, and outlined the following four sessions. The topics covered in the first session were defining stress, sources of stress, psychological signs of stress, physiological signs of stress, finding one's optimum stress level, the importance of paying attention to signs of over-stress, a personal evaluation that included client goals and individual stressors, and relaxation exercises.

Session two discussed the correlation between stress and illness, reducing negative effects of stress, replacing maladaptive coping behaviors, and changing attitudes toward situations.

Session three included an examination of attitude changes, healthy life-styles, more relaxation techniques, and analyzing individual work/play/sleep patterns.

Session four covered specific stresses inherent in the following life periods: childhood, adolescence, young adulthood, middle age, and aged. Also, we elaborated on the handling of over-stress arising from home, work and social situations.

Session five included a discussion of physical exercises to use when faced with stressful situations, listing in point form of "things to remember" in dealing with stress, role-playing difficult situations using the video, and evaluating of the program to find out whether people achieved their goals.

Defining stress is an important aspect of the program since many people are not aware that they are experiencing a physiological or psychological response to stress. Individual differences are also important. Some people thrive on being busy, whereas others have a much lower tolerance for a busy schedule. Similarly, different people have various methods for handling stress. One person relaxes by doing physical activities, whereas another person prefers to do relaxation exercises or read.

The correlation between stress and illness was also discussed. Emphasis was placed on the ability of the individual to influence his or her health in a positive manner by dealing effectively with stress and by using healthy coping behaviors such as relaxation, yoga, or physical exercise, as opposed to doing such things as overeating and over-smoking. A healthy life style is an important tool in dealing with stress. Such techniques as

assertiveness training can be useful, as can attitude change. For example, a person can learn to say "I would like to get this done," instead of "I must get this done."

Having a balance between work, play and sleep is also important. One exercise used in the course is a "life pie." Clients are asked to divide the pie according to how much time they spend at work, play and sleep over a 24-hour period. These are then divided further into whether these activities are physical or mental. In this way, they can look at how much time is spent in each area and can evaluate where changes are needed to achieve a balanced life style.

The course also deals with the effects of change on stress level. Although Hans Selye's stress scale is outdated, it is discussed briefly, and the importance of not having too much change at one time is emphasized. If, for instance, someone had just changed residences as well as recently married, it might not be a good time to change jobs as well. Even positive events can be stressful when they involve change, and limiting the number of changes occurring at the same time is an important factor in preventing over-stress. It is also important to consider stresses specific to different aspects of life. Home, work and social situations each present certain problems. Stresses arising from home life and social situations are primarily related to skill and comfort in interpersonal relationships. Although work stresses involve these areas, they also involve pressures specific to the job. Stresses arising from any one area can affect the individual's ability to function in another.

The following procedures are used to evaluate how individuals deal with stress. In each instance, clients are asked to identify what they find stressful, and to consider how they are currently dealing with these stresses. Are they doing such things as over-smoking, overeating , or overdrinking to cope, or are they using more healthy methods? If their usual methods seem inadequate, more useful ways of dealing with stress can be pointed out. Particular attention should be paid to the individual's own stress tolerance. Is he or she a "racehorse" or a "turtle"? What is fun for one person may be stressful for another.

Skills such as diaphragmatic breathing, relaxation exercises and yoga can be taught as alternatives to unhealthy coping behavior. Other behaviors, such as assertiveness training, leading a generally healthy and balanced life style, and using breaks in the day's routine for relaxation and exercise, are useful as well. Limiting change when under stress is also an important technique, as is being assertive and direct about needs and sharing feelings. A list of specific stresses with possible solutions can then be generated, providing the client with a number of alternatives. The more alternatives the individual has available, the less likely [he or she is] to be overwhelmed by stressful situations.

It is also important to be aware that different life stages give rise to certain specific stresses. A child just starting school, for example, will experience stress as a result of the necessity to leave home, make friends, and function independently, whereas the adolescent will be more concerned with the issues needed to [be dealt] with as he or she changes from child to adult. The child or adolescent who is under stress may demonstrate it by stuttering, nail-biting, poor eating and sleeping, or rebellious behavior. If this type of behavior is apparent, it is useful to find out what specific stress is occurring and to look at more positive ways of dealing with it.

Likewise, the young adult, the middle-aged and the elderly [each] have their own set of problems. The young adult will have to make career choices and become emotionally and financially independent. The adult in the middle years will be likely to experience such things as the "empty nest syndrome," accepting the problems of aging and perhaps looking after aging parents. Again, it is important to evaluate the specific stress and to adapt healthy methods of dealing with it. The middle years can be used as a time to re-evaluate life roles and goals and to set new goals for the next thirty years.

Perhaps no age group has more problems of stress than the elderly. Loss of physical or mental ability, loss of friends, power, independence and role in society all contribute to the difficulties of the older citizen. Stresses can be identified and alternate solutions generated for each problem. Planning ahead of time for change of life style can be particularly useful as it enables the individual approaching retirement to cushion the effects of change by developing interests away from work, building a network of friends and developing a variety of interests.

In evaluating techniques for handling stress, several things become apparent. A variety of techniques are needed because specific situations require different skills. In addition, it was evident that different methods work for different people. When clients evaluated the stress management program, no specific technique was seen by the group as being most helpful. Individual groups found different things useful. Some found relaxation exercises and yoga most helpful, whereas others found sharing feelings, being assertive and leading a more balanced life-style most important.

A number of stress management techniques can be adapted for use in the general hospital setting. Health care teaching needn't take a great deal of staff time and can pay off in extra dividends for the patient. First, he needs to evaluate his life-style. Get him to do a "life pie" to assist him in his evaluation. Is his life balanced between work, play and sleep? Does he get adequate exercise and rest? What stresses is he presently under and what is he doing about [them]? What changes are happening in his life and can some of these be postponed? Will there be any long-term effects of illness and what stress management techniques can he use in view of this illness? The person with coronary difficulties, or the patient with a permanent physical disability, who formerly used vigorous physical exercise as a form of relaxation, will need to look at alternate methods of coping with stress. Relaxation exercises and yoga can be taught, and patients could be given cassette tapes to listen to and follow. Teaching the patient to cope with the physical aspects of illness is also important. Talk to the patient and try to ascertain how he or she views that illness. Keeping the stresses of different life periods in mind and helping to evaluate the patient's life-style can be useful in identifying the stresses a patient may be under, and can help in planning the nursing care.

In summary then, there are certain general principles in stress management. These are as follows:

1. We need to re-evaluate our life patterns and to take control over our lives.
2. Stress weakens psychological resistance as well as immunological response.
3. Be aware that your emotional and physical health affect each other.
4. Avoid excessive simultaneous life changes. Be aware of which pace of life is appropriate for you and pay attention to yourself.
5. If feeling uncomfortable, stop to consider why and make any appropriate changes.
6. Maintain a steady pace at work and play. Avoid great swings in activity levels. Pace yourself.
7. Remember to equalize stress through variety in daily activities.
8. Live at a tempo and direction best suited to yourself. Remember, "One man's work is another man's play."
9. Adopt a healthy life-style and a positive attitude.
10. Work on clear communication to decrease tension in interpersonal situations. Don't be afraid to make your needs known.
11. Learn a variety of coping techniques so that if one doesn't work you can use another.
12. Note those around you who cope well and try mimicking their behaviors.
13. Remember, it's not stress in itself that is harmful but rather, what you do or don't do to deal with it.

References

1. Rosenman, R., and Friedman, M., *Type A Behavior and Your Heart*, Fawcett Crest 1978.

2. Selye, Hans, *The Stress of Life*, McGraw-Hill, 1976.

3. Selye, Hans, *Stress Without Distress*, New American Library, 1971.

4. Pelletier, Kenneth, *Mind as healer, mind as layer: A wholistic approach to preventing stress disorders*, Dell Publishers, 1977.

5. Holmes, T., and Rahe, "*The Social Readjustment Rating Scale*" Journal of Psychosomatic Research 2, (1967).

Chapter 48

A Stress Management Program: Inpatient-to-Outpatient Continuity

Cyndi Courtney, OTR
Barbara Escobedo, OTR

Recent statistics indicate that 75% of all medical complaints are stress related, including ulcers, stomach disorders, headaches, hypertension, insomnia, aches and pains, and many psychiatric disorders (Charlesworth & Nathan, 1984).

Uniform terminology (Hopkins & Smith, 1983) defines *situational coping* as the skill and performance to handle stress and deal with problems in a manner that is functional to self and others. This includes

- Setting goals and managing activities of daily living to promote optimal performance.
- Testing goals and perceptions against reality.
- Perceiving changes and need for changes in self and the environment.
- Directing and redirecting energy to overcome problems.
- Initiating, implementing, and following through with decisions.
- Assuming responsibility for self and consequences of actions.
- Interacting with others: dyadic and group. (Hopkins & Smith, 1983, pp. 899-907)

According to Selye (1980), the stress syndrome has three stages: (a) the alarm reaction (the fight or flight response), (b) resistance (the body's increasing adaptation to constant stress and illness), and (c) exhaustion (energy depletion that may result in serious illness or death). Occupational therapists treat patients at each of these stages.

Program Description

In 1983, the University of Texas Medical Branch hospitals (Galveston, Texas) incorporated a stress management program into their existing occupational therapy program, because of the mental health medical team's increased emphasis on the role of stress in illness. The program was part of a 12-bed open milieu therapy unit that emphasized family therapy. The stress management program was designed to develop and improve situational coping skills in adult psychiatric patients. Upon discharge, patients with a continued need to practice these skills are followed in the outpatient setting. The outpatient occupational therapy clinic receives referrals from throughout the hospital, but particularly from the inpatient psychiatry units at the time of discharge.

The following criteria were established for a patient's referral to the stress management program:

1. Recent experience of stressful life events.
2. Low stress tolerance.
3. Maladaptive methods of stress reduction.
4. Attention span of at least 45 min.
5. Functional verbal skills.
6. Insight into own behavior.

Information for criteria 1, 3, 5, and 6 was gained through interviews with patients; information for criterion 2 and additional information for criteria 1, 3, and 6 was gained through a review of charts; and information for criterion 4 was identified by a task performance evaluation.

Although evaluations are used to determine which occupational therapy groups are most applicable for a referred patient, the evaluation for the stress management program will be the focus of this paper. Before a patient begins the program, his or her medical chart is reviewed to determine current and past stressors and to identify parts of the stress management program that may be contraindicated. For example, isometric exercises are contraindicated for patients with hypertension and circulatory problems, deep breathing exercises are contraindicated for patients with chronic obstructive pulmonary disease, and visual imagery exercises are contraindicated for actively hallucinating patients.

The IPAT Anxiety Scale (Krug, Scheier, & Cattell, 1975), a standardized measure, is used initially to assess anxiety; it is also helpful for reassessment. An initial interview is used to evaluate the effectiveness of the patient's social and interpersonal skills and the extent of insight into his or her behavior. The lack of social and interpersonal skills is often a contributor to high stress in work, family, and everyday social encounters (Charlesworth & Nathan, 1984). A task performance evaluation (Mosey, 1981) is used to assess concentration, attention span, comprehension, and the ability to follow directions. A sensorimotor screening (Hopkins & Smith, 1983) is used to identify areas of muscle tightness, tone, conditioning, and strength. The Interest Check List (Matsutsuyu, 1969), Assertiveness Questionnaire (Bower & Bower, 1976), and Time Utilization Schedules (Larrington, 1970) are used to determine the patient's satisfaction with his or her life situation and to assess the balance of work, play, and sleep activities. Blood pressure and pulse readings (Brunnet & Suddarth, 1982) can be taken before and after each session to evaluate the patient's response to the stress management program as well as the program's overall effectiveness.

After all of the evaluations are completed, a treatment plan, which may include the stress management program, is established. Goals that emphasize the development of adaptive methods of dealing with life stressors are identified. Individual goals are established, which might include (a) an improved ability to identify common life stressors, (b) an improved ability to identify personal life stressors and physical or emotional effects, and (c) an improved ability to achieve a relaxation response during stress management sessions and to integrate these techniques into daily life.

At the University of Texas Medical Branch at Galveston, occupational therapy patients are seen both individually and in task-oriented groups. Inpatient programming emphasizes the remediation of stress-related symptoms and group oriented activities. The inpatient program consists of five treatment groups: exercise, assertiveness training, occupational therapy task, relaxation training, and stress management.

Exercise Group

Charlesworth and Nathan (1984) stated that exercise provides a way of releasing muscle tension and general physical arousal accumulated in response to stress. At the University of Texas Medical Branch, the exercise group is a progressive walking-jogging-running program that meets for 45 minutes five times a week. A 15-minute warm-up exercise focuses on stretching and muscle preparation. The patients then go outside and walk, jog, or run for an assigned length of time and at an assigned speed. Pulses are taken before and after the exercises to determine tolerance to the physical activity, improved endurance, and whether more demanding exercise is appropriate.

Assertiveness Training Group

The assertiveness training group emphasizes improved methods of communication to express feelings, wants, and needs effectively, either verbally or nonverbally. This group focuses on activities that help clarify and encourage the practice of appropriate verbal and nonverbal communication. The treatment modalities that are used include group expression and self-expression through media, the identification and labeling of emotions, training in social skills, role-playing with feedback regarding communication styles, and training in assertiveness techniques (Bower & Bower, 1976). This group meets for 1 hour twice a week.

Occupational Therapy Task Group

The occupational therapy task group uses arts and crafts as treatment modalities. This group, which meets for 1 hr five times a week, gauges the patient's ability to perform tasks within a social context and to deal with the related stressors. It is also used as a training modality for leisure skills and time management.

Relaxation Training Group

The relaxation training group focuses on decreasing

muscle tension and improving the ability to relax by teaching patients to use relaxation techniques. This group meets for 30 minutes twice a week. Patients are first taught appropriate breathing techniques and are encouraged to practice deep breathing, as opposed to shallow breathing. They then progress to slow rhythmic movements of the head, neck, shoulders, and arms. Progressive muscle relaxation techniques in which successive muscle groups are tensed and relaxed are performed. This technique helps the patient distinguish between muscle tension and relaxation. Autogenic techniques are also incorporated into the exercises; they promote vasodilation through the suggestion of heavy and warm feelings in the extremities. Autogenic techniques are especially beneficial for headache sufferers (Charlesworth & Nathan, 1984). Visual imagery exercises that focus on a favorite memory or pleasant place also are used (Charlesworth & Nathan, 1984). Autogenic training or visual imagery techniques are not recommended for patients who are extremely agitated or who have distorted perceptions of reality. A therapy set is included before and after an exercise to explain the rationale behind the technique and to encourage patients to include the activity in their behavioral repertoires (Peloquin, 1983, 1988).

Stress Management Group

Inpatient treatment. The stress management group meets for 1 hour once a week and is the keystone of all of the programming. Patients in this group are encouraged to identify their personal life stressors, their symptoms of stress, and the ways in which stress has affected their physical and emotional well-being. Specific stress management techniques are taught, and the patients are given homework to encourage them to practice these techniques outside of the group structure. Specific topics include time management and goal setting techniques; nutrition and exercise education; activities to improve attitudinal and behavioral awareness, such as values clarification (Simon, Howe, & Kirschenbaum, 1978); thought stopping; rational emotive therapy techniques (Ellis, 1975); positive self-talk (Lazarus, 1981); and role-playing. Although the importance of improved communication, exercise, and relaxation techniques as means for dealing with stress and stress-related symptoms are discussed, these topics are covered more thoroughly in the other groups. The attitudinal and behavioral awareness activities are usually covered when the patients have almost completed the program. Patients with low IQs or limited insight may have difficulty comprehending this material; we therefore recommend the use of the other treatment modalities for this population.

One example of an activity used in the stress management group is the Life Events Scale (Holmes & Rahe, 1967), which measures the psychological stress of life events and changes. The patient uses this scale to identify personal life stressors and how they may relate to his or her illness.

Tips for reducing stress (Woolfolk & Richardson, 1978) are also used. These tips help to educate patients about various attitudinal and behavioral changes necessary for stress reduction.

Outpatient treatment. As patients improve and are discharged from the hospital, outpatient occupational therapy is often prescribed as part of their follow-up treatment. Outpatient therapy is more individualized than group treatment. Electromyograms and skin temperature biofeedback may be used to provide objective data on relaxation responses (Danskin & Crow, 1981). Outpatient programming continues with the therapist and patient working on relaxation techniques and perfecting the ability to achieve a relaxation response. Patients are frequently given a home program that incorporates daily relaxation and stretching exercises. They are also given audiocassettes that include those techniques that the patient may have found to be particularly beneficial or especially relaxing. Patients keep logs of their daily stressors and their reactions to those stressors; they also rate their ability to induce relaxation as a response to a stressor. This log is reviewed with the occupational therapist and provides the patients with feedback of their progress and their ability to induce relaxation and lessen their anxiety levels.

The individual sessions focus eventually on time management and goal setting. Patients are given activity configuration tasks (Larrington, 1970) and are instructed to analyze how they use their time daily to meet their responsibilities and their goals. Values clarification exercises (Simon et al, 1978) are used to assist with goal setting. Patients are asked to arrange their daily schedules to accomplish the short term goals that may contribute to the achievement of long-range plans. In arranging their daily schedules, the patients are taught the importance of regular exercise, good nutrition, relaxation, and leisure activities. Treatment modalities similar to those used in the inpatient program are also used.

This treatment is given for 2 hours a week for approximately 4 to 6 weeks, depending on the patient's progress with the home practice program. Treatments become less frequent as patients become more proficient in handling their daily life stresses.

Case Study

The following case study illustrates the use of a stress management program and its results. Ms. J., a 32-year-old divorced black woman, became an inpatient after she attempted suicide with a drug overdose. She had been living with her mother, grandfather, and brother and raising two teenagers. Her youngest child, age 15 years, was pregnant. The patient had had several previous psychiatric admissions since she was 16 years old and had made previous suicide attempts. The patient was hypertensive, had migraine headaches, and was obese. Her condition was diagnosed as major depression (American Psychiatric Association, 1987), and it was later found that she had characterological problems indicative of a mixed personality disorder.

The initial occupational therapy evaluation included an interview, cognitive assessment, and observation of interpersonal skills in a group setting. Ms. J. refused to cooperate with a full sensorimotor assessment.

Test results revealed that Ms. J. had much anger concerning family problems. Although she had good functional verbal skills, it was noted that she resisted communicating clearly with others, which often led to conflicts with family members and co-workers. Her daily schedule did not indicate a balance of work, rest, and play activities, but rather included as much as 20 hours of work per day in a convenience store. She reported having few social contacts outside of her family, often speaking to no one and having, as she stated, "blow-ups." During these periods, she would act impulsively and often drive aimlessly or contemplate wrecking her car. She had no cognitive deficits on the task performance evaluation and no observable gross motor deficits on the sensorimotor evaluation (of which she did not complete the fine-motor, cross-midline, and imitating movement sections). She complained of feeling anxious and of having a poor self-concept. She appeared tense, angry, withdrawn, and resistive to group and, on occasion, dyadic interactions. Her insight was fair in that she recognized her behavior as self-destructive.

On the inpatient unit, some of the initial treatment goals devised for Ms. J. were as follows:

1. Increase ability to structure the day to include a balance of work, play, and leisure.
   (a) Be punctual for all scheduled appointments.
   (b) Develop a daily schedule to be followed on overnight and weekend passes.
2. Improve ability to identify and express emotions constructively.
   (a) Identify three occasions when she felt angry.
   (b) Identify situations in which she felt uncomfortable expressing herself.
3. Improve feelings of self-worth.
   (a) Realistically assess quality of work on three occasions.
   (b) Make three positive statements about herself.

4. Improve ability to work comfortably in a group situation.
   (a) Initiate one conversation with a peer.
   (b) Ask for help from a peer on two occasions.
5. Improve ability to deal with stress more functionally.
   (a) Identify three current life stressors.
   (b) Identify how these stressors affect her physical and emotional well-being.

The patient's program included exercise, relaxation, occupational therapy tasks, and participation in assertiveness and stress management groups to assist with the achievement of the specified goals.

Ms. J. was initially resistive to treatment. She often refused to attend groups and participated poorly when she did attend. After 2 months, however, progress on goals was noted. She was attending all appointments on a regular basis. She was developing varied leisure interests and showing an improved understanding of time management and the ability to balance work and leisure. She appeared less anxious and angry and was able to verbalize feelings of anger to staff and family in an assertive manner. She agreed to become involved in exercise and relaxation groups, with good results. Her interactions with peers and staff increased. Ms. J. initiated discussions in the clinic without prompting from the therapist (the second author). She identified her stressors and related these to her behavioral patterns, including her migraine headaches and explosive outbursts.

After 6 months of inpatient treatment, Ms. J. had successfully achieved her goals, with the exception of improving her feelings of self-worth and competency. Although her self-concept had improved since her admission, she continued to make derogatory comments concerning her self-worth and her ability to handle the environmental demands outside of the hospital. Ms. J. was discharged to outpatient follow-up for individual psychotherapy and occupational therapy. As an outpatient, she attended the occupational therapy task group and individual stress management sessions for a total of 3 hours weekly. She was seen by the first author over a 2-year period, with some interruption of treatment when she found employment and when her grandson was born. Treatment focused on continued relaxation training, time management and goal setting, assertiveness training, and improved attitudinal and behavioral awareness.

Ms. J. had initial setbacks in her ability to relax and to deal effectively with others in conflict situations. She began to work long hours, yet attempted to include more time for peers and socialization. She did not report experiencing her previous blow-ups and self-destructive feelings during stressful situations. She slowly improved her ability to relax and to practice assertive behaviors, and she began to establish goals for herself and to acknowledge her achievements when they were met. She moved from her mother's house and became the primary caretaker of her grandson. She found a new job that provided increased health benefits and required fewer hours. Ms. J. was able to arrange her work schedule so that her day off coincided with her therapy day. She noted positive changes in her behavior and in others' reactions to her. She stated she felt more content and better able to "get by and make it on a day-to-day basis."

Six months after discharge from the hospital, Ms. J. was discontinued from the stress management sessions. She remained in the occupational therapy task group and in psychotherapy for 1 year. She was able to practice stress management techniques independently and to achieve a relaxation response on most occasions.

Although she continues to have occasional setbacks, Ms. J. has managed to make positive major life changes. She consistently incorporates leisure and relaxation activities into her daily routine. She is active in her church and participates in a church volleyball league. Her grandson, who is now 3 years old, was found to have leukemia, and she was able to respond functionally, arranging her work hours so that she can be at the hospital as much as possible. She returned to live with her mother after her grandfather died and her brother moved out. This has decreased the financial burden of her grandson's illness and has provided her with additional caretaking support. Ms. J.'s oldest child is now 20 years old and is unemployed, but is the primary caretaker for his nephew during the day. The child's mother dropped out of school and assumes no responsibility for the child. Ms. J. reported that the communication within her family has improved. She occasionally calls the outpatient occupational therapy clinic to chat or to request new relaxation tapes. She has maintained her present job for 2½ years without readmission to the hospital.

In conclusion, this treatment program was effective in improving Ms. J.'s ability to deal with stress and to develop adaptive coping skills. Patients with characterological disorders usually respond poorly to treatment, are frequently readmitted, and are unable to maintain employment (American Psychiatric Association, 1987). This cycle appears to have been broken with Ms. J.

Summary

The number of stress-related illnesses and dysfunctions has increased. To deal with stress, a person requires situational coping skills. For 6 years, the University of Texas Medical Branch has been operating a stress management program for adult psychiatric patients that starts in the inpatient setting and continues in the outpatient setting, where the patient is again confronted by situational stressors. Many evaluations are used in the development of an inpatient treatment plan. This plan may include exercise, relaxation training, assertiveness training, traditional occupational therapy clinic modalities, and stress management training. Outpatient treatment continues to focus on techniques learned in the inpatient setting in addition to individualized programming.

References

American Psychiatric Association. (1987). *Diagnostic and statistical manual of mental disorders* (3rd ed. rev.). Washington, DC: Author.

Bower, S. A., & Bower, G. G. (1976). *Asserting yourself.* Reading, MA: Addison-Wesley.

Brunnet, L., & Suddarth, D. (Eds.). (1987). *The Lippincott manual of nursing practice* (3rd ed.). Philadelphia: Lippincott.

Charlesworth, E. A., & Nathan, R. G. (1984). *Stress management: A comprehensive guide to wellness.* New York: Atheneum.

Danskin, D., & Crow, M. (1981). *Biofeedback: An introduction and guide.* Palto Alto, CA: Mayfield.

Ellis, A. (1975). *A new guide to rational living.* North Hollywood, CA: Wilshire.

Holmes, T. H., & Rahe, R. H. (1967). The Social Readjustment Rating Scale. *Journal of Psychosomatic Research, 11,* 212-218.

Hopkins, H. L., & Smith, H. D. (Eds.). (1983). *Willard & Spackman's occupational therapy* (6th ed.). Philadelphia: Lippincott.

Krug, S. E., Scheier, I. H., & Cattell, R. B. (1975). *IPAT Anxiety Scale.* Champaign, IL: Institute for Personality and Ability Testing.

Larrington, G. (1970). *An exploratory study of the temporal aspects of adaptive functioning.* Unpublished master's thesis, Department of Occupational Therapy, University of Southern California, Los Angeles.

Lazarus, A. A. (1981). *Behavior therapy and beyond.* New York: McGraw-Hill.

Matsutsuyu, J. S. (1969). The Interest Check List. *American Journal of Occupational Therapy, 23,* 323-328.

Mosey, A. C. (1981). *Activities therapy.* New York: Raven.

Peloquin, S. M. (1983). The development of an occupational therapy interview/therapy set procedure. *American Journal of Occupational Therapy, 37,* 457-461.

Peloquin, S. M. (1988). Linking purpose to procedure during interactions with patients. *American Journal of Occupational Therapy, 42,* 775-781.

Selye, H. (1980). *Stress without distress.* New York: Lippincott.

Simon, S. B., Howe, L. W., & Kirschenbaum, H. (1978). *Values clarification: A handbook of practical strategies for teachers and students.* New York: A and W Visual Library.

Woolfolk, R. L., & Richardson, F. C. (1978). *Stress, sanity and survival.* New York: New American Library.

Chapter 49

The Day Center and its Role as a Social Network

Harriet Woodside, MA, OTR

When chronic mentally disabled persons move into supervised care settings in the community after living in a large mental hospital for two, ten, or 20 years, they usually arrive without any social links to their new home or neighborhood. If they are fortunate, they may find an old friend from their ward in the residence who can introduce them to some of the other boarders and point out the local doughnut shop. If they are especially fortunate, they will attend a day program, or they may have a conscientious case manager to help them establish new roots.

However, the deinstitutionalized often move from a ward where they had some social life and involvement in occupational and recreational programs to a new home chosen because it had a vacant bed or was in the same catchment area as the hospital they were leaving. Accustomed to having all activity occur under one roof in a highly controlled way, many of the deinstitutionalized seem to hover in the community as though waiting for something to happen.

If no comprehensive social networks are organized by members of the community or staff at the residence, it becomes the concern of the mental health professional to assist the chronic mentally disabled living in the community to find and maintain social links. While the need for social contacts for the chronic mentally disabled has often been identified, concrete descriptions of programs addressing this need are not plentiful.

I will begin by discussing the chronic psychiatric patient's need for social networks. I will then describe the Fennell Program Day Center that provides a social network for its clients.

The Importance of Friends and Family

Test and Stein (1) list the following as characteristics of the chronic psychiatric patient:

- A high vulnerability to stress
- Deficiencies in coping skills such as budgeting, using public transportation, and preparing meals
- Dependency so extreme that they perceive them-

This chapter was previously published in *Hospital and Community Psychiatry, 36*, 177-180. Copyright © 1985, the American Psychiatric Association. Reprinted by permission.

selves as helpless and requiring massive support from people and/or institutions in order to survive

- Difficulty in working in competitive jobs
- Difficulty in managing interpersonal relationships, especially close ones.

These characteristics may be the result of the disease process, the result of lasting incapacities that remain after an acute episode, the result of the process known as "institutionalization," or an intertwining of several factors. If we take these characteristics into account, it seems that most chronic psychiatric patients do not have the ability to seek social contact with others. Yet North American investigators have found that the social network is an important indicator of outcome (2), even though it is very difficult for the disabled person to maintain (3, 4).

Cross-cultural studies supply evidence that the nature and form of the social network is important to the health of the chronic mentally disabled. One major cross-cultural study has shown better outcomes for individuals with schizophrenia in developing countries, compared with outcomes in developed countries (5). In interpreting these findings, Mosher and Keith (6) point out that extended kinship networks and natural support systems protect schizophrenic patients from stress. The importance of social support systems in relieving stress for schizophrenic patients is also emphasized by other authors (7, 8).

Because the close and caring social network of communal villages like those in Nigeria or Laos does not exist in North America, our chronic mentally disabled require some substitute that will mediate their anxiety while helping them to maintain coping skills. Support for this premise comes from Linn and her associates (9), who compared ten day treatment centers. They found some to be more effective than others in reducing the symptomatology of schizophrenic patients, in changing some attitudes about the hospital, and in delaying relapse. Centers that focused on counseling their patients were less successful than those offering occupational therapy and recreational activities. Linn and her associates suggest that a nonthreatening environment offering activities rather than insight-oriented therapy is an effective model for management of the chronic schizophrenic patient. These findings imply that low-stress group programs that include tasks for the participants will meet the needs of the deinstitutionalized chronic population.

The Fennell Program Day Center

In the fall of 1980 another occupational therapist and I began planning a program for deinstitutionalized clients from the two chronic care wards (known as the Fennell Program) of Hamilton Psychiatric Hospital in Hamilton, Ontario. The day center is part of the Fennell Program community team that provides case management and program planning for 100 discharged patients.

The original goals of the day center were to improve the quality of the clients' lives, to regularly monitor their behavior, and to offer structure and support to help them maintain their present status. We did not focus on the program's potential for building and maintaining a social network.

Our clients are between 26 and 77 years of age; they have been hospitalized from two to 40 years. Of the 23 people we currently see, 12 are men and 11 are women; 19 are outpatients.

Of these outpatients, 11 have a diagnosis of schizophrenia and four have a schizoaffective disorder. The remaining four have various diagnoses, each reflecting a chronic psychiatric condition. Eighteen live in supervised board-and-care residences; one lives at home.

Their relationships with other people are generally unilateral. For example, while patients receive support and encouragement from residence staff, they rarely help each other. They constantly request cigarettes from fellow outpatients, but, because their financial resources are limited, they seldom reciprocate.

All but three have very little contact with their family. Five report friendships with other ex-patients, but only one reports having regular contact with friends who are not ex-patients or residents of the board-and-care home. Some report casual relationships with storekeepers and others in the immediate community, and all see a case manager on a regular basis. For many, the day center is the only regular activity in which they engage outside of their residence.

The day center is open two days a week from 9:30 a.m. to 3:00 p.m. It is housed in the Sunday school rooms of a centrally located church. Clients come either one or two days. The program varies greatly, and much of it is planned by the entire group.

The overall objective of the program is to provide activities that will interest the participants, although we do not expect any one activity to interest everyone. Activities include five-pin and lawn bowling, maintaining a large vegetable garden in the summer, indoor gardening in the winter, collating and stapling newsletters and information packages for community groups free of charge, cooking, and participating in birthday parties, holiday events, calisthenics, folk dancing, and simple crafts sessions. (The crafts are usually sold to add to the group's funds.) The clients also sing, watch movies rented from the local library, and take trips to places of interest in the community.

Most visitors to the day center are struck by its warm, concerned atmosphere. One client started calling the day center "the club" and thus characterized it as a place that provides a sense of belonging, interest, and friendship. There is a good deal of joking and teasing among clients and staff; unusual behavior is generally treated in an appropriate way.

This atmosphere developed slowly. It is undoubtedly strengthened by case managers who continually encourage their clients to attend. The two occupational therapists serve as role models, clearly showing concern for their clients (for example, by telephoning absent clients) and appreciation of clients' talents. As with any group, the more verbal members are helpful in stimulating and maintaining conversation and establishing a spirit of optimism. Those who have been at the day center for a while serve as role models for newcomers.

Although the church was selected for its location, facilities, and willingness to house the day center, several members of the congregation and staff have quite naturally befriended our clients. The caretaker, ministers, secretary, and some members of the congregation now chat with our clients and request their help around the church. We feel that in a small way true community integration is taking place; its natural development and reciprocity have done much to boost the self-esteem of our clients.

From the start we set the goal of maintaining, rather than rehabilitating, our clients. The entire program reflects that decision. We keep pressure and stress at a level we know the clients can tolerate and rarely insist that people participate. Instead, we try to offer a variety of activities so that all of the clients will be able to complete successfully and enjoy at least one activity.

Consequently we have not seen major improvement in skills and abilities. However, we have seen dramatic changes in our clients' level of socialization and in their desire to come to the center. It is as though we have touched their innate need to form interpersonal relationships and to give and receive meaning from others.

Discussion

When faced with the problem of creating programs that will take into account the characteristics of the chronic mentally disabled as well as the effects that their illness and long periods of hospitalization have had on them, health professionals may vacillate between despairing and attempting to design the most comprehensive and sophisticated program yet devised.

Even when we planned what we thought were low-level, and therefore possible, goals, we underestimated our clients' degree of disability. The first thing we learned was to lower our expectations to match extremely limited skill levels, poor or erratic motivation, lack of self-esteem, difficulty in expressing ideas, and years of accumulated hurts from hospital experiences and family and community rejection.

Once we gave up grand plans and focused on understanding our clients, treating them with respect and dignity, and finding projects that they could accomplish successfully and that were familiar to them, the group began running itself. It became cohesive and positive in outlook. As though soothed by gentleness and concern, clients slowly began to try new activities and to help each other. For instance, members who feared public transportation began taking the public bus to the center. Other clients attempted a new craft or volunteered when an extra partner was needed for folk dancing. These changes occurred only after a client had developed a sense of trust and a genuine liking for the day center.

Thus it is possible for chronic mental patients to function in social networks that are open and reciprocal. Each member is capable of giving as well as of receiving. The silent, most isolated members of our center are often among the first to offer part of their lunch to someone who has forgotten to bring one. In turn, the more outgoing clients acknowledge such isolation and make a point of noticing and praising a new shirt or blouse worn by a withdrawn member.

However, while the social networks of our clients have expanded, they are still largely limited to mental health professionals and ex-patients. This finding is not necessarily negative or surprising, since all individuals are generally most comfortable in the company of people with whom they share experiences and interests.

Mosher and Keith (6) note that community support systems "are intended to provide the support that has been lost because of the dissolution of extended kinship networks or discharge from hospital." It is possible to view our day center as a surrogate extended family for some clients. The staff members become parents or family leaders, and the sharing of meals and housekeeping duties adds a note of domesticity to the environment. As in a family, reciprocal roles develop that involve relating to others and carrying out activities. For example, some clients regularly perform chores or run errands without being asked. Others have become the members who provide humor, tenderness, or advice.

As has been described, the social network at the day center is slowly extending into the church and urban community. Church members who have known some of the clients for more than two years often remark that they are more outgoing and that they look happier. Through our volunteer work of collating and stuffing envelopes, we have friends at the arts council, the women's center, and other local agencies, and occasionally clients will mention that they have passed a familiar face on the street.

Thus the developing social network has had a ripple effect on many areas of our clients' lives. They now have a definable role, that of "group member," which encom-

---

passes volunteer, companion to others, and participant in sports or crafts. This role provides a needed stability and focus for each client. With the concomitant improvement in self-esteem, this role also enables clients to cope with stress more successfully. At the same time the protective nature of the group shields clients from stress.

Conclusion

From its start, the day center was led by mental health professionals backed up by a competent team of case managers. Although the literature reflects hopes that communities will offer programs to integrate and occupy discharged chronic psychiatric patients, such programs cannot be established without professional help. Our clients are still symptomatic, and they have frequent crises requiring professional support. The development of an efficacious program demands a knowledge of the clients' disease process, the ability to assess their strengths and weaknesses, and a suitable and flexible response to their needs. It also demands reconsideration of what constitutes success; we have found that success may be best measured by voluntary attendance rather than by actual participation. We hope that as the community becomes better educated and more sensitized, it will respond to the chronic mentally ill as the church did, accepting them without making many demands. However, we cannot expect the community to provide programs for them without some informed leadership.

Turner and Shifren (10) feel that a manufactured social system will create supportive relationships for the chronic mentally disabled who live in the community. Our experience indicates that such a system initially should be a protected and protective one. Once a client participates willingly, other goals, such as improving one's quality of life or becoming involved in community activities, will be more attainable. Although the security of a safe place and people who care may not improve the behavior of some clients, it does appear to cushion life's stresses and give meaning to daily existence.

References

1. Test MA, Stein LL: Community treatment of the chronic patient: research overview. Schizophrenia Bulletin 4:350-364, 1978

2. Strauss JC, Carpenter WT Jr: Predictors of outcome in schizophrenia, III: five-year outcome and its predictors. Archives of General Psychiatry 34:159-163, 1977

3. Lipton FR, Cohen CI, Fischer E, et al: Schizophrenia: a network crisis. Schizophrenia Bulletin 7:144-151, 1981

4. Pattison EM, Pattison ML: Analysis of a schizophrenic psychosocial network. Schizophrenia Bulletin 7:135-143, 1981

5. Sartorius N, Jablensky A, Shapiro R: Cross-cultural differences in the short-term prognosis of schizophrenic psychoses. Schizophrenia Bulletin 4:102-113, 1978

6. Mosher IR, Keith SJ: Psychosocial treatment: individual, group, family, and community support approaches. Schizophrenia Bulletin 6:10-41, 1980

7. Solomon K: Societal structure and prognosis. Schizophrenia Bulletin 4:314-315, 1978

8. Westermeyer J, Pattison EM: Social networks and mental illness in a peasant society. Schizophrenia Bulletin 7:125-134, 1981

9. Linn MW, Caffey EM, Klett CJ, et al: Day treatment and psychotropic drugs in the aftercare of schizophrenic patients: a Veterans Administration cooperative study. Archives of General Psychiatry 36:1055-1066, 1979

10. Turner JEC, Shifren I: Community support systems: how comprehensive? New Directions for Mental Health Services, no 2:1-13, 1979

Chapter 50

Helping Families Cope With Alzheimer's Disease

J. Paul Teusink, MD
Susan Mahler, MSW, ACSW

This chapter was previously published in *Hospital and Community Psychiatry*, *35*, 152-156. Copyright © 1984, the American Psychiatric Association. Reprinted by permission.

Alzheimer's disease is the most common of a number of diseases known as dementia. Since most medical authorities and the public do not distinguish between the presenile onset and the senile onset of this primary degenerative dementia, and refer to the majority of Alzheimer patients as one group, we shall do the same in this paper.

According to several studies cited by Wells (1), Alzheimer's disease accounts for approximately 51 percent of dementia cases, vascular disease (multiinfarct dementia) for approximately 10 percent, a combination of Alzheimer's disease and vascular disease for 8 percent, normal pressure hydrocephalus for 6 percent, alcoholism for 6 percent, and multiple other causes for less than 20 percent.

More than three million Americans are affected to some degree by Alzheimer's disease, and more than one million, or 5 percent, of the elderly over age 64 are severely affected by it (2). All mental health professionals who work with elderly patients, in general hospitals or clinics, but particularly in long-term care facilities, are frequently involved with Alzheimer patients.

Dementias are unique diseases, not only because they are not curable, but because they cause a progressive impairment of memory and orientation with generalized deterioration in intellectual functioning and eventually in physical health. Roth and Myers' definition of dementia (3) stresses the progressive failure of the patient in the activities of everyday life, the failure of memory and intellect, and the disorganization of the personality. A patient's intellectual impairment may lead to emotional changes, to deterioration in self-care, and even to delusions and hallucinations.

The tremendous burden that dementia patients create for their caretakers is therefore magnified because these patients are, in a sense, intellectually dying. In addition, many of the caretakers of Alzheimer patients are members of what has been called "the sandwich generation"—middle-aged adults whose relief at having just finished caring for their own children is shattered by the new responsibility of caring for their aging parents. It is therefore no surprise that families have strong, and often varied, reactions to the development of Alzheimer's disease in family members.

Despite the variability in family reactions that we have seen in our work with Alzheimer patients at New

York Hospital—Cornell Medical Center, we have found that the reactions of families coping with the disease may be similar to the reactions of families coping with death. Thus although the reactions of family members may seem abnormal at times, they may actually be normal steps in a process of coming to terms with this overwhelming illness.

In this paper, we will characterize what we have seen to be a normal series of responses to Alzheimer's disease, consisting of initial denial that there is anything wrong, followed by overinvolvement of the family with the patient in an attempt to compensate for the illness, anger when the compensation fails, guilt that is created by the anger, and, finally, resolution or acceptance of the problem. It is not difficult to note the similarity of the process we will describe to the mourning process described by Kübler-Ross (4), which also consists of five stages: denial and isolation, anger, bargaining, depression, and acceptance.

Because Alzheimer's disease requires such an enormous adjustment by families and because any one of the stages of acceptance can become abnormal or problematic if it is not worked through, we will provide some guidelines for working with the family members of Alzheimer patients as they go through the reaction process. We will provide a case example to illustrate how one family member went through the five stages of the process and how staff were able to help him. Finally, we will discuss some of the specific problems that the individual in the case example faced, and that many other families face, when coping with Alzheimer's disease.

The Reaction Process

Stage One—Denial

Family members will often first notice memory losses in the patient, but may explain these away by saying that they're "just senility." Although this reaction might partially be explained by the family's lack of education about aging, it may also represent a wish on the part of family members to deny what they are seeing. Some memory loss with aging is common, but when memory loss exceeds mild forgetfulness, it is a sign of abnormal cognitive functioning secondary to dementia or some other physical or metabolic disease.

Some denial may be a normal reaction to memory loss and forgetfulness, but we have seen many families who were able to carry this reaction to a remarkable extreme. At times families even fail to recognize grossly disturbed behavior and marked deterioration in memory and cognitive functioning. Their denial in this case may be aided by the common finding that recent memory fails with age while remote memory remains somewhat well preserved. Thus the family may focus on the still well-functioning remote memory and ignore the patient's inability to keep track of recent time or events.

Denial may be a way of defending against the pain of loss and the family disruption that results from illness; it may also allow the family to postpone dealing with their grief. In that case denial can make realistic assessment, decision making, and treatment planning impossible. Families that exhibit excessive denial must be helped, through education and at times through confrontation, to recognize the extent of the disability of their family member. Only then can they make realistic plans for treatment and move on to an acceptance of their loved one's illness.

Stage Two—Overinvolvement

As the deterioration of the sick family member becomes more obvious to the family, family members may become more involved with the patient in an effort to compensate for his or her losses. This may involve a realistic adjustment, such as taking over the family's financial responsibilities. When involvement with the patient's needs is carried to an exaggerated degree, however, family members may sacrifice many aspects of their personal lives, such as their social relationships, their freedom to come and go, and even their sleep. Although these families recognize that there is a problem, they may not seek help from the medical profession or other agencies; out of intense loyalty to their loved one, they feel they must deal with the illness themselves.

Certain aspects of overinvolvement seem to be culturally motivated. Our experience has shown us that in some very close Italian and Jewish families, for example, sons or daughters are raised to believe that they must care for their parents without regard to their own needs. If they do not do so, they fear they will be ridiculed by the community. Eventually, overinvolved family members may react in anger to feeling unable to shoulder the tremendous burden of caring for an Alzheimer's patient.

To deal with overinvolvement and to arrange for appropriate care, the treating professionals must be able to differentiate between a pathological reaction and a normal reaction within each family and its cultural group. The relatives can then be helped to see their overinvolvement as a hindrance rather than a help in realistically dealing with the patient's problem. One helpful approach is to confront the relatives with the specific difficulties that their overinvolvement is creating for the patient and for the rest of the family.

Stage Three—Anger

Anger among family members develops not only as a

reaction to the added physical burden of caring for a demented person and to the embarrassment caused by the frequent behavioral problems presented by that person; it also results from the feeling of having been abandoned by the still-living but now afunctional parent or spouse.

When anger predominates within a family, it is often projected or displaced onto the very people who are trying to help the family deal with their overwhelming sense of helplessness—the mental health professionals. If the professionals do not help the family to actively confront their anger and to realize that they are displacing their own painful feelings about the situation, family members may become so dissatisfied that they remove the patient from treatment or accuse staff of neglecting the patient and therefore causing the deterioration that naturally occurs with this illness. Countertransference issues in staff must be similarly addressed, since the normal reaction to being accused of neglect is defensiveness or anger, either of which will further alienate the relatives.

Stage Four—Guilt

As anger lessens, guilt may become more obvious. Some feelings of guilt among family members may be a normal reaction to recognizing feelings of anger or wishes that the demented patient would die. Family members may feel guilty for many other reasons, such as feeling that they delayed in bringing in the patient for evaluation and thus may have contributed to the illness, feeling that they were not attentive enough to their parent or spouse earlier in their lives, for unexpressed anger from past times and events, or for needing to make decisions objected to by the patient.

Mental health professionals must deal with the family members' guilt by discovering its cause and by taking corrective steps to alleviate it. One step can be simply to educate the family about the illness itself, thereby providing reassurance that the family has not harmed the patient. More extensive counseling may be needed to help the family make difficult but necessary decisions, some of which may be objected to by the patient.

Stage Five—Acceptance

Acceptance comes only after relatives have understood the disease process that is affecting their loved one, have found sufficient resources within themselves and the community to deal with the increased burden of care for the patient, have worked through their anger and guilt, and have recognized that their loved one is no longer the person they once knew. Acceptance is made more difficult by the disease's insidious onset and often long progressive course, as well as by the patient's relative preservation of normal physical vigor and appearance during the early stages of the illness.

Case Examples

Mrs. K, a profoundly demented 76-year-old Jewish widow, was transferred from a long-term-care facility to the Cornell Medical Center for an evaluation of agitated behavior including constant pacing, verbal abusiveness, and at times combativeness. Although Mrs. K had had symptoms of Alzheimer's disease for approximately one and a half years, she had worked in her family's garment manufacturing business until one year before her transfer to the center.

In the transfer summary, the nursing home complained of difficulty with the patient's 50-year-old son, who was running his mother's business. During the initial phase of his mother's hospitalization in our facility, Mr. K was unable to accept his mother's progressive deterioration and was insistent that certain signs, such as intact long-term memory, were proof that she was less impaired than he had been told. He believed that his mother's wandering stemmed from her boredom at not having work to do and from the lack of staff initiative in engaging her in activity.

Mr. K visited his mother nightly and brought her dress patterns to cut. When she was unable to perform the tasks he expected of her, he displaced his disappointment and anger onto the nursing staff in a hostile, abusive, and accusatory fashion, thus engendering staff defensiveness and resistance to empathizing with his pain. Mr. K was critical of all aspects of his mother's treatment and expected the hospital to find a miracle cure for her illness.

Engaging Mr. K in family therapy was difficult since he saw both the doctor and social worker (JPT and SM) as his adversaries. He was seen in weekly sessions, where he was encouraged to talk about his frustration at our inability to make his mother well. At the same time, we educated him about Alzheimer's disease—its manifestations, course, and treatment.

Mr. K eventually revealed his concerns that the illness was hereditary or contagious and his feelings of helplessness in caring for his mother. He had attempted to have her live with his family before placing her in a nursing home, but he and the family were unable to control her wandering and disruption of family life.

As Mr. K began to discuss his family history and his feelings about his mother, it became clear that he had a conflict-ridden, ambivalent relationship with her. Mrs. K had worked long hours in the family's business since Mr. K was a young child and had left his care to an older sibling. Mr. K had felt neglected and abandoned, and had developed angry feelings toward his mother. Having to put his mother into a nursing home reawakened these repressed feelings of anger and abandonment, and aroused concerns that he was now abandoning her. He was still unable to see his mother as anything other than the strong, capable, working woman he had known in the past, and although he was capable of running the family business, he was experiencing self-doubts. In addition, he was furious at his sibling, who lived out of town and was not involved with his mother's care.

Mr. K's reminiscences about his mother helped him to realize the source of his angry feelings and he became less critical of the staff. His lessened anger enabled him to understand the symptoms of Alzheimer's disease, to more realistically assess his mother's illness, and to mourn her loss.

When Mrs. K was discharged from our facility, we talked with the social worker in the long-term-care facility where Mrs. K would return, so that we could apprise her of Mr. K's conflicts and encourage her to provide him with continued support.

Specific Problems in Reaching Acceptance

Many of Mr. K's reactions resulted from his attempts to cope with some specific problems that arise when families must face the onset of Alzheimer's disease in a family member. By recognizing the likelihood that these problems will occur and by providing supportive guidance, mental health professionals can help ease families through the reaction process.

Role Reversal

One of the most difficult adjustments that a family member must make is to assume the patient's former family role when he or she is no longer able to function as in the past. Frequently the family member must become a parent to his or her own parent, and that adjustment can be particularly difficult when the previously dependent child must make decisions for the previously more dominant parent. The adjustment can be equally difficult when a previously dependent spouse assumes the role of the more dominant spouse.

It is important for staff to help the responsible relatives of Alzheimer's patients see that a reversal in roles is occurring and to help them accept the necessary change in their concept of themselves and their loved one. By helping relatives to express their fear, anger, and disappointment, and by showing them that there is someone who is sharing their burden, staff can help relatives be more accepting of the necessary reversal in roles.

Reactivated Interpersonal Problems

As seen in our case example, long-standing interpersonal problems between the patient and relative may be reawakened when the relative is forced to assume more responsibility and become more involved with the deteriorating patient. A son or daughter may even move to another part of the country to avoid dealing with their demanding, unsatisfied parent and with any problems that may have resurfaced.

When it becomes obvious that an immediate relative does not want to be involved with the patient, the helping professional must decide if he or she can change the relative's mind without causing further alienation. Frequently, counseling to help resolve the reactivated problems or even family therapy with the demented patient, although unlikely to improve the patient's condition, may be necessary to keep the alienated relative involved. In other cases, the professional must firmly insist that the relative has a responsibility to participate in the evaluation and disposition planning, although this approach is not always successful.

Lack of Understanding about the Illness

Most relatives of Alzheimer's patients know little or nothing about this common disease. It is unlike any other disease they have encountered. To make decisions about the patient's future, they may need considerable education about their loved one's symptoms and the progression of the illness. The doctor may need to meet with the relatives personally to reassure them that the patient does not have other illnesses that could explain his symptoms. They must be educated regarding what resources are available for the care of the patient. They may need to be encouraged to seek legal advice or to take legal responsibility for the patient should they have to make decisions that the patient opposes.

Fears about Heredity

Many family members fear that heredity may be involved in the dementia of their parent and may either directly or indirectly inquire about whether they too will be afflicted by such an illness. They may talk about their own failing memory and need reassurance and education about normal memory loss with aging and dementia. Education can therefore play an important role in working with families' reactions to this disease. For example, it may be reassuring for a family member to know that although there is a fourfold increase in dementia among first-degree relatives of Alzheimer's patients, Alzheimer's disease is still a relatively uncommon disorder. Thus a relative's chances of developing Alzheimer's disease may be increased from only 1 percent in the general population to 3.8 percent (5).

Shopping for Cures

Relatives of patients with dementia are understandably gullible about treatment promises made by unscrupulous persons or even well-meaning physicians. These persons may suggest, among other treatments, nutritional supplements, medications such as vitamins and vasodilators, and physical therapy and physical stimulation programs. Although some of these treatments may be helpful in preventing deterioration, they will also not cure dementia.

Again, families must be educated about Alzheimer's disease so that they will not develop unrealistic hopes that some new treatment will cure the dementia. Fad therapies are usually more harmful than beneficial. Improved therapies may be found in the future, but they will be the result of careful and laborious research.

Discussion

Unlike many other illnesses, Alzheimer's disease is a progressive illness. Families of Alzheimer patients must therefore endure an ongoing grief process, and they may need ongoing intervention and support to cope with the illness. Many authors (6-9) have shown that education and support can be effectively provided through relatives' discussion and support groups.

The stages of the reaction process discussed in this paper need to be recognized and addressed by mental health professionals. Although every family will cope with Alzheimer's disease in its own way, there are several common experiences and problems that most families must deal with and work through so that they can mourn their loved one, make necessary decisions for his or her care, and reestablish family equilibrium.

Mental health professionals should make the assessment of family reactions to Alzheimer's disease an important part of any thorough case evaluation (10), and family members must be helped to recognize and deal with their reactions. Until they do so, until they have been educated about the disease and know what to expect, and until they are reassured that the mental health professionals understand their needs, they will not be able to realistically plan for the care of, and make decisions for, their afflicted relative.

References

1. Wells CE: Chronic brain disease: an overview. American Journal of Psychiatry 135:1-12, 1978

2. Katzman R: The prevalence and malignancy of Alzheimer disease. Archives of Neurology 33:217-218, 1976

3. Roth M, Myers OH: The diagnosis of dementia, in Contemporary Psychiatry, no. 9. Edited by Silverstone T, Barraclough B. Ashford, Kent, England, Headley Brothers, 1975

4. Kübler-Ross E: On Death and Dying. New York, Macmillan, 1969

5. Jarrik LF: Genetic factors and chromosomal aberrations in Alzheimer's disease, senile dementia, and related disorders, in Aging, vol 7. Edited by Katzman R, Terry RD, Bick KL. New York, Raven Press, 1978

6. Hayter J: Helping families of patients with Alzheimer's disease. Journal of Gerontological Nursing 8:81-86, 1982

7. Barnes RF, Raskind MA, Scott M, et al: Problems of families caring for Alzheimer patients: use of a support group. Journal of the American Geriatrics Society 29:80-85, 1981

8. Lazarus LW, Stafford B, Cooper K, et al: A pilot study of an Alzheimer patient's relatives discussion group. Gerontologist 21:353-358, 1981

9. LaVorgna D: Group treatment for wives of patients with Alzheimer's disease. Social Work in Health Care 5:219-221, 1979

10. Farkas SW: Impact of chronic illness on the patient's spouse. Health and Social Work 5:39-46, 1980

Section VI

Program Evaluation: The Assurance of Quality in Clinical Practice

Introduction

The past few sections of this text have included numerous descriptions of well-designed, effective treatment programs. These programs are distinguished by their solid plans based on strong theoretical foundations. However, one cannot assume that a program will automatically maintain its excellence, no matter how good the initial developmental process. Patient populations change, goals are met (or unmet), and new needs arise. To respond proactively to these changes, the therapist must view program evaluation as an essential component of program development. As Grossman and Bortone emphasize in their chapter on program development in section two, program evaluation is the last stage in the program development cycle.

Program evaluation ensures that patients are receiving the highest quality of professional services. This assurance of quality of care is essential in today's health care system. Increased demands for accountability and cost-effectiveness, the growth of the consumer movement, and the rise of competition within the health care market all require the occupational therapist to become fluent and skilled in program evaluation principles and methods (AOTA, 1991; Joe, 1985; Shaw, 1985; Wilkerson, 1991). By evaluating treatment efficacy, occupational therapists can modify and adjust their programs, as needed, to increase the effectiveness and relevance of their interventions (Shaw, 1985; Wilkerson, 1991). The accumulation of treatment efficacy data can also be utilized to market model programs, obtain increased funding, expand program services, recruit and employ additional staff, maintain program accreditation, and increase staff pride and patient morale successfully (Hoffman-Grotting & Ralph, 1991; Shaw, 1985; Wilkerson, 1991).

Everyone strives to be connected with a "success."

Occupational therapy programs, with their holistic functional approach, are frequently successful in their treatment outcomes. Consequently, the professional image of occupational therapy can be greatly enhanced by program evaluation studies. Providing meaningful quality care to patient populations is an achievement occupational therapists can proudly (and frequently) report. The acquisition of program evaluation skills will empower occupational therapists with the knowledge and competence to do their jobs better and to demonstrate this enhanced effectiveness to consumers, administrative bodies, and regulatory agencies.

One of the major program evaluation approaches utilized in today's health care system is quality assurance. In chapters 51 and 52, Zusman and Joe review the historical development of quality assurance. Pertinent program evaluation terms are defined, and fundamental principles of quality assurance are described. Practical issues and clinical realities that influence the implementation of program evaluation activities in mental health practice are explored. Both authors advocate an increase in professional knowledge of program evaluation principles and techniques and support active professional involvement in quality assurance studies.

The role of the occupational therapist in program evaluation is examined further in chapter 53, by Stoffel and Cunningham. These authors present the continuous quality improvement (CQI) approach to evaluating and improving the quality of patient care in mental health. The relevance of the CQI approach to current trends in mental health practice is explored. CQI concepts and principles are described, with relevant clinical examples provided to illustrate the application of CQI to current occupational therapy practice. Suggestions and references for the implementation of CQI are provided. According to the authors, the utilization of this consumer-oriented, interdisciplinary, systems approach to program evaluation will result in substantial benefits for treatment settings, patient populations, and the profession of occupational therapy.

The significance of occupational therapy program evaluation is also highlighted in chapter 54, by Thien. In her presentation, Thien reviews three methods commonly utilized to demonstrate the effectiveness of occupational therapy treatment. She describes a treatment efficacy study conducted by an occupational therapy department and presents two data analysis methods employed in this research. While this study does have its limitations, the benefits from documenting measurable patient improvements are notable. Most significant is the concomitant increase in staff interest in documentation, program development, and program evaluation.

The ability of program evaluation studies to trigger renewed interest and enthusiasm among professional staff is clearly a worthwhile "side effect" of this process. While many will initiate program evaluation studies solely to meet administrative requirements and accreditation standards, they will often be pleasantly surprised by the energizing momentum that arises from their efforts. Documenting the efficacy of their treatment can empower therapists to challenge themselves to be their professional best. The resulting increase in quality of care and improved patient outcome can enhance professional image, decrease stagnation, and prevent burnout. Readers are urged to utilize these chapters and the references provided to develop their program evaluation skills and to ensure quality of care in their provision of occupational therapy services.

Questions to Consider

1. How do current health care issues and trends impact occupational therapy program evaluation? What effect may cost-containment and accountability demands have on program evaluation?

2. What are the areas of occupational therapy treatment most relevant for program evaluation studies? What can the occupational therapist uniquely offer to interdisciplinary program evaluations? How can the occupational therapist maximize a collaborative, client-centered approach to program evaluation?

3. How can the outcomes of program evaluations be utilized to benefit the patient? The treatment setting? The occupational therapy profession? What are the marketing implications of program evaluations?

4. Imagine you have recently been hired as the director of a community day treatment program for persons with chronic mental illness. The program's primary goal is to develop community living skills through the provision of case management and therapeutic activity groups. The program's patient population totals 35; however, daily attendance averages between 8 and 12 clients. Your clinical staff includes a Certified Occupational Therapy Assistant (COTA), a nurse, and a mental health aide. You are designing your program evaluation plan: What approach will you utilize? What will be your evaluation focus and methodology? What are potential implications of your study for program development?

References

American Occupational Therapy Association (1991). *Quality assurance in occupational therapy: A practitioner's guide to setting up a QA system using three models.* Rockville, MD: Author.

Hoffman-Grotting, K., & Ralph, V. J. (1991). Enhancing the program's image and performance by comparing and using quality assurance and program evaluation information. *Occupational Therapy in Practice, 2*(2), 16-25.

Joe, B. (1985). Quality assurance. In J. Bair & M. Gray (Eds.), *The occupational therapy manager* (pp. 252-265). Rockville, MD: American Occupational Therapy Association.

Shaw, K. J. (1985). Program evaluation. In J. Bair & M. Gray (Eds.), *The occupational therapy manager* (pp. 235-249). Rockville, MD: American Occupational Therapy Association.

Wilkerson, D. L. (1991). Program and outcome evaluation: Opportunity for the 1990s. *Occupational Therapy Practice, 2*(2), 1-15.

Chapter 51

Quality Assurance in Mental Health Care

Jack Zusman, MD

Quality assurance is the general term for a burgeoning field of health care operations that monitor the quality of health care services, including mental health services. Every facility accredited by the Joint Commission on Accreditation of Healthcare Organizations must have a significant quality assurance operation. A number of federal and many state health care financing programs require participating facilities to maintain a quality assurance program.

In many facilities, quality assurance activities encompass the related fields of utilization review, which focuses on the manner in which resources are used, and risk management, which attempts to limit institutional liability. Peer review of health care, in which independent third parties monitor the quality of medical services, usually to determine whether they should be reimbursed, is considered by many to be part of quality assurance. Quality assurance activities also overlap considerably with those of medical staff services, whose central activity is to make decisions related to medical staff credentials and privileges.

New professional organizations and new classes of professionals have evolved to perform all of these functions. Many mental health professionals and most psychiatrists now interact in a variety of ways with quality assurance specialists. Yet relatively few seem to be aware of the definitions, processes, and problems of quality assurance or the direction in which it is moving. This paper reviews some of the more important aspects of quality assurance activities in relation to mental health services.

Early Development

Quality assurance was probably first introduced to modern health care through the work of Ernest Codman early in the 20th century (1). Concerned about the varying treatment provided by different hospitals, Codman devised a method of measuring hospitals by their results. In 1913 his approach was incorporated into the objectives of the newly established American College of Surgeons.

The "minimum standard," as the college's criteria came to be known, laid out in just a few hundred words the facilities and services required for hospitals to provide high-quality care. The standard became the foundation of the college's hospital accreditation program, which was subsumed in 1951 after many years of successful operation by the newly formed Joint Commission on Accreditation of Hospitals, now the Joint Commission on Accreditation of Healthcare Organizations.

In the 1970s concerns about increasing malpractice liability stimulated interest in quality assurance. It was assumed that the increase in medical malpractice lawsuits and the increasingly larger claims awarded must have been due to poor quality care. Stringent quality assurance was regarded as the most obvious preventive measure. (Of course, studies have made it clear that the liability crisis is not due mainly to a decrease in the quality of care; therefore, intensive quality assurance efforts may reduce the liability crisis but will certainly not resolve it.)

In 1972, hoping to control the massive costs of the Medicaid and Medicare programs, Congress passed legislation authorizing the establishment of professional standards review organizations (PSROs) to conduct utilization reviews of federally financed hospital treatment. The PSROs, later modified and renamed peer review organizations, set guidelines for the hospitals and monitored their internal utilization review programs.

Peer review became the term or catchword for a whole new approach to case review. In the past quality of care had been monitored through traditional, informal clinicopathologic conferences about individual cases or mortality review. In contrast, the new peer review system consisted of rapid screening of large numbers of cases by nonphysician reviewers or even screening by computer using predetermined criteria. Clinical peer review methodology has now spread far beyond its original application in utilization review and is used in all of the quality-assurance-related areas.

Quality Assurance in Mental Health Care

The development of quality assurance programs has been slower in the mental health field than in the medical field. In 1951 the American Psychiatric Association published an extensive list of standards for psychiatric hospitals (2), which presumably represented professional consensus about the characteristics considered necessary for the provision of high-quality care. It was not until 1969, however, that the first discussion of the application of quality assurance to mental health issues and services appeared in the literature. In it, Zusman and Ross (3) articulated some proposals for the development of quality assurance in mental health based on a three-year analysis of quality assurance efforts in general medical care.

In 1970 the Joint Commission developed accreditation standards specifically for psychiatric facilities, substance abuse programs, and community mental health programs. The successors to these first standards are now contained in the *Consolidated Standards Manual* (CSM) (4), which, except for a few differences, resembles the better-known *Accreditation Manual for Hospitals*, which contains standards for acute hospitals (5). (The Joint Commission recently decided to use the *Accreditation Manual for Hospitals* rather than the *Consolidated Standards Manual* to evaluate acute care psychiatric hospitals. Other mental health facilities will continue to be evaluated using the consolidated manual.)

Peer review programs developed in the late 1960s and early 1970s by the American Psychiatric Association and the American Psychological Association to evaluate psychiatric care provided under the Civilian Health and Medical Program of the Uniformed Services, or CHAMPUS, have had a major impact on peer review and quality assurance in mental health (6,7). CHAMPUS, which provides medical benefits to military dependents, instituted coverage for psychiatric care in 1966.

Further accelerating the progress of quality assurance in mental health care were federal laws enacted in 1975 and 1980 requiring community mental health centers to conduct program evaluation (8). Though the activities mandated under the laws are program evaluation and not quality assurance, they were closely related to quality assurance and piqued interest in the organization of quality assurance programs and useful techniques for conducting quality assurance activities. (Program evaluation has a much longer and far more complex history than quality assurance and will not be discussed further here.)

Fundamental Principles

Though many aspects of the quality assurance process can be carried out in an objective manner, quality assurance is fundamentally subjective. Unlike the concentration of sodium in the blood or the size of a patient group, quality has no inherent, physical characteristics.

Quality is a socially defined value, and the desirability of any treatment practice is determined by consensus. Those who monitor quality, whether health care professionals themselves or those they designate to speak for them, reach a mutual agreement about how good or bad care will be recognized and measured. They are free to change their minds or even redefine quality without violating any laws of nature or scientific principles. For example, even the conviction that the preservation of life is an element of good medical care is changing. Some have questioned whether life is necessarily a positive medical outcome in the context of extreme disability or permanent absence of consciousness.

Though quality is subjective, the quality assurance field has succeeded in developing very elaborate procedures that organize the decision-making process and reduce random variations, biases, and uncertainties. The field has widely adopted the three-part evaluation process proposed by Donabedian (9) addressing structure, process, and outcome.

Evaluation of structure involves examining whether the institution possesses the tools presumed by authorities to be necessary to provide care. These tools include adequate technical equipment, space, and record keeping. The presence of these tools is assumed to be associated with high-quality care, or, perhaps more accurately, their absence is assumed to make it impossible to provide high-quality care. Evaluation of process involves examining how the tools are used. For example, records are reviewed to determine whether appropriate medications were provided for various syndromes or whether psychological tests were interpreted correctly. Again, proper use of the tools is assumed to be associated with high-quality care.

Outcome evaluation is the most direct measure of the quality of care, since a good outcome is considered indicative of good care. This assumption may not be without exceptions, however, since a poor outcome does not necessarily mean care was poor.

Each of these three approaches has serious inherent problems. While common sense would argue that procedures done with the right tools and in the right manner will result in predictable outcomes, the reality may not bear out that assumption. Indeed, one study found that outcome did not correlate with the use of proper tools and procedures (10).

Measuring outcome is associated with a different set of problems, particularly in the field of mental health, as it is very difficult to measure psychiatric outcome objectively. Differing outcomes may reflect the nature of the patient and the illness as much as they do the care provided. In addition, mental illnesses are commonly intermittent and produce variable effects, even when they are untreated, making it difficult to associate outcome at any one time with the effectiveness of a particular treatment. Regardless of these drawbacks, outcome is considered "the gold standard" in the evaluation of health care. Even measures of structure or process are evaluated in relation to outcome.

Practical Application

An institution's first step in developing a quality assurance program is to prepare a plan describing what it hopes to achieve, how it will organize its quality assurance effort, and how it proposes to define quality. It should also list the specific standards and criteria it will use to measure quality, called indicators and criteria by the Joint Commission, or at least describe how it plans to establish them. The plan should also include procedures for providing feedback to the staff about the quality assurance review or for following up problems. The Joint Commission has identified seven key characteristics of quality assurance programs and nine steps that can be used by any service to set up a quality assurance system (11).

In hospitals, responsibility for operating the quality assurance program rests with the medical staff. In non-hospital facilities the professional staff is responsible. Usually the work of the system is carried out by a staff committee, often called the quality assurance committee. The committee commonly assigns day-to-day work to one or more support staff provided by the facility. The principal member of the support staff is frequently given the title of quality assurance coordinator. In large facilities the work may be subdivided, with each department or clinical area having its own quality assurance subcommittee and perhaps its own support staff. These subcommittees report to the overall quality assurance committee.

The quality assurance committee prepares the institution's quality assurance plan. It establishes the criteria the support staff will use to screen out cases that are likely to have problems. Cases that "drop out" of the screening process or incidents that are so problematic that they must be reviewed every time they occur, such as inhospital suicides, are presented to the quality assurance committee for peer review. In many cases the peer reviewers will decided that treatment was adequate and the review process will end. Others will require further investigation. The committee has the responsibility to ask clinicians involved in those cases to explain the questionable aspects of care.

The quality assurance committee reports to the medical or professional staff either directly or through an executive committee. Their report serves two purposes: it recommends what action is necessary to address lapses in care, and it educates all staff members to the quality assurance issues and needs of the facility. Particularly because of their educational function, the work of the quality assurance committee and their reports deserve to have a prominent place among staff activities. Unless quality assurance is a concern of all the professionals participating in providing care, rather than an unpleasant process reluctantly accepted to achieve accreditation or licensure, it cannot be effective.

All quality assurance activities and reports must be documented in order to verify the quality assurance process for accrediting and licensing bodies and, perhaps more important, to facilitate follow-up of problem cases and practitioners.

Quality assurance is a continuous process in which all patients or problems are eligible for scrutiny. At one time the Joint Commission required that hospitals audit only a particular number of cases, a practice that restricted quality assurance efforts. Currently the Joint Commission emphasizes the need to continuously carry out the procedures necessary to upgrade care.

Utilization review and risk management are frequently associated with the quality assurance process, for several reasons. The screening and review processes used in all three areas are very similar. In some institutions, the same support staff conduct the first-level screening in all three areas.

Utilization review focuses on the manner in which the institution's resources are used in treatment. The primary concern of utilization review is ensuring that resources are not wasted and, to a lesser extent, that they are adequate. Of course, since it is difficult to provide high-quality care with inadequate resources and since by some definitions of quality waste of resources is synonymous with poor-quality care, there is a close theoretical link between utilization review and quality assurance.

Risk management focuses on protecting the institution from legal liability or financial losses associated with negligence lawsuits. Risk management activities generally consist of a system in which staff report incidents that lead or could have led to patient injury or institutional liability and do not usually involve formal screening of all cases. Nevertheless, review of these cases often provides important information for improving care.

Another major facet of quality assurance is credentialing and privileging, since one way to ensure high-quality care is to permit only professionally competent individuals to provide care. Credentialing is usually conducted by a committee of the medical or the professional staff, commonly called the credentials committee, which determines whether an individual meets the requirement for staff membership based on the individual's education, training, licensure, clinical experience, and other factors.

The privileging process involves determining the procedures the institution is equipped to offer, establishing the training and experience necessary to perform each procedure, and evaluating each staff member's competence to conduct the procedures. The procedures that individual staff members are authorized to perform are compiled into a list of privileges. The quality assurance process directly influences credentialing and privileging by generating statistics and case reviews that should help to determine who gets what privileges.

Unlike the field of surgery, which can easily list and monitor distinct procedures, the mental health field has had difficulty specifying staff privileges in a meaningful way. For example, the essential elements of the various psychotherapies are hard to describe objectively, and questions about the kind of training and quantity of training necessary to provide a particular therapy remain unsettled. Furthermore, the means of preventing unprivileged professionals from performing a particular form of therapy are also unclear. A recent report from the American Psychiatric Association suggesting an approach to providing privileges in psychiatric units holds some promise for resolving these difficult issues (12).

Practical Problems

Perhaps the most basic problem with quality assurance efforts is the lack of evidence that they actually improve quality. Of course, there is overwhelming consensus that quality assurance activities do improve care. Like many other aspects of mental health care, and general medical care, its value remains unproved, but few if any individuals would wish to eliminate the process. In any case, no one seems to have demonstrated objectively that patients are any better off in an institution with a quality assurance program than they would be in an institution without one. One study implied that quality assurance did not improve the quality of care (13).

The lack of studies evaluating the effectiveness of quality assurance activities means no quality assurance model or approach is clearly better than any of the others. Quality assurance professionals, who depend on data in their everyday work, are in the strange position of having to depend on consensus or personal preference in selecting approaches to monitor the quality of care.

A second problem with quality assurance efforts involves difficulties in determining a threshold of quality, the minimal acceptable level of quality below which it becomes necessary to take action to bring about improvement. Experience suggests that each institution's threshold level is determined by a host of factors, including the consensus of professionals in the community, the auspices and orientation of the facility, the extent of the resources of the facility, and even the social backgrounds of the patients. Research on these determinants is a critically important but neglected area.

A third problem with the practice of quality assurance is the reluctance of professionals to take action against colleagues who do not appear to be practicing within an acceptable standard. In part their reticence may be traced to a recognition that the quality assurance process and the quality standards are not objective or necessarily reliable. The decision to jeopardize, or possibly even end, someone's career is difficult to make when it is not based on firm criteria.

Another reason for the reluctance to report colleagues, however, seems to relate to the desire to preserve social relationships. This desire makes professionals unwilling to recognize that a close co-worker and possibly a friend is not performing acceptably and must be penalized, or to risk incurring the hostility of one's small group of colleagues as a result of taking action against one of its members.

A final practical problem in quality assurance encountered very frequently is the failure of quality assurance leaders and administrators to distinguish between the professional quality assurance process and general across-the-board quality measures. Across-the-board measures focus on all of the products and activities of the institution, including the professional ones. These measures, which resemble industrial quality control factors, involve, for example, the temperature of the food served to patients, the timeliness of chart completion, the timeliness of billing, the cleanliness of the floors, and the time patients spend waiting for x-rays.

All of these aspects of institutional performance are important to monitor and attempt to improve, but they are not the items on which professional staff quality assurance committees should spend their expensive and very limited time. Professional quality assurance must focus on the quality and appropriateness of clinical care and on issues related to professional judgment, not on the many routine processes an institution carries out.

Finding More Information

Surprisingly, there are few books and practical articles about quality assurance and even fewer about quality assurance in mental health. Nevertheless enough publications are available to place the beginner in the field on the right track. The Joint Commission publishes a number of pamphlets on quality assurance (14). It also offers brief training courses and educational audiotapes and videotapes (15). Thus it probably offers the most comprehensive and practical material available.

A number of other documents provide examples of quality assurance plans along with a small amount of explanatory text (16,17). Several commercially published monographs have been devoted to quality assurance, but they tend to be more theoretical than practical and tend not to focus on mental health (18, 19). An exception is a new book by Stricker and Rodriguez (20). The literature on industrial quality control is fairly broad and old but is of limited use to the health care professional because of its technical complexities (21).

Conclusions

Quality assurance is a field that can only grow larger and more important as third-party payers, government, and national organizations become more involved in control of medical care. Every health care professional ought to have some exposure to the concepts and practice of quality assurance. Every health care profession should involve some of its practitioners in quality assurance efforts, both to represent the unique point of view of the quality assurance field and to interpret the quality assurance field to the profession. Finally, every professional's education should include training in the principles of quality assurance.

References

1. Roberts J, Coale JG, Redman RR: A history of the Joint Commission on Accreditation of Hospitals. JAMA 258:936-940, 1987

2. Standards for Hospitals and Clinics. Washington, DC, American Psychiatric Association, 1951

3. Zusman J, Ross E: Evaluation of the quality of mental health services. Archives of General Psychiatry 20:352-357, 1969

4. Consolidated Standards Manual/87. Chicago, Joint Commission on Accreditation of Hospitals, 1986

5. Accreditation Manual for Hospitals/88. Chicago, Joint Commission on Accreditation of Hospitals, 1987

6. Shepherd G: A brief history of the American Psychiatric Association's involvement in peer review, in Psychiatric Peer Review: Prelude & Promise. Edited by Hamilton J. Washington, DC, American Psychiatric Press, 1985

7. Claiborn W, Biskin B, Friedman L: CHAMPUS and quality assurance. Professional Psychology 13:40-49, 1982

8. Mattson M: Quality assurance: a literature review of a changing field. Hospital and Community Psychiatry 35:605-616, 1984

9. Donabedian A: Explorations in Quality Assessment and Monitoring, vol 1: The Definition of Quality and Approaches to its Assessment. Ann Arbor, Mich, Health Administration Press, 1980, p 79

10. Brook R, Appel F: Quality of care assessment: choosing a method for peer review. New England Journal of Medicine 288:1323-1329, 1973

11. Joint Commission on Accreditation of Hospitals: Monitoring and evaluation of the quality and appropriateness of care: a hospital example. Quality Review Bulletin 12:326-330, 1986

12. Task Force on Medical Staff Bylaws: Credentials and Privileges for Psychiatrists in Hospital-Based Services. Washington, DC, American Psychiatric Association, 1986

13. Repp A, Barton L: Naturalistic observations of institutionalized retarded persons: a comparison of licensure decisions and behavioral observations. Journal of Applied Behavior Analysis 13:333-341, 1980

14. Publications Catalog. Chicago, Joint Commission on Accreditation of Hospitals, 1987

15. Education Programs, 1988 Annual Calendar. Chicago, Joint Commission on Accreditation of Hospitals, 1987

16. Guide to Quality Assurance. Washington, DC, National Association of Private Psychiatric Hospitals, 1987

17. Quality Assurance in a Psychiatric Setting. Portland, Ore, Brown-Spath and Associates, 1987

18. Williamson J, Hudson J, Nevins M: Principles of Quality Assurance and Cost Containment in Health Care: A Guide for Medical Students, Residents, and Other Health Professionals. San Francisco, Jossey-Bass, 1982

19. Meisenheimer G: Quality Assurance: A Complete Guide to Effective Programs. Rockville, Md, Aspen, 1985

20. Stricker G, Rodriguez AR: Handbook of Quality Assurance in Mental Health. New York, Plenum, 1988

21. Groocock J: The Chain of Quality: Market Dominance Through Product Superiority. New York, Wiley, 1986

Chapter 52

Quality Assurance

Barbara E. Joe, MA

Program evaluation is a critical step in occupational therapy service delivery. It is often implemented after assessment and treatment of a group of patients/clients so that data about the effectiveness and efficiency of occupational therapy with a specific population can be determined. This chapter discusses one approach to program evaluation—quality assurance.

As demands for accountability have grown, quality assurance has come into its own as a necessary and recognized component of health care. Yet because it is a relatively recent addition to the health care lexicon, many occupational therapy personnel—clinicians and students alike—lack a clear understanding of its role and importance in the health care system. *Peer review, patient care evaluation, audit, outcome assessment, health accounting*—all of these increasingly familiar terms are encompassed under the more general rubric of *general assurance*.

Quality assurance lies at the heart of the basic purpose of health care. That purpose, generally stated, is to improve human well-being, function, and longevity. The existence of, or the desire to avoid, a health problem (as defined by society and by patients/clients) is what leads patients/clients to seek care. Quality assurance is a system of enhancing the benefits that are the *raison d'etre* of intervention. People would not submit to treatment or pay its costs, even indirectly, unless they expected benefits. How health care achieves and increases these benefits is what quality assurance is all about.

Quality assurance is a problem-solving system. It is like the system used with individual patients/clients, but it applies to aggregates of patients/clients with similar diagnoses and characteristics. Quality assurance asks and answers questions such as the following: Is the care being provided to a given group of patients/clients having the expected or desired effect? If so, to what extent? If not, what changes are likely to produce the intended outcomes? Are these changes feasible? Is this an area in which expenditures of effort and resources are apt to produce considerable improvement, or might these be better directed to some other, more fruitful area? If a plan for improvement has been implemented, has it actually been successful?

All the basic elements of quality assurance are implied in the above questions:

This chapter was previously published in S. C. Robertson (Ed.), *Mental health focus: Skills for assessment and treatment* (pp. 1-178—1-185). Rockville, MD: The American Occupational Therapy Association, Inc. (AOTA). Copyright © 1988, AOTA.

1. Identification of a problem through an apparent failure to achieve a standard of quality based on the desired or expected outcomes of the care provided.
2. Verification of the problem through measurements showing that desired outcomes are not being achieved.
3. Formulation of a plan to achieve such outcomes that is both feasible and cost-effective.
4. Implementation of the plan for improvement.
5. Measurement to determine if the problem has been solved (i.e., if the standard of quality has been met).

This process, with its emphasis of measurement, provides checks at two critical junctures. First, there is initial measurement to make sure the problem identified actually exists. This may seem obvious, yet such initial measurement often shows that the standard is already being achieved. Therefore, there is no problem after all. Second, when a problem has been verified, a measurement is made *after* the intended improvement to make sure the problem has actually been solved. Unless this final step is included, it may be blithely assumed that a new procedure has taken care of the problem when actual measurement would reveal this not to be so. In such cases the improvement action must be reformulated, or, in rare instances, the standard itself must be revaluated to make sure it is achievable.

Historical Perspectives and Present Regulations

Early Pioneers

Before the elements of quality assurance are explored in greater depth, it is instructive to look at how a concern with health care quality evolved, from a set of implicit and unquestioned beliefs in the value of health care, to the explicit, formal, and objective system called quality assurance.

Throughout history and in much of the world today, folk remedies have predominated, and only the wealthy have enjoyed the privilege of medical treatment. Even among the latter, probably few questioned whether the treatment they were receiving actually worked.

Society has come a long way from the days when healers had magical status and absolute authority, yet the patient's/client's trust in the practitioner contributes to health improvement. Although health care today remains art as well as science, science has been in the ascendancy ever since the sixteenth century, when Harvey, Willis, and other prominent physicians shocked their contemporaries by dissecting the human body to discover its workings firsthand.

In the 1860s, Florence Nightingale (Huxley, 1975) observed and reported on the deficiencies of health care services provided to those wounded in the war. The first person to collect and compare mortality statistics from different hospitals, she saw the death rate in military hospitals during the Crimean War plunge from 42 percent to 2.2 percent (p. 117). Her efforts were continued by Abraham Flexner, a physician whose 1910 report on the poor quality of medical education (Flexner, 1910) was instrumental in closing 60 of 155 U.S. medical schools then in existence. Another key pioneer was E. A. Codman, who in 1912 initiated "end-result" assessment to improve hospital care (Codman, 1914).

On November 15, 1912, The Third Clinical Congress of Surgeons of North America put forth a resolution that was both prophetic and revolutionary: "Some system of standardization of hospital equipment and hospital work should be developed, to the end that those institutions [that] have the highest ideals may have proper recognition before the profession, and those of inferior equipment and standards should be stimulated to raise the quality of their work" (as quoted in Davis, 1960, p. 476). Several years later, the American College of Surgeons initiated the process of hospital accreditation. Of 692 hospitals covered in their first survey, only 90 (12.9 percent) were approved (Graham, 1982).

Quality Assurance Requirements of the Joint Commission on Accreditation of Hospitals

The Joint Commission on Accreditation of Hospitals (JCAH) was established in 1951. Most states now mandate JCAH accreditation for licensure, and most third-party and government payers require it for reimbursement.

The quality assurance program of JCAH has been evolving over the years. In 1955, JCAH first began to stress the importance of medical audits. By 1974, hospitals were required to audit medical records and make quarterly reports. In 1981, judging that the audit system was producing good medical records but not necessarily better care, JCAH began urging the introduction of additional monitors (measures of important outcomes of patient/client care) and a focus on problem resolution.

The JCAH has included the following elements in its guidelines for quality assurance plans: problem identification, priority setting, problem assessment, problem resolution, and problem-monitoring follow-up (Joint Commission on Accreditation of Hospitals, 1980). Also included are concerns about how the quality assurance plan is developed and carried out, such as designating responsibility, assuring representation of all disciplines involved in patient care, and establishing quality assurance reporting procedures (Joint Commission on Accreditation of Hospitals, 1980).

Quality assurance, according to the most recent JCAH policy statements, is concerned with monitoring and evaluating the quality and appropriateness of patient care. Quality assurance covers all clinical activities, using continuous monitors or indicators selected according to criteria identified in the literature or by experts and professional associations. Data sources can include patient records, as in the audit days, but should go beyond them. JCAH gives the following examples of data sources for monitoring quality assurance: medical records, incidence reports, laboratory reports, generic screening, patient bills, staff surveys, patient surveys, direct observation, and credentialing reports. The most essential monitors should be selected first, such as those dealing with life and death. Monitors may be continually added, and those no longer needed may be discarded. Quality assurance monitors in health care must have a direct impact on patient care; thus, administrative concerns are excluded unless such an impact can be demonstrated.

In addition to measuring important aspects of patient care, monitors must be comprehensive in scope, ongoing, and continuous, according to JCAH. Routine, systematic monitoring initially identifies problems and subsequently verifies that remedies continue to be effective. In sum, quality assurance monitors must be important, routine, and comprehensive, and must directly affect patient care. Dealing with discrete problems no longer satisfies JCAH's quality assurance standards. However, when the monitoring process picks up a problem, if appropriate, it may be dealt with separately by a special quality assurance study (Roberts & Walczak, 1984; Joint Commission on Accreditation of Hospitals, 1984).

Designing a quality assurance monitor requires designation of the activity, its objectives, measurable criteria, data sources, frequency of monitoring, and responsibility for monitoring and reporting. Specific reporting intervals are not mandates by JCAH, but must be appropriate to the situation.

In occupational therapy, monitors could assess whether or not treatment goals are being met. Cost and efficiency concerns such as promptness, frequency, and length of treatments could be included, as long as they were also related to treatment outcomes. Standards could be established for such variables as functional ability at discharge, or discharge dispositions for various diagnoses, or groups of patients. Failure to achieve the standards would signal the need for improvement. These standards have implications not only for patient/client well-being, but for cost, with higher function and discharge to home likely to be related to cost savings.

Peer Review

In 1965 the federal government began requiring JCAH accreditation for hospitals participating in Medicare. It initiated another formal check on health care quality in 1972 with the establishment of professional standards review organizations (PSROs). These were groups of locally organized physicians and other health care representatives authorized to perform a continuous form of peer, nonbureaucratic, grass roots review of the quality of care being provided to Medicare patients/clients. Organized medicine initially opposed PSROs as an infringement on professional prerogatives. However, many physicians eventually swung behind the program, which was designed to improve care, correct deficiencies, and contain costs.

Professional standards review organizations were an innovative idea intended both to protect patients/clients and to assure that federally financed care was appropriate in quality and cost. Proponents estimated savings beyond the program's cost of $144 million per year (Kurtz, 1981). However, opponents disputed these claims and characterized PSROs as a costly and complicated layer of bureaucracy.

Eventually, cost pressures led to the Peer Review Improvement Act of 1982, a reformulation of peer review that called for the replacing of PSROs by peer review organizations (PROs). According to federal regulations, each state was required before the end of 1984 to designate a single PRO to act on its behalf in monitoring the quality of care for Medicare beneficiaries under a two-year contract with the federal Health Care Financing Administration (HCFA). The law gave preference in designing PROs to physician-sponsored organizations. Other professions, including occupational therapy personnel, can volunteer to serve on state PRO advisory boards.

Peer review organizations' quality objectives must be expressed in numerical or percentage terms. They include reduction of unnecessary surgery, patient/client deaths, inappropriate admissions, and readmissions due to prior substandard care.

It is too soon to evaluate the specific contributions of PROs. However, a comment about PSRO from quality assurance theoretician Avedis Donabedian (1982) may also pertain to PROs: "In time, the records of the PSROs may create historical archives into which the antiquary of quality assessment may wish, mole-like, to burrow" (p. 375).

Other Quality Assurance Mechanisms

Some commentators include credentialing, licensure, and practice standards or protocols under quality assurance because the aim of these measures is to assure or improve the quality of care. In addition, program evaluation, the system used by the Commission on Accreditation of Rehabilitation Facilities (CARF) is sometimes considered a tool or a method of quality assurance (Michnich, Shortell, & Richardson, 1983).

In practice, quality assurance and program evaluation are sometimes merged. Some occupational therapy departments use program evaluation as their monitoring system for identifying quality assurance problems, and a number of rehabilitation programs have both program evaluation and quality assurance programs in place.

States may require either JCAH or CARF accreditation for rehabilitation programs, and sometimes both. States may also have their own requirements related to quality of care, usually adapted from the standards and procedures of these two accrediting bodies.

Definitions and Distinctions

Measuring Quality

According to quality assurance expert John W. Williamson (1982), health care "demands a continual objective appraisal of outcomes so as to seek and achieve the highest benefit consistent with the patient's needs within constraints set by society and current health care technology. This continual reassessment of the outcomes of one's performance (that is, quality assurance) is an indispensable and integral part of providing care" (p. 275). Failing to take time for quality assurance, Williamson (1982) maintains, "is equivalent to a pilot's being too busy flying the plane to have time to check his compass to see where he is in relation to where he wants to be" (p. 275).

The term *quality* ultimately rests not on objective facts but, as Williamson (1982) indicates, on values, the values of health care practitioners, patients/clients, and society. Sometimes there is agreement on these values, such as the value of a life saved or a death postponed. Sometimes there is a disagreement, such as whether abortion is a desirable medical procedure. In other cases, values about the continuance of life conflict with values about its quality. Does the maintenance of physical life through extraordinary measures take precedence over maintaining a "meaningful" life, and how is the latter defined?

In quality assurance, determinations such as these must be made by a broad spectrum of professionals, along with patient/client representatives. There should be a fairly high consensus on what constitutes quality and therefore on what constitutes a problem, because lack of agreement, by definition, puts the existence of a problem in doubt and undermines solution.

However, once standards of quality are established—such as what percentage of stroke patients can be expected to improve one level in activities of daily living after a given number of treatments—measurement of how well these standards are being achieved can be fairly

objective, a matter of numbers and statistical sampling. Although quality assurance measures are objective, "subjective" feelings of well-being and satisfaction—whether expressed by patients/clients or staff—can be surveyed (for example, through questionnaires). Quality assurance makes certain that quality, once defined, is measured, improved, and then maintained.

The term *quality assurance*, with its implication of promises for the future, is perhaps more accurately rendered as *quality confirmation*. This is because the judgment that patient/client outcomes actually meet standards of quality can only be made after measurement of the results of a particular health care intervention.

Cost-Effectiveness as a Component of Quality

Usually a distinction is made between health benefits and costs, the latter referring to the individual's or society's sacrifice in providing such benefits. Quality assurance attempts to blend these sometimes antagonistic themes into a single formulation, transforming Bentham's "greatest good for the greatest number" into "the best care at the least cost." According to the Institute of Medicine, quality assurance is a system "to make health care more effective in improving the health status and satisfaction of a population within the resources which society and the individual have chosen to spend for that care." (National Academy of Sciences, 1976).

The cost component is not something new in quality assurance; it has always been part of the quality equation. However, it is now receiving renewed emphasis and is an explicit concern. As Donabedian (1982) has expressed it, "Quality consists in a precise matching of services to needs, without excess or deficit" (p. 116). He contends that "the net benefit to health must exceed the monetary cost incurred in obtaining that benefit. Unfortunately, our estimates of the benefits, harm, and cost of care are often very imprecise" (p. 5). Donabedian (1982) goes on to argue that "the schemes of management used in actual practice may embody more efficient strategies than those incorporated in norms that presuppose almost unlimited resources" (p. 139), and that even when "attention to cost may lower the standards of care below the optimal...one could argue that the new standards merely represent an attempt to optimize the attainment of a broader set of social objectives" (p. 204).

Williamson (1982), the father of a problem-oriented approach to quality assurance, defines quality assurance in terms of both effectiveness and efficiency, thereby recognizing "that quality assurance encompasses both the traditional concept of quality (that is, a high degree of effectiveness in providing care) and cost-containment (that is, an efficient use of resources)" (p. xvii).

Williamson (Ostrow, Williamson, & Joe, 1983) also

distinguishes between *efficacy*, which is the benefits of health care intervention under ideal or experimental conditions, *effectiveness*, which refers to health care benefits under the ordinary circumstances of clinical practice, and *efficiency*, which means the extent to which health care benefits are achieved with a minimum of unnecessary expenditure and effort.

Relation to Research

Although quality assurance relies on research in setting standards and borrows some of its measurement techniques, quality assurance is not research. As a practical matter, most clinicians are not able to set up controlled trials, to control variables, to collect data on sufficient numbers for valid research, or to draw conclusions applicable beyond their own organization. However, as part of their regular clinical duties, they are able to conduct quality assurance that has no control groups as such, though patients/clients measured *before* and *after* an improvement action do function as a type of control for themselves.

This does not make quality assurance just a poor cousin of research. The basic difference between quality assurance and research is one of purpose, not of technique. Research shows *what* happens, whereas quality assurance is concerned with *making* a particular thing happen. In very crude terms, research shows what is possible, and quality assurance applies research findings in actual clinical situations.

For example, research shows that early occupational therapy intervention results in earlier hospital discharge and greater functional improvement for stroke patients (Garraway, Akhtar, & Prescott, 1980; Smith, Garraway, & Smith, 1982). A hospital desiring to achieve earlier discharge and better functional gains for stroke patients initiates early occupational therapy services, then determines whether it has actually achieved the results research has shown to be possible. Even in the absence of research data, quality assurance can show measurable improvement in meeting preestablished standards in a given setting and can also point the way to areas for further research.

Criteria, Norms, Standards, and Outcomes

It is easy to become entangled in a semantic tie-up over the distinction between *criteria*, *norms*, and *standards*. The 1974 PSRO *Program Manual* (American Medical Association, 1974) defines *medical care criteria* as predetermined elements of care developed by professionals, based on professional expertise and the literature, which in turn define quality care. *Norms* are numerical or statistical measures of usual or observed performance, that is, statements of what is actually occurring apart from any evaluation of quality. *Standards* are professionally developed expressions of the permissible range of variation from either criteria or norms (American Medical Association, 1974). Therefore, standards, like criteria, carry a quality or value component, whereas norms are merely statements of averages.

C. M. Jacobs (1976), commenting on JCAH's Performance Evaluation Procedure (PEP), defines a criterion as an element of care of major consequence and a standard as a percentage that attaches to each criterion. In a recent book Donabedian (1982) skirts the issue of distinguishing between standards and criteria, but seems to favor concentration on criteria, reserving the term *standard* for a broader measure, based on percentage or numerical measurement, of a cluster of criteria. Along these lines, quality assurance theoretician Nancy Graham (1982) defines criteria as the important elements of health care being measured and monitored, with standards being numerical or percentage expressions of the acceptable level or range of criteria expression. Thus, among quality assurance experts criteria seem to be items that define the broader standards, which are expressed in percentage terms.

Donabedian (1982) goes on to point out that "criteria sets can be distinguished by whether they consist primarily of elements of structure, process, or outcome" (p. 90). Observing that the lines between these three types of criteria are fuzzy and sometimes arbitrary, Williamson (1978) has attempted to clarify matters, at least between process and outcome standards or criteria, by defining outcomes broadly as "any characteristics of patients, health problems, providers, or their interaction in the care process that results from care provided or required, as measured at one point in time" (p. 26).

Overcoming Obstacles to Quality Assurance

There has been resistance to quality assurance on several grounds. One has been the fear of malpractice suits or, conversely, the fear of lawsuits from colleagues judged to be providing substandard care (Fifer, 1983). Other significant barriers have been health professionals' expectations of autonomy (Rosenberg, 1975), habitual and established systems of behavior and interaction, psychological inflexibility, investment in current procedures, the financial impact of change, and entrenched official policies (Luke & Boss, 1981).

Rachelle Kaye, who calls quality assurance "a strategy for planned change," observes that there are three stages in the change process: unfreezing of current attitudes and behaviors, change, and "refreezing" (Kaye, 1983, p. 157). The latter represents a new equilibrium. However, in quality assurance, as in life, this equilibrium is only temporary. Solution of one problem leads to discovery of another, and the process of change goes on.

An example from occupational therapy bears this out. A quality assurance study identified, measured, and then solved the problem of occupational therapists failing to respond to referrals within twenty-four hours. Once the standard response time had been routinely achieved, a new problem was discovered and tackled through quality assurance: initial evaluations being given patients/clients within the specified time limit were not always complete; that is, standards for quality evaluations were not being met.

Quality assurance, therefore, like health care itself, is evolving. Occupational therapy personnel are continually adding to the course of development and to the body of knowledge and practice in this vital area.

Summary

Quality assurance is an expression of the new demand for accountability and cost containment in health care. It offers a method for solving either treatment or cost problems for aggregates of patients/clients with similar diagnoses and characteristics. There are five basic elements in quality assurance:

1. Identification of a problem through an apparent failure to achieve a standard of quality based on the desired or expected outcomes of the care provided.
2. Verification of the problem through measurements showing that desired outcomes are not being achieved.
3. Formulation of a plan to achieve such outcomes that is both feasible and cost-effective.
4. Implementation of the plan for improvement.
5. Measurement to determine if the problem has been solved.

The quality assurance program of the JCAH has been evolving over the years. According to the most recent JCAH policy statements, quality assurance is concerned with monitoring and evaluating the quality and appropriateness of patient care. Data sources used in monitoring can include patient records, incident reports, laboratory reports, generic screening, patient bills, staff surveys, patient surveys, direct observation, and credentialing reports. Designing a quality assurance monitor requires designation of the activity, its objectives, measurable criteria, data sources, frequency of monitoring, and responsibility for monitoring and reporting.

Monitors must have a direct impact on patient care. They must also be comprehensive in scope, ongoing, and continuous. Dealing with discrete problems no longer satisfies JCAH's quality assurance standards. However, when the monitoring process picks up a problem, it may be dealt with separately by a special quality assurance study.

Quality assurance attempts to blend the sometimes antagonistic themes of health benefits and low costs into a single formulation, "the best care at the least cost." Unlike research, which shows what happens, quality assurance is concerned with making a particular thing happen. There are many established methods of quality assurance. A given health care situation might be most appropriately measured by one method, whereas another aspect of care might best be measured by a different method. Many of the approaches are not sufficient in themselves for full-scale quality assurance activities, but are effective as problem-solving tools within a broader plan.

There has been resistance to quality assurance on several grounds: fear of lawsuits, health professionals' expectations of autonomy, habitual and established systems of behavior and interaction, psychological inflexibility, investment in current procedures, the financial impact of change, and entrenched official policies.

References

American Medical Association. (1974, March 17). *PSRO program manual.* (Chap. 7). Chicago, IL: Author.

Codman, E. A. (1914). The product of a hospital. *Surgery, Gynecology, and Obstetrics.*

Davis, L. (1960). *Fellowship of surgeons. A history of the American College of Surgeons.* Springfield, IL: Charles C. Thomas Publisher.

Donabedian, A. (1982). *Explorations in quality assessment and monitoring, vol. 2. The criteria and standards of quality.* Ann Arbor, MI: Health Administration Press.

Fifer, W. (1983). Integrating quality assurance mechanisms. In R. D. Luke, J. C. Krueger, & R. E. Modrow (Eds.), *Organization and change in health care quality assurance* (pp. 217-230). Rockville, MD: Aspen Systems Corp.

Flexner, A. (1910). *Medical education in the United States and Canada.* New York: Carnegie Foundation, Merrymount Press.

Garraway, W. M., Akhtar, A. J., Prescott, R. J., et al. (1980). Management of acute stroke in the elderly: Preliminary results of a controlled trial. *British Medical Journal,* April 12, 1040-1043.

Graham, N. (1982). Criteria development. In N. Graham (Ed.), *Quality assurance in hospitals* (pp. 43-53). Rockville, MD: Aspen Systems Corp.

Graham, N. (1982). Historical perspective and regulations. In N. Graham (Ed.), *Quality assurance in hospitals.* Rockville, MD: Aspen Systems Corp.

Huxley, E. (1975). *Florence Nightingale.* (p. 117). New York: Putnam.

Jacobs, C. M., Christoffel, T. H., & Dixon, N. (1976). *Measuring the quality of patient care. The rationale for outcome audit.* Cambridge, MA: Ballinger Publishing Co.

Joint Commission on Accreditation of Hospitals. (1980). *The QA guide.* (pp. 177-181). Chicago, IL: Author.

Joint Commission on Accreditation of Hospitals. (1984). *Accreditation manual for hospitals.* Chicago, IL: Author.

Kaye, R. (1983). Quality assurance: A strategy for planned change. In R. D. Luke, J. C. Krueger, & R. E. Modrow (Eds.), *Organization and change in health care quality assurance* (pp. 157-169). Rockville, MD: Aspen Systems Corp.

Kurtz, H. (1981, November 5). Three medical study units in area lose funds. *The Washington Post.*

Luke, R. D., & Boss, R. W., (1981). Barriers limiting the implementation of quality assurance programs. *Health Science Research, 16,* 305-314.

Michnich, M. E., Shortell, S. M., & Richardson, W. C. (1983). Program evaluation resource for decision making. In R. D. Luke, J. C. Krueger, & R. E. Modrow (Eds.), *Organization and change in health care quality assurance* (pp. 263-279). Rockville, MD: Aspen Systems Corp.

National Academy of Sciences, Institute of Medicine. (1976). *Assessing quality in health care: An evaluation.* Washington, DC: Author.

Ostrow, P. C., Williamson, J. W., & Joe, B. E. (1983). *Quality assurance primer.* Rockville, MD: American Occupational Therapy Association.

Roberts, J. S., & Walczak, R. M. (1984). Toward effective quality assurance: The evaluation and current status of JCAH QA standard. *Quality Review Bulletin, 10*(1), 11-15.

Rosenberg, E. W. (1975). What kind of criteria? *Medical Care, 13,* 966-975.

Smith, M. E., Garraway, W. M., Smith, D. L., et al. (1982). Therapy impact on functional outcome in a controlled trial of stroke rehabilitation. *Archives of Physical Medicine and Rehabilitation, 63,* 21-24.

Williamson, J. W. (1978). *Assessing and improving health care outcomes: The health accounting approach to quality assurance.* Cambridge, MA: Ballinger Publishing Co.

Williamson, J. W., Barr, D. M., Fee, E., et al. (1982). *Teaching quality assurance and cost containment in health care.* San Francisco, CA: Jossey-Bass Publishers.

Chapter 53

Continuous Quality Improvement: An Innovative Approach Applied to Mental Health Programs in Occupational Therapy

Virginia Carroll Stoffel, MS, OTR
Susan M. Cunningham, MS, OTR

A value intrinsic to health care professionals is the desire to influence improvement in patients. For occupational therapists, the guiding objective that propels our day-to-day activities is facilitating optimal patient functioning. Yet how do we really know that we have, indeed, contributed to improvement in function? Frequently, we only hope that we have used appropriate treatment techniques and, consequently, that we will see visible results in the patient's behavior. If we have used the appropriate treatment techniques correctly and have obtained the desired result, then we may subjectively feel confident in our ability to provide quality patient care. In many mental health settings, however, we still do not have a systematic means by which to focus our review of patient care, to collect meaningful data, to determine how we can improve occupational therapy mental health services, and, consequently, to improve patient outcomes.

The issues of professional accountability and making determinations about effectiveness have been germane to all health care professionals. The need for a formal process to review and evaluate the quality of patient care provided was an important issue for the American College of Surgeons in 1917. At that time, the minimum standard was established for review of medical staff performance in hospitals. The minimum standard contained the first formal requirements for the review and evaluation of the quality of patient care for physicians.[1] Since that time there has been a proliferation of standards through organizations such as the Joint Commission on Accreditation of Healthcare Organizations (Joint Commission). Mechanisms for evaluating the quality and appropriateness of care have evolved from retrospective audits to the hospital-wide, systematic, problem-focused monitoring and evaluation approach to quality assurance. Occupational therapists, particularly those working in hospital-based settings, should be familiar with the current quality assurance mechanisms for evaluating processes and outcomes of care.

This article describes a practical approach to evaluating and improving the quality of patient care in mental health occupational therapy programs. Clinical examples are provided for clear illustration of the continuous quality improvement (CQI) process. We suggest that each and every registered occupational therapist and certified occupational therapy assistant be actively involved for the CQI process to be effective under the direction of a supportive, facilitative supervisor or director. When such activities become an integral part of the daily activities of each occupational therapy staff member, CQI will become a reality.

CQI, as developed by Deming[2,3] and Juran,[4,5] may be seen as the evolving approach to quality monitoring in health care in the 1990s. This approach espouses development of a system to measure, direct, and improve the quality of services on a continuous basis. Such an approach can be used by occupational therapists in all settings. In mental health settings, occupational therapists may find CQI to be a particularly helpful process. Frequently, the mental health environment is not conducive to clear articulation of the occupational therapist's role and to demonstration of the outcome of occupational therapy services to consumers and other professionals because of the various functions performed by the occupational therapist and the other mental health professionals. Because CQI is formulated on an interdisciplinary systems approach to the quality of care, the contributions of all professionals working in the system are examined to identify opportunities for improved patient outcomes. As the CQI approach takes hold throughout the health care industry, the occupational therapist in mental health will probably spend less time trying to explain his or her rationale for treatment and more time demonstrating contributions through group problem-solving techniques and other improvement approaches inherent in CQI.

Trends in Mental Health Occupational Therapy Practice

In the 1990s the role of occupational therapy personnel working in mental health settings is in a state of flux. Numerous concerns have been reported in the literature. Bonder[6] and Kielhofner and Barris[7] reported shortages of occupational therapy personnel in mental health. The report of the Ad Hoc Commission on Occupational Therapy Manpower,[8] further clarified by Silvergleit,[9] noted a decline in the percentage of registered occupational

therapists and an increase in the percentage of certified occupational therapy assistants working in mental health between 1973 and 1982. The reasons behind such a shift in personnel have not been fully explored. Possible contributing factors may include better utilization of both levels of occupational therapy personnel, cost-saving measures, and the flow of therapists into other practice arenas. A CQI approach could provide data, more systematically measure outcomes in care, and lead to action that could affect the utilization of human and material resources in mental health settings.

The Ad Hoc Commission's report[8] also noted other factors influencing changing practice trends in mental health. They include the continued movement of mental health consumers from institutions into the community, the increase of occupational therapy personnel in case manager roles, and continued emphasis on skilled and accountable clinical management. Given these trends, the need to gather data to analyze systematically the impact of community-based care compared to institutionally based care for specific mentally ill groups is indicated. Monitoring the outcomes of case management programs staffed by occupational therapists lends support to this emerging role. CQI is a tool for clinical management that will enhance program accountability as well as improve patient care.

Given the state of change in the mental health practice arena, Cottrell[10] examined the level of perceived competence among occupational therapists practicing in mental health. She reported that 90% of the respondents perceived their ability to adapt to their role changes and changes in the mental health system as being good to excellent. Additionally, 97% reported that they felt good to excellent about their ability to describe the occupational therapy role in psychiatry to multidisciplinary staff. When asked about their ability to conduct a quality review of their mental health program, however, one of four saw their competence as fair to poor. CQI could offer occupational therapists a philosophy and methodology for systematically collecting data, analyzing information, and making decisions regarding opportunities to improve care.

Definition of Terms

How can CQI and quality assurance be distinguished? Essentially, the distinction lies in a philosophic shift from seeking out the bad apples to promoting quality and excellence. Quality assurance, as practiced during the last decade, assumes that there will be defects and that ongoing inspection will identify these defects so that the service can be restructured to eliminate defects or problems. For example, in quality assurance typically we conduct audits of medical records to determine whether all the essential elements are documented rather than assess the data to identify opportunities for improvements in the quality of care provided.

The attitude toward customers (patients) approach, as suggested by Berwick,[11] differs as well. The mindset of the supplier (in this case, the health care provider) toward the customer has traditionally been "I know what the customer wants," and the resources are allocated toward remaking or redoing the product to match the supplier's perception of what the customer wants. Applying this concept to occupational therapy, a therapist may say "Mr. Jones needs assertiveness and relaxation training. I will place him in these groups." Instead of the patient being involved in the program development and selection process, he or she is slotted into existing programs on the basis of the resources or convenience of the staff.

CQI acknowledges that there may be defects in the products or services. This approach, however, is highly sensitive to customer needs and constantly strives to receive customer input to improve and to meet the customer expectations. For example, the therapist could ask "Mr. Jones, what would you like to do in occupational therapy today?", "How can I help you meet your goals?", or "What are your suggestions for improving the assertiveness training program?"

CQI, rather than honing in on an individual practitioner's deficiencies, emphasizes improving systems, which lessens the employee's defensiveness and negativity toward the self-assessment process. Berwick[11] suggests that by focusing on systems all personnel can continuously seek ways to improve rather than seek out the bad apples in the inspection-oriented approach. Additional differences in the approaches or mindset between quality assurance and CQI are illustrated in the example below.

Sally, a registered occupational therapist working on a day hospital unit, has a history of not monitoring potentially dangerous tools such as scissors and knives in her task groups. Given the nature of the client tasks and the fact that the clients go home each day, she feels justified in having her clients take responsibility for keeping track of their own tools and materials. Because the occupational therapy program also serves acute inpatients who may be suicidal, Sally's approach to this issue is clearly at odds with that of her co-workers, who see her as being irresponsible and unsafe.

An inspection-oriented approach might identify Sally's behavior as not reaching the 100% standard of providing a safe and secure environment, and Sally might be dealt with by her supervisor in a disciplinary manner. Sally could feel coerced and misunderstood and that her professional integrity is being challenged.

A CQI approach might ask "How is Sally facilitating individual responsibility with her clients? What are the risks in expecting clients to monitor tools? How can the task group be run in a safe and secure manner while responsibility is promoted on the part of the client?" With this approach, Sally and her co-workers can grow from their collective wisdom and arrive at a decision that demonstrates respect for their professional concerns while at the same time recognizing the different needs of the different patient groups. The supervisor now acts in a facilitative manner.

In other words, a focus for monitoring is determined by identifying the important functions of the service being provided, describing how these key functions should be performed in a quality situation, and measuring the difference between what is and what should be on an ongoing basis.

Understanding CQI can be enhanced by further examination of its concepts. *Continuous* means an ongoing and planned approach. This is accomplished through monitoring. Monitoring is the systematic and ongoing collection and organization of data related to the indicators of quality and appropriateness of important aspects of care and the comparison of cumulative data with thresholds for evaluation related to each indicator.[1] *Quality* addresses two components: process and outcome.[1] Quality as related to process answers the question "Am I doing the appropriate thing effectively?" In other words, is the occupational therapist providing the appropriate therapeutic approach or technique in a correct manner? For example, when working with a manic patient, is the therapist following appropriate protocols for dealing with stimulus-sensitive patients? Quality as related to outcomes addresses the results of care. That is, what is the patient able to do as a result of the therapeutic interventions provided? Processes and outcomes are related by virtue of the fact that appropriate and effective application of processes will probably have an impact on outcomes.[12] *Improvement* is defined by Juran[4] as the organized creation of beneficial change or the attainment of unprecedented levels of performance. He likens improvement to breakthrough.

In summary, CQI provides the philosophic framework for designing systems to improve care by systematically monitoring the quality of the processes and the outcomes of care.

Where to Begin

Here are several suggestions that might help create the environment that is necessary for CQI to flourish:

- Make a commitment to educating yourself and your staff about CQI.
- Attend CQI workshops, train your staff and co-workers in CQI techniques (e.g., pareto analysis and fishbone diagrams) and use them regularly

in your department (see the reference list at the end of this [chapter]).

- Be sensitive to the overall organization. Take care to control what you can control by integrating this approach in your own department. The ideal environment is for the total organization to espouse the CQI climate.
- Involve all staff.
- Provide encouragement to one another, and foster teamwork.
- Become adept at setting up data collection systems so that the data can be translated into meaningful information.
- Hone in on what you are doing well in your program, and celebrate your successes as a group.

Additionally, staff can build on their current quality assurance activities. Two resources, *The Joint Commission Guide to Quality Assurance*[1] and "Getting Started: Perspectives on Initiating a Quality Assurance Program,"[13] provide information to carry out the 10-step, data-driven monitoring and evaluation process suggested by the Joint Commission. The 10 steps for monitoring and evaluation used in quality assurance are applicable to the CQI process as well. The 10-step process in CQI will shift to a more internal continuous improvement mindset rather than being used to fulfill requirements for meeting quality assurance standards as the primary objective.

Case Example

The following case example illustrates how the data-driven process can help in making decisions that will lead to CQI.

An occupational therapy department meeting was initiated to identify important aspects of care that could be the focus for improved patient care. The staff generated a list of items that included patient assessment, treatment planning, timely initiation of therapy, attendance, safety issues, patient satisfaction with the treatment program, and matching the occupational therapy groups with the patients' functional abilities.

The staff decided that they were concerned about patient assessment because they were uncomfortable with the timeliness and availability of assessment information in the medical record. Questions were generated that would help identify specific activities carried out by the therapists that could be systematically reviewed as they related to quality assessment. They asked the question "What needs to take place in the patient assessment for quality care to occur?" The following activities were identified and correlated with the existing department standards for patient assessment:

1. The patient is assessed within 48 hours of admission.

2. The assessment is conducted by a registered occupational therapist.
3. The assessment is conducted with the department protocol for initial assessment battery.
4. Results of the assessment are documented in the patient's medical record within 72 hours of admission.
5. Appropriate referrals to other disciplines are made for additional testing (e.g., psychologic testing, chemical dependency consultation).

A system was designed for data collection; for the purposes of this discussion, we will assume that data had been collected and aggregated over a 3-month period. A total of 30 patients were monitored, and the following characteristics emerged:

1. In 50% of the cases the patient was assessed within 48 hours.
2. All assessments were conducted by a registered occupational therapist.
3. In 5% of the cases the assessment was not conducted with the department-specific protocol.
4. In 30% of the cases the results were documented within 72 hours of admission.
5. Only two cases indicated a need for referral, and the referrals did occur in both cases.

When evaluating this information, it would be easy to conclude that the therapists are not doing their jobs and that irresponsibility is at the root of the situation. A CQI mindset will focus on the system to explain the problems and the opportunities for improvement. The staff would again meet to engage in a group problem-solving process. With the data noted above, the group identified numbers 1 and 4 as priority issues because these two aspects of the evaluation process fell significantly below the norms for the established protocol.

The next step was to identify possible contributing factors that might lead the group to potential solutions. Possible contributing factors for number 1 included the following:

1. The referral was written after 5 pm on Friday and not received until Monday morning.
2. A record number of admissions occurred within a 2-day period (Monday and Tuesday).
3. Because the department protocol for the initial assessment battery takes 2 hours for each patient, the therapists were not able to complete it within 48 hours.
4. There may be workload problems (i.e., balancing scheduled treatment groups with limited assessment time).
5. Patients could have refused to do the assessment.
6. Patients could have been unavailable during the

48 hours because of scheduling conflicts with other disciplines conducting their assessments.

Possible contributing factors generated by the group for number 4 included all the points listed for number 1 plus the following:

1. Therapists may not see the written assessments as priorities in comparison to other job tasks.
2. Therapists may value verbal more than written reporting.
3. Therapists may find written documentation cumbersome.
4. Therapists may experience difficulty in gaining access to the patient's medical record.

Once the group felt that they had identified all the contributing factors, they rank ordered the factors that they felt were most significant to the issue. For example, the highest ranked contributing factors for number 1 included the record number of admissions on Monday and Tuesday and the fact that the assessment process was too long (conclusions). Potential solutions (recommendations) to these problems included reallocating the personnel resources so that a registered occupational therapist could devote time exclusively to the evaluation team, flexibility to allow for admission rates, streamlining the assessment to a 30-minute screening or small group process, and changing the 48-hour standard to reflect more accurately the ability of the available staff.

For number 4, the highest ranked factor was that the therapists found the documentation system cumbersome (conclusion). Possible solutions (recommendations) could be providing inservice training about the importance of written and verbal assessment reports for team communication, reimbursement, and accreditation; building in a reward system for timely completion of documentation; and experimenting with other documentation formats such as checklists, dictation of assessments to a dedicated stenography pool, or computerized documentation. The group noted that some improvement could occur with number 4 if the solutions for number 1 were put into place because the two factors interrelate.

Once a solution is identified, there is a tendency to implement it and to assume that it will alleviate the problem and improve the situation. It is important, however, to proceed to the next step in the CQI process, which is to continue to monitor on the basis of the actions to improve, so that it can be determined whether the improvement actually occurs. This process can continue to be fine tuned until the team feels comfortable with the assessment and its level of efficiency and effectiveness, having evaluated the results of the action taken.

The acronym CRAE (conclusion, recommendations, action, evaluation) is helpful for remembering the steps toward improvement (Table 1).

CQI is dependent on the involvement of all staff. By being involved, each staff member will experience greater

---

Table 1. Format Used in Making Improvements (Acronym: CRAE)

Important Aspect of Care Monitored: Timely Documentation of Patient Assessment

Information element 1: In 50% of cases, the patient was assessed in 48 hours.
Conclusions (results of information analysis)
- Record numbers of admissions on Monday and Tuesday.
- Assessment process too long.

Recommendations (proposed solutions)
- Reallocate personnel resources (e.g., OTR doing assessments only).
- Streamline assessment to 30 minutes.
- Conduct assessments in small groups.
- Change 48-hour standard to a more realistic time frame based on resource availability.

Information element 4: In 30% of cases, the results were documented within 72 hours of admission.
Conclusions:
- Documentation too cumbersome.
    Recommendations
- Inservice training about the importance of documentation for communication, reimbursement, and accreditation.
- Reward for timely completion.
- Design more efficient assessment formats (e.g., checklists).
- Dictate assessments to a dedicated stenography pool.
- Use computerized documentation.

Actions (solution implementation)
- Choose proposed solution(s) from above and implement until enough data are collected to make judgments regarding effectiveness of actions.

Evaluation
- Evaluate results of action taken and determine whether to accept solution (conclude monitoring) or to try another proposed solution until acceptable improvement is evidenced.

---

improvement in his or her own work process, which in turn positively affects the quality of care provided to patients.

* * *

CQI offers a systematic process by which occupational therapists can measure, direct, and improve the quality of patient services. To date CQI has been integrated into several well-known hospitals, such as Hospital Corporation of America; Humana, Inc; Massachusetts General Hospital; and New England Medical Center.[14] CQI is in the planning stages for inclusion in future Joint Commission standards. CQI is practical, useful, and powerful, as evidenced by its success in Japanese industry and more recently in American industry.[15]

The potential for effecting constructive change can take many forms. Occupational therapists who incorporate the CQI approaches may find that they can enhance productivity by focusing on priority activities through team efforts. Department cohesiveness may be fostered. Mental health patients will be encouraged to take more responsibility for their own care in a service environment where their input will be more respected and will have more impact, thus reinforcing their own ability to function. Staff time can be spent more effectively on a focused approach to improving services and systems rather than the staff feeling out of control or lacking ability to solve problems. Clinical and administrative decisions will be based on objective data rather than on hunches and speculation. Most important, a CQI approach promoted in the occupational therapy mental health setting will equip occupational therapists to improve and upgrade continually the quality of services provided.

CQI as a management style that values data for the purpose of continuous improvement will evolve over time. By incorporating CQI approaches now, occupational therapists will proactively prepare themselves for the inevitability of CQI being implemented in health care organizations throughout America. One benefit of adopting interdisciplinary group problem solving for quality improvement endeavors is that occupational therapists will enhance their credibility in the mental health arena.

References

1. Joint Commission on Accreditation of Healthcare Organizations. *Joint Commission Guide to Quality Assurance*. Chicago: Joint Commission; 1988.

2. Deming WE. *Quality, Productivity, and Competitive Position*. Cambridge, Mass: Massachusetts Institute of Technology Center for Advanced Engineering Study; 1982.

3. Deming WE. *Out of the Crisis*. Cambridge. Mass: Massachusetts Institute of Technology Center for Advanced Engineering Study; 1982.

4. Juran JM. *Juran on Leadership for Quality: An Executive Handbook*. New York: Free Press; 1989.

5. Juran JM, Gryna FM Jr, Bingham RS Jr. eds. *Quality Control Handbook*. New York: McGraw-Hill; 1979.

6. Bonder BR. Occupational therapy in mental health: Crisis or opportunity? *Am J Occup Ther*. 1987;41:495-499.

7. Kielhofner G, Barris R. Mental health occupational therapy: Trends in literature and practice. *Occup Ther Ment Health*. 1984;4:35-49.

8. Masagatani G, Olson T, Reed K, et al. *Occupational Therapy Manpower: A Plan for Progress*. Rockville, Md: American Occupational Therapy Association;1985.

9. Silvergleit IT. Clarifies figures from manpower commission. *Am J Occup Ther*. 1987;41:759. Letter.

10. Cottrell RF. Perceived competence among occupational therapists in mental health. *Am J Occup Ther*. 1990;44:118-124.

11. Berwick DM. Sounding board: Continuous improvement as an ideal in health care. *N Engl J Med*. 1989;320:53-56.

12. *The Joint Commission 1991 Accreditation Manual for Hospitals*. Oakbrook Terrace, Ill: Joint Commission; 1990.

13. Brinson MH. Getting started: Perspectives on initiating a quality assurance program. *Ment Health Spec Interest Sect Newslett*. 1987;10:4.

14. James BC. *Quality Management for Health Care Delivery*. Chicago: Hospital Research and Educational Trust; 1989.

15. Walton M. *The Deming Management Method*. New York: Dodd, Mead; 1986.

Chapter 54

Demonstrating Treatment Outcomes in Mental Health

Martha H. Thien, MOT, OTR/L

Traditionally, outcome measures of psychiatric rehabilitation have focused on recidivism and vocational adjustment. In an article relevant to the practice of occupational therapy, Anthony, Cohen, and Vitalo (1978) found positive outcomes to be related to the patient's level of skilled activity in the areas of social relationships, coping, and work and job-seeking behaviors. They recommended that patient gains in skills and satisfaction with services be included as types of outcome measures in evaluation of psychiatric rehabilitation services. They also felt that patients' critical skill areas should be identified and evaluated at the beginning and end of rehabilitation services.

The quality assurance and program evaluation consultants for the American Occupational Therapy Association report annually on their own activities in this area. The most frequently reported outcome measures used by this group are (a) progress toward treatment goals, (b) patient satisfaction questionnaires, and (c) patient rating scales. Each of these types of measurement can be applied to outcomes in mental health.

This article briefly reviews these three methods of demonstrating treatment effectiveness in occupational therapy. The experience of one occupational therapy department is discussed to illustrate the use of a rating scale analysis to answer important clinical and management questions.

Progress Toward Goals

The establishment of goals and objectives is an integral part of the treatment planning process. If properly devised and constructed, goals and objectives provide an indication of the quality of care by linking treatment to desired outcomes. This type of goal writing is often elusive and must be consistently scrutinized and reinforced with practice.

In order to collect outcome data derived from treatment goals, the clinician will want to be specific about the expected behavioral performance, the criterion or standard for acceptable performance, and the conditions under which this performance can be expected to occur (Denton, 1987). Numerically stated goals increase the ease of data collection (Kuntavanish, 1987). Finally, it will be helpful if the outcome goal is a statement of the desired level of performance on an assessment instrument or rating scale used by the clinician. For example, the patient will improve five points on the safety subtest of the Scorable Self-Care Evaluation (SSCE) within 1 week; or, at discharge, the patient will attend to task in work skills group with no more than 15 minutes lost concentration (improvement on the Comprehensive Occupational Therapy Evaluation [COTE] Scale).

Patient Satisfaction Questionnaires

The second method of collecting outcome data, measurement of patient satisfaction, has not been widely used as an indicator of quality care. However, patient satisfaction with health care is becoming more important in view of recent trends toward consumerism and self-responsibility. In a recent address to the Third International Symposium on Quality Assurance in Health Care, Dr. Hannu Vuori (1987) of the World Health Organization concluded that patient satisfaction is an essential criterion of good health care in nontechnical matters.

Psychiatric Occupational Therapy: A Workbook of Practical Skills (Denton, 1987) contains a helpful discussion of self-report instruments, their uses and limitations. For the purpose of quality assurance data collection, those instruments that yield numerical data will be more useful than questionnaires that require short answers or checklists that do not measure frequency, duration, or intensity. Anchored rating scales, which are frequently used for self reports, ask the patient to rate a range of responses and can easily be transferred to numerical form. Patient satisfaction questionnaires may be administered at the beginning and end of treatment, as well as at a postdischarge interval to measure outcome and transfer of skill from the treatment setting to the community. An example of this type of instrument can be found in *Improved Productivity in an Acute-Care Psychiatric Occupational Therapy Program* (Ostrow & Kaufman, 1981).

Behavior Rating Scales

Behavior rating scales represent the final method for collecting data that I will discuss. Scales that rate the patient's level of skill performance at the beginning and end of treatment are used and reported by clinicians in physical rehabilitation settings to demonstrate outcomes of treatment (Kuntavanish, 1987). This method of data

collection can be used to measure psychiatric rehabilitation outcome. As with patient satisfaction surveys, the most useful scales for data collection will have numerical ratings.

In two of the three types of outcome measures discussed, data is gathered from documentation. In order to enhance this process, documentation must be standardized and data must be objective, numerical or convertible to numerical form, and consistently collected (Kuntavanish, 1987). Narrative documentation does not always meet these requirements. One of the first problem-solving actions taken as a result of documentation review is likely to be the correction of sloppy and inadequate documentation habits.

Broadlawns Medical Center is a county-supported general hospital with adult and adolescent inpatient and outpatient psychiatric programs. In order to simplify and standardize the documentation process, the occupational therapy service recently adopted a form containing a rating scale based on the COTE scale, similar to the one described by Ostrow and Kaufman (1981).

A documentation review was undertaken for all adult patients with occupational therapy referrals who were discharged in May 1987 to evaluate occupational therapy treatment outcomes. A data collection form was designed to record initial and discharge ratings, number of initial deficits, number of deficits showing improvement, and goals and objectives set in the treatment plan. Information about treatment goals was collected in order to determine if behaviors reflected in the rating influenced the treatment planning process.

Forty-one records were reviewed by the six occupational therapy staff members and one student during the weekly staff meetings. Given the average length of stay and the frequency of documentation requirements, 20 of the records reviewed were expected to have two or more ratings in order to evaluate treatment outcomes. Thirteen records had two ratings and improvement was demonstrated by a decrease in total rating points in 11 cases. Improvement ranged from 1 to 19 points.

More detailed data analysis options for this type of data collection are possible. The clinician can look at the average number of points of improvement from initial to discharge rating and percent of deficits showing improvement. Results can then be compared to a standard such as percent of cases in which improvement is expected.

A *Client-Oriented System of Mental Health Service Delivery and Program Management* (Carter and Newman, 1976) describes the use of an outcome matrix to analyze data collected at the beginning and end of a time period, as in initial and discharge ratings. The matrix consists of an equal number of intersecting rows and columns. Each row on the left margin corresponds to a score at initial evaluation, with "most dysfunctional" at the top and "most functional" at the bottom; each column across the top corresponds to a score at discharge with function increasing from left to right (see Figure 1).

Figure 1. Comparison of Outcome with the Number of Treatments

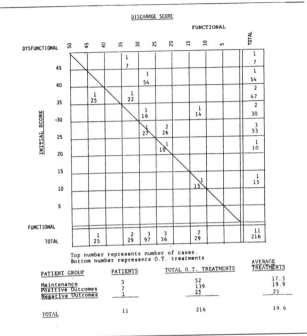

Each case is located on the outcome matrix by finding the box formed by the intersection of the initial and discharge scores, similar to locating distance between two cities on a mileage table. Cases that fall in the boxes along the diagonal from upper left to lower right represent maintenance, that is, no change from initial to discharge score. Cases that fall in the boxes above and to the right of the diagonal are positive outcomes; those in the boxes below and to the left of the diagonal represent negative outcomes. Thus, the number of cases that deteriorated, maintained, or improved is easily seen in the display. If the clinician or manager goes one step further and computes the number of total service hours delivered (or costs) for each of these groups, the relationship between amount of service (or cost) and outcome can be determined for groups of patients. This type of analysis provides information that is useful for allocating resources and in making decisions about appropriateness of service.

In another method of data analysis, patients are listed down the left margin, while columns across the top represent each behavior rated by the scale (see Figure 2). For each patient, the number of points of change from evaluation to discharge is entered in the box for each behavior. The total amount of change for each behavior is entered at the bottom of the column. The manager or clinician can determine which behaviors are being most

Figure 2. Occupational Therapy Outcomes in the Treatment of Specific Task Behaviors

Task Behavior

Patient	16		17		18		19		TOTAL		#TX
	DC	C	DC	C	DC	C	DC	C	DC	C	
A	1	-1	3	0	1	0	2	-1	7	-2	
B	0	-2	0	-3	--	--	1	-1	1	-6	
C	1	-2	4	0	2	-2	2	-1	9	-5	
D	1	-2	2	-1	2	+1	2	-1	7	-3	
Total	3	-7	9	-4	5	-1	7	-4	24	-16	
# Rated	4		4		3		4				
# Improved	4		2		1		4				
# Unimproved/Worse	0		2		2		0				

DC = Discharge rating 16 – Concentration, 17 – Problem solving
18 – Follow directions, 19 – Activity neatness
C = Amount of change, admission to discharge; a decrease in rating represents improvement.

effectively changed by current treatment methods. Since the scale groups behaviors by categories, such as self-care and task, treatment outcomes for categories of behaviors can also be measured. Again the relationship between outcome and amount of service or cost can be determined. This type of outcome monitoring by behavior helps the clinician make decisions about changing treatment techniques for targeted behaviors, consider discontinuing types of services that do not show improvement, and monitor to see if new types of treatment are producing expected outcomes.

Perhaps the simplest and most gratifying conclusion from this study was that patients improved and that improvement can be measured and evaluated. Occupational therapy treatment cannot be assumed to be solely responsible since improvement from admission to discharge is expected in most inpatient settings regardless of the treatment regimen. However, the behaviors and skills reflected on the rating scale are those typically addressed in psychiatric occupational therapy, and occupational therapy contributed a significant number of visits to the treatment of these patients.

While the study revealed many documentation problems, a beneficial result has been increased staff interest in documenting, evaluating, and improving treatment outcomes. Staff are also interested in revising the scale to enhance the sensitivity, accuracy, and reliability of ratings. Continued quarterly monitoring of outcomes is planned, although sampling may change to include different groups of patients and specific aspects of patient behavior.

In summary, treatment outcomes can be measured and evaluated in psychiatric occupational therapy settings using several methods. However, standardized objective documentation and numerical data are essential to the process. A study of occupational therapy outcomes in an acute adult inpatient program using a rating scale showed improvement in skills and behaviors typically treated in occupational therapy. Data analysis may vary according to the type of information desired and its intended use. Based on this experience, it is recommended that other psychiatric occupational therapy settings undertake some form of outcome study.

References

Anthony, W. A., Cohen, M. R., & Vitalo, R. (1978). The measurement of rehabilitation outcome. *Schizophrenia Bulletin, 4*(3), 365-383.

Carter, D. E., & Newman, F. L. (1976). *A client-oriented system of mental health service delivery and program management: A workbook and guide*. Harrisburg, PA: Department of Public Welfare, Commonwealth of Pennsylvania.

Denton, P. L. (1987). *Psychiatric occupational therapy: A workbook of practical skills*. Boston: Little, Brown.

Kuntavanish, A. A. (1987). *Occupational therapy documentation*. Rockville, MD: American Occupational Therapy Association.

Ostrow, P. C., & Kaufman, K. L. (1981). Improved productivity in an acute-care psychiatric occupational therapy program: A quality assurance study. In *Productivity improvements in physical and occupational therapies*. Chicago: American Hospital Association.

Vuori, H. (1987). Patient satisfaction—An attribute or indicator of the quality of care? *Quality Review Bulletin, 13*(3), 106-108.

Section VII

Neuroscientific and Research Considerations for Occupational Therapists

Introduction

A comprehensive presentation of occupational therapy practice in mental health would be seriously remiss if it did not address neuroscientific and research considerations relevant to the treatment of mental illness in the current health care system. The explosion of contemporary neuroscience research and technological advances, the developing acceptance of neurophysiological etiologies for many mental illnesses, and the increased demand for quality and accountability in multidisciplinary treatment are all trends that require occupational therapists to become knowledgeable in neuroscience and research terminology, principles, and practices (Allen, 1985; Barris, Kielhofner, & Watts, 1983; Bonder, 1991; Fine, 1980; King, 1983). The chapters in this section introduce readers to critical neuroscience and research concepts and their clinical applications, and facilitate active integration of this knowledge with daily occupational therapy practice.

Chapter 55, by Brown and Mann, provides a comprehensive review of the vital role neurotransmitters play in major mental illnesses. General aspects of neural transmission, specific nerve tracts, and neurotransmitters that have been implicated as etiological factors in affective disorders and schizophrenia are identified and described. The synthesis, receptor location, and pharmacologic responses of the three primary neurotransmitters (dopamine, norepinephrine, and serotonin) are discussed. This presentation provides the necessary foundation for understanding the relevance of neuroscience to the etiology and pharmacologic treatment of mental illness.

Issues related to pharmacologic treatment are expanded upon in chapter 56, by Keith, Starr, and Matthews. The authors specifically discuss the effects of psychotropic medications on the symptoms of schizophrenia. They emphasize a team approach to maximize the efficacy of pharmacologic treatment for persons with schizophrenia. The limitations of psychotropic medications in managing the negative symptoms of schizophrenia are clearly described. The authors' emphasis on a collaborative, psychoeducational approach and their call for psychosocial interventions to maximize the effectiveness of psychotropic medications are clearly relevant to occupational therapy practice in mental health.

The potential for occupational therapy to enhance the treatment efficacy of psychotropic medications is directly explored in chapter 57, by Smith. Smith discusses the therapeutic and adverse side effects of psychotropic medications and the functional impact of these potential effects on occupational therapy's evaluation and intervention. A hypothetical treatment group is presented to substantiate the need for occupational therapists to be cognizant of the functional effects of pharmacologic treatment. The occupational therapist who is knowledgeable about psychotropic medications can make a significant contribution to the psychiatric treatment team by sharing skilled observations of the functional effects of these medications on the patient's activity performance and social interactions (Allen, 1985; Fisher, 1991).

In addition to being knowledgeable about the functional effects of psychotropic medications, occupational therapists need to be aware of the functional effects of electroconvulsive therapy (ECT). ECT may be viewed by some as a controversial treatment method; however, ECT does have an established reputation as a safe and effective form of treatment for severe affective disorders (Kaplan & Sadock, 1985). Chapter 58, by Coffey and

Weiner, provides a clear overview of current medical standards for the therapeutic use of ECT. Although this chapter was written for medical practitioners directly involved with the administration of ECT, the occupational therapist will find the discussion of indications, contraindications, and adverse effects of ECT informative and relevant. The impact of these issues on a patient's functional performance needs to be considered by the occupational therapist when planning and implementing evaluation procedures and intervention methods.

The next five chapters in this section provide thoughtful presentations on mental health research relevant to occupational therapy practice. In chapter 59 Barris begins by providing a brief overview of medical research on schizophrenia. The focus, findings, limitations, and implications for occupational therapy of major research studies are discussed. Barris argues that occupational therapists can develop an important and complementary role to the medical researcher, which will lead to an increased recognition of the need for and value of occupational therapy interventions.

The utilization of medical research and theory as a basis for occupational therapy intervention is further explored in chapter 60, by MacRae, which specifically focuses on hallucinations. MacRae reviews historical and contemporary definitions and etiological theories for hallucinations. An overview of research on intervention techniques and symptom management is provided. MacRae argues that the limitations inherent in etiological theories and intervention research can be countered by utilizing a functional model to determine deficits caused by hallucinations and to plan appropriate occupational therapy intervention. The clinical application of this functional model is explored through the presentation of two case studies.

Chapter 61, by Reisman and Blakeney, focuses specifically on occupational therapy research on sensory integrative (SI) treatment in schizophrenia. A literature review of SI research provides the background for a presentation of the authors' recent research study on the treatment efficacy of SI interventions for patients with chronic schizophrenia. The study's sample, instruments, procedures, and results are described. The authors' discussion of the study's limitations and implications clearly warrants critical thought. Further research on the efficacy of SI treatment for chronic schizophrenia is advocated by the authors and can prove to be an exciting research avenue for occupational therapists.

Sensory integrative treatment for psychiatric patients also provides the foundation for the next research study, described by Van Schroeder and Chung in chapter 62. They review the effectiveness of an interdisciplinary treatment approach for monitoring the extrapyramidal side effects of psychotropic medications in patients with chronic mental illness. They conclude that the combination of SI treatment and medication reduction was a cost effective way to prevent tardive dyskinesia and to increase patients' functioning and psychiatric status.

The efficacy of an interdisciplinary treatment approach is further validated by chapter 63, which presents an American Occupational Therapy Association (AOTA) data brief summarizing an historically significant research study on the aftercare of patients with chronic schizophrenia. The results of this study indicate that the most effective aftercare treatment provided psychotropic medications and a day program that had a great amount of occupational therapy services. These findings validate the vital role occupational therapy plays in improving the functional status of patients with mental illness in a cost-effective, therapeutic manner.

The interdisciplinary nature of several chapters in this section highlights the need for occupational therapists to become informed, active members of the mental health treatment team. A unilateral, circumscribed view of occupational therapy in mental health does not benefit the patient or the profession. While it is vital for occupational therapists to become proficient in their own unique professional roles, it is equally essential for them to become fluent in the languages and practices of related disciplines. The ability to communicate and demonstrate the value of occupational therapy in a manner congruent with the language and philosophy of other professions enhances occupational therapy's contribution and worth to the treatment team and leads to improved quality of care for the patient (Barris, Kielhofner, & Watts, 1983; Fine, 1980). It is hoped that this strong introduction to neuroscience and research will enable readers to engage in informed dialogues with other professionals, to make relevant contributions to interdisciplinary treatment programs, and to participate actively in treatment efficacy research. Readers are urged to seek and utilize the numerous continuing education opportunities available in neuroscience and research. The American Occupational Therapy Association (AOTA), the American Occupational Therapy Foundation (AOTF), and the American Psychiatric Association (APA) are invaluable resources for references, publications, workshops, and conferences on these areas (see reference and resource listings at the end of this text for further detail). In addition, the reader is referred to section IX in this text for guidelines and suggestions on professional career development and clinical research. The utilization of a diversity of resources to expand their knowledge base can place occupational therapists at the forefront of current clinical applications and future advances in neuroscience and research.

Questions to Consider

1. How does an understanding of neuroscience enhance the occupational therapist's ability to evaluate and intervene with persons with mental illnesses? What are the implications of neurophysiological etiologies for mental illness on the patient's performance components and on occupational performances?

2. What are the functional effects of psychotropic medications and ECT? How do these medical interventions interfere with or enhance the patient's ability to engage in functional activities and social relationships?

3. How can occupational therapists modify their evaluation and intervention activities and adapt the treatment environment to maximize the therapeutic effects and minimize the adverse side effects of psychotropic medications and ECT?

4. What information is vital for the occupational therapist to share with the treatment team about the effects of psychotropic medications and ECT on functional performance? How can an occupational therapist facilitate a collaborative approach to the medical management of mental illness with the psychiatrist, patient, and patient's family? What information can an occupational therapist appropriately share with a patient and his or her family to enhance compliance with the medical management of mental illness?

5. How do current trends in the medical research of mental illness relate to occupational therapy practice? How can an occupational therapist become an effective partner in medical research? What are the unique contributions an occupational therapist can make to treatment efficacy studies?

6. How might an occupational therapist utilize MacRae's functional model for hallucinations in a research study? What are the implications of this model for clinical practice?

7. What are the benefits and limitations of sensory integrative (SI) treatment for persons with chronic schizophrenia? What are potential research designs for examining the efficacy of SI intervention?

8. How do the characteristics of aftercare programs affect the treatment outcome of persons with chronic mental illness? What can occupational therapy uniquely offer to multidisciplinary day treatment programs? How can occupational therapists research the effectiveness of their interventions in day treatment?

References

Allen, C. K. (1985). *Occupational therapy for psychiatric diseases: Measurement and management of cognitive disabilities.* Boston: Little, Brown.

Barris, R., Kielhofner, G., & Watts, J. H. (1983). *Psychosocial occupational therapy: Practice in a pluralistic arena.* Laurel, MD: RAMSCO.

Bonder, B. R. (Ed.). (1991). *Psychopathology and function.* Thorofare, NJ: Slack.

Fine, S. B. (1980). Psychiatric treatment and rehabilitation: What's in a name? *Journal of the National Association of Private Psychiatric Hospitals, 11*(5), 3-13.

Fisher, P. J. (1991). Psychotropic medications. In B. Bonder (Ed.), *Psychopathology and function* (pp. 155-183). Thorofare, NJ: Slack.

Kaplan, H. I., & Sadock, B. J. (1985). *Modern synopsis of comprehensive textbook of psychiatry/IV* (4th ed.). Baltimore: Williams & Wilkins.

King, L. J. (1983). Occupational therapy and neuropsychiatry. *Occupational Therapy in Mental Health, 3*(1), 1-12.

Chapter 55

A Clinical Perspective on the Role of Neurotransmitters in Mental Disorders

Richard P. Brown, MD

J. John Mann, MD

This chapter was previously published in *Hospital and Community Psychiatry*, *36*, 141–150. Copyright © 1985, the American Psychiatric Association. Reprinted by permission.

The brain is probably the most complex and phylogenically advanced organ in man. Its physical inaccessibility has rendered it difficult to study, but progress has suddenly accelerated over the last 20 years. Therefore mental health professionals should be familiar with the current state of knowledge and directions of future research, since findings in the neurosciences are having a more immediate clinical impact than ever before.

Researchers estimate that they have identified fewer than 5 percent of the brain's neurotransmitters, chemicals that facilitate the transmission of impulses between neurons.

We are only beginning to appreciate the complexity of these neurotransmitters, their receptors, the interaction of transmitter-receptor-effector complexes, and the interactions between several transmitter systems. At times neuropsychopharmacologists have been in the fabled position of the blind wise men: each feeling a part of the elephant and imagining the part to be like the whole. However, in conjunction with studies of individual neurons and transmitters, new techniques such as positron emission tomography, autoradiography, and immunocytochemistry are permitting preliminary studies of the neuronal wiring of the human brain.

This [chapter] will first review certain general aspects of neural transmission and salient aspects of specific nerve tracts in the brain; it will then discuss theoretical models of affective disorders and schizophrenia and the mechanisms of action of antipsychotic and antidepressant medications.

Mechanisms of Neural Transmission

The basic functional unit of the nervous system is the nerve cell, which transmits through its specialized parts electrochemical excitation to other neurons. From the nerve cell body there are two principal outgrowths: the dendrites, numerous extensions that receive information by their receptors, and the axons, which transmit messages to the presynaptic terminal. The synapse is a narrow gap separating two neurons at a transmission point. Neurotransmitter chemicals are released from the presynaptic nerve terminal to diffuse across the synaptic cleft and combine with the postsynaptic receptor (see Figures 1 and 2).

Figure 1.

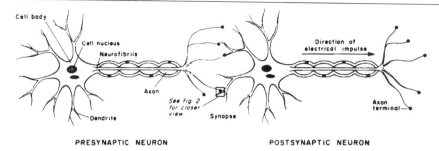

PRESYNAPTIC NEURON   POSTSYNAPTIC NEURON

Neurotransmitter precursors produced in the cell body are carried by neurofibrils to axon terminals, where neurotransmitters are synthesized. An electrical impulse traveling from the cell body down the axon to the terminals causes a release of transmitter into the space called the synapse.

This process may be affected by drugs at several points including release (for instance, tranylcypromine enhances the release of the neurotransmitter norepinephrine); combination with the receptor (antihypertensive drugs can block alpha- and beta-catecholamine receptors); response of the receptor to stimulation by the neurotransmitter (chronic antidepressant therapy reduces the responsivity of beta receptors); and termination of the signal by reuptake of the transmitter into the presynaptic neuron (blocked reuptake by tricyclic antidepressants).

Figure 2.

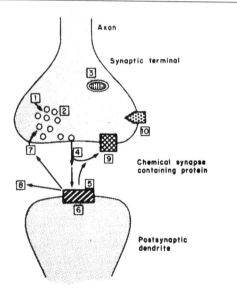

Close-up of synapse: 1. Transmitter synthesis. 2. Storage vesicles. 3. Intra-cellular organelles, such as mitochondria. 4. Release. 5. Postsynaptic receptor. 6. Postsynaptic receptor processes (see Figure 3). 7. Reuptake into presynaptic terminal. 8. Inactivation. 9. Autoreceptor. 10. Receptor for transmitter feedback from adjacent neuron (such as opiate regulation of dopamine turnover).

Amine neurotransmitters are synthesized in neurons from precursors circulating in the bloodstream. At norepinephrine and serotonin nerve terminals, uptake systems in the cell membrane transport the precursor into the nerve cell from the extracellular space and blood stream. Amine transmitters may be made in the cell body or the terminals. Terminal vesicles may also contain enzymes that convert one neurotransmitter into another.

The precursors of neuropeptide transmitters, which are larger molecules than amines, are carried from the cell body, where they are synthesized, down the axon through tubes called neurofibrils. Transmitters are then usually stored in vesicles that are located at the nerve terminal. These vesicles protect the transmitters from intracellular catabolic enzymes, such as monoamine oxidase.

When an action potential arrives at the presynaptic nerve terminal, the stored transmitter is released by diffusion through special channels or by exocytosis. In exocytosis a vesicle merges with the presynaptic membrane and empties its contents into the synapse. Both processes are calcium-dependent.

The transmitter molecules move to occupy specific postsynaptic receptors. Through the action of a coupling protein at certain receptors the enzyme adenyl cyclase is activated. This enzyme converts adenosine triphosphate into cyclic adenosine monophosphate (cAMP). Cyclic AMP can mediate a number of effects intracellularly; for instance, it acts as a cofactor for protein kinase enzymes, which phosphorylate proteins in the postsynaptic membrane. This action, in turn, creates an open pore through which sodium and potassium ions may flow to cause depolarization.

Cyclic AMP activates beta-adrenergic receptors, some serotonin (5-HT$_1$) receptors, histamine receptors, and dopamine (D$_1$) receptors. However, other substances activate different receptors. For example, gamma-aminobutyric acid (GABA) activates a system of receptors that rapidly open chloride channels, and muscarinic acetylcholine receptors are linked to the enzyme phospholipase C to control calcium channels.

The neuron is only semipermeable to ions. Ion pumps actively maintain a lower concentration of sodium and a higher concentration of potassium inside the cell compared with concentrations outside the cell. These ionic concentration gradients result in polarization of the axonal membrane and a resting electrical potential across the cell membrane.

At the nerve terminal, transmission to the next neuron generally takes place by release of a chemical transmitter across the synaptic cleft. Interaction of excitatory transmitters with postsynaptic receptors leads to changes in membrane ionic permeability that allow ions to flow down their concentration gradients, which results in depolarization (see Figure 3). If the depolarization exceeds a certain threshold level, an action potential is generated and moves down the axon to its terminal. Inhibitory transmitters have the reverse effect and lower the resting membrane potential, thereby raising the threshold for an action potential.

After release the neurotransmitter must be inactivated by enzymes in the synaptic cleft (acetylcholinesterase inactivates acetylcholine) or by reuptake into the presynaptic terminal (norepinephrine and serotonin are inactivated by reuptake). The latter process has the advantage of allowing the neuron to reuse the transmitter.

It is not easy to prove that a chemical is a neurotransmitter. The reader should consult basic textbooks for a more detailed description of experimental criteria (1, 2). It can be even more difficult to distinguish neurotransmitters from neuromodulators. Neuromodulators are substances that act on or within neurons to change the responsiveness of the transmission process—perhaps by altering transmitter synthesis or release, receptor sensitivity, or second-messenger activity.

Neuropeptides and classical neurotransmitters may be present and released from the same neurons. For example, some recent research has focused on the interaction of dopamine and the cotransmitter neuropeptide cholecystokinin, and serotonin and the cotransmitter neuropeptide substance P. Other examples of neuromodulation include the action of prostaglandins on noradrenergic or dopaminergic neurons and of autoreceptors on adrenergic nerve terminals. A recent paper by Snyder (3) provides an in-depth review of research into neurotransmitter receptors in the past decade.

Biogenic Amine Neurotransmitters

The neurotransmitters of principal interest in affective disorders and schizophrenia have been the biogenic amines norepinephrine, dopamine, and serotonin (1, 2). The basic aspects of synthesis, location, receptors, and pharmacologic response of these neurotransmitters will be discussed in this section.

Norepinephrine

Norepinephrine (noradrenaline) is a catecholamine neurotransmitter in the central nervous system and in sympathetic (postganglionic) nerves of the peripheral

Figure 3.

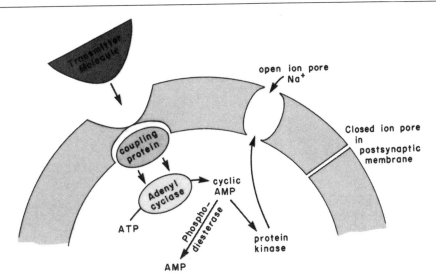

A simplified model of one kind of receptor-coupling-effector complex to induce membrane permeability changes. Cyclic AMP is often referred to as a second messenger.

nervous system. Norepinephrine is also released from the adrenal medulla.

Most norepinephrine neurons originate in the brain stem from the locus ceruleus, the nucleus where the cell bodies are located. One of the two main pathways is the dorsal bundle. Arising in the locus ceruleus of the pons, the dorsal bundle runs a considerable distance to terminate in the neocortex, limbic system, hippocampus, cerebellum, thalamus, and dorsal hypothalamus (see Figure 4). The other pathway is the ventral tract, which travels from the pons to the hypothalamus and limbic system. These ventral tracts are implicated in control of movement, alertness, emotion, pleasure, the sleep cycle, and other basic vegetative functions such as hunger, thirst, temperature regulation, and reproduction. Other pathways in the medulla or lower brain stem influence blood pressure and spinal reflexes.

Alpha and beta receptors for norepinephrine are classified by relative affinities for drugs. Postsynaptic or alpha$_1$ receptors are stimulated by the agonists norepinephrine, phenylephrine, and epinephrine, and are blocked by phentolamine and the antihypertensive drug prazosin. Beta receptors are most sensitive to epinephrine and isoproterenol and are blocked by the antihypertensive and antiarrhythmic drug propranolol.

The functions of these subtypes of adrenergic receptors in the brain are unclear at this time. However, it appears that adrenergic receptors are so widespread that they may generally modulate other neurons. When norepinephrine is released from adrenergic nerve terminals, it stimulates neurons in the surrounding area like water from a sprinkler system spraying over a crop.

One general metabolic function that may be stimulated by norepinephrine stimulation is neuronal glucose turnover. Presynaptic alpha$_2$ receptors act as autoreceptors (see Figure 1) to provide feedback inhibition on the presynaptic neuron and to assist in turning off the signal by inhibiting further release of norepinephrine. The pharmacology of some drugs that affect norepinephrine transmission is summarized in Table 1.

Dopamine

Neurotransmission of dopamine principally occurs in the central nervous system, although it may also occur at some sites in the autonomic nervous system. Synthesis follows the same path as described above for norepinephrine; however, dopamine neurons lack the enzyme dopamine beta hydroxylase (DBH), which converts dopamine into norepinephrine.

There are three main dopamine systems in the brain (see Figure 5). The extrapyramidal pathway begins in the substantia nigra of the midbrain and ends in the caudate nucleus and putamen of the basal ganglia. Although this pathway is best known for fine coordination of movement, it is also implicated in attention and other mental processes, particularly in animals.

The midbrain-to-forebrain mesolimbic system appears to be involved in emotion and memory. The tuberoinfundibular system connects the hypothalamus to the pituitary for control of the hypothalamic-pituitary endocrine system. Table 2 presents in summary form the drugs that affect dopamine transmission.

There are many kinds of dopamine receptors, including the D$_1$ and D$_2$. The D$_1$ receptor is linked to adenylate cyclase; the D$_2$ receptor is not. The D$_2$ receptor appears to be involved in neuroendocrine control of growth hormone and prolactin, the movement disorder in drug-induced Parkinsonism, and the antipsychotic action of dopamine

Figure 4. The Dorsal-Bundle Pathway of Norepinephrine Neurons

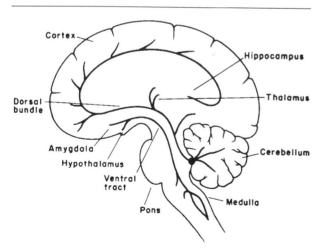

Figure 5. The Three Main Dopaminergic Tracts in the Brain

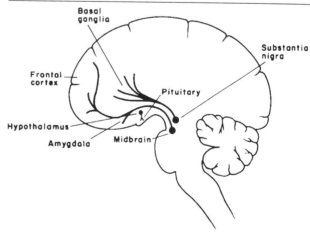

Table 1. Drugs That Affect Norepinephrine Transmission

Transmission Stage	Drug	Effect	Use
Synthesis	Alpha-methyl-dopa	False transmitter	Hypertension
	Alpha-methyl-p-tyrosine	Blocks tyrosine hydroxylase	Research
	Disulfiram	Blocks dopamine beta hydroxylase	Alcoholism
Storage	Reserpine	Depletes norepinephrine, dopamine, serotonin from vesicles	Hypertension, animal model of depression
	Phenelzine Other MAOIs	Increases norepinephrine in presynaptic terminal, prevents norepinephrine metabolism	Antidepressant
Release	Amphetamine Tyramine	Causes release of norepine-phrine (and dopamine)	No therapeutic use
	Guanethidine	Blocks norepinephrine release	Hypertension
	Bretylium		Antiarrhythmic
Receptor	Phenylephrine	Alpha receptor agonist	Decongestant
	Clonidine (dose-related)	Alpha receptor agonist	Hypertension, research in anxiety
	Phentolamine Phenoxybenzamine	Alpha blockers	Hypertension
	Isoproterenol Terbutaline Salbutamol Clenbuterol	Beta activation	Asthma, potentiate antidepressants?
	Propanolol	Beta blocker	Hypertension
	Tricyclics MAOIs Electroconvulsive therapy	Decrease in beta receptor number	Antidepressants
Uptake	Cocaine Tricyclics[1]	Inhibits uptake	

[1] These drugs also inhibit serotonin uptake in many cases.

antagonists. However, the clinical implications of these receptor subtypes are only beginning to be explored.

It should be noted that dopamine neurons may influence or be influenced by other transmitters such as norepinephrine, serotonin, GABA, and opiate peptides, and modulators such as prostaglandins. Disturbance in the balance between dopamine and acetylcholine systems in the basal ganglia is thought to account for the appearance of Parkinsonian symptoms during treatment with antipsychotics; degeneration of dopaminergic neurons in the substantia nigra causes the most common form of Parkinson's disease.

Serotonin

Serotonin (5-hydroxytryptamine or 5-HT) is an indoleamine. It is made from the amino acid L-tryptophan in a two-step process. Tryptophan hydroxylase is the first, and rate-limiting, enzyme in the process; it can be blocked by parachloro-phenylalanine.

The storage and release of serotonin are similar to those processes described for norepinephrine and dopamine. The locations of its pathways are more diffuse and its function is less well understood than those of norepinephrine and dopamine.

However, a major component of serotonergic neurons begins in the raphe nuclei of the pons and projects to the thalamus, hypothalamus, hippocampus, cortex, limbic forebrain, and basal ganglia. These neurons are implicated in mood, cognition, eating, slow-wave sleep, motor activity, and release of hormones such as prolactin and adrenocorticotropic hormone. Drugs that affect serotonin transmission have become increasingly im-

Table 2. Drugs That Affect Dopamine Transmission

Transmission Stage	Drug	Effect	Use
Synthesis	L-Dopa	Increases dopamine	Parkinson's Disease
Storage	Reserpine	Depletes dopamine	Hypertension
	MAOIs Phenelzine Deprenyl	Increases dopamine storage, storage, prevents metabolism	Antidepressant
Release	Amphetamine Mazindol Ritalin	Releases dopamine	Stimulant, anorectic
Receptor	Apomorphine	Activates receptors	Emetic
	Bromocriptine		Parkinson's Disease
	Chlorpromazine	Blocks receptors	Antipsychotic, antiemetic, sedative
Uptake	Amphetamine Mazindol	Inhibits uptake	Stimulant

portant in psychiatry and are presented in Table 3.

At least two serotonin receptors have been proposed. The 5-HT$_1$ receptor is preferentially bound by serotonin, appears in many brain regions, and is involved in spinal cord function. The 5-HT$_2$ receptor is affected by many antidepressants including electroconvulsive therapy (ECT); it is blocked by certain antipsychotics and the class of antidepressants that includes mianserin and ketanserin.

Serotonin neurons in the limbic forebrain have a significant interaction with norepinephrine neurons (4). Without intact serotonin neurons, antidepressants such as desipramine (which acts purely on norepinephrine neurons) and ECT would be unable to decrease postsynaptic beta-adrenergic receptor sensitivity, a condition implicated in the antidepressant effect.

Neurotransmitters and Depression

The somatic treatments for depression have many different effects on neurotransmission (5-7). We still do not understand which of these effects account for their therapeutic action. Even if one or several linked biological abnormalities in depression are found to be normalized by antidepressant treatments, the origin of such biological abnormalities may remain unclear. Nevertheless, past and current theories provide a context that enables us to better understand directions of future research and development of more specific treatment approaches.

Affective disorders were first linked to disturbance of monoamine transmission in the 1950s through a series of parallel observations. Researchers noted that reserpine, prescribed for hypertension, produced serious

Table 3. Drugs That Affect Serotonin Transmission

Transmission Stage	Drug	Effect	Use
Synthesis	L-tryptophan	Increases synthesis	Antidepressant
	Para-chlorophenyl-alanine	Blocks trytophan hydroxylase	No therapeutic use
Storage	Reserpine	Depletes serotonin	Hypertension
	MAOIs	Increases storage, prevents serotonin metabolism	Antidepressent
Release	Fenfluramine	Releases serotonin	Research in autism, anorectic
Receptor	LSD	Stimulates receptors	Hallucinogen
	Methysergide Cyproheptadine	Blocks receptors	Migraine
	Ketanserin	Blocks serotonin (5-HT$_2$)	Research
Uptake	Tricyclics Trazodone Fluoxetine	Inhibits uptake	Antidepressant Antidepressant Experimental antidepressant

depression in some patients. The drug was also found to deplete norepinephrine, dopamine, and serotonin. Furthermore, it was observed that amphetamines elevated mood and indirectly potentiated dopamine and norepinephrine neurons (see Table 1). Iproniazid, which produced mood elevation in patients treated for tuberculosis, was found to elevate monoamine concentrations by blocking the enzyme monoamine oxidase (MAO).

On the basis of these observations, the classic amine hypothesis was constructed. This hypothesis proposed that clinical depression resulted from deficiencies in norepinephrine and/or serotonin and therefore from decreased neuronal activity; in contrast, mania was associated with an excess of these amines. Pharmacologic studies suggested depression could be treated by increasing synaptic levels of norepinephrine and/or serotonin. This goal could be achieved by inhibiting reuptake through acute treatment with tricyclic antidepressants or by decreasing catabolism through inhibition of MAO.

Many subsequent observations have not been consistent with this simple, attractive theory. The reuptake-blocking effects of tricyclic antidepressants or MAO inhibitors occur within minutes to hours; the clinical effect may be observed in patients only after several weeks of treatment. The same degree of reuptake inhibition in depressed patients may be associated with a wide range of antidepressant effects.

At the same time, equally effective tricyclic antidepressants vary widely in their ability to inhibit norepinephrine and/or serotonin reuptake, and certain new atypical antidepressants, such as iprindole, trazodone, and mianserin, do not significantly inhibit amine reuptake or inhibit MAO but effectively treat depression. Conversely, amphetamine and cocaine inhibit reuptake but are not effective antidepressants.

These and other deficiencies of the classic theory led researchers to examine postsynaptic processes, such as the coupling of receptors with adenylate cyclase. The most consistent observation is that chronic but not acute treatment with virtually all clinically proven antidepressants reduces functional beta-receptor sensitivity, and usually also reduces the number of beta-adrenergic receptors in animal cortex.

This subsensitivity, or downregulation, of beta receptors has been assumed to be the result of chronic exposure of adrenergic receptor sites to increased levels of norepinephrine. However, some newer antidepressants, such as iprindole, do not directly affect norepinephrine reuptake or metabolism and may act more directly on the postsynaptic cell to reduce beta-receptor sensitivity. No such uniform pattern has been demonstrated for alpha-adrenergic, serotonergic, cholinergic, dopaminergic, or histaminic receptors.

Some antidepressants, such as mianserin, may exert part of their effect on beta-adrenergic receptors by blocking presynaptic alpha$_2$-adrenergic receptors (7). If these autoreceptors are prevented from inhibiting presynaptic neuronal firing and norepinephrine release, higher synaptic levels of norepinephrine could induce subsensitivity in postsynaptic beta-adrenergic receptors.

Somewhat inconsistent results have been obtained for the 5-HT$_2$ group of serotonin receptors. The degree of down-regulation of 5-HT$_2$ receptors is greater than that seen for beta receptors after chronic but not acute exposure to some antidepressants. However, while most antidepressants down-regulate 5-HT$_2$ receptors, ECT actually increases their sensitivity.

If reduction of beta-receptor sensitivity is the major common therapeutic effect of antidepressants, then it could be theorized that depression itself is due to a disorder of a beta-receptor function, such as supersensitivity. Evidence for such a primary receptor abnormality is the subject of studies currently under way.

Recent studies have demonstrated a link between the noradrenergic and serotonergic systems. Desensitization of beta receptors in rats medicated by antidepressants or ECT requires an intact serotonergic system. Consistent with this observation was the report that the antidepressant effect of tricyclics or MAO inhibitors could be reversed by giving patients parachlorophenylalamine, which depletes serotonin. When administered to animals, this drug reverses or prevents the desensitization of beta receptors by tricyclics (see Figure 6).

Although the theory that antidepressants work through 5-HT$_2$ receptors or by desensitizing beta receptors has a simple elegance, it is based largely on pharmacologic studies in animals. Other experimental approaches have produced inconsistent results (5).

Electrophysiological studies have suggested that chronic antidepressant treatment leads to decreased beta-adrenergic responsivity in some areas of the brain, but that it also increases serotonergic and alpha-adrenergic responsivity. Studies of animal behavior (behaviors believed to be related to activity of serotonergic and alpha-adrenergic pathways) tend to show increased serotonergic and alpha-adrenergic function after tricyclic antidepressant treatment.

Neuroendocrine studies (for example, cortisol response to methyl-amphetamine or growth hormone response to clonidine) suggest a pretreatment abnormality in the functioning of alpha-adrenergic receptors in some depressed patients that improves after treatment. To further resolve these findings, our laboratory and others have attempted to develop neuroendocrine models of beta-adrenergic and serotonergic receptor

Figure 6.

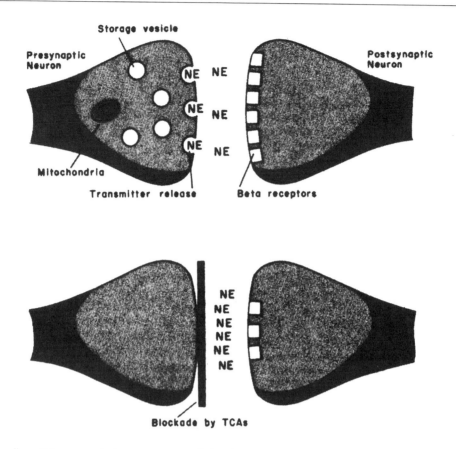

Treatment with tricyclic antidepressants increases synaptic levels of norepinephrine (NE) and eventually reduces the number of postsynaptic receptors.

function and to combine these studies with assays of serotonin and alpha- and beta-adrenergic receptors on blood cells of depressed and healthy subjects.

The study of the neurochemical basis of depression is further complicated by the probability that there are several subgroups of depressive disorders. A "hyperadrenergic" group is apparently marked by elevated urinary levels of cortisol and 3-methoxy-4-hydroxyphenylglycol (MHPG), the metabolite of norepinephrine; elevated MHPG in spinal fluid; and elevated blood levels of norepinephrine, cortisol, and possibly epinephrine (8,9).

Although the high norepinephrine levels of these depressive disorders serve to down-regulate peripheral beta receptors, they probably do not comparably downregulate central beta receptors. Drugs that produce further down-regulation of beta receptors could thereby be antidepressants.

A second group of depressive disorders is marked by apparently normal levels of peripheral adrenergic activity. This group may be accompanied by either unstable control of norepinephrine function (amplified by other-

wise normal fluctuations of serotonin activity) or perhaps deficient serotonergic function (10).

In fact, impaired serotonergic function has been linked to suicidal behavior, not only among depressive patients but among other diagnostic groups. There have been few studies of central serotonergic function in depression other than studies of 5-hydroxyindoleacetic acid (5-HIAA) in cerebrospinal fluid. The data indicate that there may be a subgroup of depressed patients with reduced levels of 5-HIAA in cerebrospinal fluid (11), and that among patients with schizophrenia, alcoholism, and depression, reduced levels correlate with increased suicidal behavior (12,13).

Studies of suicide victims conducted by our laboratory and others have found reduced levels of 5-HIAA in cerebrospinal fluid and fewer imipramine-binding sites in the brain; these studies also found a corresponding increase in 5-HT_2 binding sites in the victims' brains (14-16). Other findings include reduced platelet serotonin uptake in patients with melancholia (17) and reduced platelet imipramine-binding in depressive patients (18). Generally neuroendocrine-challenge tests have shown reduced serotonergic function after administration of oral fenfluramine (19) and intravenous L-tryptophan (20), but increased cortisol response to oral 5-hydroxytryptophan in both depressed patients and patients who have panic attacks correlated with suicidal tendencies (21).

A third hypoadrenergic group of depressed patients with low levels of urinary MHPG may also exist (10). These patients appear to respond preferentially to the most potent norepinephrine reuptake blockers—desipramine, imipramine, and maprotiline. An approach aimed at the biochemical subclassification of depression may aid treatment selection, since it may explain why some clinically similar patients respond differently to noradrenergic drugs, such as desipramine or maprotiline, than they do to serotonergic drugs, such as trazodone.

Other interesting possibilities include evidence implicating not only norepinephrine or serotonin but dopamine in bipolar depression and mania (22,23). Clinical links between depression and anxiety have long been established. Recently GABA has been implicated in nonepisodic anxiety and depression in humans. The interaction of GABA with norepinephrine and serotonin systems is being studied in animal models of depression and in animals treated with antidepressants (24).

Neurotransmitters and Schizophrenia

No single theory is adequate to explain the etiology and pathophysiology of the heterogeneous syndrome of schizophrenia (25-28). However, the central theory is the dopamine hypothesis. This hypothesis proposes that acute positive symptoms of schizophrenia (such as delusions, hallucinations and thought disorder) are caused by excessive dopaminergic activity in the mesolimbic and mesocortical dopamine tract.

Excessive dopaminergic activity could be due to increased dopamine synthesis, increased dopamine release or turnover, or an increase in the number or activity of dopamine receptors. The neurochemical correlates of the negative symptoms (such as poverty of speech, blunted affect, and avolition) are less clear and could be due to decreased dopamine turnover and/or release, perhaps at the frontal lobe or sites other than the areas that influence positive symptoms (for example, the limbic system).

The bases for this theory were developed during the 1950s and 1960s. In 1952 Delay and Deniker noted the specific antipsychotic activity of chlorpromazine (25). In 1958 it was noted that amphetamine could induce a paranoid psychosis similar to acute schizophrenia. This effect was later shown to be related to dopamine release and thus could be prevented by neuroleptics.

In 1963 Carlsson and Lindquist discovered that neuroleptics enhanced presynaptic turnover of dopamine and increased dopaminergic neuronal firing (25). They suggested this might be due to dopamine-receptor blockade. In the 1970s it was shown that clinical potencies of the antipsychotics correlated with their ability to bind to the D_2 receptor. Although some evidence exists that elevated brain levels of transmitters, such as norepinephrine, may play a role in schizophrenia, it is widely accepted that the therapeutic effect of neuroleptics partly depends on their ability to block postsynaptic dopamine receptors.

More recently it has been found that certain antipsychotics, particularly thioridazine, are quite potent calcium-channel blockers. However, the converse does not apply since drugs such as verapamil, a calcium-channel blocker used as an antiarrhythmic, are not dopamine-receptor antagonists.

The possible implications of this newly discovered property of the antipsychotics is that blockade of the calcium channel may contribute to the side effect of erectile impotence (through interference with vas deferens contraction), the arrhythmogenic side effect of antipsychotics, and perhaps part of the antipsychotic or antimanic action of these drugs.

Is there a primary lesion in dopamine neurotransmission in schizophrenia? If so, does it occur during synthesis, metabolism, release, receptor, or postreceptor processes? Among schizophrenic patients no abnormality, such as in tyrosine hydroxylase, has yet been found in the synthesis steps. Our laboratory and others have shown that the repeated finding of low platelet MAO activity among schizophrenic patients is actually an artifact of previous neuroleptic treatment.

Studies of dopamine, its receptors, its metabolite homovanillic acid (HVA) in the cerebrospinal fluid, and postmortem dopamine levels have been inconclusive. One postmortem study of schizophrenic patients found no evidence of increased dopamine turnover (26). More recently, however, another group has found increased dopamine concentration in the basal ganglia and limbic forebrain of young patients; this concentration was not related to previous neuroleptic treatment (29).

Assays of dopamine receptors in postmortem brain samples from schizophrenic patients have consistently shown increased concentrations of D_2 but not D_1 receptors (26,29). These effects can be produced by antipsychotics, however. We still cannot determine whether D_2 receptors are increased in the brains of schizophrenic patients who are not currently receiving medication, because of our uncertainty over how long the effects of prior medication persist.

Poor prognosis and increasing severity of schizophrenic negative symptoms have been associated with lower levels of HVA and evidence of cerebral atrophy. At least two studies (30,31) have shown an association between large ventricles and lower levels of HVA in cerebrospinal fluid. One of these studies found decreased HVA associated with decreased 5-HIAA in subjects with large ventricles.

Crow (26) divided schizophrenia into Type I and Type II. Type I schizophrenia was characterized by positive symptoms such as hallucinations, delusions, incongruent mood, thought disorder, and catatonia. These patients responded to neuroleptics. Patients with Type II schizophrenia showed negative symptoms, neurostructural changes, and nondopaminergic pathology, and responded poorly to neuroleptics.

There is considerable evidence that noradrenergic hyperfunction is also associated with schizophrenia (31, 32). Antipsychotic drugs perturb brain norepinephrine function. Four groups have shown that schizophrenic patients had increased levels of norepinephrine in the limbic forebrain at autopsy. Two groups have found increased levels of norepinephrine in the cerebrospinal fluid of schizophrenic patients. Another study showed that clinical response to neuroleptics was associated with a decrease in cerebrospinal fluid levels of norepinephrine.

Decreased activity of the enzyme DBH has been associated with a better response to neuroleptics (33). In another study DBH levels correlated positively with enlarged ventricles and decreased levels of HVA in cerebrospinal fluid (30). A clonidine challenge of norepinephrine function found decreased activity of central inhibitory presynaptic alpha$_2$-adrenergic receptors in schizophrenic patients (32). Using a peripheral platelet model for these central receptors, another group found decreased alpha-adrenergic receptor function in schizophrenic men (34).

Abnormal serotonin transmission has been suggested as an etiological factor in schizophrenia, but no consistent findings have emerged (26). Because LSD psychosis bears some resemblance to schizophrenia and LSD blocks serotonin receptors, investigators have postulated that the serotonergic system plays a role in schizophrenia. However, other serotonin antagonists do not produce psychosis (2,35).

Various studies have reported both increased and decreased levels of 5-HIAA in cerebrospinal fluid. Serotonin receptors in schizophrenic patients have shown no consistent, replicable abnormality (35). Both low levels of 5-HIAA in cerebrospinal fluid (36) and increased blood levels of serotonin (37) have been found in separate studies of schizophrenic patients with enlarged ventricles. Such studies need further replication to determine whether a deficit in serotonin neurotransmission applies to all or only a subset of schizophrenic patients.

Investigators have speculated that other putative neurotransmitters or neuromodulators (usually modulators of dopamine and/or norepinephrine activity) play a role in psychosis. Examples of such substances include opioid peptides, GABA, prostaglandins, acetylcholine, histamine, phenethylamines, cholecystokinin, vasoactive intestinal peptide, and somatostatin (38-40). However, no consistent evidence has yet emerged that links these transmitters and neuromodulators with abnormal function in schizophrenic patients or with the therapeutic actions of antipsychotic drugs.

Overall, the evidence links schizophrenia with disturbance of monoaminergic transmission, particularly dopaminergic. Damage to these tracts by genetic, viral, and/or autoimmune processes could lead to the clinical syndrome of schizophrenia; in some cases such damage could cause the increased gliosis found in neuropathological examination of periventricular regions (41) and the neuronal cell loss with compensatory increase in apparent ventricular size as revealed by computer tomography (31).

Conclusions

Knowledge of these general aspects of neural transmission will enable the clinician to fit further scientific advances into an organized context. Future studies in some depressive subtypes may identify correctable defects at a molecular level. Schizophrenia research has thus far been unable to transcend the dopamine hypothesis, which appears to explain only part of the disorder's psychopathology and the action of antipsychotics. Further research into schizophrenia may benefit most from a creative synthesis of advances in neurophysiology, neurochemistry, and neuroradiologic imaging (with a dash of serendipitous clinical observation).

Receptor techniques have been particularly fruitful in suggesting a possible common mechanism of action for somatic antidepressant treatments. This mechanism, delayed down-regulation of beta receptors, requires the presence of an intact serotonergic system. Such findings need to be confirmed in depressed human subjects and may disclose the biochemical basis of depressive disorders.

Thus laboratory studies are having a greater impact on clinical practice, by furthering our understanding of how psychotropic drugs work and by revealing potential neurochemical substrates of the major psychiatric syndromes. Mental health professionals will find it increasingly important to follow these laboratory developments in coming years.

References

1. Shaw DM, Kellam AMP, Mottram RF: Brain Sciences in Psychiatry. London, Butterworth Scientific, 1982

2. Kruk ZL, Pycock C: Neurotransmitters and Drugs, 2nd ed. Baltimore, University Park Press, 1983

3. Snyder SH: Drug and neurotransmitter receptors in the brain. Science 224:22-31, 1984

4. Sulser F: Deamplification of noradrenergic signal transfer by antidepressants: a unified catecholamine-serotonin hypothesis of active disorders. Psychopharmacology Bulletin 19:300-304, 1983

5. Brown RP, Mann JJ: Current theories of antidepressant action and the biochemical basis of depression. Journal of Clinical Psychiatry (in press)

6. Charney DS, Menkes DB, Heninger GR: Receptor sensitivity and the mechanism of action of antidepressant treatment. Archives of General Psychiatry 38:1160-1180, 1981

7. Hauger RL, Paul SM: Neurotransmitter receptor plasticity: alterations by antidepressants and antipsychotics. Psychiatric Annals 13:399-407, 1983

8. Schatzberg AF, Orsulak PJ, Rosenbaum AH, et al: Toward a biochemical classification of depressive disorders, V: heterogeneity of unipolar depressions. American Journal of Psychiatry 139:471-475, 1982

9. Carroll BJ, Feinberg M, Greden JF, et al: A specific laboratory test for the diagnosis of melancholia. Archives of General Psychiatry 38:15-22, 1981

10. Schildkraut JJ, Orsulak PJ, Schatzberg AF, et al: Toward a biochemical classification of depressive disorders, I: differences in urinary excretion of MHPG and other catecholamine metabolites in clinically defined subtypes of depression. Archives of General Psychiatry 35:1427-1433, 1978

11. Traskman L, Asberg M, Bertilsson L, et al: Monoamine metabolites in CSF and suicidal behavior. Archives of General Psychiatry 38:631-636, 1981

12. Banki CM, Arato M: Amine metabolites and neuroendocrine responses related to depression and suicide. Journal of Affective Disorders 5:223-232, 1983

13. Ninan PT, van Kammen DP, Scheinin M, et al: CSF 5-hydroxyindoleacetic acid levels in suicidal schizophrenic patients. American Journal of Psychiatry 141:566-569, 1984

14. Stanley M, Virgilio J, Gershon S: Tritiated imipramine binding sites are decreased in the frontal cortex of suicides. Science 216:1337-1339, 1982

15. Stanley M, Mann JJ: Increased serotonin$_2$ binding sites in frontal cortex of suicide victims. Lancet 1:214-216. 1983

16. Stanley M, Mann JJ, Gershon S: Alterations in pre- and postsynaptic serotonergic neurons in suicide victims. Psychopharmacology Bulletin 19:684-687, 1983

17. Kaplan RD, Mann JJ: Altered platelet serotonin uptake kinetics in schizophrenia and melancholia. Life Sciences 31:583-588, 1982

18. Briley MS, Langer SZ, Raisman R, et al: ^{3}H-Imipramine binding sites are decreased In platelets of untreated depressed patients. Science 209:303-305, 1980

19. Murphy DL, Siever LJ, Mueller EA, et al: Serotonergic challenges with fenfluramine, L-tryptophan, and m-chlorphenylpiperazine in humans and monkeys: effect on plasma prolactin and cortisol. Absracts of the annual meeting of the American College of Neuropsychopharmacology, San Juan, Puerto Rico, Dec 1983

20. Heninger GR, Charney DS, Sternberg DE: Serotonergic function in depression. Archives of General Psychiatry 41:399-402, 1984

21. Meltzer HY, Perline R, Tricou BJ, et al: Effect of 5-hydroxytryptophan on serum cortisol levels in major affective disorders. Archives of General Psychiatry 41:379-387, 1984

22. Halaris AE: Evidence in support of a role of dopamine in affective illness. Psychopharmacology Bulletin 18:31-34, 1982

23. Randrup A, Munkvad I, Fog R: Mania, depression, and brain dopamine: overview. Psychopharmacology Bulletin 18:35-36, 1982

24. Sherman AD, Henn F: Is there a locus of antidepressant activity? in Depression and Antidepressants. Edited by Friedman E, Mann JJ, Gershon S. New York, Plenum Press (in press)

25. Haracz JL: The dopamine hypothesis: an overview of studies with schizophrenic patients. Schizophrenia Bulletin 8:438-469, 1982

26. Crow TJ: Two dimensions of pathology in schizophrenia: dopaminergic and nondopaminergic. Psychopharmacology Bulletin 18:22-29, 1982

27. Deutsch SI, Davis KL: Schizophrenia: a review of diagnostic and biological issues, II: biological issues. Hospital and Community Psychiatry 34:423-437, 1983

28. Sayed Y, Garrison JM: The dopamine hypothesis of schizophrenia and the antagonistic action of neuroleptic drugs: a review. Psychopharmacology Bulletin 19:283-288, 1983

29. MacKay AVP, Iversen LL, Rossor M, et al: Increased brain dopamine and dopamine receptors in schizophrenia. Archives of General Psychiatry 39:991-997, 1982

30. Van Kammen DP, Mann LS, Sternberg DE, et al: Dopamine-beta-hydroxylase activity and homovanillic acid in spinal fluid of schizophrenics with brain atrophy. Science 220:974-977, 1983

31. Nyback H, Berggren B-M, Hindmarsh T, et al: Cerebroventricular size and cerebrospinal fluid monoamine metabolites in schizophrenic patients and healthy volunteers. Psychiatry Research 9:301-308, 1983

32. Sternberg DE, Charney DS, Heninger GR, et al: Impaired presynaptic regulation of norepinephrine in schizophrenia. Archives of General Psychiatry 39:285-289, 1982

33. Sternberg DE, van Kammen DP, Lerner P, et al: Schizophrenia: dopamine betahydroxylase activity and treatment response. Science 216:1423-1425, 1982

34. Kafka MS, van Kammen DP: Alpha-adrenergic receptor function in schizophrenia. Archives of General Psychiatry 40:264-270, 1983

35. Whitaker PM, Crow TJ, Ferrier IN: Tritiated LSD binding in frontal cortex in schizophrenia. Archives of General Psychiatry 38:278-280, 1981

36. Potkin SC, Weinberger DR, Linnoila M, et al: Low CSF 5-hydroxyindoleacetic acid in schizophrenic patients with enlarged cerebral ventricles. American Journal of Psychiatry 140:21-25, 1983

37. Delisi LE, Neckers LM, Weinberger DR, et al: Increased whole blood serotonin concentration in chronic schizophrenic patients. Archives of General Psychiatry 38:647-650, 1981

38. Meldrum B: GABA and acute psychoses. Psychological Medicine 12:1-5, 1982

39. Domino E: Quo vadis: biology of schizophrenia. Psychopharmacology Bulletin 18:21-22, 1982

40. Rotrosen J, Miller AD, Mandio D, et al: Prostaglandins, platelets, and schizophrenia. Archives of General Psychiatry 37:1047-1054, 1980

41. Stevens JR: Neuropathology of schizophrenia. Archives of General Psychiatry 39:1131-1139, 1982

Chapter 56

A Team Approach to Pharmacologic Treatment of Chronic Schizophrenia

Samuel J. Keith, MD

Shirley Starr

Susan Matthews

Our therapeutic approach to the schizophrenic patient involves interaction between the patient, the family or significant other, and the clinician. In describing this model, we will provide examples that illustrate the pharmacologic aspects of treating schizophrenia because they are relatively uncomplicated.

We do not mean to imply, however, that our therapeutic principles should be confined only to the pharmacologic component of treatment. On the contrary, we feel they apply equally well to the psychosocial dimensions of treatment. Our separation of the pharmacologic and psychosocial treatment modalities is artificial and for illustrative purposes only. We will also present a conceptual organization for schizophrenia that makes use of the available clinical armamentarium and the mechanisms available for delivering these treatments.

The approach to schizophrenia that we have found most helpful was first presented by Strauss and associates (1) in 1974. Drawing from the Hughlings Jackson evolution-dissolution theory, they developed a compelling data base of precursors and prognostic factors that divided problems associated with schizophrenia into three groups: positive symptoms, negative symptoms, and disorders of interpersonal relationships.

Positive symptoms referred to symptoms that characterize schizophrenia by their presence—hallucinations and delusions—or the category A symptoms as defined in the third edition of the *Diagnostic and Statistical Manual of Mental Disorders* (DSM-III). Negative symptoms referred to those symptoms that characterize schizophrenia by their absence—lack of goal-directed behavior, blunting of affect, and verbal paucity—similar to DSM-III symptom categories B (deteriorating from a prior level of functioning) or C (the prodromal or residual symptoms).

Disordered interpersonal relationships referred to patterns of asociality, withdrawal, and lack of close personal ties, a more specific explication of DSM-III dysfunction criteria. A subtle but significant emphasis of the report by Strauss and associates was the importance of both the negative symptoms and the impaired interpersonal relationships in the "premorbid" or "prepositive" symptom-onset states. Thus Strauss and associates laid the groundwork for distinguishing negative symptoms that precede the onset of the diagnosable disorder from the defect stage that may result from a gradual withdrawal from functioning and is a residual of the disorder. Their data supported the following conclusions:

Positive symptoms:

- Develop over a short period of time and are state specific.
- Represent a reaction to either biological or socioenvironmental factors.
- Contribute little to overall prognosis.

Negative symptoms:

- Develop over an extended period of time before or after the appearance of the positive symptoms.
- Represent either the source of chronicity (for example, poor premorbid adjustment) or the result of chronicity (for example, deteriorating course).
- Contribute considerably to overall prognosis.

Disordered interpersonal relationships:

- Develop over an extended period of time, frequently in the premorbid state, but may become acute with the onset of positive symptoms or of their prodrome or may deteriorate over the course of the disorder.
- Represent an interactive process between inherent social skills of the patient, the destructive impact of the positive symptoms, and the environmental response patterns.
- Account for important aspects of prognosis in terms of predicting future social functioning, but also interact with positive and negative symptoms in determining the pattern of the patient's eventual outcome.

Application of our current treatment modalities and delivery mechanisms to this conceptual framework offers the possibility of achieving realistic treatment expectations and the rationale for the best possible delivery mechanism.

Before we discuss psychopharmacologic principles for the treatment of schizophrenia, it is important to consider why the modality is used. Well-designed, rigorous clinical trials of neuroleptics have produced an impressive body of data supporting their efficacy. Few clinicians would question that positive symptoms are profoundly affected by pharmacologic treatments. Further, controlled studies of maintenance chemotherapy have demonstrated a decided advantage over placebo treatment in preventing the recurrence of positive symptoms (2).

The distinct advantage of neuroleptic therapy is the ability to control the flagrant psychotic symptoms of schizophrenia. Patients who respond to neuroleptics (unfortunately, a small but significant group of people do not respond) have the potential to become free of psychotic symptoms. At this point in our understanding of schizophrenia, such a reduction of positive symptoms becomes a sine qua non for any treatment directed at the negative symptoms or disordered interpersonal rela-

tionships. We take this position even though we fully acknowledge that positive symptoms are the least enduring and the least prognostic aspect of schizophrenia.

Positive symptoms are the most characteristic, dramatic, and frightening aspect of the illness because they are clearly incongruous with normal behavior and experience. We can conceptualize negative symptoms and disordered interpersonal relationships as being at the lowest functioning end of a spectrum of normal behavior. Therapists who do not share our concept of schizophrenia feel that these negative symptoms are clearly under volitional control, representing "laziness" or some equally undesirable attribute of the patient. Thus the patient is blamed for having these symptoms, and the family is placed under increasing pressure to motivate the patient to overcome them.

A Comprehensive Treatment Strategy

We believe both positive and negative symptoms are inherent in schizophrenic disorders. The latter, however, are not responsive to our current medications, whereas positive symptoms are usually alleviated by such treatment, indicating that a dichotomous approach is necessary in developing a comprehensive treatment strategy for schizophrenia.

The reduction of positive symptomatology is an absolutely necessary first step in treatment. Although a few dedicated and talented clinicians work in settings where regressed behavior and florid symptomatology are accepted as relevant to therapeutic recovery (see Mosher [3], for example), most of us find it difficult to address issues of negative symptoms and social competence in the presence of florid symptoms. In two previous reviews (4,5) we have emphasized that recovery from schizophrenia is not synonymous with recovery from positive symptomatology. Unless we find new drugs that directly affect negative symptoms and disordered interpersonal relationships and that do not simply create a baseline state, without which improvement is unlikely to occur, we must rely on psychosocial interventions to provide the necessary impetus for improvement. In our approach to the schizophrenic patient, we emphasize that all aspects of the disorder require treatment. Blame, guilt, and disparagement have no place in this therapeutic compendium.

The results achieved through the pharmacologic treatment of positive symptoms are impressive. The management of these acute symptom periods is relatively well understood: a therapeutic dosage of neuroleptic medication will generally bring these symptoms under control in a short period of time. Indeed, if the pharmacological treatment of schizophrenia were as straightforward and uncomplicated as may have been implied by our presentation thus far, we would have difficulty justifying our initial premise that the treatment of schizophrenia requires an interactive process involving the patient, the family, and the clinician.

We know now that the benefits gained through our current pharmacologic treatments are not without a price. The disadvantages of this treatment modality include side effects and the risk of interference with improvement in negative symptoms and interpersonal relationships.

Of the many side effects involved with the administration of neuroleptics, the short-term effects may be uncomfortable and lead to patient noncompliance; nevertheless, they are generally tolerable and treatable. Twenty percent of patients treated with neuroleptics are at risk of developing long-term tardive dyskinesia, however. Disguised onset and lack of effective treatment make tardive dyskinesia the subject of intense investigation and innovative pharmacologic strategies.

The second disadvantage, interference with improvement in negative symptoms and interpersonal relationships, is less well established by scientific evidence and rests with clinical impressions. For example, on a clinical basis, the psychomotor retardation frequently observed in patients receiving neuroleptics is not only a drug side effect but also a component of the negative symptom complex. And the patient's family members consider the negative symptoms of schizophrenia a major problem (6). Thus the avoidance of iatrogenic symptoms must assume therapeutic primacy.

Several new strategies have been developed to offset the undesirable aspects of pharmacologic treatment. All involve the reduction of dosage. Kane and associates (7) have tested a one-fifth dosage strategy, Carpenter and associates (8) are testing an approach called targeted medication, and Herz and associates (9) are using a strategy called intermittent medication.

Each group of researchers is exploring the potential benefits of lowering the overall level of medication in an attempt to find the best compromise between the prevention of relapse, the reduction of side effects, and the improvement in negative symptoms and interpersonal relationships. Just as full medication (standard or high dose) has its unwanted aspects, these newer reduced-dosage strategies also have disadvantages. The disadvantages can be remedied, but only through the cooperation of the patient, the family, and the clinician.

A Therapeutic Alliance

In both full-medication and reduced-dosage strategies the major risk is patient relapse, an exacerbation of positive symptoms. The risk of relapse can be reduced through the early identification of prodromal signs; in such preventive measures the interaction of the patient, the family, and the clinician becomes crucial. The clinician can use his or her broad base of knowledge to identify general areas that should be considered in predicting relapse. Clinical experience with a wide range of patients, familiarity with the relevant literature on early signs of relapse, and an ability to communicate with the patient and family are critical to the success of treatment. Yet the skills of the clinician must be supplemented by the family's support.

While the clinician is an expert in the treatment of schizophrenia and the conditions involved in relapse, the family must use its specific knowledge of the patient to adapt the clinician's therapeutic recommendations to particular situations. Thus the family provides an important source of information and also adds the perspective of interested observers.

Although the patient may periodically be able to provide information, he or she will be unable to provide information during the onset of psychosis. Yet the patient should not become the forgotten element in our proposed therapeutic alliance. Quite the contrary, the patient's assistance must be elicited in providing necessary information so that all parties will contribute to the recovery process. Only the patient has direct access to the subtle inner workings of his (or her) mind where the initial signs of psychosis begin. The clinician and family must rely on inferences from observed behavior until the patient is able to trust them and describe the disruptions in the functioning of his (or her) mind.

We feel this concept of the treatment of schizophrenia must be presented to everyone involved when the treatment program begins. The patient, the family, and the clinician must understand that the treatment is the responsibility of all parties, that there will be progress and setbacks during the course of the disorder, and that no one will be called on to accept responsibility or blame. When setbacks occur, the current treatment methods must be examined and modified with input from all members of the treatment alliance. Such interaction should help to avoid or at least reduce the frequently seen, but often denied, demoralization of the patient, the family, and the clinician.

We have presented a conceptual organization for schizophrenia that permits an understanding of the relative importance of differing treatment modalities. This approach minimizes the likelihood of "blaming" behavior on the part of anyone involved in the treatment program. Too often we have observed the destructive effects of blaming: the loss of patient morale, the feeling of failure on the part of the family, and the feeling of inadequacy on the part of the clinician. None of these effects can possibly contribute to positive outcomes.

Our proposed team approach to the treatment of schizophrenia requires the active participation of the patient, the family, and the clinician. The importance of this approach in maintaining positive symptom remission by pharmacologic treatment may be most dramatically exemplified through the new reduced-dose strategies. These strategies have the advantage of reducing the likelihood of side effects and the possible detrimental impact on negative symptoms of full-dose strategies. However, they also increase the risk of relapse, and thus heighten the need for early intervention. The team approach appears to be the most efficient way to ensure early intervention.

As the patient, the family, and the clinician negotiate the initial treatment contracts, they should keep these principles in mind. The requirements are that we combine an ability to educate with an ability to learn, a giving of support with an acceptance of support, and a need to understand with a need to be understood.

References

1. Strauss JC, Carpenter WT Jr, Bartko JJ: Speculations on the processes that underlie schizophrenic signs and symptoms, III. Schizophrenia Bulletin 1:61-69, 1974

2. David JM, Schaffer CB, Killian GA et al: Important issues in the drug treatment of schizophrenia. Schizophrenia Bulletin 6:70-87, 1980

3. Mosher LR: Research design to evaluate psychosocial treatments of schizophrenia, in Psychotherapy of Schizophrenia. Edited by Rubenstein D, Alanen YO. Amsterdam, Excerpta Medica Foundation, 1972

4. Keith SJ, Matthews SM: Group, family, and milieu therapies and psychosocial rehabilitation in the treatment of the schizophrenic disorders, in Psychiatry Update, vol 1. Edited by Grinspoon L. Washington, DC, American Psychiatric Press, 1982

5. Williams JBW, Spitzer RL (eds): Psychotherapy Research: Where Are We and Where Should We Go? New York, Guilford, 1984

6. Schulz PM, Schulz SC, Dibble E, et al: Patient and family attitudes about schizophrenia: implications for genetic counseling. Schizophrenia Bulletin 8:504-513, 1982

7. Kane JM, Rifkin A, Woerner M, et al: Low-dose neuroleptics in outpatient schizophrenics. Psychopharmacology Bulletin 18:20-21, 1982

8. Carpenter WT Jr, Stephens JH, Rey AC, et al: Early intervention vs continuous pharmacotherapy of schizophrenia. Psychopharmacology Bulletin 18:21-23, 1982

9. Herz MI, Szymanski HV, Simon J: An intermittent medication for stable schizophrenic outpatients: an alternative to maintenance medication. American Journal of Psychiatry 139:918-922, 1982

Chapter 57

Effects of Psychotropic Drugs on the Occupational Therapy Process

Doris A. Smith, MEd, OTR

Since the late 1950s the majority of mental health clients who have received occupational therapy were also receiving one or more psychotropic drugs. What effect have these drugs had on patients and on the occupational therapy evaluation and treatment process?

Some of these effects will be explored here, along with a brief review of the therapeutic and side (adverse) effects of the antipsychotic (neuroleptic or major tranquilizer) drugs. A hypothetical group of patients will be described to illustrate some of the behaviors, activities, settings, and media that the occupational therapist should consider as he/she evaluates, plans, and carries out treatment with a client (clients) who is (are) taking an antipsychotic drug.

Psychotropic drugs include any drug that affects psychic function and behavior. Antipsychotic, antidepressive, antimanic, and antianxiety drugs comprise the four major groups of psychotropic drugs currently in use. Until the introduction of these new drugs in the mid-1950s, there had been a steady increase in hospitalized mental patients until there were approximately 560,000 patients in state and local government hospitals in the U.S. in 1955 (Freedman, et al., 1976, pp. 943-4). Twelve years later, in 1967, due mainly to drug therapy, this population had decreased to 426,000 (Freedman, et al., 1976, p. 944), and by 1974 it declined to 216,000 (Ethridge, 1976, p. 624). This decline has continued due to improvements in drug therapy, client's subsequent responsiveness to other therapies (including occupational therapy), increases in community mental health services, new mental health codes, and recent judicial and legislative decisions which have recognized the individual's right to treatment and to the least restrictive environment for treatment.

Although psychotropic drugs rarely produce a cure, they usually benefit the patient by diminishing the symptoms of the disorder. For example, the schizophrenic patient receiving an antipsychotic drug usually shows less of the following symptoms: thought disorder, blunted affect, withdrawal, hallucinations, delusions, hostility, and resistiveness, with no loss and usually marked improvement in cognitive functions (Freedman, 1976).

This improvement has enabled the patient who is receiving drug therapy to be more responsive to occupational therapy. This ability to respond has been noted in the literature. Kline and Davis (1973, p. 54) wrote, "Not only did drugs come into widespread use, but such other modalities as psychotherapy and group, family, occupational and recreational therapies were used to a greater extent, mostly because patients on drug therapy were able to take part in and benefit from these therapies." Freedman, et al. (1976, p. 943) in their textbook for psychiatrists note that "The fact that clinically significant therapeutic effects could be produced by a drug created an atmosphere that emphasized positive treatment and led to the vigorous application of milieu therapy, psychotherapy, group therapy and occupational therapy."

Despite the positive effects on 70% to 80% of patients who receive psychotropic drugs (Clark, et al., 1979) and the increased demand for occupational therapy and increased ability of patients to respond to our services, there are many disturbing side effects that we observe in our patients who receive drug therapy. What can occupational therapists do when they observe the negative effects of drugs?

Three recent books (Bockar, 1976; Goldsmith, 1977; and Irons, 1978) written for mental health professionals emphasized the need for awareness of side effects of psychotropic drugs so that these can be reported to the physician. Goldsmith (1977, pp. vii-viii) says the mental health worker "...should be prepared to refer a patient for medication and to monitor drugs' actions between contacts with the prescribing physician." He goes on to say "...their observations may be crucial to the doctor who makes these decisions." Bockar (1976), in her introduction, states as the purpose of her book a need for a developing awareness by nonmedical psychotherapists of the effects of drugs, because the M.D. prescribing the drugs rarely sees the patient, and the patient and M.D. need the shared observations of the nonmedical professional to obtain the best treatment. One book, *Occupational Therapy*, refers to psychotropic drugs and that one (Hopkins and Smith, 1978, p. 296) devotes one paragraph and a small inset (listing four major medication groups and possible side effects) to this subject. Tiffany, who authored this chapter, says, "The therapist who works with clients who are receiving medication needs to be aware of the possibility of side effects. In addition to the fact that side effects may be extremely troublesome and upsetting to the client, it is essential that they be monitored closely, so that changes in medication will be made when necessary."

Noting and reporting side effects that occur in one's clients is an important contribution that a therapist should and does make, but there are other important considerations for the therapist working with a client or group of clients who are on psychotropic drugs. These center around the following questions. How does this drug affect the person's ability to function in daily activities and in relationships with others? How do specific drugs, such as mellaril, thorazine, haldol, valium, cylert,

tofranil, with both the therapeutic and side effects, influence the behaviors and syndromes that the therapist observes during evaluations? How will the drug affect goals for the client, and activities, settings and media that will be selected for treatment? How can the occupational therapist design treatment to capitalize on the therapeutic effects of the drug the client is receiving and diminish the negative side effects?

These questions will be explored here relative only to the antipsychotic drugs, although these are questions that can apply to any of the other psychotropic drugs.

The antipsychotic drugs, also known as neuroleptics, major tranquilizers, and antischizophrenic drugs, have the capacity to modify affective states without seriously impairing cognitive function. The major gains from these drugs are noted within the first six weeks, and gains can continue up to 12 to 18 months. Some of the positive effects are a decrease in psychotic thinking; there is a decrease in projection, delusions, suspiciousness, perplexity, ideas of reference, and hallucinations. There is a normalization of psychomotor behavior; the hyperactive client is less active and the retarded, slow patient is more alert. The client becomes more responsive (with more affect) and cooperative with increased interest in and response to the environment and other people.

The major toxic reactions to these agents are the extrapyramidal syndromes: Parkinsonism, akasthesia, and tardive dyskinesia. According to Sovner (1978, p. 2) recent studies indicate that tardive dyskinesias (abnormal movements of any part of the body) occur in 40% to 55% of patients who have received moderate to high doses of antipsychotic drugs for a year or more. Therefore, tardive dyskinesia is a syndrome that one is likely to observe when working with clients who receive antipsychotic drugs.

In a pamphlet published by Sandoz Pharmaceuticals to alert persons to signs of tardive dyskinesia, Dr. Sovner (1978, pp. 3 & 9) states that one may first observe tardive dyskinesia during a drug holiday, since antipsychotic drugs tend to suppress its clinical signs. It is also most apparent when the client is emotionally aroused and is least apparent during sleep. Early detection is crucial since the earlier the drug dose is reduced or discontinued, the more likely there will be a resolution of this syndrome or a decrease in its severity. A simple method called the "AIMS examination procedure" is described in this pamphlet and is a measure that can be used in the occupational therapist's assessment. There is also reference to a 17-minute film (p. 1) produced by Sandoz Pharmaceuticals. This pamphlet has other information that should be useful for therapists who are working with clients on antipsychotic drugs.

Some other side effects observed in clients who are on neuroleptics that could interfere with daily activities and interpersonal interactions are motor retardation, drooling, tremor, akasthesia (restlessness, inability to sit still, and pacing), akinesia (apathy, blunted affect), dry mouth and throat, weight gain, increased appetite, sedation and drowsiness (especially on large doses), visual changes, sensitivity to the sun, orthostatic hypotension, changes in sexual functions, food aspiration and choking, and many others. These effects vary from individual to individual and vary in intensity or occurrence with different types or compositions of antipsychotic drugs. The books referred to above for allied health professionals, those by Bockar, Goldsmith, and Irons, provide assistance in identifying these differences relative to both therapeutic and side effects of individual drugs.

In order to illustrate the effects that psychotropic drugs can have on the occupational therapy process, a hypothetical group of twelve schizophrenic clients will be considered; each is receiving an antipsychotic drug. Not all of the drugs they are receiving are the same, so it is possible that each person will experience different therapeutic and/or side effects. Also, each person potentially can respond in a unique and unusual manner to a drug. Some may not receive any therapeutic benefits or experience any side effects. For purposes of this discussion, generalizations about these drugs will be made. In actual practice, however, it would be advisable to use a drug reference to identify and determine the potentials (reported effects) of each specific, individual drug in order to enhance the therapeutic effects and to alert the therapist to possible side effects. This will enable the therapist to diminish and sometimes avoid the potential side effects of these drugs.

Relative to the group of twelve clients, assessment of each individual indicates that each of them has many characteristics and manifestations that King described in her article "A Sensory Integrative Approach to Schizophrenia" (1973). These include S-curve posture, immobile shoulder girdle, shuffling gait, weak grip, and internally rotated, adducted and flexed extremities. Following King's recommendations for stimulation of the client's vestibular, proprioceptive and tactile systems, parachute and ball activities will be used. It would seem ideal to conduct these activities out-of-doors where there is adequate space and to design the activities so that each person can bend, turn the head, push and pull against objects, lift the arms overhead and do bilateral activities. What should be considered by the therapist relative to these activities and the drugs the clients are taking?

Because of therapeutic effects of drugs, one might expect that the clients will be able to understand the directions that are given and be receptive to most communication with them. They will probably not be too withdrawn or hostile or involved in their delusions and hallucinations to participate when requested.

Relative to possible side effects of drugs and the activities described above, the therapist should be alerted to some or all of the following considerations:

1) Is the activity near a source of liquid to counteract the dry mouth and throat that so frequently is a side effect? Can water or a low calorie, nonstimulant (non-caffeine) refreshment be provided before and perhaps midway in the activity so that the clients will not be as likely to leave for a Coke or coffee or become uncomfortable because they have a need to relieve this dryness?

2) Are any of the clients on neuroleptics that make them more sensitive to the sun? If so, perhaps sunscreen preparations, long sleeves, a hat, or having the activity indoors will be necessary to adapt to or avoid this possible side effect. The therapist can also minimize the time these persons are out in the sun and observe them closely for reactions to the sun.

3) Will clients be required to bend, to turn their heads, and to lift their arms overhead suddenly as they participate in the parachute and ball activities? These are all activities appropriate to Lorna Jean King's recommendations, but sudden postural changes do occur in them and may result in severe discomfort, dizziness, or even fainting due to orthostatic postural hypotension. This side effect, which is a sudden drop in blood pressure, can occur in patients on neuroleptics. (It is also a serious side effect in patients who take antidepressive drugs.)

4) Will light, soft balls be used to enable clients who have blurred vision and contracted or dilated pupils (any of these can occur with neuroleptics) to be able to follow the flying object and have a chance to catch or hit or kick the ball? This would enable the client to be successful in meeting the objective of the activity, and would provide the success and fun that can lead to continued participation in activities.

5) Will the activity be short enough or allow enough moving about to accommodate to and perhaps interrupt akasthesia, which is restlessness, inability to sit or stand still, and constant pacing? This symptom or side effect often occurs early in drug therapy even before the therapeutic effects occur.

These are only a few of the many possible therapeutic and side effects of drugs and adaptations of activity that should be considered in planning an activity for a client or group of clients who are on neuroleptics. It is possible for occupational therapists, through careful observation and thorough assessment of their clients, to design treatment goals and activities that can enhance the therapeutic effects of psychotropic drugs and to diminish the side effects. Frequently, the therapeutic effects of a drug outweigh the side effects, and the patient will be continued on the drug. When this occurs, it is a challenge to the occupational therapist to enable the client to adapt to these effects and be able to benefit from all forms of therapy and learn to participate more effectively in daily activities and interactions with people.

This [chapter] has explored only a few of the effects of the antipsychotic (neuroleptics) drugs that should be considered by the occupational therapist. There are similar and different effects that occur with the other psychotropic drugs—the antidepressive, antimanic, antianxiety, and cerebral stimulant drugs that should be considered when the occupational therapist evaluates a client and develops and carries out a plan for treatment.

References

Bockar, J. A., *Primer for the Non-Medical Psychotherapist.* Spectrum Publications, New York, 1976.

Clark, M. et al., Drugs and Psychiatry: A New Era, *Newsweek* November 12, 1979. p 98-104.

Ethridge, D. A., The Management View of the Future of Occupational Therapy in Mental Health, *American Journal of Occupational Therapy*, Vol. 30:10, 1976, p. 623-628.

Freedman, A. M., Kaplan, H. I., and Sadock, B. J., *Modern Synopsis of Psychiatry/II.* Williams and Wilkins Company, Baltimore, 1976.

Goldsmith, W., *Psychiatric Drugs for the Non-Medical Mental Health Worker*, Charles C. Thomas, Springfield, Illinois, 1977.

Hopkins, H. L. and Smith, H. D., *Willard and Spackman's Occupational Therapy*, (5th ed.), New York: J. B. Lippincott Company, 1978.

Irons, P. D., *Psychotropic Drugs and Nursing Intervention*, New York: McGraw-Hill Book Company, 1978.

King, L. J., A Sensory-integrative Approach to Schizophrenia, *American Journal of Occupational Therapy*, Vol. 28, 1974, p 529-536.

Kline, N. S. and Davis, J. M., Psychotropic Drugs, *American Journal of Nursing*, Vol. 73:1, 1973, p 54-62.

Sovner, R., *Tardive Dyskinesia: Diagnosis and Management*, Sandoz Pharmaceuticals, 1978 (pamphlet)

Chapter 58

Electroconvulsive Therapy: An Update

C. Edward Coffey, MD

Richard D. Weiner, MD, PhD

"ECT? You mean shock therapy? Do they still do that?"

These questions, which continue to be raised by patients and their families, as well as by our nonpsychiatric colleagues, reflect the ongoing controversy that surrounds electroconvulsive therapy (ECT). Yet despite this history of controversy, ECT has survived, and it has done so primarily because it remains a profoundly effective treatment that continues to evolve into a safer (if not more acceptable) form of therapy.

In 1988 the 50th anniversary of the discovery of ECT was celebrated by international conferences, scientific symposia, and special publications (1). Frequently during those 50 years, panels of scholars have carefully considered whether a role for ECT still exists in contemporary psychiatric practice. One of the most recent of these evaluations was undertaken in June 1985 by a National Institute of Mental Health and National Institutes of Health Consensus Development Panel (2). In agreement with virtually all previous such investigations, the panel concluded that ECT is, when administered properly, a safe and effective procedure for which there continues to be an established clinical need.

Given what appears to be a growing acceptance of this treatment modality, an update on the current practice of ECT and its role in contemporary psychiatry is timely and relevant. This [chapter] will review the historical evolution and present use of ECT, its indications, contraindications, and adverse effects, and what we currently understand about its mechanism of action. We will describe modern ECT technique and will offer recommendations for education and training in this treatment modality, based primarily on recent recommendations by the American Psychiatric Association's task force on ECT (3). Many additional references are available for readers desiring a more comprehensive discussion of this topic (4-6).

Evolution and Present Use

The historical roots of ECT lie in the misconception by early-20th-century neuropsychiatrists that epilepsy and schizophrenia were incompatible (1,7). In 1935 Lazlo Meduna, a Hungarian neuropsychiatrist, used intramuscular injections of camphor oil to elicit seizures in patients with schizophrenia and reported marked improvement in their psychoses. However, camphor was a painful and extremely unreliable technique for inducing seizures, leading Ugo Cerletti and Luciano Bini to develop a technique of seizure induction using an electrical rather than a pharmacologic stimulus. In 1938 they reported the first application of "electroshock therapy," which within two years would largely supplant pharmacoconvulsive therapy and become the dominant form of somatic therapy for major mental disorders.

Eventually, with the development of antidepressant and antipsychotic drug therapy in the mid-1950s, the use of ECT began to wane. This decline may have begun to plateau in recent years, however, with the awareness of the limitations of available psychopharmacologic therapies. Indeed, use of ECT may actually be increasing, as suggested by the growing number of ECT devices, utilization surveys, and citations in the scientific literature (8).

Economic pressures in this era of cost containment and limited insurance coverage may also encourage the use of ECT, especially in view of a recent study in which depressed patients treated with ECT had significantly shorter hospital stays than depressed patients treated with pharmacotherapy and thus realized considerable economic savings (9). Further economic savings may be achieved by administering a course of ECT on an outpatient basis, a practice we find quite feasible for clinically stable patients with social support networks capable of carrying out the appropriate pre- and post-ECT treatment instructions.

Surveys of ECT usage in the 1970s suggested that in this country the therapy was administered primarily by private and university hospitals, typically to white, middle-aged, depressed women (10,11). This pattern of usage appears to continue today. In a recent survey of the southern United States, McCall (12) found that ECT was administered by 89 percent of the university hospitals, 57 percent of the VA hospitals, and 44 percent of private hospitals, but by only 19 percent of state hospitals. Furthermore, state hospitals had discontinued the use of ECT at a higher rate than the other institutions, and no state hospital established since 1970 offered ECT as a treatment option. These data suggest that the poor may have limited access to one of the most effective treatment options in psychiatry.

Clinical Indications for ECT

Major Depression

The primary indication for ECT is major depression, which probably accounts for up to 90 percent of referrals for ECT in this country. Numerous carefully controlled scientific studies have demonstrated that ECT is superior to placebo (sham ECT) in establishing a therapeutic remission—overall response rates with ECT may be 80 percent or greater (5). In studies comparing the efficacy of ECT with that of antidepressant medications, groups receiving ECT have always shown better or at least comparable levels of improvement.

The presence of delusions and a history of favorable response to ECT have been suggested as good prognostic signs, but in fact there are no established clinical or laboratory predictors of response to ECT. Even the presence of melancholic or "endogenous" symptoms may be unrelated to outcome from ECT (13,14). Likewise, some patients with clinical features traditionally felt to predict a poor response to ECT (for example, anxiety, hypochondriasis, long-standing dysthymia, and personality traits of inadequacy, dependency, and "hysteroid dysphoria") may nevertheless show enough clinical improvement with ECT to justify its use when an adequate trial of antidepressant drug therapy has failed.

Need for Faster Onset of Action

ECT has been shown to have a faster onset of action than antidepressant drug therapy and thus should be considered as a first-line therapy when rapid remission is needed, as in patients with severe suicidal potential, catatonia, or marked malnutrition and dehydration (2,5). Although it is a common clinical belief that patients undergoing ECT may be at increased risk of suicide early in the treatment course because they recover their energy before their suicidal impulses are resolved, recent data indicate that suicidal ideation improves significantly faster than energy is recovered, and after fewer ECT treatments (15). Indeed, the Consensus Development Panel stated that "the immediate risk of suicide (when not manageable by other means) is a clear indication for consideration of ECT" (2). Finally, ECT should also be considered as an initial intervention when its anticipated side effects are less than those associated with drug therapy—for example, in the elderly, in patients with heart block, and during pregnancy.

Acute Mania

ECT is also a very effective treatment for acute mania, and recent controlled studies indicate that it may be at least as effective as lithium and may act more rapidly (5,16-18). Thus ECT should be considered for patients with extreme mania who require a rapid remission.

Schizophrenia

Although there is no evidence that ECT is more effective than drug therapy in schizophrenia, schizophrenic patients with catatonia or prominent affective symptoms (as in schizoaffective disorder) may show a good response to ECT treatments. Recent reports that the combination of ECT and neuroleptic medications may be efficacious for drug nonresponders suggest the need for further studies of the use of ECT in schizophrenia (19,20).

Other Disorders

There is no evidence that ECT is effective in the

treatment of other mental disorders such as anxiety, somatoform, or characterologic disorders, although an associated depressive illness may respond to ECT. A variety of organic mental syndromes, including catatonia and delirium from many different causes, may improve with ECT (5). Finally, several reports have suggested that the neurobiological changes associated with ECT may directly benefit a variety of underlying systemic disorders, including intractable epilepsy, certain endocrinopathies, and Parkinson's disease (5, 21).

Relative Contraindications

We believe that there are no absolute contraindications to ECT, only conditions for which there is increased risk. Of greatest concern are patients with increased intracranial pressure secondary to intracerebral masses, along with individuals with markedly fragile myocardial vascular status and those with leaky or otherwise unstable aneurysms. As with any therapy, the potential benefits of ECT must be weighed against the risks of treatment; this comparison is especially critical for patients with those conditions. Still, modifications in treatment technique can often attenuate the risks (21). In addition, it is important to remember that other treatment alternatives, including taking no action at all, carry their own associated morbidity and mortality.

Adverse Effects of ECT

Mortality

The mortality from ECT is quite low, ranging from .002 percent to .004 percent per treatment and from .01 percent to .03 percent per patient (4). These rates compare very favorably with the .01 percent mortality rate from childbirth in the U.S. and are at the bottom of the reported range for anesthesia induction alone (.003 percent to .04 percent).

Cardiovascular Complications

These complications are the main cause of morbidity and mortality associated with ECT, with risk varying as a function of the patient's baseline medical status. The stimulation of the sympathetic nervous system that occurs during the seizure increases pulse, blood pressure, and myocardial oxygen consumption (21,22). Premature ventricular contractions may also be seen during the period of tachycardia (22). Although often quite marked, these changes are typically transient and rarely require intervention unless they persist well beyond seizure termination or are associated with clear evidence of ischemia on electrocardiogram.

For the most part, the risk of cardiac ischemia and arrhythmias can be greatly diminished by optimization of the patient's cardiac status before ECT and by appropriate ECT technique (that is, administration of oxygen before treatment and judicious use of antihypertensive therapy during treatment) (21). Vagalmediated arrhythmias (bradycardia, sinus arrest, and arterial premature contractions) may occur immediately after the electrical stimulus is administered or around the time of seizure termination or both. The occurrence of these vagatonic [sic] arrhythmias can be diminished by the administration of anticholinergic medication, such as atropine or glycopyrrolate, before ECT treatment.

Systemic Effects

Headaches, nausea, and muscle aches and soreness occasionally occur after ECT, but usually respond to supportive management. Other systemic adverse effects—for example, oral trauma, musculoskeletal injuries, bladder rupture, and skin burns—are extremely rare and should not occur when adequate ECT technique is used.

Encephalopathic Effects

The encephalopathic side effects of ECT include transient electroencephalogram (EEG) slowing, a brief period of confusion in the immediate postictal period, and anterograde and retrograde amnesia. The severity and duration of these effects vary considerably among individuals, but are heavily influenced by ECT technique, including the number and frequency of the induced seizures, the anatomic location of the stimulating electrodes, and the electrical intensity of the ECT stimulus (23).

Regardless of severity, both EEG slowing and postictal confusion typically disappear within days to weeks after completion of the ECT course (24, 25). Anterograde amnestic effects also improve rapidly after completion of treatments. Retrograde memory disturbances tend to resolve more slowly, however, and in some cases (for example, with bilateral stimulus electrode placement) a modest degree of spotty memory loss, particularly for autobiographical material, may persist for months or even years. Still, it is uncommon for patients to perceive such effects as problematic (26-29).

Finally, recent studies using computed tomography (CT) and magnetic resonance imaging (MRI) have revealed a surprisingly high prevalence of structural brain abnormalities, such as cortical atrophy and subcortical hyperintensity, in elderly patients referred for ECT (30-36). The potential impact of these brain changes on both the therapeutic and the adverse cognitive effects of ECT is an area in great need of investigation, especially given the frequent use of this treatment modality for elderly depressed patients.

The alterations in cerebral functioning associated with ECT have raised the concern that this treatment may produce structural brain damage. However, neuropathological studies in animals indicate that brain damage does not occur when seizures are induced under conditions that approximate standard clinical ECT practice—that is, when the seizures are relatively brief and infrequent and are modified by oxygenation and muscle relaxation (23, 37). In addition, recent noninvasive human studies—anatomic brain imaging (as by MRI) as well as plasma assays for metabolic byproducts of neuronal injury—have also failed to demonstrate any such effects (36, 38), although measures like this can reflect changes only at the macroscopic level.

Mechanism of Action

The mechanism of action for a therapeutic response to ECT is intimately related to the presence of a generalized seizure. Neither the motor component (convulsion) of the seizure nor its amnestic side effects are related to the beneficial effects of ECT. However, recent data indicate that even eliciting a generalized seizure of a certain minimum duration may not be sufficient to produce a therapeutic effect (39). Identifying markers that distinguish therapeutic from nontherapeutic ECT seizures is an area of active research interest.

The neurobiological mechanisms that underlie the antidepressant effects of the ECT seizure are unknown. Animal studies indicate that electrically induced seizures result in a variety of alterations in neurotransmitter, neuropeptide, and neuroendocrine function, and that many of these changes are similar to those produced by antidepressant drugs (39-41). It remains unclear, however, whether any of these changes are related to the therapeutic effects of ECT treatments in humans.

ECT Technique

Pre-ECT Evaluation

The evaluation of a patient for ECT consists of the demonstration of an appropriate clinical indication and an assessment of pertinent risk factors (4, 5, 21, 42). The pre-ECT work-up must include, therefore, a complete medical and psychiatric history and examination, with a focus on areas of particular relevance to anticipated beneficial or adverse effects with ECT. The laboratory evaluation of patients referred for ECT should routinely include serum electrolytes, hemoglobin or hematocrit or both, and electrocardiogram. Further procedures, such as spine and chest x-rays, EEG, and brain CT or MRI, should be ordered when specifically indicated. Each case should also be reviewed by an anesthesia provider.

Additional consultations should be requested when clinically appropriate, to ensure that the patient's medical status has been optimized.

In general, psychotropic medications should be discontinued before ECT both because there is no evidence that their concurrent use augments the antidepressant efficacy of ECT and because they may produce major adverse effects (as when lithium is combined with ECT) or may interfere with the ability to induce therapeutic seizures (as with benzodiazepines) (43, 44). Finally, ECT is a procedure for which voluntary informed consent is required. Accordingly, an important responsibility of the ECT treatment team is to provide enough information to allow the patient to make an informed decision about ECT versus alternative therapies (45).

Treatment Procedure

The ECT treatment involves a series of electrically induced seizures, usually three per week, administered by a skilled team of personnel (psychiatrist, anesthesia provider, and appropriate nursing staff) granted privileges by their facility to administer ECT. The seizures themselves are induced by the application of a controlled electrical stimulus to the patient's scalp following administration of anticholinergic premedication (when indicated), oxygen, ultrabrief general anesthesia (usually methohexital), and muscle relaxation (usually succinylcholine). Stimulus dosage levels, as well as the location of stimulus electrodes, are chosen on the basis of both beneficial and adverse effects (see below).

Seizure activity is monitored physiologically by EEG to help assure therapeutic potency and to detect the occurrence of prolonged seizures. Similarly, cardiovascular response is monitored to help minimize adverse systemic effects. For patients who are responding to ECT, the treatment course ends when the patient reaches a plateau in therapeutic response, usually by six to 12 treatments.

The most recent modifications in ECT technique have focused on electrode placement, the stimulus wave form, and intensity of the stimulus dosing. Traditionally, the two stimulus electrodes used for ECT have been placed bilaterally over frontotemporal regions (bilateral ECT). Beginning in the 1940s there were claims that unilateral stimulation—placement of both stimulus electrodes over the nondominant cerebral hemisphere—may be associated with fewer cognitive side effects (46). Since then, numerous controlled studies comparing unilateral placement over the nondominant hemisphere (47) and bilateral electrode placement have shown that unilateral ECT is associated with significantly fewer cognitive side effects, including disorientation, disturbances of verbal and nonverbal memory function, and pathologic EEG changes (5, 48, 49).

Despite the pronounced cognitive advantages of unilateral over bilateral ECT, concerns continue to be expressed that, at least for some patients, the therapeutic response to unilateral ECT may be less rapid, potent, or enduring than that achieved with bilateral ECT (5, 50). Still, other researchers have found a therapeutic equivalence between unilateral and bilateral ECT (51). Some of the reported differences in efficacy may be related to technical factors—for example, to stimulus dosing (discussed below), adequacy of skin-electrode contact, and precise location of the nondominant-hemisphere electrodes (the D'Elia technique, with high centroparietal and frontotemporal locations, is preferred) (52). Because no consensus yet exists within the field on this issue, a variety of clinical practices are followed, including starting all patients on unilateral ECT and then switching nonresponders to bilateral ECT, or starting severely ill patients on bilateral ECT and then switching those who develop substantial cognitive deficits to unilateral ECT.

Another recent modification in ECT technique has been the use of the brief pulse electrical stimulus wave form. This stimulus consists of an undulating alternating current that in the U.S. cycles 60 times per second. Largely because of convenience, ECT devices initially incorporated the use of the sine wave stimulus. Beginning in the 1940s, research interest developed in the use of interrupted patterns of electrical stimulation because they were capable of eliciting a seizure with much lower stimulus intensity (53).

Since then, data have established that the brief pulse stimulus appears to be as therapeutically effective as the sine wave stimulus and that it produces less confusion, amnesia, and EEG slowing (28, 54). For these reasons, the pulse stimulus is now generally preferred for routine use and is the stimulus administered by ECT devices produced by all of the major manufacturers in this country (ElCoT, Mecta, Medcraft, and Somatics).

A final issue pertinent to electrical parameters with ECT is stimulus dosing. The threshold for an ECT seizure varies widely across individuals, covering more than a tenfold range. Seizure threshold is higher in males and in the elderly and with bilateral electrode placement (55). In addition, seizure threshold typically rises over the ECT course, reflecting the inherent anticonvulsant effect of this therapy. Recent data indicate that both the therapeutic and the adverse cognitive effects of ECT may be related to the extent to which the ECT stimulus is above the seizure threshold. Thus stimuli that are barely above seizure threshold may be less therapeutic than stimulation moderately above the threshold, particularly with unilateral nondominant ECT, while stimulation grossly above the threshold may be associated with increased cognitive side effects (39, 56).

In theory, then, a "moderately suprathreshold" stimulus dosage would appear to be optimal. Clinically, two general approaches are currently used to achieve this level. In the first, stimulus parameters are chosen empirically at the initial treatment to reflect a relatively high probability (such as 80 percent) that an adequate seizure will be induced. Depending on the ictal response (see below), stimulus parameters are then adjusted up or down at successive treatments.

The second approach involves actually estimating the seizure threshold at the time of the first treatment. This determination is made by starting at intensity levels that are likely to be subthreshold and then increasing stimulus intensity in steps until an adequate ictal response takes place (55). This stimulus intensity defines the "seizure threshold." For the second ECT treatment, dosage levels at a fixed level above this setting are chosen—for example, 100 percent greater with unilateral nondominant electrode placement, and 50 percent greater with bilateral placement.

Stimulus parameters for brief pulse devices include pulse width, frequency of pulses, peak pulse current, and duration of the entire pulse train, although some devices have only a single intensity control (intensity is usually proportional to duration). In general, a given percentage increase in one parameter has an effect equivalent to an identical increase in another.

Although the therapeutic potency of ECT depends on the production of an adequate ictal response, the criteria for an "adequate" seizure are still largely empirical. Currently, most practitioners require a seizure of at least 25 to 30 seconds; if a seizure does not occur or is too brief the ECT stimulus intensity is increased and the patient is restimulated within 30 to 60 seconds. In addition to the seizure-duration criterion, some practitioners also focus on the "quality" of the ECT seizure. If the EEG seizure pattern is substantially lower in amplitude or regularity, for example, a higher stimulus intensity might be used at the next ECT treatment. Pharmacologic augmentation, as with caffeine, may also be used to enhance seizure duration or quality (57, 58).

Management After ECT

After the successful treatment of a major depressive episode, whether by ECT or pharmacotherapy, early relapse is common unless some form of continuation therapy is employed (59). To prevent such a relapse after ECT, patients are typically placed on antidepressant medication for at least six months.

However, continuation pharmacotherapy may be problematic with patients who do not tolerate the side effects of the medications, and recent data suggest that continuation drug therapy after ECT may not be efficacious for patients who initially failed to respond to adequate drug therapy (60). In such cases, continuation therapy with outpatient ECT may be recommended (61). The precise timing of continuation ECT varies considerably, but we find that weekly treatments for the first month after remission, followed by a gradual tapering to monthly treatments, is an effective protocol (61). When risk of relapse remains high after six months, further maintenance ECT is indicated.

The management of patients who have failed to respond to ECT is also problematic. Some practitioners consider a repeat course of ECT, using high-intensity stimuli and bilateral electrode placement, while others prefer combination drug therapy. Combining psychotropic medications with ECT in such situations is a possibility that remains to be evaluated.

Education and Training in ECT

It should be clear from this overview that contemporary ECT practice is a complex technology that involves much more than simply "pushing a button on a black box." The ECT specialist must be able to identify indications and risk factors for the therapy, provide an appropriate informed consent procedure for patients and their families, make technical decisions about ECT technique (for example, selection of anesthetic, muscle relaxant, electrode placement, stimulus wave form, and dosing), determine the "adequacy" of the ECT seizure using EEG monitoring, and manage the physiologic changes in cardiac, pulmonary, and cerebral function that accompany the treatments.

Unfortunately, educational programs in many medical schools and residencies do not provide adequate training in ECT technique. In addition, physicians may be granted board certification in psychiatry without any experience or practical knowledge of ECT (62). In a recent survey, psychiatry department chairmen and residency training directors ranked the ability to administer ECT as 42nd among 48 skills necessary for a psychiatrist (63). (It was ranked ahead of conducting play therapy but well below developing liaison relationship with nurses.)

To assure that ECT is carried out in a safe and effective fashion, those involved in its administration, including psychiatrists, nursing personnel, and anesthesia providers, should receive adequate training. In addition, facilities providing ECT should exercise control over the competence of practitioners by means of local privileging. Educational experiences related to ECT should be incorporated into medical and nursing school curricula. Exposure to ECT during psychiatric residency training should include both didactic presentations and practical experience supervised by faculty members who are clinically privileged in ECT. Opportunities for postgraduate continuing medical education in ECT, including practically oriented courses, symposia, and fellowships, should be offered. Currently, postgraduate programs as well as advanced residency training are provided by the departments of psychiatry at Duke University Medical Center and at the State University of New York at Stony Brook.

Acknowledgments

The authors' research was supported by grants from the National Institute of Mental Health (MH-41803, MH-30723, and MH-40159) and the North Carolina United Way.

References

1. Commemorative issue, Convulsive Therapy 4(1):1-113, 1988.

2. Consensus Conference: electroconvulsive therapy. JAMA 254:2103-2108, 1985

3. APA Task Force on ECT: The Practice of ECT: Recommendations for Treatment, Training, and Privileging. Washington, DC, American Psychiatric Press, 1990

4. Abrams R: Electroconvulsive Therapy. New York, Oxford University Press, 1988

5. Weiner RD, Coffey CE: Indications for use of electroconvulsive therapy, in American Psychiatric Press Review of Psychiatry, vol 7. Edited by Frances AJ, Hales RE. Washington, DC, American Psychiatric Press, 1988

6. Weiner RD: Electroconvulsive therapy, in Comprehensive Textbook of Psychiatry, 5th ed. Edited by Kaplan HI, Sadock BJ. Baltimore, Williams & Wilkins, 1989

7. Fink M: Meduna and the origins of convulsive therapy. American Journal of Psychiatry 141:1034-1041,1984

8. Fink M: Is ECT usage decreasing? Convulsive Therapy 3:171-173, 1987

9. Markowitz J, Brown R, Sweeney J, et al: Reduced length and cost of hospital stay for major depression in patients treated with ECT. American Journal of Psychiatry 144:1025-1029, 1987

10. Asnis GM, Fink M, Saferstein S: ECT in metropolitan New York hospitals: a survey of practice, 1975-1976. American Journal of Psychiatry 135:479-482, 1978

11. Morrissey JP, Steadman HJ, Burton NM: A profile of ECT recipients in New York State during 1972 and 1977. American Journal of Psychiatry 138:618-622, 1981

12. McCall WV: Physical treatments in psychiatry: current and historical use in the southern United States. Southern Medical Journal 82:345-351, 1989

13. Zimmerman M, Coryell W, Stangl D, et al: An American validation study of the Newcastle Scale, III: course during index hospitalization and six-month prospective follow-up. Acta Psychiatrica Scandinavica 73:412-415, 1986

14. Prudic J, Devaand DP, Sackeim HA, et al: Relative response of endogenous and nonendogenous symptoms to electroconvulsive therapy. Journal of Affective Disorders 16:59-64, 1989

15. Rich CL, Spiker DG, Jewell SW, et al: Response of energy and suicide ideation to ECT. Journal of Clinical Psychiatry 47:31-32, 1986

16. Small JG: Efficacy of electroconvulsive therapy in schizophrenia, mania, and other disorders, II: mania and other disorders. Convulsive Therapy 1:271-276, 1985

17. Small JG, Klapper MH, Kellams JJ, et al: Electroconvulsive treatment compared with lithium in the management of manic states. Archives of General Psychiatry 45:727-732, 1988

18. Mukerjee S, Sackeim HA, Lee C: Unilateral ECT in the treatment of manic episodes. Convulsive Therapy 4:74-80, 1988

19. Small JG: Efficacy of electroconvulsive therapy in schizophrenia, mania, and other disorders, I: schizophrenia. Convulsive Therapy 1:263-270, 1985

20. Small JG, Milstein V, Klapper MH, et al: ECT combined with neuroleptics in the treatment of schizophrenia. Psychopharmacology Bulletin 18:34-35,1982

21. Weiner RD, Coffey CE: Electroconvulsive therapy in the medically ill, in Principles of Medical Psychiatry. Edited by Stoudemire A, Fogel B. New York, Grune & Stratton, 1987

22. Dec GW Jr, Stern TA, Welch C: The effects of electroconvulsive therapy on serial electrocardiograms and serum cardiac enzyme values: a prospective study of depressed hospitalized inpatients. JAMA 253:2525-2529, 1985

23. Weiner RD: Does ECT cause brain damage? Behavioral and Brain Sciences 7:1-53, 1984

24. Weiner RD, Rogers HJ, Davidson JRT et al: Effects of ECT upon brain electrical activity, in Electroconvulsive Therapy: Clinical and Basic Research Issues. Edited by Malitz S, Sackeim HA. New York, New York Academy of Sciences, 1986

25. Daniel WF, Crovitz HF: The recovery of orientation after electroconvulsive therapy: a review. Acta Psychiatrica Scandinavica 66:421-428, 1982

26. Daniel WF, Crovitz HF: Acute memory impairment following electroconvulsive therapy. Acta Psychiatrica Scandinavica 67:1-7, 1983

27. Squire LR: Memory functions as affected by electroconvulsive therapy, in Electroconvulsive Therapy: Clinical and Basic Research Issues. Edited by Malitz S, Sackeim HA. New York, New York Academy of Sciences, 1986

28. Weiner RD, Rogers HJ, Davidson JRT, et al: Effects of stimulus parameters on cognitive side effects. Ibid

29. Freeman CPL, Cheshire KE: Attitude studies on electroconvulsive therapy. Convulsive Therapy 2:31-42, 1986

30. Coffey CE, Hinkle PE, Weiner RD, et al: Electroconvulsive therapy of depression in patients with white matter hyperintensity. Biological Psychiatry 22:629-636, 1987

31. Coffey CE, Figiel GS, Djang WT, et al: Leukoencephalopathy in elderly depressed patients referred for ECT. Biological Psychiatry 24:143-161, 1988

32. Figiel GS, Coffey CE, Weiner RD: Brain magnetic resonance imaging in elderly depressed patients receiving electroconvulsive therapy. Convulsive Therapy 5:26-34, 1989

33. Coffey CE, Figiel GS, Djang WT, et al: Subcortical white matter hyperintensity on magnetic resonance imaging: clinical and neuroanatomic correlates in the depressed elderly. Journal of Neuropsychiatry and Clinical Neurosciences 1:135-144, 1989

34. Coffey CE, Figiel GS: Neuropsychiatric significance of subcortical encephalomalacia, in Psychopathology and the Brain. Edited by Carroll BJ. New York, Raven, 1990

35. Coffey CE, Figiel GS, Djang WT, et al: Subcortical hyperintensity on magnetic resonance imaging: a comparison of normal and depressed elderly subjects. American Journal of Psychiatry 147:187-189, 1990

36. Coffey CE, Figiel GS, Djang WT, et al: Effects of ECT on brain structure: a pilot prospective magnetic resonance imaging study. American Journal of Psychiatry 145:701-706, 1988

37. Meldrum BS, Vigouroux RA, Bierley JB: Systemic factors in epileptic damage: prolonged procedures in paralyzed artificially ventilated baboons. Archives of Neurology 29:82-87, 1973

38. Hoyle NR, Pratt RTC, Thomas DGT: Effect of electroconvulsive therapy on serum myelin basic protein immunoreactivity. British Medical Journal 288:1110-1111, 1984

39. Sackeim HA: Mechanisms of action of electroconvulsive therapy, in American Psychiatric Press Review of Psychiatry, vol 7. Edited by Frances AJ, Hales RE. Washington, DC, American Psychiatric Press, 1988

40. Lerer B, Shapira B: Neurochemical mechanisms of mood stabilization: focus on electroconvulsive therapy, in Electroconvulsive Therapy: Clinical and Basic Research Issues. Edited by Malitz S, Sackeim HA. New York, New York Academy of Sciences, 1986

41. Fink M: A neuroendocrine theory of convulsive therapy. Trends in Neuroscience 3:25-27, 1980

42. Elliot DL, Linz DH, Kane JA: Electroconvulsive therapy: pretreatment medical evaluation. Archives of Internal Medicine 142:979-981, 1982

43. Standish-Barry HMAS, Deacon V, Snaith RP: The relationship of concurrent benzodiazepine administration to seizure duration in ECT. Acta Psychiatrica Scandinavica 71:269-270, 1985

44. Small JG, Kellams JJ, Milstein V: Complications with electroconvulsive treatment combined with lithium. Biological Psychiatry 15:103-112, 1980

45. Culver CM, Ferrell RB, Green RM: ECT and special problems of informed consent. American Journal of Psychiatry 137:586-591, 1980

46. Friedman E, Wilcox PH: Electrostimulated convulsive doses in intact humans by means of unidirectional currents. Journal of Nervous and Mental Disease 96:56-63, 1942

47. D'Elia G (ed): Unilateral Electroconvulsive Therapy. Acta Psychiatrica Scandinavica Suppl 215, 1970

48. Lancaster NP, Steinert RR, Frost I: Unilateral electroconvulsive therapy. Journal of Mental Science 104:221-227, 1958

49. Squire LR, Slater PC: Bilateral and unilateral ECT: effects on verbal and nonverbal memory. American Journal of Psychiatry 135:1316-1320, 1978

50. Abrams R: Is unilateral electroconvulsive therapy really the treatment of choice in endogenous depression? in Electroconvulsive Therapy: Clinical and Basic Research Issues. Edited by Malitz S, Sackeim HA. New York, New York Academy of Sciences, 1986

51. D'Elia G, Raotma H: Is unilateral ECT less effective than bilateral ECT? British Journal of Psychiatry 126:83-89, 1975

52. Weiner RD, Coffey CE: Minimizing therapeutic differences between bilateral and unilateral nondominant ECT. Convulsive Therapy 2:261-265, 1986

53. Liberson WT: Brief stimulus therapy: physiological and chemical observations. American Journal of Psychiatry 105:28-39, 1948

54. Weiner RD: EEG related to electroconvulsive therapy, in EEG and Evoked Potentials in Psychiatry and Behavioral Neurology. Edited by Hughes JR, Wilson WP. Boston, Butterworth, 1983

55. Sackeim HA, Decina P, Prohovnik I, et al: Seizure threshold in ECT: effects of sex, age, electrode placement, and number of treatments. Archives of General Psychiatry 44:355-360, 1987

56. Sackeim HA, Decina P, Kanzler M, et al: Effects of electrode placement on the efficacy of titrated, low-dose ECT. American Journal of Psychiatry 144:1449-1455, 1987

57. Coffey CE, Figiel GS, Weiner RD, et al: Caffeine augmentation of electroconvulsive therapy. American Journal of Psychiatry (in press)

58. Coffey CE, Weiner RD, Hinkle PE, et al: Augmentation of ECT seizures with caffeine. Biological Psychiatry 22:637-649, 1987

59. Prien RF, Kupfer DJ: Continuation drug therapy for major depressive episodes: how long should it be maintained? American Journal of Psychiatry 143:18-22, 1986

60. Sackeim HA, Brown RP, Devanend DP, et al: Should tricyclic antidepressants or lithium be standard continuation treatment after ECT? An alternative view. Convulsive Therapy 5:180-183, 1989

61. Clarke TB, Coffey CE, Hoffman GW, et al: Continuation therapy for depression using outpatient electroconvulsive therapy. Convulsive Therapy 5:330-337, 1989

62. Fink M: New technology in convulsive therapy: a challenge in training. American Journal of Psychiatry 144:1195-1198, 1987

63. Langsley DG, Yager J: The definition of a psychiatrist: eight years later. American Journal of Psychiatry 145:469-475, 1988

Chapter 59

Review of Current Research on Schizophrenia

Roann Barris, EdD, OTR

Current research on schizophrenia can be grouped into two major categories. The first consists of studies that have focused on identifying characteristics that predispose individuals to become schizophrenic; the second is more concerned with comparing approaches to the treatment and maintenance of persons with schizophrenia. Unfortunately, the link between these two groups of studies is often tenuous, for reasons that will become clear later in this article.

The first group of studies is typified by research seeking to identify or confirm the existence of biochemical or structural abnormalities in persons with schizophrenia. Examples of research in this area include studies of enzyme activity (1-4), structural abnormalities or asymmetries within the brain and brain stem (5-8), and genetic studies (9-10). Although some of these studies appear to advance an etiological understanding of schizophrenia, more often than not findings are inconclusive or contradictory (10).

Another focus of research concerned with predisposing traits has concentrated on the family environment. Although, in the past, the mother has frequently been the subject of family studies, recent research has been more concerned with identifying communication patterns and effective styles that characterize the family as a whole (11). These studies suggest that certain deviant communication patterns, as well as high levels of expressed emotion within the family, relate to a later onset of schizophrenia and to relapses in identified patients (11-12).

The second area of research has attempted to compare various treatment programs in terms of their cost, their effectiveness in reducing or preventing hospitalizations, and their contribution to the psychosocial functioning of schizophrenic persons. Findings in this area are not always encouraging, at least not within a medical model framework. First, these studies show that despite an increased understanding of the biological etiology of schizophrenia, treatment with neuroleptics remains a very inexact science (13-16). The problem is compounded by the fact that many patients discontinue their medications. Yet even among those who do not, relapse rates are quite high (16). Second, these studies indicate that there is an ongoing need for treatment of some sort

(17-18). Although schizophrenia is not curable, it may be controllable (14-18). However, gains that may be made while the individual is in a treatment program are likely to be lost if treatment is discontinued (18). Nevertheless, outcome studies have also found that changes in daily functioning do result from treatment when daily living skills are specifically targeted for treatment (18). These studies also indicate that, contrary to the approach espoused by the psychoeducational model, group treatment may not be the most efficacious treatment modality for persons who are unable to "connect" with others and whose cognitive deficits center around an inability to form abstractions and to distinguish between relevant and irrelevant information (18-19). Cost comparison studies of treatment also suggest that rehospitalization and wage loss as a result of unemployment (20) are major factors affecting direct costs. Since work or a substitute role may enable schizophrenic persons to remain outside the hospital for a longer period of time (using less costly outpatient services), these studies emphasize the need for developing employment opportunities or alternative work experiences for persons with schizophrenia (20).

On the surface, the implications of these studies for occupational therapy seem straightforward. If treatment gains can be made in those areas that are targeted for treatment and if independent daily living is a desired goal, then it follows that treatment must focus on the development of life skills or survival skills (e.g., strategies for coping with daily life and stressful events) and on the use of these skills in the context of certain roles (i.e., worker and family member).

However, there is a more critical implication of the existing research which relates to the absence of a connection between etiologically-based research and treatment-based research. The connection between the two types of research is missing because there is an inherent contradiction in the medical model approach to the study of schizophrenia. The contradiction lies in the fact that the research focuses on underlying biological mechanisms while simultaneously acknowledging the problems that schizophrenic persons have in daily life. Since these problems generally continue to exist after the more acute symptomatology is brought under control, studies of brain structure and enzyme production ultimately offer the clinician and the client little in the way of new knowledge for coping with these problems of daily living. Furthermore, because occupational therapists are more likely to make their contributions to the remediation of daily living deficits than to the remediation of neurological deficits, biological explanations of schizophrenia overly restrict a conceptualization of the role of occupational therapy with chronic schizophre-

nia. However, occupational therapists can delineate an important and complementary role to that of the medical model professional by developing a theoretical explanation of (a) the occupational dysfunction that characterizes schizophrenic persons and (b) the relationship of occupational dysfunction to symptomatology and to the patients' need for and continued use of medical services.

One example is the work done by Oakley (21). Using the model of human occupation (22) as a theoretical framework, Oakley administered a battery of assessments that yielded information on the subjects' personal causation, temporal orientation, valued goals, internalized roles, and task skills. This information was then used as the basis for a global rating of system organization or degree of occupational dysfunction. Oakley found that although system organization correlated with symptomatology, the two measures were not synonymous. Moreover, Oakley found that system organization was a better predictor than symptomatology of adaptive behavior, as measured by the Adaptive Behavior Scale. Although this research was limited in scope and design, it illustrates a viable approach to the study of schizophrenia. What is especially significant about this approach is that it contains clear implications for occupational therapy treatment. The implications are that time management, goal-setting, habit training, and the development of role-related behaviors are not merely ancillary or splinter forms of treatment; they are critically and directly relevant to a reduction of socially maladaptive behaviors in schizophrenic persons.

The conclusion to draw from this review is that we can—and should—couch research in terms of occupational therapy frameworks so that we can use our increased knowledge to point directly to the need for occupational therapy intervention.

References

1. Baron M, Asnis L, Gruen MA, Levitt M: Plasma amine oxidase and genetic vulnerability to schizophrenia. *Arch Gen Psychiatry* 40:275-279, 1983

2. Linnoila M, Ninan PT, Scheinin M, Waters RN, Chang W, Bartko J, van Kammen DP: Reliability of norepinephrine and major monoamine metabolite measurements in CSF of schizophrenic patients. *Arch Gen Psychiatry* 40:1290-1294, 1983

3. Sternberg DE, van Kammen DP, Lerner P, Ballenger JC, Marder SR, Post RM, Bunney WE, Jr: CSF dopamine B-Hydroxylase in schizophrenia. *Arch Gen Psychiatry* 40:743-747, 1983

4. Ferrier IN, Johnstone EC, Crow TJ, Rincon-Rodriguez I: Anterior pituitary hormone secretion in chronic schizophrenics. *Arch Gen Psychiatry* 40:755-761, 1983

5. Morstyn R, Duffy FH, McCarley RW: Altered P300 topography in schizophrenia. *Arch Gen Psychiatry* 40:729-734,1983

6. Rieder RO, Mann LS, Weinberger DR, van Kammen DP, Post RM: Computed tomographic scans in patients with schizophrenia, schizo-affective, and bipolar affective disorder. *Arch Gen Psychiatry* 40: 735-739

7. Reveley AM, Reveley MA: Aqueduct stenosis and schizophrenia. *J Neurol Neurosurg Psychiatry* 46:18-22, 1983

8. Tsai LY, Nasrallah HA, Jacoby CG: Hemispheric asymmetries on computed tomographic scans in schizophrenia and mania. *Arch Gen Psychiatry* 40:1286-1289, 1983

9. Abrams R, Taylor MA: The genetics of schizophrenia: A reassessment using modem criteria. *Am J Psychiatry* 140:171-175, 1983

10. Deutsch SI, Davis KL: Schizophrenia: A review of diagnostic and biological issues. II. Biological issues. *Hosp Community Psychiatry* 34:423-437, 1983

11. Parker G: Re-searching the schizophrenic mother. *J Nerv Ment Dis* 170:452-462, 1982

12. Goldstein MJ: Family interaction: Patterns predictive of the onset and course of schizophrenia. In *Psychosocial Intervention in Schizophrenia*, H Stierlin, LC Wynne, M Wirshing, Editors. Berlin: Springer-Verlag, 1983

13. Wilson HS: *Deinstitutionalized Residential Care for the Mentally Disordered: The Soteria House Approach*. New York: Grune Stratton, 1982

14. Sheehan S: *Is There No Place on Earth for Me?* New York: Vintage, 1982

15. Kieth SJ, Starr S, Matthews SM: A team approach to pharmacologic treatment of chronic schizophrenia. *Hosp Community Psychiatry* 35:802-805, 1984

16. Barter JT, Queirolo JF, Ekstrom SP: A psychoeducational approach to educating chronic mental patients about community living. *Hosp Community Psychiatry* 35:793-797, 1984

17. Lamb HR, Peele R: The need for continuing asylum and sanctuary. *Hosp Community Psychiatry* 35:798-801, 1984

18. Stein MA, Test LI: Community treatment of the chronic patient: Research overview. *Schizophr Bull* 4:350-364, 1978

19. Ciompi L: How to improve the treatment of schizophrenics: A multicausal illness concept and its therapeutic consequences. In *Psychosocial Intervention in Schizophrenia*, H Stierlin, LC Wynne, M Wirshing, Editors. Berlin: Springer-Verlag, 1983

20. Muller CF, Caton CLM: Economic costs of schizophrenia: A postdischarge study. *Med Care* 21:92-104, 1983

21. Oakley F, Kielhofner G, Barris R: An occupational therapy approach to assessing psychiatric patients' adaptive functioning. *Am J Occup Ther* 39:147-154, 1985

22. Kielhofner G, Burke JP: A model of human occupation, Part I: Conceptual framework and content. *Am J Occup Ther* 34:572-581, 1980

Chapter 60

An Overview of Theory and Research on Hallucinations: Implications for Occupational Therapy Intervention

Anne MacRae, MS, OTR

The purpose of this paper is to provide a theoretical background for the understanding of hallucinations and to discuss the role of occupational therapy in the management of such symptoms. Although it is well documented that hallucinations exist with a variety of both transitory and chronic psychotic disorders, very little is known about the impact of hallucinations on an individual's ability to function. Since maximum involvement in Activities of Daily Living (ADL) is often a key to quality of life for those with chronic mental illness (Klasson & MacRae, 1985; Malm, May & Dencker, 1981) this is a key area for treatment. The identification of coping mechanisms for hallucinations which improve ADL function has implications for both the treatment of individuals with chronic mental illness and for the training of clinicians in the field of mental health.

The topic of hallucinations has been widely addressed in the psychiatric and psychological literature but virtually ignored in the occupational therapy literature. The medical orientation commonly used in psychiatry and psychology places much emphasis on clinical symptomatology, while occupational therapy (OT) is more likely to focus on the disruption of the occupational performance areas of work, leisure and self-care rather than on specific symptoms (Rogers, 1982). In some cases,

> it is difficult if not impossible to separate medically defined pathology from the kind of disorder that occupational therapy recognizes. For instance, the schizophrenic person exhibits pathological symptoms such as hallucinations and extreme anxiety and at the same time may show a dearth of interests, poorly formed or contradictory values, a lack of life goals, and disruption of many occupational performance components. (Barris, Kielhofner & Watts, 1988, pp. 43-44)

The lack of discussion in the OT literature regarding

psychiatric symptoms is unfortunate because the occupational therapy focus on function could provide valuable information on not only how to attempt symptom management but also when it is appropriate to do so. Included in this paper is a discussion of the functional deficits associated with hallucinations and specific suggestions for appropriate occupational therapy intervention.

Historical Definitions of Hallucination

A basic definition of hallucinations as false perceptions can be traced back to Aristotle who differentiated "true" from "false" perceptions of sight, hearing and smell (Brieire de Boismont, 1853/1976). Hallucinations however can only be inferred from the writings of the ancients, as their descriptions are intertwined with cultural and religious issues. One theory, articulated by Jaynes (1979), is that hallucinations were the norm among ancient peoples because they could not differentiate thoughts as their own and therefore attributed them to the gods. Jaynes' theory is highly speculative, however there is a general consensus in the literature that perceptual distortions were not only considered acceptable, they were socially and religiously significant in many pre- and post-Christian cultures (Hume, 1988; Slade & Bentall, 1988; West, 1975). There remains considerable disagreement as to whether these phenomena were indeed hallucinations or events that fall into perhaps broader categories of sensory deception or mental imagery. Pre-Christian and some non-Western cultures generally considered perceptual distortions as positive events even when they did have some frightening aspects. Usually, they were seen as direct communications with the gods. However, Western culture, beginning with Christianity, viewed such phenomena as essentially evil. Johnson (1978) suggests that the irrational behavior and vivid hallucinations of several Roman leaders, including Tiberius, Caligula and Nero, account for this shift in attitude. The association between hallucination and evil was further strengthened by the demonological theories of Augustine, Thomas Aquinas and Ignatius of Loyola (Sarbin & Juhasz, 1975).

The actual term "hallucination" is believed to have originated in the 1830's and is generally credited to Esquirol of France (Briere de Boismont 1853/1976; Field and Ruelke, 1973; Reed, 1972; Slade and Bentall, 1988; West, 1975), but repeated translations and interpretations of this original work have not been in agreement as to its meaning. Even now, "after nearly two centuries of clinical investigation of hallucinations and a voluminous literature there are still misconceptions and contradictions at the level of description, classification and theory" (Lothane, 1982, p. 335).

Contemporary Definitions of Hallucination

There are three specific parameters of the concept of hallucination which appear to create the most controversy. These include the type of experience, the source of the phenomena and the relationship to disease.

Type of Experience

It is generally accepted that the hallucinatory experience is in the realm of sensory perception rather than ideation (Aggernaes, 1972; Reed, 1972; West, 1975). Probably the most commonly used definition in the Western world is from The Diagnostic and Statistical Manual-III Edition-Revised (DSM-III-R) which defines hallucination as "A sensory perception without external stimulation of the relevant sensory organ" (American Psychiatric Association [APA], 1987, p. 398). There is however some strong disagreement with the current accepted definition. Lothane (1982) states that the inclusion of sensory perception as the key element of the definition is both a distortion of Esquirol's original definition and fundamentally incorrect. Rather, Lothane views hallucinations as "multifaceted complex human mental activity" (p. 347), very much rooted in ideation and authored by the hallucinator.

Although the APA definition is the most common reference, there is a myriad of different views as to the exact role of thought or ideation in the hallucinatory experience. La Barre states "Since all men are accustomed to believe their senses, it is the sensory form of its presentation that gives hallucination its psychic conviction" (1975, p. 10). Horowitz (1975a) includes both the cognitive and perceptual components of hallucinations in definition but avoids a sharp distinction between them by referring to hallucinations as the result of faulty information processing. This particular controversy of sensorium verses ideation may simply be one of semantics, in that the appearance or quality of hallucinations is distinctly different from their actual etiology. In other words, there is no doubt that hallucinations are experienced as sensory phenomena, however the disturbance is essentially an inaccurate interpretation of the sensorium and is therefore a perceptual process which, in turn, is part of cognition (Lezak, 1983).

Source of the Phenomena

Traditionally, in psychiatry, true hallucinations were limited to phenomena perceived to have originated from the environment or outside the head. This strict interpretation of the hallucinatory experience is based on the notion that only phenomena that are perceived as externally generated mimic true perception. Using this criterion, sensory deceptions thought to be internally generated would be classified as pseudo-hallucinations, dreams, illusions or other forms of imagery.

The rigid definition of hallucination has drawn much criticism in the literature. The DSM-III-R does not adhere to the concept of source as a limitation because it has not been shown to be clinically significant (APA, 1987). Aggernaes (1972) raises a practical consideration, reporting that hallucinators are not always able to identify whether a phenomenon is originating from the environment or from their own minds, therefore this criterion leads to doubtful identification of hallucinations. Horowitz (1975b) believes that there is a qualitative difference between hallucinations and pseudo-hallucinations based not only on perceived source but degree of vividness and a belief in the reality of the phenomena. However, he does not propose clear parameters for definition, rather the concepts of hallucination and pseudo-hallucination are "only points along a dimension of experience" (Horowitz, 1975b, p. 166).

A study conducted by Junginger and Frame (1985) on the auditory hallucinations of people with schizophrenia concluded that there is no significant difference in the perceived reality of voices thought to originate outside or inside the head. Therefore, these investigators state that the perceived source of the experience should probably be abandoned as a criterion for diagnosis or definition.

Relationship to Disease

The term hallucination is typically associated with a mental disorder (Reed, 1972; Starker, 1986), but it also occurs in many physical disorders and may occur when no state of illness is present. Mosak and Fletcher (1973) state that "although it is characteristic of psychosis, neurotics also occasionally hallucinate, as might normal individuals in situations of monotony or reduced sensory input" (p. 177). The APA (1987) acknowledges the occurrence of hallucinations in intensely religious experiences but rules out the term's usage for the "false perceptions that occur during dreaming, while falling asleep (hypnagogic) or when awakening (hypnopompic)" (p. 398). Special consideration is given to children under the age of six because it is generally recognized that a part of normal development includes occasional hallucinations involving communication from imaginary friends (Bender, 1970).

Numerous studies conclude that hallucinations can indeed fall within the range of normal experience with 5-15% of the population having experienced the phenomena without benefit of drugs or mental illness (Bentall & Slade, 1985). In fact, some authors believe the experience to be far more frequent than Bentall and Slade suggest. Hartmann (1975) states "Actual hallucinatory activity is extremely common, and the ability to hallucinate is probably ubiquitous" (p. 71).

Not only is there a general association between pathology and hallucinations but it is also widely believed that specific types of hallucinations, such as auditory, visual or tactile, might be indicative of particular disorders. However, a study of 117 psychiatric inpatients conducted by Goodwin, Alderson, and Rosenthal (1971) [sic] showed no correlation between diagnosis and types of hallucinations. In fact, these researchers concluded that most people who report a particular form of hallucination have had past experiences with hallucinations involving other sensory modalities. Multi-sensory hallucinatory experiences were also documented by Lemberg (1978) in a case study of a woman with psychotic paranoia. Lemberg concluded that "hallucinatory processes across sensory modalities...may be more common than previously believed" (p. 466).

Bliss, Larson and Nakashima (1983) are highly critical of the assumption of pathology in the presence of hallucinations. Based on a study of 45 patients with auditory hallucinations, they concluded that the diagnosis of schizophrenia is often made solely because of the presence of hallucinations and is therefore frequently inaccurate. Hopefully this type of misdiagnosis has decreased since the development of the specific criteria of the DSM-III.

The exact relationship between mental illness and hallucinations remains unclear; however, the concept that hallucinations are exclusively a psychopathological symptom has become obsolete. Hallucinations can be related to many normal and abnormal organic, psychological, biochemical, pharmacological or physiopathological processes (Keup, 1970).

Theories of Etiology

Just as there is no consensus as to the definition of hallucination, there is also a lack of agreement regarding the etiology of hallucinations. The psychodynamic and the biological theories attempt to explain hallucination as a single universal phenomena. However, some theorists have found it fruitful to research the specific sub-classifications of hallucinations in order to discover their cause. For example, there are many studies proposing etiological theories about the auditory hallucinations of people with schizophrenia (Bick & Kinsbourne, 1987; Collicutt & Hemsley, 1981; Green & Preston, 1981; Heilbrun & Blum, 1984; Inouye & Shimizu, 1970; Inouye & Shimizu, 1972; Junginger & Frame, 1985; Junginger & Rauscher, 1987). Such theories are not generalizable to other classifications of hallucinations or to the non-schizophrenic population.

Psychodynamic theory explains hallucinations in terms of their content and the individual's motivation for them. Lothane (1982) states "hallucinations come about as a result of a dynamic shift in psychological functions and forces; emerge from their latent to the manifest form through the dynamics of hallucination-work, homologous to dream-work; are motivated and meaningful" (p. 344). Mosak and Fletcher (1973) support an Alderian point of view of hallucinations, stating that their purpose is to enhance self esteem, circumvent logic and avoid responsibility. In specific reference to the hallucinations of children, Bender (1970) states "they are always a window to the inner life of the child and reveal the child's psychodynamic problems to the observer and may serve the function of substitute interpersonal relationships in deprived children" (p. 100). From a psychodynamic perspective, the individual is involved on some level in the creation of the hallucinations, responsible for their content and utilizes the phenomena to dissociate from an often painful reality (Lemberg, 1978; Lothane, 1982; West, 1975).

The biological theories of hallucinations are many and varied. It is well known that endocrine abnormalities, organic lesions, toxic metabolic stressors and certain pharmacologic substances can induce hallucinations (APA, 1987; Johnson, 1978). This information has not led to any generalizable theory of hallucinations. Much study has been devoted to the belief that hallucinations can be traced to a specific location of dysfunction in the brain. The cerebral cortex, (particularly the left hemisphere), temporal lobes, cerebellum, brain stem and reticular activating system (RAS) have all been implicated.

Rather than strict adherence to a specific theory of hallucinations, it is perhaps more productive to utilize a working model. Although current researchers fail to agree on the terminology or specific details of such a model, there does seem to be a general consensus that a cognitive or information processing approach is most useful. One reason for general acceptance is that such a model does not conflict with psychodynamic or biological explanations. Rather it is concerned with how information is encoded, transformed and interpreted (Horowitz, 1975b).

Horowitz's (1975a) cognitive model consists of four constructs: Hallucinations "(1) occur in the form of images, (2) are derived from internal sources of information, (3) are appraised incorrectly as if from external sources of information, and (4) usually occur intrusively" (p. 789). Inherent in this model is the assumption that there are predisposing factors that create a situation where the erroneous appraisal of information occurs. Slade (1976) presents a four factor model in which he postulates that the interaction of a stressful event, environmental stimulation, a basic genetic predisposition, and reinforcement produces hallucinations. This is very much in line with current theories regarding the etiology of schizophrenia but has been scantily studied with specific reference to hallucinations. Heilbrun and Blum (1984) conducted a study with 44 patients and concluded that cognitive vulnerability, especially premature judgement, is a predisposing factor to the development of auditory hallucinations. In conclusion, a general broad based definition of hallucination coupled with a cognitive model incorporating both psychodynamic and biologic theories would seem to be the most useful and clinically significant approach to the study of hallucinations.

Management of Hallucinations

The traditional medical approach for controlling hallucinations is the administration of antipsychotic drugs (Slade & Bentall, 1988). While these agents are extremely helpful in some cases, their effectiveness is not universal and the side effects can be quite detrimental. Drugs are, at best, only partly successful in controlling the hallucinations associated with psychotic disorders; they often reduce the more florid symptoms of a dysfunction but do not necessarily totally eliminate hallucinations (Falloon & Talbot, 1981; Hogarty, Goldberg, Schooler & Ulrich, 1974; Slade and Bentall, 1988; Wallace et al., 1980). It appears, however, that some people can remain quite functional despite ongoing hallucinations while others cannot. Some studies and subjective reports suggest that maintenance of function in the presence of hallucinations may be due to the development of coping mechanisms for minimizing the disruption of the intrusive experiences (Breier & Strauss, 1983; Falloon & Talbot, 1981; Fisher & Winkler, 1975; Green & Kinsbourne, 1989; Romme & Escher, 1989).

There are several methods that have been evaluated for controlling hallucinations either without the use of psychopharmaceuticals or in addition to them. Attempted techniques have included humming (Green & Kinsbourne, 1989), use of earplugs (Birchwood, 1986; Done, Frith & Owens, 1986, James, 1983), varying auditory input by the use of stereo headphones (Hemsley & Slade, 1981), increasing auditory input by the use of stereo headphones (Feder, 1982), and aversion therapy (Alford & Turner, 1976; Weingaertner, 1971). All of these techniques have met with some success but results have not been consistently replicated. Researchers agree that further investigation is needed both on specific techniques and on the phenomenon of hallucinations in general. A major limitation of all of these studies is that the locus of control is with the researcher or clinician. It is possible that the inconsistent findings are related to the level of involvement of the individuals being studied. Another approach to the study of this problem is to discover the coping mechanisms initiated and directed by persons with hallucinations.

Breier and Strauss (1983) conducted a study in which

20 persons hospitalized for psychotic disorders were given semi-structured interviews with the purpose of assessing the ability to self control psychotic symptoms. "Subjects described three major kinds of special control mechanisms: self-instruction, decreased involvement in activity, and increased involvement in activity" (p. 1143). Their conclusion is that self control measures, although not always effective, do have a significant role to play in the management of psychotic disorders and deserve further study. A case study conducted by Fisher and Winkler (1975) also supports the value of self control measures, but credits success of these techniques to the subjects' belief in their effectiveness.

Falloon and Talbot (1981) conducted in depth interviews with 40 out-patients diagnosed as having chronic schizophrenia with persistent auditory hallucinations. Each patient was interviewed with open ended questions several times over a six month period. This study showed that a wide variety of "common sense" strategies such as relaxation, exercise and leisure activity, are indeed used by hallucinating patients, but the effectiveness of such techniques is highly individual. "Successful coping appeared to result from systematic application of widely used coping strategies" (Falloon & Talbot, 1981, p. 329).

Functional Deficits Associated with Hallucinations

Since the etiology of hallucinations is unclear, it is often difficult to judge the effectiveness of clinical intervention. This problem can be partially alleviated by focusing on functional deficits rather than abstract theories of etiology. The San Jose State University (SJSU) psychosocial OT clinic uses a model, developed by this author, in which observable behaviors are correlated with the class of hallucination. The goal of such a model is to assist the clinician in determining if intervention is appropriate. A deduction can then be made regarding types of treatment modalities for symptom management.

Table A lists five classes of hallucinations. The following is a more extensive description of these classifications and a discussion of their significance for treatment.

Class I

This classification includes individuals who not only deny the presence of hallucinations but exhibit no behaviors that might be indicative of their presence. It is not important whether hallucinations ever existed, are in remission, or are completely controlled by medication. The implication is simply that no intervention (other than the possibility of continued medication) is required at this time.

Class II

Although hallucinations do exist, there is no evidence of significant functional limitations. In fact, it is possible that the hallucinations actually incur some benefits for the individual by providing a creative outlet, companionship or entertainment, as some patients have reported (Falloon & Talbot, 1981). In these situations, treatment would not be necessary and might be counter-productive. Individuals who experience hallucinations of this classification generally only do so when they are not in social situations or in environments requiring their attention. Typically the individual is lonely and bored when the hallucinations begin. If this is a limited and intermittent phenomenon, then the situation is relatively benign. However, if the frequency or subjective distress related to the hallucinations increases, then intervention is appropriate. Occupational therapy treatment may include social skills training and structured activity groups. In several controlled comparison studies, these interventions have been shown to reduce positive symptomatology (Hogarty et al., 1986; Liberman, Mueser & Wallace, 1986).

Class III

Significant functional impairment is directly related to the content of the hallucinations. Typically the hallucinations are auditory in nature. Occupational therapy interventions consist of social skills training, including community awareness and mobility, assertiveness training and communication skills, as well as structured activities to enhance a sense of self esteem. Patients with a poor self esteem often develop a maladaptive cycle in which they feel ineffective and controlled by external factors and therefore lose their motivation to interact with their environment or explore and master potential life roles in work, play and self care (Barris, Kielhofner & Watts, 1988). It has been occasionally observed in the SJSU psychosocial OT clinic that poor self esteem can also manifest itself as grandiose behavior accompanied by poor judgment and lack of safety awareness. Social skills training with extensive perceptual checks for reality orientation and activities to enhance a positive, yet realistic, self image remain appropriate modalities.

Class IV

Regardless of content or sensory expression, these hallucinations have a quality of intrusiveness into one's daily activities. It is not unusual for individuals to feel out of control, yet it is often possible for the hallucinator to be re-directed by another person or to learn specific coping strategies to decrease intrusiveness. Interven-

Table A. Model of Functional Deficits Associated with Hallucinations

Classification		Observable Behavior
Class I	No hallucinations	None
Class II	Intermittent hallucinations with minimal or no functional deficits.	Phenomena reported upon questioning or in appropriate settings. May appear withdrawn.
Class III	Intermittent or persistent hallucinations with functional deficits related to the content of the phenomena.	Evidence of poor self esteem such as frequent self deprecating remarks, poor posture, lack of social interaction, and poor motivation.
Class IV	Intermittent or persistent hallucinations with functional deficits directly related to the intrusiveness of the phenomena.	Inappropriate behavior while apparently responding to internal stimuli. Inappropriate affect such as giggling not related to the outside environment. Conversations with self. Poor attention to task on hand. However, can be re-directed to task and surroundings.
Class V	Persistent hallucinations with profound functional deficits. Generally acute.	Inability to appropriately respond to the external environment.

Anne MacRae, MS, OTR

tion techniques are quite variable and should be specifically tailored to the individual. Typically, modalities involve the altering of environmental stimuli either by increasing involvement in a specific task or by filtering and limiting stimuli through conscious relaxation.

Class V

This classification is reserved for the severe and persistent hallucinations generally only seen in an acute episode of a psychotic disorder. Treatment is geared toward the stabilization of the patient. Typically, a new medication or increased dosages of the patient's current medication is utilized. Environmental modification to create a non-stressful atmosphere with minimal demands or stimuli may also facilitate the stabilization process.

Application of the Model

Although many psychotic patients may experience Class II hallucinations, occupational therapy intervention is most likely going to occur with the presence of Class III and IV hallucinations because of the degree of associated functional deficits. In order to clarify the model presented in Table A, two short case studies using these classifications are presented. Case Study I is an example of Classification III, where the individual's functioning level is most affected by the content of his hallucinations. Case Study II describes an individual experiencing Class IV intrusive hallucinations with resulting functional deficits. In both cases, the treatment modalities attempted and the results of treatment are discussed.

Case Study I

Denis is a thirty-seven year old man diagnosed with Schizophrenia, Paranoid Type, Chronic. His initial hospitalization occurred in 1973 while he was away at college. Symptoms included depression, anxiety and self deprecating auditory hallucinations. Treatment has included repeated hospitalizations for stabilization and ongoing psychotropic medications including Navane and Trilafon. Several attempts at group therapy and vocational training have ended in failure as the client was unable to complete programs or otherwise comply with regime.

In the Fall of 1989, Denis was referred to the SJSU

psychosocial OT clinic. Based on formal and informal evaluations, it was determined that presenting problems included: (1) Low self esteem, (2) Inability to follow through with commitments, (3) Poor daily structure, and (4) Self isolative behavior. Interestingly, a formal assessment of functional living skills showed Denis to have the necessary skill proficiency and cognitive awareness to perform Activities of Daily Living (ADL). History and observation however showed that Denis' self care, in the areas of health and hygiene, was erratic; involvement in leisure activities was minimal; and work performance was non-existent.

Initially, Denis had poor attendance in clinic and was resistant to participation in clinic activities. However, he responded positively to the consistent encouragement provided by the student therapist and clinic supervisor and his attendance markedly improved. The primary goal of initial treatment was to provide a success experience both by engaging Denis in short term activities with minimal frustration and by completing a semester in clinic. This goal was satisfactorily met, however there was no change in Denis' behavior or activity level outside of clinic.

During the formal evaluation sessions, Denis refused to discuss the symptoms of his illness and was resistant to any form of interview. However, by the second semester of enrollment in clinic, he agreed to in-depth interviews with the clinic supervisor and revealed that "the voices" talked to him almost daily and discouraged him from attempting any changes in his life. The auditory hallucinations were always derogatory and Denis recognized that they negatively affected his self esteem and increased his fear of failure. Clinic activities continued to be geared towards providing success experiences but treatment expanded to include a gradual increase in easy to complete projects outside of the clinic and the use of specific techniques to counteract the hallucinations. Denis was instructed to make a conscious effort to make positive statements about himself on a daily basis and rehearsed this technique with his student therapist twice per week throughout his third semester of clinic. In addition, it was suggested that Denis engage in one of his planned activities, such as taking a walk, as soon as the voices began. By the end of the third semester of clinic attendance, Denis stated that the clinic strategies resulted in a decrease in the frequency of hallucinations from daily to approximately 2 or 3 times per week. Denis also reported a subjective feeling of being better able to cope with the remaining hallucinations. Moreover, Denis showed a more positive, relaxed affect and an increase in socialization and spontaneous expression. His overall activity level has increased to include daily exercise and some community outings. Long term goals include the exploration of volunteer work.

Case Study II

Jose is a bi-lingual (English/Spanish) 22 year old man who immigrated from El Salvador at the age of 14. He is unemployed, has never completed high school and presently lives in a residential care home. He is diagnosed as having Schizoaffective Disorder with an Axis II diagnosis of Dependent Personality Disorder. Jose has had repeated hospitalizations since the age of 16 for acute psychotic episodes with occasional assaultive behavior. He has been medically maintained on lithium carbonate and Prolixin.

Jose has been enrolled in the SJSU psychosocial OT clinic for several semesters. A functional skills assessment showed Jose to be dependent in all ADL except basic personal hygiene. He also displayed significant deficits in memory, attention span and problem solving. Through repeated interviews and observation, it was determined that Jose experienced visual, auditory, tactile and somatic hallucinations. He did not have an understanding of the nature of his hallucinations and vacillated between thinking they were either spiritual visitations or from his imagination. The content of the hallucinations usually involved the presence of spirits but also involved sexual activity and generalized sensations. The visual hallucinations were characterized as frightening or disturbing and the tactile hallucinations were painful and/or uncomfortable. The one description of a somatic hallucination (electricity in the body) was perceived as enjoyable. Jose admitted to auditory hallucinations but he did not perceive them to be "voices" or sounds from the external environment. He perceived these communications as an internal process which he credited to the "telepathy of the spirits." These communications were puzzling rather than demanding or frightening.

Although the *content* of the hallucinations did not appear to directly affect Jose's level of function, observation and patient self report confirmed that the *intrusive nature* of the hallucinations did interfere with ADL performance. With Jose's cooperation, the OT student therapists attempted to decrease the intrusiveness of the hallucinations by instituting a program using a variety of coping strategies. These included the reciting of a word with special significance, going to sleep, participating in clinic activities, and dialoguing with himself to increase reality orientation.

The combination of techniques met with success in that Jose reported a reduction in the intrusiveness of the hallucinations and the clinic staff observed an increase in Jose's ability to attend to the task on hand. However, Jose does not initiate the techniques independently. He appears to need a highly structured environment and verbal cueing for the techniques to be effective. This may be a manifestation of his dependent personality or attributable to his evident cognitive deficits, rather than any specific quality of the hallucinations. Consequently, part of Jose's treatment plan includes staff training at his residential care home.

Discussion

Psychotic illness is a complex phenomenon with a myriad of different symptoms and functional deficits. Hence, it is often difficult to determine the effectiveness of any intervention strategy. By focusing on a specific type of symptom, such as hallucinations, and determining the associated functional deficits, the clinician may better determine the type of intervention required. It is hoped that the model presented in this article can be used as a guideline for further clarification and research regarding the impact of symptomatology on individuals' functional levels as well as for the development of specific intervention strategies.

References

Aggernaes, A. (1972). The experienced reality of hallucinations and other psychological phenomena. *Acta Psychiatrica Scandinavica, 48*, 220-238.

Alford, G. S. & Turner, S. M. (1976). Stimulus interference and conditioned inhibition of auditory hallucinations. *Journal of Behavior Therapy and Experimental Psychiatry, 7*, (2),155-160.

American Psychiatric Association (1987). *The diagnostic and statistical manual, (3rd ed., revised)*. Washington, DC: Author.

Barris, R., Kielhofner, G., & Watts, J. H. (1988). *Occupational therapy in psychosocial practice*. Thorofare, New Jersey: Slack.

Bentall, R. P., & Slade P. D. (1985). Reality testing and auditory hallucinations: a signal detection analysis. *The British Journal of Clinical Psychology, 24*, 159-169.

Bick, P. A. & Kinsbourne, M. D. (1987). Auditory hallucinations and subvocal speech in schizophrenic patients. *American Journal of Psychiatry, 144*, 222-225.

Bender, L. (1970). The maturation process and hallucinations in children. In W. Keup (Ed.) *Origin and mechanisms of hallucinations*. (pp. 95-102). New York: Plenum Press.

Birchwood, M. (1986). Control of auditory hallucinations through occlusion of monaural auditory input. *British Journal of Psychiatry, 149*, 104-107.

Bliss, E. L., Larson, E. M., & Nakashima, B. A. (1983). Auditory hallucinations and schizophrenia. *The Journal of Nervous and Mental Disease, 171*, 30-33.

Breier, V. & Strauss, J. (1983). Self control in psychotic disorders. *Archives of General Psychiatry, 40*, 1141-1145.

Brieire de Boismont, A. (1976). *Hallucinations.* (Reprint of the 1853 edition). Philadelphia: Lindsay and Blakiston.

Collicutt, J. R., & Hemsley, D. R. (1981). A psychophysical investigation of auditory functioning in schizophrenia. *The British Journal of Clinical Psychology, 20*, 199-204.

Done, D. J., Frith, C. D., & Owens, D. C. (1986). Reducing persistent auditory hallucinations by wearing an earplug. *British Journal of Clinical Psychology, 25*, 151-152.

Falloon, I. & Talbot, R. (1981). Persistent auditory hallucinations: coping mechanisms and implications of management. *Psychological Medicine, 11*, 329-339.

Feder, R. (1982). Auditory hallucinations treated by radio headphones. *American Journal of Psychiatry, 139*, (9),1188-1190.

Field, W. & Ruelke, W. (1973). Hallucinations and how to deal with them. *American Journal of Nursing, 73*, 638-640.

Fisher, E. B. & Winkler, R. (1975). Self control over intrusive experiences. *Journal of Consulting and Clinical Psychology, 6*, 911-916.

Goodwin, D., Alderson, P. & Rosenthal, R. (1970). Clinical significance of hallucinations in psychiatric disorders. *Archives of General Psychiatry, 24*, 76-80.

Green, M. F., & Kinsbourne, M. (1989). Auditory hallucinations in schizophrenia: does humming help? *Biological Psychiatry, 25*, 630-633.

Green, P. & Preston, M. (1981). Reinforcement of vocal correlates of auditory hallucinations by auditory feedback: a case study. *British Journal of Psychiatry, 139*, 204-208.

Hartmann, E. (1975). Dreams and other hallucinations: An approach to the underlying mechanism. In R. K. Siegal & L. J. West (Eds.) *Hallucinations: behavior, experience, and theory* (pp. 71-80). New York: John Wiley.

Heilbrun, A. & Blum, N. (1984). Cognitive vulnerability to auditory hallucination impaired perception of meaning. *British Journal of Psychiatry, 144*, 508-512.

Hemsley, A. M. & Slade, P. D. (1981). The effects of varying auditory input on schizophrenic hallucinations. *British Journal of Psychiatry, 139*,122-127.

Hogarty, G., Anderson, C., Reiss, D., Kornblith, S., Greenwald D., Javna, C., & Madonia M. (1986). Family psychoeducation, social skills training and maintenance chemotherapy in the aftercare treatment of schizophrenia. *Archives of General Psychiatry, 43*, 633-642.

Hogarty, G., Goldberg, S., Schooler, N., & Ulrich R. (1974). Drugs and sociotherapy in the aftercare of schizophrenic patients. *Archives of General Psychiatry, 31*, 603-608.

Horowitz, M. (1975). A cognitive model of hallucinations. *The American Journal of Psychiatry, 132*, 789-795.

Horowitz, M. (1975). Hallucinations: An information processing approach. In R. K. Siegal & L. J. West (Eds.) *Hallucinations: behavior, experience, and theory* (pp. 163-196). New York: John Wiley.

Hume, A. (1988). Let me whisper in your ear. *Nursing Times, 84*, 39-41.

Inouye, T. & Shimizu, A. (1970). The electromyographic study of verbal hallucination. *The Journal of Nervous and Mental Disease,151*, 415-422.

Inouye, T. & Shimizu, A. (1972). Visual evoked response and reaction time during verbal hallucination. *The Journal of Nervous and Mental Disease, 155*, 419-426.

James, D. (1983). The experimental treatment of two cases of auditory hallucinations. *The British Journal of Psychiatry, 143,* 515-516.

Jaynes, J. (1979). *The origins of consciousness in the breakdown of the bicameral mind.* Harmondsworth: Penguin.

Johnson, F. (1978). *The anatomy of hallucinations.* Chicago: Nelson-Hall.

Junginger, J. & Frame, C. (1985). Self-report of the frequency and phenomenology of verbal hallucinations. *Journal of Nervous and Mental Disease, 173,* 149-155.

Junginger, J. & Rauscher, F. (1987). Vocal activity in verbal hallucinations. *Journal of Psychiatric Research, 21,* 101-109.

Keup, W. (Ed.) (1970). *Origin and mechanisms of hallucinations.* New York: Plenum Press.

Klasson, E. & MacRae, A. (1985). A university based occupational therapy clinic for chronic schizophrenics. *Occupational Therapy in Mental Health, 5,* 1-11.

La Barre, W. (1975). Anthropological perspectives on hallucination and hallucinogens. In R. K. Siegal & L. J. West (Eds.) *Hallucinations: behavior, experience, and theory* (pp. 9-52). New York: John Wiley.

Lemberg, R. (1978). Multi-sensory hallucinatory experiences: a diary account. *American Journal of Psychotherapy, 32,* 457-468.

Lezak, M. (1983). *Neuropsychological assessment.* (2nd ed.) New York: Oxford.

Liberman, R., Mueser, K., & Wallace, C. (1986). Social skills training for schizophrenic individuals at risk for relapse. *American Journal of Psychiatry, 143,* 523-526.

Lothane, Z. (1982). The psychopathology of hallucinations—a methodological analysis. *British Journal of Medical Psychology, 55,* 335-348.

Malm, U., May, P., & Dencker, S. (1981). Evaluation of the quality of life of the schizophrenic outpatient: A checklist. *Schizophrenia Bulletin, 7,* (3), 477-487.

Mosak, H. & Fletcher, S. (1973). Purposes of delusions and hallucinations. *Journal of Individual Psychology, 29,* 176-181.

Reed, G. (1972). *The psychology of anomalous experience.* London: Hutchinson & Co.

Rogers, J. (1982). Order and disorder in medicine and occupational therapy. *American Journal of Occupational Therapy, 36,* 29-35.

Romme, M. & Escher, A. (1989). Hearing voices. *Schizophrenia Bulletin, 15,* 209-216.

Sarbin, T. & Juhasz, J. (1975). The social context of hallucinations. In R. K. Siegal & L. J. West (Eds.). *Hallucinations: behavior, experience, and theory* (pp. 241-256). New York: John Wiley.

Slade, P. D. (1976). Towards a theory of auditory hallucinations: outline of a hypothetical four-factor model. *The British Journal of Social and Clinical Psychology, 15,* 415-423.

Slade, P. & Bentall, R. (1988). *Sensory deception.* Baltimore: Johns Hopkins University Press.

Starker, S. (1986). From image to hallucination: Studies of mental imagery in schizophrenic patients. In A. Sheikh (Ed.) *International review of mental imagery* (pp. 192-215). New York: Human Sciences Press.

Wallace, C., Nelson, C., Liberman, R., Lukoff, D., Elder, J., & Ferris, C. (1980). A review and critique of social skills training with schizophrenic patients. *Schizophrenia Bulletin, 6,* (1), 42-63.

Weingaertner, A. (1971). Self administered aversive stimulation with hallucinating hospitalized schizophrenics. *Journal of Consulting and Clinical Psychology, 36,* 422-429.

West, L. J. (1975). A clinical and theoretical overview of hallucinatory phenomena. In R. K. Siegal & L. J. West (Eds.) *Hallucinations: behavior, experience, and theory* (pp. 287-312). New York: John Wiley.

Chapter 61

Exploring Sensory Integrative Treatment in Chronic Schizophrenia

Judith E. Reisman, PhD, OTR
Anne B. Blakeney, MSOT, OTR, FAOTA

The purpose of this study was to investigate the effect of sensory integrative treatment activities on psychiatric status and physical functioning in persons with chronic schizophrenia. Sensory integration may be defined as "the nervous system's process of assimilating and organizing sensory information for functional use. An individual's ability to interact with the environment is influenced by how effectively and efficiently that person is able to process and use information from the tactile, vestibular, proprioceptive, visual, auditory, olfactory, and gustatory systems" (American Occupational Therapy Association, 1982, p. 831). There is accumulating evidence that many persons with schizophrenia have signs of sensory integrative dysfunction (e.g., Endler & Eimon, 1978; Huddleston, 1978; Leach, 1960; Myers, Caldwell & Purcell, 1973). They are not able to process and use sensory information well.

In a discussion of clinical research, Kazdin (1984) differentiates between an experimental criterion, which determines "if an intervention has a reliable or veridical effect on behavior" and a therapeutic criterion, in which "the intervention needs to make an important change in the client's everyday functioning" (p. 285). Although it is important to document changes in sensory integrative status as a result of treatment employing sensory integrative techniques, the real goal of occupational therapy is functional improvement, or the therapeutic criterion. Ayres (1972, 1979) emphasized the value of sensory integrative treatment for its ability to influence brain functioning which in turn facilitates purposeful interaction with the environment. This study's focus, therefore, was on both psychiatric status as well as sensory integrative function.

Review of Literature

Since King's (1974) first publication outlining the rationale and application of sensory integrative techniques with the chronic schizophrenic population, there have been several researchers who have attempted to test her hypothesis. In a review of occupational therapy with schizophrenic patients, Hayes (1989) concluded that sensory integrative treatment did not have an impact on sensory integrative functioning but resulted in improved motivation and affect; however, her conclusions are drawn upon an incomplete review and analysis of the studies available. Levine, O'Connor and Stacey (1977) involved six schizophrenic patients in daily sessions for a six week period and observed changes in the raw scores of sensory integration measures adapted from those used with children. They concluded that there was a need for further efficacy studies in this area and for the development of standardized tests of sensory integrative status in adults. In the absence of such a tool, Crist (1979) was not able to quantify changes in body image using a modification of the Goodenough Harris Draw-a-Man Test. However, she reported many subjective observations of improved ability to function in the treatment group as well as a decrease in some of the characteristics of sensory integrative dysfunction. As the investigator stated, without standardized measurement tools, these observations can only be used as indicators of areas for future research.

Bailey (1978) focused on the effect of sensory integrative treatment on increasing verbalizations in chronic schizophrenics, an observation reported by King (1974) and other therapists (Blakeney, Strickland & Wilkinson, 1983). While Bailey's study lends partial empirical support to increased verbalizations following sensory integrative treatment, her study was hampered by measures which turned out to be insensitive to many of the language changes observed clinically in her study population.

Rider (1978) was the first therapist to use a standardized tool designed specifically for the adult psychiatric population. She hypothesized that "given adequate stimulation, these posture and movement patterns (of schizophrenia) can be altered, and if so, there may be corresponding change in psychological organization evidenced by a decrease in psychotic behavior" (p. 452). Using the NOSIE-30 (Honigfeld, Gillis & Klett, 1966) and other measures of physiological status, Rider tested her treatment group before and after six weeks of sensory integrative treatment and again after a six week no-treatment period (post-posttreatment). While no change was seen in the positive factors of the NOSIE-30, there was a significant post-treatment drop in negative factors. Unfortunately, it was not maintained on two of the three

factors in the post-posttreatment testing. An important limitation of this study was the fact that subjects were not matched to King's (1974) physiological criteria associated with chronic schizophrenia.

Crist, Thomas and Stone (1984) compared the effects of prevocational and sensorimotor training on two groups of clients with chronic schizophrenia. They found that the total patient sample showed significant change on eight of 54 measures of coordination, strength and perceptual motor performance, as well as on part of the Psychotic Inpatient Profile, and attributed the changes primarily to the prevocational group. The unexpected finding that prevocational training produced a significant result must be tempered by the study's small number of subjects (N = 4/group) and mixture of diagnoses and experimental treatment settings for each group. In addition, the description of the sensorimotor activities leads one to believe that while the therapists used the accepted continuum of passive to active to adaptive activity (Gilfoyle, Grady & Moore, 1981), this was applied to the entire group in a lesson plan format instead of adjusting for individual differences or rates of change. The authors were careful to call their treatment sensorimotor and not sensory integration, so this approach is acceptable in that context, but the two treatments should not be taken as equivalent.

A final study compared the effect of sensory integrative activities versus more sedentary craft and grooming activities on two groups of patients with chronic schizophrenia (Blakeney et al., 1983). As in the Rider (1978) study, Blakeney et al., chose the NOSIE-30 as well as tests of physical status (gait, grip, Object Manipulation Speed Test [King, 1978]) to measure possible treatment effects. Following six weeks of treatment, the sensory integration group showed a significant improvement on the NOSIE-30 total score and on the factor, manifest psychosis. There were no changes in gait, grip or Object Manipulation Speed Test scores, but as in the other studies, the researchers report observations of change in appearance, verbalization, affect and socialization.

Tickle-Degnen (1988) applied two models of analysis to sensory integration research which may be helpful in understanding the study designs. The first is the synchronic, "a model of immediate response that describes what sensory integration does during the moment of treatment delivery," and the second is the diachronic, "a model of change that describes the effect of sensory integration over successive periods of time" (p. 427). Tickle-Degnen (1988) maintains that the latter model is useful in determining effectiveness of therapy over multiple sessions and, therefore, appropriate for single-subject research. Perhaps the model may also be useful in looking at investigations of groups in which performance is sampled over successive time periods.

This study was designed using the diachronic model. Patients were tested before, during and after the application of sensory integrative treatment to determine whether treatment would result in improved psychiatric status and sensory integrative function. The following hypotheses were tested:

1. Sequenced sensory integrative treatment produces changes in psychiatric status (NOSIE-30) and sensory integrative function (grip strength, speed of manipulation, thumb-finger opposition, diadochokinesis, eye pursuits and balance).
2. Sensory integration treatment activities produce cumulative changes, i.e., scores from multiple periods of measurement reflect a linear trend.

Subjects

Five subjects in a large state psychiatric institution met the criteria for inclusion in the study. All subjects had a DSM-III (American Psychiatric Association, 1980) diagnosis of chronic, undifferentiated schizophrenia, characterized by multiple admissions with short periods of community living. All subjects received psychotropic medication which remained unchanged in type and amount during the 17 weeks of the study. All displayed an S-curve posture, an inability to differentiate head and trunk movement, and a shuffling gait as described by King (1974). The subjects attended occupational therapy for the sensory integrative treatment sessions in lieu of the regularly scheduled craft-oriented occupational therapy. Each subject gave informed consent before participating.

There were three men and two women in the group. Age of subjects ranged from 21 years to 61 years. Four of the subjects were 46 years old or younger. It was decided to include the oldest subject because he met the study criteria and because of the growing evidence for plasticity of the aging nervous system (e.g., Black, Greenough, Anderson & Isaacs, 1987). All subjects had their first hospital admission in their adolescence or twenties. Ideally, a second group of subjects should have served as a control. Unfortunately, this was not possible due to staffing limitations.

As Huddleston (1978) and Rider (1979) [sic] point out, most chronic schizophrenic patients have received a variety of treatments, but show little significant or lasting improvement. The subjects in this study were no exception, having been scheduled for programs such as craft-oriented occupational therapy, art therapy, behavior modification and psychotherapy, with little change noted in psychiatric status.

Instruments

King (Posthuma, 1983) recommends the use of the NOSIE-30 in psychiatric occupational therapy research, stressing the importance of correlating assessment in occupational therapy with assessment of psychiatric status. Accordingly, the NOSIE-30 was the first instrument chosen for this study. In addition to yielding a total score, one may obtain scores on three positive factors—social competence, social interest and neatness, and three negative factors—irritability, manifest psychosis and psychomotor retardation. The instrument has been found sensitive to change and has good interrater reliability ($r = 0.73$ to 0.89) (Honigfeld et al., 1966). It has the added advantage in occupational therapy research of being scored by nursing staff. During this study, staff were instructed to administer the NOSIE-30 to other patients as well as study subjects. This ensured that they were blind to the subjects' research status. The separation of scoring personnel from treatment personnel decreases potential bias which could occur by therapists unconsciously inflating scores when looking for behavior change as a result of their treatment.

Two other measures from the Blakeney et al. (1983) study were chosen, the Object Manipulation Speed Test (King, 1978) and grip strength using the Jamar dynamometer in the second position. Gait was not included because of the lack of numeric scores in the original study.

There are many studies (e.g., Falk-Kessler, Quittman & Moore, 1988) documenting soft neurological signs in psychiatric populations, but no consistent and objective method for identifying these signs. The Schroeder, Block, Campbell Adult Psychiatric Sensory Integration Evaluation (SBC) (Schroeder, Block, Trottier & Stowell, 1983) provides an initial point of patient observation; however, the SBC is not yet normed. An attempt was made to quantify observations of sensory integrative function for the purposes of this study.

Thumb-finger opposition, diadochokinesis and ocular pursuits were measured (right, left and bilateral) using the procedure outlined by Schroeder et al. (1983). Subjects placed their hand over one eye for monocular pursuits. The scoring system of the SBC, however, was not used. Instead, the five point scale below was developed with categories related to amount of assistance required, in addition to quality of performance.

1. Inadequate; simply could not complete the task even when walked/guided through it.
2. Inadequate; could only complete task if walked/guided through it.
3. Shows minimal competence; could almost mimic task but had difficulty completing it.
4. Adequate; could complete task after some help

was given through demonstration, guidance or more verbal direction.

5. Adequate; could initiate and perform task on verbal command without further guidance.

In addition, a balance beam task was added in which subjects were scored using the above scale to rate their ability to walk forward, backward and sideways on the beam. Subjects were simply instructed to "Walk down the beam. Do the best you can." These measures of sensory integrative function were chosen based on unreported observations made during the Blakeney et al. (1983) study in which videotaped records showed marked improvement in performance of these tasks.

Procedure

Subjects were tested in the week before treatment began and again in four one-week periods. These test sessions were interspersed between four successive three-week treatment periods and after the last treatment period (see Table 1). Beginning in week two, subjects were provided a program that followed a sequence of progressive application of activities within a sensory integrative context. In general the activities were designed to follow the treatment principles outlined by King (1974) and Ayres (1972, 1979), specifically, that the activity be pleasurable and that the focus be on the activity and not on the underlying sensory input or motor act that is occurring.

setting, (but) patients were encouraged to pursue a particular activity individually, if they demonstrated a desire to do so...This allowed for flexibility within the group and for individual adaptive responses" (p. 402).

Treatment activities were introduced in a sequence. Levine et al. (1977) reported a design which focused on a specific type of sensory stimulation each week, for example, vestibular input, although each activity tended to be multi-sensory in nature. The concept of using a hierarchy of activities is appealing because it provides a predictable structure within the flexible, patient-directed activities appropriate for sensory integration treatment. Those activities likely to be most familiar and least threatening to patients were introduced first, progressing to activities that were less familiar and more physically and/or socially challenging.

The first three weeks of treatment (Rx 1) had a primarily visual and auditory focus. Patients were assisted to sit on the floor. This kept the stable base most were used to from long term sitting and yet provided a different set of sensations than a chair gives. Brightly colored streamers were introduced for tracking and to give visually-mediated vestibular input to each person. Patients threw large colored nerf balls and bean bags at targets, thus tying together visual, tactile and proprioceptive input while balance was maintained. Instrumental, folk and march music stimulated clapping and "moving to the music" while seated for links between auditory, proprioceptive and vestibular input.

Table 1. Study Design of Test (T) and Treatment (Rx) Weeks

Week	1	2-4	5	6-8	9	10-12	13	14-16	17
Test/Rx	T 1	Rx 1	T 2	Rx 2	T 3	Rx 3	T 4	Rx 4	T 5

Ottenbacher (1982), in his meta-analysis of studies related to sensory integration, defines sensory integration therapy as only those procedures that employ sensory stimulation and adaptive responses involving total body movement. In addition, the sensory stimulation procedures have to include some combination of vestibular, proprioceptive or tactile stimulation and be based on the theoretical work of Ayres. Desk activities, speech training, reading lessons and specific perceptual motor skills training are not considered sensory integration. The treatment activities in this study meet the criteria defined by Ottenbacher (1982). As in the Blakeney et al. (1983) study, the "activities were carried out in a group

The second set of treatment weeks (Rx 2) added a stronger proprioceptive focus to the activities. Patients marched and jumped to the music, bounced on large balls, rolled and crawled over a simple obstacle course, played parachute games, jumped rope, and pushed/pulled their arms and legs in games with each other, the parachute or with bungy cords. The tactile element was strengthened by the increased variety of objects and textures, and strong linear vestibular input was provided through the up-and-down and back-and-forth head motions most of the games required.

Angular vestibular stimulation was added in the third set of treatments (Rx 3) through individual swinging and spinning, as tolerated, as well as modified dancing to the music and more parachute games. It is important to emphasize that all previous activities were continued. The new activities were an expansion of a gradually increasing repertoire of pleasurable activities from which patients could choose.

The last treatment period (Rx 4) had more concentration on the tactile system. Applying lotion and powder while swinging, brushing body areas with differently textured brushes, walking barefoot over different surfaces, and deep pressure touch in the form of "group hugs" were favorite activities. The increased social comfort of the group is reflected in their ability to enjoy the last mentioned activity.

The ratio of staff to patients in each treatment session was 3:5. One therapist was consistently present each day and other therapists participated several times a week on a regular schedule. Each session lasted for one hour five days per week. All patients had nearly perfect attendance because they were brought to the clinic by one of the therapists. The only absences were due to physical illness.

Results

A single factor repeated measures analysis of variance was performed on the scores from each of the tests (Abacus Concepts, 1986; Currier, 1990). The change in scores over time was the statistically and therapeutically relevant factor, since a significant result here would indicate that the behaviors and abilities of the patients were changing over the course of the treatments. The analysis of variance was followed by a trend analysis (Steel & Torrie, 1980) in order to support or reject the second hypothesis. Both linear and quadratic components of the trend were examined.

A significant ($F = 12.27$; $p < 0.0001$) increase in the total scores on the NOSIE-30 was found (see Table 2.)

Table 2. Mean Scores on the NOISIE 30 and Factors.

Test	Total*	COM*	INT*	NEA*	IRR*	PSY*	RET
1	84.8	9.2	22.4	14.0	23.6	22.8	12.4
2	93.6	11.2	21.2	14.0	18.2	16.4	13.2
3	88.8	10.0	21.6	13.2	21.2	17.6	15.2
4	116.8	19.6	24.0	16.0	15.2	11.6	12.0
5	134.8	21.6	26.4	16.4	9.2	5.6	10.8

* $p \leq 0.05$ level   COM: Social competence, INT: Social interest, NEA: Neatness, IRR: Irritability, PSY: Manifest psychosis, RET: Psychomotor retardation

Four of the six factors also showed a significant improvement. These were the positive factors of social competence ($F = 4.86$; $p < 0.01$) and social interest ($F = 2.98$; $p < 0.05$) and the negative factors of irritability ($F = 3.98$; $p < 0.02$) and manifest psychosis ($F = 16.53$; $p < 0.0001$). It should be noted that an elevation in scores is considered improvement on positive factors and a decline in scores is considered improvement on negative factors. The positive factor of neatness and the negative factor of psychomotor retardation did not show a significant change.

Both linear and quadratic components were found in the analysis of trend in the total scores of the NOSIE-30 (see Figure 1.). The linear trend ($F = 40.94$; $p < 0.005$) indicates that, on the average, scores improve as amount of treatment time increases. The quadratic component ($F = 5.05$; $p < 0.05$) indicates a decline in improvement at the third testing period. Suggestions for why this decline was present will be presented in the discussion below. Analysis of trend in the four NOSIE-30 factors reaching significance in the main analysis revealed a significant linear, but not a quadratic trend.

Figure 1. Curvilinear Relationship of Mean Scores: NOISIE-30.

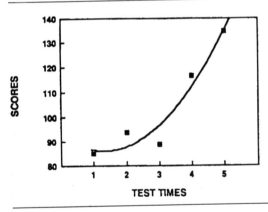

On the measures of physical function (see Table 3), there was a significant change in thumb-finger opposition for the left hand ($F = 12.51$; $p < 0.0001$), right hand ($F = 12.7$; $p < 0.0001$) and for bilateral function ($F = 3.22$; $p < 0.04$). There was also a significant change in diadochokinesis for the left hand ($F = 8.92$; $p < 0.001$), right hand ($F = 10.67$; $p < 0.0002$) and for bilateral function ($F = 8.95$; $p < 0.0005$). Binocular eye pursuits showed a significant improvement ($F = 3.33$; $p < 0.04$), but neither eye when tested alone showed a significant change. Lastly, ability to walk the balance beam forward and sideways showed a significant change ($F = 3.08$; $p < 0.05$ and $F = 5.97$; $p < 0.02$, respectively). Missing data (subject refusal) precluded analysis of the balance beam backwards task. There was no significant change in scores

Table 3. Mean Scores on Tests of Physical Function.

Test	TF-L*	TF-R*	TF-B*	DI-L*	DI-R*	DI-B*	EP*	BB-F*	BB-S*
1	1.4	1.0	1.0	1.4	1.6	1.4	2.0	2.8	1.3
2	1.2	1.2	1.0	1.4	1.6	1.6	2.8	3.0	1.3
3	2.4	2.2	2.0	2.2	2.2	2.2	1.6	4.0	3.3
4	2.4	2.2	2.4	3.4	3.6	3.2	3.2	3.4	3.3
5	3.4	3.8	2.4	3.4	4.0	3.6	3.4	4.6	5.0

* $p \leq 0.05$ level   TF-L, R, B: Thumb-finger opposition—left, right, bilateral; DI: Diadokokinesis; EP: Eye pursuits; BB-F, S: Balance beam—forward, sideways

of grip strength or the Object Manipulation Speed Test. As in the NOSIE-30 factors, there was a significant linear, but not a quadratic trend in the physical function scores.

Discussion

The results demonstrate that there is a relationship between involvement in sensory integrative activities and improvement in psychiatric and physical status. The change in the NOSIE-30 total scores replicates the finding of Blakeney et al. (1983). The average improvement of 50 points in the 17 weeks of the study is encouraging for anyone who has worked with patients with chronic disabilities. In addition, the improvement in four of the six factors of the test provides some evidence that the improvement in the total score is based on generalized improvement in several areas of behavior and is not confined to marked improvement in a single factor. It is interesting to note that the factor showing greatest improvement was that of manifest psychosis, the only one reaching significance in the original Blakeney et al. (1983) study. It is also heartening to see that just a small increase in number of treatment weeks seemed to enable most patients to achieve significant improvement in the other factors that were improved but did not reach statistical significance in the Blakeney et al. (1983) study. As in that study, the factor of neatness was highly resistant to change. Perhaps this is a higher level function more dependent on adequate body concept or perhaps it reflects habits acquired in institutional living.

The lack of change in grip strength and object manipulation speed also replicates the earlier findings of Blakeney et al. (1983). The newly added measures of thumb-finger opposition, diadochokinesis, eye pursuits, and balance beam tasks all showed improvement. The refusal of subjects in the initial test periods to attempt walking backwards on the balance beam is probably related to their reliance on vision to assist in maintenance of balance. This greater challenge to balance was rejected by some until they had achieved better integration partway through the study.

The frustration many researching therapists have felt over clearly observable changes in patients while their tests of these same patients did not reach quantitative significance may be partly the result of choosing the wrong measures. Schizophrenia and sensory integrative dysfunction are complicated neurological problems. The measures of grip strength and speed of manipulation, which showed no change in this study, have been studied repeatedly by others (e.g., Mather & Putchat, 1983; Neuchterlein, 1977) and may be tapping the brain dysfunction which is hypothesized to result in the schizophrenic process (Andreason et al. 1988; Chapman, 1966; Corbett, 1976). Perhaps these abilities represent medication side effects and are resistant to sensory integrative treatment at least when applied for this period of time.

In contrast to the usual time spent in clinical treatment of chronic schizophrenics, most studies on the use of sensory integration intervention have a relatively short treatment period. This leads to discouraging results. In general, however, the significant linear trend in the data of this study supports the hypothesis that amount of treatment time is directly related to improvement.

Now that the biological bases of schizophrenia are becoming well documented (Andreason et al. 1988; Henn & Nasrallah, 1982; Wyatt, Alexander, Egan & Kirch, 1988), occupational therapists working in mental health may be able to view their efforts similarly to those therapists who work with other brain damaged individuals in the physical disabilities specialty area. We may expect multiple periods of progress with plateaus and even short regressions over an extended period of treatment.

This pattern of response may explain the quadratic trend in the NOSIE-30 data in which a dip or leveling of scores was seen in the middle of the study. The dip occurred just after strong proprioceptive input and linear vestibular input was emphasized. Perhaps some of the patients seemed more irritable and resistant to cooperation on the ward because they were now more alert and active. While absence of positive behavior had been a concern, the emergence of new behaviors may have made patient management more difficult for ward staff. This phenomenon has been observed when working with children with sensory integrative dysfunction. Some of the passive children begin to "feel their oats" and pass through a period of early aggressiveness before learning the elements of living in a social world.

While children with learning disabilities and other disorders associated with sensory integrative dysfunction are often treated individually, adults with chronic schizophrenia are often treated in groups. In part, this reflects differences in availability of staff and funding resources between the clinics and schools that serve children and the long term care facilities that serve chronic adults. However, it is recommended that sensory integrative treatment be provided in a group setting when working with most adult patients. Adults, even those with such a severe disability as schizophrenia, are often able to "rally" and benefit from observing and helping others in a group until they are able to participate more actively on their own behalf. In addition, individual treatment, especially of such an explicit sensory nature, may be embarrassing or misinterpreted by some of these adults.

King (1974) stated that "...anything that affects the body will inexorably affect the mind and vice versa" (p. 530). This study began with the explicit intent of providing schizophrenic patients with activities which would have an impact on their sensory integrative functioning and in turn improve their psychiatric status. Tickle-Degnen (1988) elaborates on this logic. She states that what mediates the effectiveness of therapy is a combination of observable (for example, behavior change) and nonobservable (for example, brain change) factors. "Since brain change...is a nonobservable factor in living organisms, it is difficult to establish support for its role in the mediation of the effects of sensory integration therapy. Brain change can be inferred only from indirect observable variables..." (p. 430). As she points out, it is difficult to understand and even accept the links in a theory when several of the factors are not observable, but "it is not appropriate to conclude on the basis of this difficulty that the theory is not correct" (p. 430).

Individual patient changes emerged within the group during the study period. One of the changes observed but not measured occurred in the area of speech. Two of the five subjects demonstrated dramatic improvements in speech clarity and ability to converse. One of the younger patients was initially unable to speak intelligibly. When spoken to directly, he responded only with garbled sounds. He made few attempts to talk. His speech performance progressed from these unintelligible sounds to short outbursts of clearly understood phrases which were echolalic. This was followed by a period in which he could respond appropriately to questions, but perseverated in his responses. At the conclusion of the study, he was able to initiate and carry on a conversation with appropriate interactions and oral motor control. He had, in essence, gained functional communication skills.

The oldest patient was thought to be mute by hospital staff when the study began. As treatment progressed, he began to respond to daily greetings by the therapist and eventually engaged in conversation, stating preferences for his favorite activities and staff members. At the midpoint of the study, he experienced a severe ear infection and was observed to stop talking altogether. He resumed appropriate speech patterns a short time after his treatment for the infection had ended.

These improvements in speech appear to support similar gains reported in the Blakeney et al. (1983) study. This remains one of the more difficult areas to quantify and measure, as demonstrated by Bailey (1978). It is, however, one of the areas in which impressive gains are often noted by therapists during sensory integrative treatment.

We are cautioned by King (Posthuma, 1983) that sensory integration is only the foundation of treatment for chronic schizophrenic patients and that occupational therapists still need to provide treatment in the areas of activities of daily living, leisure skills, community living skills and work skills. Improvement in psychiatric status results in increased readiness to participate in these higher level groups. As Ayres states, "The goal of sensory integration is to enhance the brain's ability to learn how to do...things. If the brain develops the *capacity* to perceive, remember, and motor plan, the ability can then be applied toward mastery of all...tasks, regardless of specific content" (1972, p. 2). Facilitating improved sensory integration without providing training or retraining in practical living skills is therapeutically purposeless.

Limitations

Clinical research is admittedly difficult to accomplish because there are so many factors which are difficult to control. This study contains some of the limitations of sensory integration research in schizophrenia outlined by Hixson and Mathews (1984), in particular, small sample size and lack of a control group. In addition, the occupational therapists involved in treatment delivery tested the physical function in the subjects. Care must, therefore, be taken in interpreting the significant improvement found in the physical measures. One may feel some confidence, however, that measures that tap reflex activity, such as eye pursuits and balance, and unconscious coordination, such as thumb-finger opposition and diadochokinesis, are likely to be less affected by rater bias than measures that tap psychological functioning.

Obtaining well matched control groups for patients with schizophrenia is difficult. Patients experience the disease of schizophrenia individually and uniquely. The result is that patients with the same diagnosis display many levels of function in a variety of areas.

Although the lack of a control group is a limitation in this study, a strength of the study is that patients were carefully matched to the criteria established by King (1974) for sensory integrative dysfunction in chronic schizophrenics. Therapists conducting research in this area and attempting to test King's hypotheses must be aware of the need for this careful selection of subjects.

Conclusion

The benefits of the sensory integration approach are threefold: one, it paves the way for a non-invasive treatment of a hard-to-treat population; two, it provides a vehicle for preventive mental health through early intervention of sensory integration problems in younger clients (Hixson and Mathews, 1984); and three, the improved brain functioning makes higher level training and treatment more possible (Ayres, 1972; King, 1974). The finding of highly significant effects in a group which typically has experienced but not responded to many treatments over the years is encouraging. As the same results accrue across researchers and subjects, the converging evidence begins to attain some validity, and therapists may plan sensory integrative treatment for persons with chronic schizophrenia with more confidence.

References

Abacus Concepts (1986). *Statview 512+* (Computer program). Calabasas, CA: BrainPower, Incorporated.

American Occupational Therapy Association. (1982). Occupational therapy for sensory integrative dysfunction. *American Journal of Occupational Therapy, 36*, 831.

American Psychiatric Association. (1980). *Diagnostic and statistical manual of mental disorders* (3rd ed.). Washington, DC: Author.

Andreason, N. C., Shore, D., Burke, J. D., Grove, W. D., Lieberman, J. A., Oltmann, T. F., Pettegrew, J. W., Pulver, A. E., Siever, L. J., Tsuang, M. T., & Wyatt, R. J. (1988). Clinical phenomenology. *Schizophrenia Bulletin, 14*, 345-363.

Ayres, A. J. (1972). *Sensory integration and learning disorders.* Los Angeles: Western Psychological Services.

Ayres, A. J. (1979). *Sensory integration and the child.* Los Angeles: Western Psychological Services.

Bailey, D. M. (1978). The effects of vestibular stimulation on verbalization in chronic schizophrenics. *American Journal of Occupational Therapy, 32*, 445-450.

Black, J. E., Greenough, W. T., Anderson, B. T., & Isaacs, K. R. (1987). Environment and the aging brain. *Canadian Journal of Psychology, 41*, 111-130.

Blakeney, A. B., Strickland, L. R., & Wilkinson, J. H. (1983). Exploring sensory integrative dysfunction in process schizophrenia. *American Journal of Occupational Therapy, 37*, 399-406.

Chapman, J. (1966). The early symptoms of schizophrenia. *British Journal of Psychiatry, 112*, 225-251.

Corbett, L. (1976). Perceptual dyscontrol: A possible organizing principle for schizophrenia research. *Schizophrenia Bulletin, 2*, 249-265.

Crist, P. A. H. (1979). Body image changes in chronic, nonparanoid schizophrenics. *Canadian Journal of Occupational Therapy, 46*, 61-65.

Crist, P. A. H., Thomas, P. P., & Stone, B. L. (1984). Pre-vocational and sensorimotor training in chronic schizophrenia. *Occupational Therapy in Mental Health, 4*, 23-37.

Currier, D. P. (1990). *Elements of research in physical therapy* (3rd ed.). Baltimore: Williams & Wilkins.

Endler, P. B., & Eimon, M. C. (1978). Postural and reflex integration in schizophrenic patients. *American Journal of Occupational Therapy, 32*, 456-459.

Falk-Kessler, J., Quittman, M. S., & Moore, R. (1988). The SCSIT: A potential tool for assessing neurological impairment in adult psychiatric outpatients. *Occupational Therapy Journal of Research, 8*, 131-146.

Gilfoyle, E. M., Grady, A. P., & Moore, J. C. (1981). *Children adapt.* Thorofare, NJ: Charles B. Slack.

Hayes, R. (1989). Occupational therapy in the treatment of schizophrenia. *Occupational Therapy in Mental Health, 9*, 51-68.

Henn, F. A., & Nasrallah, H. A. (1982). *Schizophrenia as a brain disease.* New York: Oxford.

Hixson, V. J., & Mathews, A. W. (1984). Sensory integration and chronic schizophrenia: Past, present and future. *Canadian Journal of Occupational Therapy, 51*, 19-24.

Honigfeld, G., Gillis, R. D., & Klett, C. J. (1966). NOSIE-30: A treatment-sensitive ward behavior scale. *Psychological Reports, 19*, 180-182.

Huddleston, C. I. (1978). Differentiation between process and reactive schizophrenia based on vestibular reactivity, grasp strength, and posture. *American Journal of Occupational Therapy, 32*, 438-444.

Kazdin, A. E. (1984). Statistical analyses for single-case experimental designs. In D. H. Barlow & M. Hersen (Eds.), *Single case experimental designs* (2nd ed.) (pp. 285-324). New York: Pergamon Press.

King, L. J. (1974). A sensory integrative approach to schizophrenia. *American Journal of Occupational Therapy, 28*, 529-536.

King, L. J. (1978). Object Manipulation Speed Test. Phoenix: Greenroom Publications.

Leach, W. (1960). Nystagmus: An integrative neural deficit in schizophrenia. *Journal of Abnormal and Social Psychiatry, 60*, 305-309.

Levine, I., O'Connor, H., & Stacey, B. (1977). Sensory integration with chronic schizophrenics: A pilot study. *Canadian Journal of Occupational Therapy, 44*, 17-21.

Mather, J. A., & Putchat, C. (1983). Motor control of schizophrenics—I. Oculomotor control of schizophrenics: A deficit in sensory processing, not strictly in motor control. *Journal of Psychiatric Research, 17*, 343-360.

Myers, S., Caldwell, D., & Purcell, G. (1973). Vestibular dysfunction in schizophrenia. *Biological Psychiatry, 7*, 255-261.

Neuchterlein, K. H. (1977). Reaction time and attention in schizophrenia: A critical evaluation of the data and theories. *Schizophrenia Bulletin, 3*, 373-428.

Ottenbacher, K. (1982). Sensory integration therapy: Affect or effect. *American Journal of Occupational Therapy, 36*, 571-578.

Posthuma, B. W. (1983). Sensory integration in mental health: Dialogue with Lorna Jean King. *Occupational Therapy in Mental Health, 3*, 1-10.

Rider, B. A. (1978). Sensorimotor treatment of chronic schizophrenics. *American Journal of Occupational Therapy, 32*, 451-455.

Schroeder, C. V., Block, M. P., Trottier, E. C., & Stowell, M. S. (1983). *Schroeder, Block, Campbell Adult Psychiatric Sensory Integration Evaluation.* Kailua, HI: Schroeder Publishing.

Steel, R. G. D., & Torrie, J. H. (1980). *Principles and procedures of statistics: A biometrical approach* (2nd ed.). New York: McGraw-Hill.

Tickle-Degnen, L. (1988). Perspectives on the status of sensory integration theory. *American Journal of Occupational Therapy, 42*, 427-433.

Wyatt, J. D., Alexander, R. C., Egan, M. F., & Kirch, D. G. (1988). Schizophrenia, just the facts. What do we know, how well do we know it? *Schizophrenia Research, 1*, 3-18.

Chapter 62

Occupational Therapy Impacts the Care of Patients at Risk for Tardive Dyskinesia

Carolyn Van Schroeder, OTR
Richard Chung, MD

In an outpatient clinic responding to 64,000 patients' visits a year, the mental health clinic is a busy place, with 14,000 visits of its own.

This article deals with the occupational therapist's concerns about the number of psychiatric patients who appeared to be experiencing physical problems that interfered with everyday functioning. It relates how an interdisciplinary team responded to this problem and the needs documented in an occupational therapy service audit. It also reviews the effectiveness of the treatment group that was devised for this problem by a psychiatrist and an occupational therapist.

The initial step was to use an audit procedure as part of the Occupational Therapy Quality Assurance Program. As part of the occupational therapy evaluation process, the Bay Area Functional Performance Evaluation (BAFPE) (1) was administered to psychiatric patients. If patients showed evidence of sensory integrative dysfunction while performing the tasks required on the evaluation, they were scheduled for further evaluation with the Schroeder, Block, Campbell Adult Psychiatric Sensory Integration Evaluation (SBC) (2,3). Results indicated a number of patients showed dysfunction of a moderate to severe degree on both the physical assessment and abnormal movement sections. The results were summarized in an audit format and discussed with the mental health clinic staff. The incidence of abnormal movements of moderate to severe intensity in 9 of the 11 patients screened with the SBC indicated a need for reviewing medication use, type, and dosage. The results also indicated a need for improved physical function and for periodic reevaluation to check for the presence of developing tardive dyskinesia.

Abnormal movements are a concern for occupational therapists working in the mental health field, because they are a disturbing remnant of antipsychotic medications and can interfere with a person's ability to function effectively. Before the advent of neuroleptics, spontaneous movement disorders, such as stereotypes and mannerisms, were described among psychiatric patients (4). After the introduction of antipsychotic agents, a variety of drug-induced movement disorders, such as parkinsonism, akathisia, dystonia, and tardive dyskinesia, were also identified among psychiatric patients. Recently, clinicians have been cautioned against overdiagnosing tardive dyskinesia and urged to establish a differential diagnosis of movement disorders (5).

Occupational therapists treating chronic patients must fully understand the symptoms and disabilities that result from tardive dyskinesia and be conversant with present-day nomenclature to effectively enter into a dialogue on the subject with treating psychiatrists and other health care practitioners. Classical tardive dyskinesia is characterized by hypersensitivity of dopamine receptors and cholinergic deficits, whereas atypical tardive dyskinesia is characterized by dopaminergic deficits and excess cholinergic activity (6). Studies in adult and elderly psychiatric patients have revealed a wide variety of clinical manifestations of the condition, supporting the view that tardive dyskinesia is a syndrome that encompasses distinct clinical entities, each with a different pathogenesis, symptomatology, and response to drug therapies (7).

The audit recommended convening a committee consisting of a psychiatrist, a nurse, a pharmacist, and an occupational therapist. The committee's task was to develop a procedure that the mental health clinic could use to ensure timely evaluation, to review treatment, and to create ongoing monitoring of patients who receive antipsychotic medications and who may be at risk for extrapyramidal side effects and tardive dyskinesia.

As a result of the committee's work, each service took the responsibility to develop educational and informational quality assurance procedures that would benefit clinic procedure, the present patient care, and patients' future health and well-being.

Pharmacy obtained and issued drug information sheets for patients, which list precautions and side effects and explain when to call the doctor.

Nursing developed health education, information, screening procedures, and classes, in addition to drug logs or flow sheets for patients' charts. In addition, psychiatric nurses implemented their own quality assurance program and audit procedures for the identified problems.

The occupational therapist and psychiatrist developed a procedure for the mental health clinic entitled "Management of Prolonged Neuroleptic Therapy." This procedure was based on the recommendations made by the American Psychiatric Association's Task Force Report 1980 (8). In addition, a Drug Side Effect Checklist for antipsychotics, tricycle antidepressants, and lithium was created (9). An educational approach was implemented through the use of in-services, distribution of information and videotapes, and the presentation of successive quality assurance/audit reports documenting the progress in handling this multifaceted problem.

The occupational therapist instituted two separate sensory integration treatment groups to handle the existing problem. One group entitled "Coordination Plus" was scheduled for patients scoring .90 or more (moderate to severe dysfunction) on only the Physical Assessment section of the SBC evaluation (10).

Another group entitled "Tardive Dyskinesia Sensory Integration Treatment" (TD/SI) met once a week for one hour. The psychiatrist and the occupational therapist continued to evaluate the client at periodic intervals. The physician's role in this group was to monitor, adjust, change, and/or discontinue the medication. The Brief Psychiatric Rating Scale (BPRS) was used to monitor psychiatric status, and the Abnormal Involuntary Movement Scale (AIMS) was used to track abnormal movements every week (11,12).

The occupational therapist engaged the patients in sensory integrative treatment based on their SBC evaluation results and monitored the drug side effect checklists. Patients were administered the SBC evaluation on a pre-, middle-, and post-test basis during 9 to 13 months of treatment.

Results of the TD/SI treatment group are presented

Table 1. Summary Data Sheet

Subject	SBC SI Physical Assessment Scores Pre	Post	SBC Abnormal Movement Scores Pre	Post	AIMS Scores Pre	Post	Equivalent Amount Prolixin mg/d Pre	Post	Amount Cogentin mg/d Pre	Post	Other Medication mg/d Pre	Post	SI Treatment Time Total	Months
1	1.27	0.91	5	5	4	3	60.0	5.0	4	2			8	
2	1.60	0.53	4	3	9	1	5.0	2.0			100	100	7	
											Trazadone			
3	1.26	1.09	5	2	6	1	15.0	9.0			50	50	10	
											Benadryl			
4	1.43	1.17	5	6	9	3	17.4	9.4	0	1			13	
5	1.13	0.63	5	5	11	9	22.5	11.0	6	4			10	
GPR X	1.34	0.87	4.8	4.2	7.8	3.4	23.98	7.28	2	1.4			9.6	
Group % Improvement	35%		12%		56%		70%		30%					

SBC, Schroeder, Block, Campbell Adult Sensory Integration Evaluation; AIMS, Abnormal Involuntary Movement Scale.

Psychosocial Occupational Therapy: Proactive Approaches

on five representative cases as part of a follow-up audit occurring one and one-half years after the initial audit (see Table 1). Group percentage improvement scores showed an increase in function in all areas as a result of medication reduction and sensory integration treatment.

SBC Physical Assessment scores improved by 35%, SBC Abnormal Movement Scores improved by 12%, and AIMS Involuntary Movement Scale Scores improved by 56%. Prolixin equivalent dosages of antipsychotic medications were reduced by 70% and Cogentin by 30%. Patients were in treatment one hour a week for an average of nine months.

The increase in functioning that occurred in the chronic psychiatric patients who were maintained on long-term neuroleptics can be attributed to this interdisciplinary treatment approach. In addition, this approach appears to be a cost-effective way to monitor abnormal movements and patients at risk for tardive dyskinesia. The combination of medication reduction and sensory integrative treatment resulted in a significant patient benefit which was measured by an increase in functioning and psychiatric status.

References

1. Bloomer J, Williams S: *Bay Area Functional Performance Evaluation*. CA: Consulting Psychologists Press, 1979

2. Schroeder CV, Block MP, Campbell E: *SBC Adult Psychiatric Sensory Integration Evaluation*. Kailua, HI: Schroeder Publishing, 1983

3. Schroeder, C: *Perceptual Motor Functioning Screening*, Kailua, HI: Schroeder Publishing, 1982

4. Marsden DC, Tarsy D, Baldessarini RJ: Spontaneous and drug induced movement disorders in psychotic patients. In *Psychiatric Aspects of Neurological Disease*, DF Benson, D Blumer, Editors. New York: Grune and Stratton, 1975

5. Granacher RP: Differential diagnosis of tardive dyskinesia overview, *Am J Psychiatry* 138:1288-1297, 1981

6. Casey DE, Senney D: Pharmacological characterization of tardive dyskinesia. *Psychopharmacology* 54:1-8, 1977

7. Wolf, ME, Mosaim AN: Identifying subtypes of tardive dyskinesia. *Hospital and Community Psychiatry* 35:828-830, 1984

8. Task Force on Late Neuroleptic Effects of Antipsychotic Drugs: Tardive dyskinesia: Summary of a task force report of the American Psychiatric Association. *Am J Psychiatry* 137:1163-1172, 1980

9. Appleton WS: Fourth psychoactive drug usage guide. *Clinical Psychiatry* 43:12-17, 1982

10. Schroeder CV, Summary Sheet, *SBC Adult Psychiatric Sensory Integrative Evaluation*. Kailua, HI: Schroeder Publishing,1984

11. Overall TE, Gorham DR: The brief psychiatric rating scale. *Psychological Reports* 10:799-812, 1962

12. *Abnormal Involuntary Movement Scale*. East Hanover, NJ: Sandoz Pharmaceuticals, 1978

Acknowledgment

The authors thank Dr. Michael Imura for his assistance.

Chapter 63

Study Suggests Occupational Therapy Benefits Schizophrenics

While biochemical theories of brain function and drug treatment of mental disorders are considered state-of-the-art, there is evidence that drugs cannot do the complete job alone. Researchers have found that day treatment including occupational therapy adds significantly to the benefits of anti-psychotic drugs in the care of chronic schizophrenics. This conclusion was reported in a nation-wide study conducted by researchers from three medical schools.

In this study, reported by Linn and others (1979), 162 schizophrenic patients were referred to day treatment centers at time of discharge from ten Veterans Administration hospitals located throughout the United States. These patients were randomly assigned to either day treatment plus drugs or to outpatient drug management, with the latter receiving drugs only.

The study was designed to learn whether the day treatment centers added significantly to the benefits of antipsychotic drugs alone in the post-hospital care of schizophrenic patients. Various criteria, such as relapse rate, social functioning, symptoms, attitudes, and cost, were established to determine treatment effectiveness and were measured every six months over a two-year period. The findings support day treatment as a cost-effective adjunct to drug therapy. In addition, occupational therapy was found to be a significant component of successful outpatient day treatment programs for schizophrenic patients.

Improved Social Function, No Extra Cost

In an analysis of changes over time between day treatment and drugs-only groups, social functioning shows statistically significant change in favor of day treatment center patients. This result fits with day treatment center goals:

1. To improve or maintain abilities to interact successfully with family and others;
2. To provide patients a place to socialize and engage in production activities; and
3. To offer a sheltered environment that sustains patients sufficiently so they can live outside an institution.

During the two-year study, day treatment center patients show marked and continuously improving function while drugs-only patients improved only slightly (Figure 1).

Specific Results

While social functioning showed significant (p < .02) change in favor of day treatment patients, it is important to note that day treatment did not increase costs; that is, there were no statistically significant differences between day treatment and drugs-only programs in terms of costs. According to the study's authors, day treatment "can help prevent relapse, enhance functioning and decrease symptoms," providing high quality care that is "less costly."

Figure 1. Changes in Social Functioning

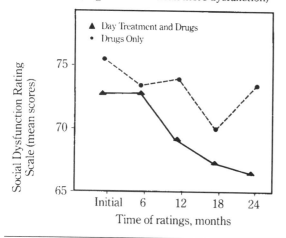

Characteristics of Successful Centers

There were differences among the ten hospitals involved in the study. Through post-hoc groupings, two types of centers emerged: six hospitals with good results for schizophrenic patients and four with poorer results in terms of relapse rate, social functioning, symptoms, and attitudes. Patients in both types of centers were similar in base-line data and personal characteristics, but the hospitals differed in their use of occupational therapy.

Good result centers used significantly more occupational therapy (p < .05) while centers with poor results for chronic schizophrenics had more professional counseling and counseled more of their patients (Figure 2). The authors' conclusion is that "the less intensely personal and more objective-focused activities of occupational therapy produced better outcomes than the intensive interpersonal stimulation often encountered in group therapy."

Figure 2. Utilization of Occupational Therapy in Treatment Program

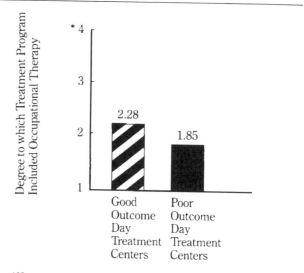

Reduced Symptoms and Relapse Rate in Centers with More Occupational Therapy

After two years, good result day treatment centers had about a 20% lower relapse rate than drugs-only centers (Figure 3). Furthermore, symptom levels, as measured by the Brief Psychiatric Rating Scale, suggested that good result day treatment centers were able to maintain hospital discharge levels over time (Figure 4).

Study Significance

The results of this study could be useful to cost-conscious legislators, consumers, and third-party payers because day treatment improved psychosocial functioning, while the cost of care was not statistically different from drug therapy only.

When centers were analyzed individually, it was found that patients in good-result centers showed higher participation in occupational therapy (p < .05), which suggests that inclusion of occupational therapy in day treatment programs for schizophrenic patients is beneficial as well as cost-effective.

Policymakers will be interested to know that for the large number of patients with chronic schizophrenia discharged from psychiatric hospitals, this study's findings support the value of day treatment as a cost-effective alternative or addition to other types of community care, and emphasize the important role of occupational therapy within these settings. For physicians,

Figure 3. Cumulative Relapse Rates for Treatment Groups.

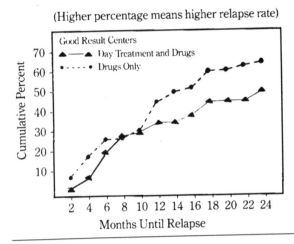

(Higher percentage means higher relapse rate)

financial managers, and hospital administrators, the outcomes of this study would favor establishment of occupational therapy outpatient services and programs for schizophrenic patients. The authors of the study conclude, "what we are suggesting is a less costly method of care which, for once, is not synonymous with a lower quality of care."

Figure 4. Changes on Brief Psychiatric Rating Scale (BPRS)

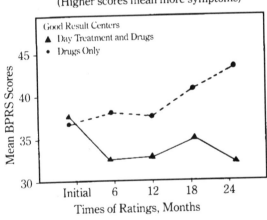

(Higher scores mean more symptoms)

Reference

Linn, M. W., Caffey, E. M., Klett, C. J., Hogarty, G. E., & Lamb, R. (1979). Day treatment and psychotropic drugs in the aftercare of schizophrenic patients. *Archives of General Psychiatry, 36*, 1055-1066.

Section VIII

Psychosocial Considerations for the Nonpsychiatric Client: Expanding Occupational Therapy's Role

Introduction

All occupational therapists learn early in their professional education that occupational therapy is concerned with the whole person. This holistic approach requires the occupational therapist to consider the patient's physical, psychological, cognitive, and social interaction skills within the patient's unique physical, familial, and sociocultural environments (Mosey, 1986; Slaymaker, 1986). Unfortunately, this holistic view of practice is often dichotomized into the practice areas of physical disabilities and mental health (Buckner, 1991; Slaymaker, 1986). Academic coursework and clinical fieldwork are frequently represented as either a physical disabilities or a mental health learning experience. While this split may be realistic for presenting many content areas (i.e., diagnostic criteria, specific evaluation, and intervention methods), it is vital for occupational therapists to remember the continual need for a holistic approach in all areas of practice (Fine, 1991; Prendergast, 1991; Schwartzberg, 1991; Slaymaker, 1986). People do not easily fit into either a physical disabilities or a mental health cubbyhole. We are not simply round or square pegs. We have innumerable dimensions and great depth. These facets do not disappear upon clinical diagnosis.

The adolescent with a spinal cord injury, the parent with multiple sclerosis, the artist with Acquired Immune Deficiency Syndrome (AIDS), the retired executive with hemiplegia—all face major disruptions in their lives and uncertain futures. These traumatic changes cannot be addressed purely from a physical perspective. While muscle strength, range of motion, sensation, and perception are vitally important to evaluate and treat, they alone are not sufficient. One also needs to consider the patient's age, personality, coping style, values, interests, and goals in order to design a meaningful and relevant treatment program and to be able to motivate the patient to participate in this program (Mosey, 1986; Pedretti, 1990; Versluys, 1989). The adolescent may want to explore school and career options, while the parent may be more concerned with maintaining a familial role within the home (Versluys, 1989). The artist with AIDS may view maintaining a modified, productive work schedule that utilizes creative skills as vital, while the retired executive may want to develop avocational interests to fill the "empty" days (Kielhofner, 1977).

These psychosocial issues must be considered to ensure that occupational therapy uses its full potential to help each patient attain and maintain a satisfying quality of life (Mosey, 1986; Pedretti, 1990; Prendergast, 1991; Versluys, 1989). The chapters in this section review important psychosocial considerations for the occupational therapist working with the non-psychiatric client. A number of viable occupational therapy program ideas for non-psychiatric treatment settings are also described.

In chapter 64, Vargo reviews the psychological effects of physical disabilities. He discusses the strong influence of society on the perception of disability and introduces the sociological concept of the "ideology of normality"; that is, "in our culture to be valued is to be normal" (Vargo, 1978, p. 436). Those with a disability must battle this ideological bias and common misconceptions about disabilities in order to adjust to and cope with their different level of ability. Vargo identifies three stages of adjustment to disability and provides several humanistic suggestions for the occupational therapist to help those affected to overcome the potentially debilitating psychological effects of their disabilities. His emphasis on the therapeutic use of self, and his stand that the *process* of treatment is as important as the *content* of treatment, embody occupational therapy's holistic tradition.

In chapter 65, Watanabe and Watson maintain this holistic viewpoint by presenting a psychiatric-consultation liaison program for an acute physical disabilities setting. This program provides multidisciplinary services to medically or surgically ill patients who are also experiencing psychological or emotional problems. Displaced anger, social withdrawal, impaired memory, poor judgment, and anxiety may become problematic for the client with physical illness and for the medical/surgical staff unaccustomed to dealing with psychosocial issues. The psychiatric-consultation-liaison team provides early detection of potential problems, educates and supports the staff, and assists the client in developing effective coping strategies.

Versluys continues this theme of utilizing psychosocial methods with the physically disabled by applying role theory to occupational therapy practice in physical rehabilitation. In chapter 66, she examines the tremendous impact a physical disability can have on a person's occupational, familial, and avocational roles. Guidelines for evaluation are provided in a comprehensive manner. The patient, the family, personal factors, and sociocultural influences are all considered in role assessment. Treatment is directed at maintaining, transforming, and/or reassigning valued roles utilizing a practical, educational approach. A number of role-focused groups are presented by Versluys to assist the patient in acquiring and/or maintaining the functional role skills that are vital to a satisfying quality of life.

Quality of life issues and functional role skills are also relevant to the next two chapters, which focus on sexuality and the disabled. When one becomes physically disabled one does not concurrently lose one's sexuality. Sensuality, physical attraction, self-esteem, sexual validation, and feeling loved are all vital components of sexuality (Burton, 1990; Mosey, 1986). As professionals concerned with the functioning of the whole person, occupational therapists need to consider sexuality within their therapeutic programs (Mosey, 1986; Pedretti, 1990; Versluys, 1989). Chapter 67 emphasizes the need for occupational therapists to assess their own views on sexuality and the disabled. Freda encourages occupational therapists to explore these issues and to increase their knowledge base through self-analysis, team collaboration, and continuing education. She urges occupational therapists to share their knowledge of sexuality, task analysis, and activity adaptation with their clients. She also emphasizes the need to develop an open therapeutic relationship that enables clients to approach the occupational therapist with their concerns regarding their sexuality.

Asrael, in chapter 68, also emphasizes the need for occupational therapists to address the sexuality needs of the physically disabled. She presents the PLISSIT model as a guide for occupational therapy intervention in response to a patient's sexuality concerns. Asrael emphasizes that a nonjudgmental, relaxed, and responsive approach can be beneficial to the patient throughout all stages of this model.

The next two chapters in this section deal with a disease that definitely requires a nonjudgmental, responsive, and holistic approach. AIDS is a disease whose physiological aspects cannot be separated from its psychosocial considerations (Pizzi, 1990a; Pizzi, 1990b). In chapter 69, Schindler reviews information regarding the clinical picture of AIDS: its transmission, diagnosis, and clinical course. She provides an important discussion of the effect of AIDS on the person's life roles and tasks. She identifies issues that may influence the person's adjustment to the AIDS diagnosis and course of the illness. Schindler presents a conceptual framework for occupational therapy evaluation and intervention. She provides descriptive case examples to substantiate the relevance of occupational therapy to the person with AIDS.

The role of occupational therapy in working with the AIDS population is expanded upon in chapter 70, which describes a day treatment program for persons with AIDS. Linda Gutterman provides an overview of the program's holistic philosophy, which strives to empower each patient with the ability to direct his or her own life. Health education and health promotion activities are provided on an individual and group basis by the occupational therapist. Assessment guidelines, intervention strategies, and case examples provided by Gutterman emphasize the value of a holistic approach in maintaining well-being and promoting health for persons with AIDS.

The ability of a day treatment program to support health and wellness is also discussed in chapter 71, by Neustadt, who describes an adult day care program that provides coordinated, comprehensive health care services to elderly persons who are physically ill, medically fragile, or disabled. These supportive services enable the elderly to remain in the community, preventing premature institutionalization. Neustadt discusses program philosophy, goals, and activities. Case examples are provided to highlight the vital role day treatment plays in maintaining functional independence and increasing quality of life.

The relevance of psychosocial issues to occupational therapy's ability to increase and maintain the quality of life and functional independence of persons with disabilities cannot be ignored. The chapters in this section validate the need for a holistic approach with non-psychiatric clients. It is my hope that readers will take the principles and ideas presented by each author and integrate them into their own practice. Questions for further consideration of these issues are provided at the conclusion of this introduction to assist in this integrative thought process.

Reference and resource lists, including numerous sources that can be utilized to meet the psychosocial needs of the physically disabled, are provided at the end of this text. Self-help groups and major health organizations are identified. In addition, I have included many vocational and leisure resources for the disabled that can be utilized to enhance significantly the quality of life for the person with a disability. These resources can be invaluable to the therapist who must deal with increased demands for treatment efficacy and decreased length of treatment stays. Realistically, a therapist may need to prioritize treatment and may be unable to deal directly with all of a client's needs. However, it is still imperative for the therapist to consider all aspects of the person and to make the appropriate referrals to ensure that all of the client's needs will be met. It is unconscionable for the occupational therapist to work solely on dressing and feeding skills with a client, then to discharge the client with a note indicating "no further services needed" once independence in these self-care skills is achieved. This type of evaluation is certainly inaccurate, as a client to whom this occurred responded, "Now I am all dressed up with no place to go." Days of inactivity resulted in depression, social isolation, and diminished self-worth, leaving the client with significant functional impairments and a poor quality of life. Appropriate referrals to a self-help group and vocational counseling and a list of leisure resources and technological aids empowered the client to regain control of his life and to pursue productive endeavors. The omission of these referrals had denied the client the full benefit of occupational therapy. Ethically, we owe it to our patients, ourselves, and our profession to preserve our holistic heritage, regardless of practice preference or area of specialization (Fine, 1991; Prendergast, 1991; Schwartzberg, 1991; Slaymaker, 1986).

Questions to Consider

1. Think of your current lifestyle: your roles, daily activities, values, interests, and goals. Now, imagine you are diagnosed with Multiple Sclerosis (MS). Your symptoms include fatigue, diminished endurance, decreased muscle strength, incoordination, and blurred vision.

   a. What would be your reaction to this diagnosis? How would the significant people in your life react to your acquired disability?

   b. How would your life change? What effect would your symptoms have on your current lifestyle?

   c. What would be important psychosocial issues facing you as you adjusted to a physical disability?

   d. What role adjustments and activity adaptations would you need to make due to your decreased functional abilities? How would MS impact your ability to perform work, leisure, and family role tasks?

   e. What impact would MS have on your view of yourself as a sexual, lovable person?

   f. How would the course of MS, with its exacerbations and remissions, affect your future goals?

   g. What are your physical and sociocultural environmental concerns, constraints, and supports? What resources would you utilize to assist you in adjusting to a disability?

   h. How would you like to be approached by an occupational therapist? What treatment activities and programs would be most relevant, interesting, and valuable to you? What would you want to work on in occupational therapy to attain and maintain a satisfying quality of life?

2. Imagine you are working in a busy, inpatient physical rehabilitation setting. You want to approach patients holistically, but you feel restricted by reimbursement constraints, strict documentation standards, and a limited length of treatment time.

   a. Why bother? Why is it important to consider psychosocial issues with a non-psychiatric, physically disabled patient population?

   b. What are the psychosocial reactions and behavioral manifestations that may be exhibited by a person with a physical disability? How might these influence the occupational therapy evaluation and intervention process?

   c. How would incorporating psychosocial issues into your evaluation procedures assist you in setting relevant goals and planning appropriate treatment for your patients with physical disabilities?

   d. What are the psychosocial issues that can influence a patient's motivation to engage in a treatment program? How can an occupational therapist increase a patient's interest and motivation to engage in physical rehabilitation?

   e. How can a busy, overworked occupational

therapist meet all of a client's needs and goals? How do you prioritize needs and goals? How do you work on two things at the same time?

f. What resources are available to assist you in meeting patients' psychosocial needs while in your treatment setting? What are the aftercare support services and professional resources available for referral to a client upon discharge from your setting? How can you ease the discharge process and the transition back home and into the community? How can you ensure that your clients are leaving your setting with the skills and knowledge needed to empower them to pursue satisfying and productive lives?

References

Buckner, M. K. (1991, July 11). A shrinking area of practice [Letter to the editor]. *OT Week*, p. 54.

Burton, G. (1990). Psychosocial aspects and adjustment during various phases of neurological disability. In D. A. Umphred (Ed.), *Neurological rehabilitation* (2nd ed.) (pp. 163-180). St Louis: Mosby.

Fine, S. B. (1991, August 22). Holistic approach includes mental health [Letter to the editor]. *OT Week*, p. 46.

Kielhofner, G. (1977). Temporal adaptation: A conceptual framework for occupational therapy. *American Journal of Occupational Therapy, 31*, 235-242.

Mosey, A. C. (1986). *Psychosocial components of occupational therapy.* New York: Raven Press.

Pedretti, L. W. (1990). Psychosocial aspects of physical dysfunction. In L. W. Pedretti & B. Zoltan (Eds.), *Occupational therapy: Practice skills for physical disabilities* (3rd ed.) (pp. 18-39). St. Louis: Mosby.

Pizzi, M. (1990a). The transformation of HIV infection and AIDS in occupational therapy: Beginning the conversation. *American Journal of Occupational Therapy, 44*, 199-203.

Pizzi, M. (1990b). The model of human occupation and adults with HIV infection and AIDS. *American Journal of Occupational Therapy, 44*, 257-264.

Prendergast, N. D. (1991, August 22). Holistic approach includes mental health [Letter to the editor]. *OT Week*, p. 46.

Schwartzberg, S. L. (1991, August 15). The future of mental health in the profession [Letter to the editor]. *OT Week*, p. 54.

Slaymaker, J. H. (1986). A holistic approach to specialization. *American Journal of Occupational Therapy, 40*, 117-121.

Versluys, H. P. (1989). Psychosocial accommodation to physical disability. In C. A. Trombly (Ed.), *Occupational therapy for physical dysfunction* (3rd ed.) (pp. 13-37). Baltimore: Williams & Wilkins.

Chapter 64

Some Psychological Effects of Physical Disability

J. W. Vargo, PhD

This chapter was previously published in the *American Journal of Occupational Therapy, 32*, 31-34. Copyright © 1978, The American Occupational Therapy Association, Inc.

A large body of research literature exists in the area of the psychological aspects of physical disability. Comprehensive reviews of the literature are presented by Janis and Leventhal (1) and by Pulton (2). The focus of this paper is on what happens to people who become physically disabled, the mechanisms through which psychological effects occur, and some suggestions as to what occupational therapists can do to help people with physical disabilities overcome some of the debilitating psychological effects of the disabilities.

Disability versus Handicap

Hamilton (3) distinguishes between disability and handicap. He defines a disability as a medically diagnosable impairment of some physical function(s). Disability, then, is a condition that is observable and can be diagnosed by use of modern technology. A disability is in evidence when some part of the body is not functioning as it normally should. A handicap, on the other hand, refers to a psychosocial relationship, and is a function of the interaction between individuals and their total environment. Most disabilities are handicaps, but not all; for example, people who wear glasses or contact lenses have physical disabilities. Their eyes do not work as they should; that is, they do not have 20/20 vision. But this disability does not handicap their lives very much. They can manage very well in their day-to-day activities despite the fact that they have less than perfect vision. On the other hand, some people are handicapped but not disabled. A female living in North American society operates under a handicap that is not imposed on males. With the advent of the women's movement in recent years, the handicapping effect of being female in our society has become readily apparent.

The point is that a disability is usually a handicap but not automatically so, and the reason this distinction is an important one is that it highlights the notion of societal responsibility in determining who is perceived as handicapped and who is not.

Stages

A number of authors, including Wright (4), have acknowledged that a person suffering a traumatic disability goes through three stages similar to those faced by dying people as outlined by Elizabeth Kubler-Ross (5).

Denial

In the denial stage, the individual is not emotionally prepared to accept the reality and the implications of the disability and, consequently, will deny that such a disability exists. For example, Simon (6) cites the case of the 60-year-old man who suffered a cerebral vascular accident and believed that he had found his paralyzed arm beside a railroad track. In all likelihood, this man was not psychologically prepared to accept the fact that one side of his body was paralyzed. This denial functioned to protect him from the overwhelming stress that would have been precipitated by admitting the consequences of his medical condition.

The denial stage reflects a state in which the individual is psychologically ill-prepared to accept the reality and the ramifications of the disability. Denial is protective in that it guards the ego from the threat of self-effacing stress.

Mourning

Once the individual moves out of the denial phase and realizes that the disability is indeed real, the person then moves into a stage of mourning. This stage takes one or both of two forms: hostility and depression. In the hostility phase, aggression is directed outwardly, toward life in general, and toward other people in particular. Individuals in this phase are very difficult to deal with in rehabilitation because they are often bitter, and their bitterness and resentment may be directed toward the very professionals who are doing their best to help them. In the depression phase, aggression is directed inwardly, and the individual feels dejected, despondent, worthless, and, in general, inadequate to cope with the future.

Adjustment

The third stage, which is the goal of any total rehabilitation scheme, is called *adjustment*. In this stage the individual is generally self-accepting and is capable of coping with the various aspects of the disability. During the adjustment stage, energies are directed toward achieving physical independence and learning productive strategies for dealing with the handicapping effects of the disability.

Ideology of Normality

A partial answer to why people who become disabled go through these stages rests in the notion of an *ideology of normality*. People with physical disabilities may feel personally inferior and often experience a number of misconceptions about themselves as people. Wright discussed ten such misconceptions (4, p. 172):

1. My disability is a punishment.
2. It is important to conform, not to be different.
3. Most people are physically normal.
4. Normal physique is one of the most important values.
5. Physique is important for personal evaluation.
6. A deformed body leads to a deformed mind.
7. No one will marry me.
8. I will be a burden on my family.
9. My deformity is revolting.
10. I am less valuable because I cannot get around (or see, or hear) as others do.

Manneheim (7) defined ideology as "an intense and unconscious loyalty to the status quo." In North American society there is an "unconscious loyalty" or irrational commitment to "normality." But what does it mean to be normal? The commitment is certainly not to *averageness* as the denotation of the word *normality* implies. Instead, *normality* connotes physical health, intelligence, beauty, youth, and wealth. It is not suggested here that these traits are not *desirable*; they are. However, our culture promulgates the myth that if a person is not all these things, then he/she is *ipso facto* less worthy or less human as a result.

In our culture to be valued is to be normal. In a capitalistic society, to be less than normal is to be of less value and, therefore, to be *worth less*. It seems reasonable that the feelings of hostility, depression, and inferiority are, at least in part, an inevitable and logical result of living in a society that values Economic Man. The body is treated as another commodity in the huge marketplace of values. Disability then becomes a status and the surplus people, such as the mentally retarded, the elderly, the physically disabled, and the poor, are perceived as being intrinsically inferior (8-12). In order to *truly* adjust, or to learn to cope, a person with a physical disability must consciously and conscientiously combat the ten misconceptions outlined by Wright, as well as any others that devalue him/her as a human being.

Helping the Disabled

There are four areas that can be worked on to help a person achieve Stage 3 or adjustment.

Pay Attention to Little Things

Pascal, the 17th Century mathematician-philosopher, once said "Little things console us because little things afflict us." Just as in marital conflicts, it is the minor frustrations and the irritations that snowball into irreconcilable differences; so too in rehabilitation it is the small frustrations in dealing with activities of daily life that make the rehabilitation process sometimes unbearable. In general, a person gains self-respect in learning to cope with little things in life. The occupational therapist, for example, plays a large role in helping an individual learn to cope through teaching activities of daily living (ADL) and thereby demonstrating that the client can deal with problems encountered in the task of day-to-day living. The *process* of the ADL program often is just as important as the *content*.

One of the greatest benefits of an effective ADL program is that it helps to establish the conviction that one has the ability to overcome the frustrations and anxieties in dealing with the handicaps associated with disability. The patient thereby becomes solution-oriented rather than problem-oriented.

Admit Difference

A necessary prerequisite for self-acceptance is for the individual to admit that he/she is *different* from nondisabled people. This difference, though, is to be distinguished from inferiority. One can be different and equal. The more a person tries to conceal or mask a disability, the less energy there is to be invested in more productive kinds of activities. The role of the occupational therapist in this regard, then, is to demonstrate to the person with the disability that he/she is accepted as a total person, that there is no justification for feelings of shame and guilt as a result of the disability. When a person with a disability is reacted to as a person (first) who happens to have a disability (second), many of the fears and anxieties with being different are diffused. This is accomplished via those therapist attitudes characteristic of any positive treatment relationship: genuineness, empathy, and concern for the patient as a unique human being.

De-emphasize Physique

It is necessary for a person undergoing the process of rehabilitation to reevaluate the importance of physique, and to look at physique in terms of what it allows and what it restricts. Viewed in this way, physique loses its status value and is looked at in terms of its functional qualities. One goal of rehabilitation is to help the patient achieve maximum functional independence physically. Beyond that, emotional strengths can be identified and interpersonal skill deficits can be developed through individual counseling, group therapy, or assertiveness training programs. The acquisition of interpersonal skills almost immediately de-emphasizes the value of physique in relating to others. Many people with severe physical disabilities are happily married and live otherwise fulfilling, productive lives. It should be mentioned, however, that this is a difficult goal to achieve because of society's continuing emphasis on physique and beauty. The occupational therapist's task is to prepare the patient for the challenge of discharge.

Overcome Misconceptions Associated with Disability

As mentioned previously, Wright (4) has outlined ten fears that support the notion that physical disability is a sign of personal inferiority. Each fear or misconception requires persistent counterpropagandizing in the manner advocated by Albert Ellis (13,14) and the principles consistent with cognitive behavior therapy (15,16). For example, a quadriplegic avoided venturing out into public places. He consistently told himself that it was awful to be different and that he could not stand it if people stared at him. These self-statements caused him great anxiety and prevented him from engaging in many activities of which he was physically capable. With therapist intervention, he was able to change his self-talk to more reasonable statements such as "I don't like it when people stare at me but I can stand it." In other words, he was helped to see that being stared at is unpleasant but it is not *catastrophic*. By counterpropagandizing his misconceptions, he was able to participate in public activities and experience only minimal discomfort when people did stare. Substituting rational ideas for irrational ones is a life-long task.

The occupational therapist can assist physically disabled individuals in counterpropagandizing misconceptions about themselves and to help them cope with life in the outside world. The methods of rational-emotive therapy (13,14), cognitive behavior therapy (15,16), and assertiveness training (17) are especially helpful here. As the general public becomes more exposed to people who are physically disabled, their attitudes will become more positive. It has been demonstrated that people with previous contact with the physically disabled have more positive attitudes toward them than those with no previous contact (18).

Conclusion

In these ways, then, an individual may come closer to achieving self-acceptance and to developing strategies for coping with life in a psychologically healthy and productive way. At present, public attitudes mitigate against successful psychosocial rehabilitation, but public attitudes are very difficult and slow to change. Occupational therapists cannot change the world. What they can do is to help a person use his/her physical and psychological resources to cope rationally in an irrational world.

Rehabilitation is a life-long task. The physical rehabilitation process, although extremely important, is relatively short. People with complete, traumatic spinal cord injuries, for example, usually achieve maximum physical rehabilitation within a year. Psychological adjustment comes much more slowly and more painfully. Perhaps an awareness of the stages discussed and their implications can assist in accelerating the process of truly total rehabilitation.

Acknowledgment

This paper is based on a presentation given at the Eighteenth Annual Conference of the Psychologists Association of Alberta, Calgary, Alberta, Canada, on October 30, 1976.

References

1. Janis IL, Leventhal H: Psychological aspects of physical illness and hospital care. In *Handbook of Clinical Psychology*, BB Wolman, Editor. New York: McGraw-Hill, 1360-1377, 1965

2. Pulton TW: Attitudes toward the physically disabled: A review and a suggestion for producing positive attitude change. *Physiother Canada*, 28:83-88, 1976

3. Hamilton KW: *Counseling the Handicapped in the Rehabilitation Process*, New York: Ronald Press, 1950

4. Wright BA: *Physical Disability: A Psychological Approach*, New York: Harper and Row, 1960

5. Kubler-Ross E: *On Death and Dying*, New York: MacMillan, 1970

6. Simon JI: Emotional aspects of physical disability. *Am J Occup Ther* 25:408-410, 1971

7. Manneheim K: *Ideology and Utopia*, London: Routledge and Kegan, 1936. Quoted by Scheff TJ: Schizophrenia as ideology. In *Labeling Madness*, TJ Scheff, Editor. Englewood Cliffs, NJ: Prentice-Hall, 1975, p 6

8. Kong-Ming New P, Ruscio AT, George LA: Toward an understanding of the rehabilitation system. *Rehabil Lit* 30:130-139, 1969

9. Goffman E: *Stigma: Notes on the Management of Spoiled Identity*, Englewood Cliffs, NJ: Prentice-Hall, 1963

10. Braginsky DD, Braginsky, BM: *Hansels and Gretels: Studies of Children in Institutions for the Retarded*, New York: Holt, Rinehart, and Winston, 1971

11. Braginsky BM, Braginsky DD, Ring K: *Methods of Madness: The Mental Hospital as a Last Resort*, New York: Holt, Rinehart, and Winston, 1969

12. Williams E: Models of madness. *New Society* 470:607-609, 1971

13. Ellis A: Showing the patient he is not a worthless individual. *Voices* 1:74-77, 1965

14. Ellis A: *Reason and Emotion in Psychotherapy*, New York: Lyle Stuart, 1962

15. Ellis A, Harper RA: *A New Guide to Rational Living*, Englewood Cliffs, NJ: Prentice-Hall, 1975

16. Raimy V: *Misunderstandings of the Self: Cognitive Psychotherapy and the Misconception Hypothesis*, San Francisco: Jossey-Bass,1975

17. Lange AJ, Jakubowski P: *Responsible Assertive Behavior*, Champaign, IL: Research Press, 1976

18. Merlin JS, Kauppi DR: Occupational affiliation and attitudes toward the physically disabled. *Rehabil Counseling Bull* 16:173-179, 1973

Chapter 65

Psychiatric Consultation-Liaison: Role of the Occupational Therapist

Dale Y. Watanabe, OTR/L

Linda J. Watson, OTR/L

Occupational therapy has a long and rich history in psychiatry. While contributing to the multidisciplinary treatment of psychiatric patients, occupational therapy uses functionally based activity groups within the context of the therapeutic community. Our own role as psychiatric occupational therapists is nontraditional in that we work with medically or surgically ill patients who experience psychological or emotional problems secondary to their illness. In fact, only about 2% of our patients have a diagnosed psychiatric disorder. This article will describe our involvement as psychiatric occupational therapists within the psychiatric consultation-liaison service of a large teaching hospital.

Rush-Presbyterian-St.Luke's Medical Center is a 1100-bed, private, tertiary care hospital. The Psychiatric Consultation-Liaison Service, a specialty within the Department of Psychiatry, has been in existence for approximately 12 years. Psychiatric occupational therapy has been involved in some capacity with this service for 7 years. Our involvement has grown from occasional referrals to a patient caseload requiring the services of two full-time occupational therapists. The therapists are an integral part of a multidisciplinary team consisting of six psychiatrists and two psychiatric nurses. Each discipline has the capacity to generate its own referrals or to cross-refer. Biweekly rounds are held to review the patient's treatment as provided by any one or a combination of team members. Occupational therapy receives approximately 65% of our referrals from nonpsychiatric physicians; consequently, we welcome these opportunities for clinical supervision and support.

Occupational Therapy Services

Psychiatric occupational therapists serve patients who are diagnosed with problems involving cardiology, nephrology, organ transplant, high-risk obstetrics, neurology, orthology [sic], infectious disease, pulmonary (ventilator-dependent) and oncology (in particular bone marrow transplantation and gynecologic oncology). Patients who are appropriate for referral are those exhibiting any one or more of the following:

- disturbances in interpersonal relationships—anger, withdrawal; behaviors that are demanding, attention-seeking, complaining, and/or manipulative.
- disturbances in cognition-memory, orientation, concentration, perception, and/or judgment impairment.
- disturbances in affect and attitude—agitation, anxiety, lability, mood swings, anhedonia, uncooperativeness, and/or lethargy.

While all patients may demonstrate these characteristics at some time during their hospitalization, therapy is indicated when these disturbances are severe, pervasive, and/or interfere with treatment (Pasnau, 1982). Given the acuity of the patient's medical condition and/or refusal to participate in treatment, therapy is done at bedside. A physician's referral initiates therapy.

Liaison Role

As liaisons, our role is one of troubleshooting. The primary purpose is to facilitate early detection of problem situations and help staff to develop intervention strategies. We do this informally in response to staff, patient, or family requests and formally through participation in patient staffings. It is important to assess each request for timeliness, clarity of problem, and emotional tone (Hengeveld, Rooymans, & Hermans, 1987). The milieu of the unit is evaluated with regard to its flexibility, attitudes, norms, and values (Strain & Grossman, 1975). Some questions to be considered include: How does the staff discuss patients who are medically or psychologically unresponsive? Are there underlying conflicts with this particular patient from previous admissions? How sophisticated is the staff's understanding of psychological problems and interventions? How does the staff deal with terminally ill patients when the physician chooses not to discuss a change in status with the patient or family? How open is the unit to support and intervention from an outsider (non-nurse, non-unit staff)? Are there other causes of stress, such as staffing changes or unexpected patient deaths on the unit, and how have they been dealt with?

Formal meetings and informal contacts also serve to educate and support staff. Education is an important aspect of the consultation-liaison role. Describing psychological issues in common, understandable terms and reframing the patient's behaviors as a response to stress rather than vindictiveness or malicious intent can renew and foster empathy among staff. Assisting staff in the identification of their own behaviors and attitudes that may be contributing to the problem situation and developing a workable plan from the staff perspective are significant features of the liaison role (Strain, 1981) [sic]. A supportive position with the staff is often necessary to manage conflicts, set limits, and deal with issues of death and dying.

Any staff consultation or patient referral is to be interpreted and respected as a plea for help. However, at times the request may seem hidden (Bustamente & Ford, 1981). For example, the referral may describe a patient as bored and needing something to do, but on observation, the patient appears severely withdrawn, disinterested, and lethargic and [demonstrates] self-deprecating signs indicating a possible depression. Staff members may not be able to articulate the need for therapy instead of volunteer services. Yet when questioned, they may be able to provide more specific clinical indicators of the patient's failing coping skills (Cohen-Cole & Friedman, 1983). Staff may feel protective of a patient (e.g., they prefer to see a favorite patient as bored rather than depressed) or may be responding to bias and prejudice within the milieu toward psychiatric problems (Perl & Shelp, 1982). Patients with personality disorders can split staff, and depressed patients can evoke a sense of anger and helplessness among staff. These issues may be difficult for nonpsychiatric staff to recognize (Strain, 1978).

Theoretical Orientation

The psychodynamic frame of reference and the model of human occupation provide the basis from which we assess and plan intervention strategies. Assessment begins with an understanding of the patient's fears, worries, and anxieties (Blumenfield, 1983). Illness or disability often represents a loss of dreams, hopes, and fantasies about the future. Treatment issues are primarily in the areas of control, self-esteem, independence, separation, and death and dying. Conflicts may occur regarding attitudes, values, ideals, and goals as a result of illness or disability. Problems may reflect a response to current stresses and/or unresolved conflicts from earlier periods in the patient's life (Mailick, 1985). The therapist examines the patient's use of defense mechanisms to manage stress, considering both adaptive and dysfunctional features. Patient regression is understood as an inadequate coping response to a perceived threat. Poor coping results in impaired functions in one or more of the following areas:

- ability to restrain or delay tension discharge
- frustration tolerance
- problem-solving abilities
- judgment

- anticipation of consequences
- ability to regulate energy
- self-constancy
- interpersonal relationships
- use of language to communicate needs
- reality testing
- perception
- affect
- motor control

Personality

Personality is composed of a lifelong style of relating, coping, behaving, thinking, and feeling and is adaptive and flexible within a variety of situations. However, illness and hospitalization may create stress that interferes with normal patterns of coping. Personality characteristics may become more rigid, exaggerated, and/or maladaptive. Stress may be caused by perceptions of illness, constraints of hospitalization, and heightened fears. Only a very small percentage of the patients we see meet the DSM-III, Axis II criteria for the diagnosed personality disorder.

The amplification of specific personality characteristics may cause the patient's behavior to become inappropriate and disruptive. The orderly and controlled patient may rely on knowing as much about his or her situation as possible in order to maintain control and handle anxieties. The dependent and thus overdemanding patient may become abusive in requests for nursing care and additional attention (Kahana & Bibring, 1964). The patient may overuse the call light, request special treatment, and refuse to be satisfied with the level of care given. These behaviors are often viewed by the unit staff as manipulative (Groves, 1978).

For some patients, familiar methods used to cope with stress may not be acceptable within the hospital setting. When confronted with the stress of hospitalization, coping methods become extreme. For example, the older man who normally manages his anxiety by yelling at his family will become loud and demanding when requesting care from nursing staff. Comfortable, familiar methods are employed in spite of their unacceptable nature within the hospital environment (Silverberg, 1985). In other situations, strange and uncomfortable behavior may be considered justifiable by patient and staff, given the traumatic situation and stress (Millon, 1981). This is demonstrated by a 37-year-old white male who received the sudden diagnosis of testicular cancer, resulting in the surgical removal of part of his genitals. Following recovery, the patient chose to lie in his bed in a double room totally exposed. Staff, roommates, and visitors complained to one another but not directly to the pa-

tient. When questioned, the patient initially denied that it was a problem and reported he was following what the doctor wanted. In further discussion he reported feeling ashamed, embarrassed, and emasculated and said he worried about his return to work.

Depression

Depression is quite common among the medically ill; Cavanaugh (1984) reports that one-quarter to a third of all hospitalized medically ill patients experience feelings of depression. Behaviors and cognitions associated with the depressed mood hinder the patient's ability to participate in medical care.

The degree of depression ranges from mild and transient, usually representing an adjustment disorder as a result of illness and hospitalization, to severe and incapacitating with suicidal ideation (Cavanaugh, 1986). As with all clinical states, the intensity, duration, and pervasiveness of symptomatology and the interference with normal functioning become decisive features in a diagnosis. In the medically ill, patients may refuse treatment or not comply and subsequently jeopardize their medical condition.

In a psychiatric setting, disturbances in sleep, motor activity, and appetite are significant vegetative criteria for differential diagnoses of depression. However, in a general hospital setting these criteria may be less applicable due to the requirements of the hospital regimen (e.g., special diets for specific medical conditions and testing procedures that periodically awaken the patient). Robinson (1984) provides a description of how the hospital environment influences body integration, control separation, and somatic preoccupation. Saltz and Magruder-Habib (1985) describe feelings of hopelessness, helplessness, and [a] sense of sadness or loss as key manifestations of depression in the medically ill. Often the loss may not be concrete, but may be related more to a diminished sense of self as a result of an illness. The patient may describe himself as a failure or worthless. Former roles and habits may no longer be attainable. The patient may struggle with his perception of self-worth and efficacy (Kielhofner, et al., 1985).

Loss of interest or pleasure in usual activities is a significant indicator of depression (Cavanaugh, Clark, & Gibbons, 1983). The patient may be uninterested in his hygiene, meals, and course of treatment. Loss of interest in family characterizes deepening depression. Such [was] the case with Mr. W., a 66-year-old man who was referred because of his lack of motivation. The therapist found the patient lying in bed staring at the ceiling. As the therapist entered the room, he quickly closed his eyes and appeared to be sleeping. He refused to open his eyes but would answer by shaking his head to short, superficial questions. His only comment with eyes still closed was, "What's the use? No one cares, no one understands," in response to the therapist's explanation of services and need for treatment. In the most severe cases, the patient wishes to be dead and minimally participates in rehabilitation or maintenance efforts.

Assessment

Assessment with this population is an ongoing process from initial evaluation to discharge. It not only provides a baseline of information for patient treatment but also contributes to the formulation of a differential diagnosis. A semi-structured interview format is used to gain information about premorbid functioning in the areas of work, leisure, and activities of daily living. Therapists evaluate coping skills based on current life circumstances, medical condition, social surroundings, and effectual state. Some assessments we use include the Allen Cognitive Levels Test, Oakley's Role Checklist, Johns Hopkins' Mini Mental Status, and Lewinsohn's Pleasant Events Scale. Formal assessments and task evaluations are useful but are secondary to establishing a therapeutic rapport and meeting the patients on their own level (Watson, 1986).

Case Assessment Example

Mike is a 14-year-old, obese, black male hospitalized for the third time this year for noncompliance with his diabetic diet and insulin adjustment. The referral to psychiatric occupational therapy followed an incident where the patient had persuaded his mother to sneak food to him from home. He said he ate because there was "nothing else to do around here."

On initial contact the patient reported that everything was fine. He explained that the food incident was an accident and had only happened once. He appeared defiant and questioned why staff was making "such a big deal about one little thing." Mike said he was tired and asked if the therapist would leave so he could get some rest. The therapist then asked if he'd rather do something other than talk and his response was "like what?" with a softened affect. He was offered an assortment of projects and was asked to complete some homework that included an adapted version of Black's Adolescent Role Assessment and Holland's Self-Directed Search (HSDS). The therapist returned the next morning to find Mike's woodworking magazine rack near completion. His work was of high quality. He had carefully followed directions on his own. When complimented, Mike stated he liked woodworking and had missed "doing stuff like that"

because he had been skipping school a lot. We reviewed his evaluation and ascertained that since being diagnosed as diabetic, he had received "special treatment" at home. He was excluded from any household responsibilities, and illness had become an acceptable excuse for missing school. "I sit around and eat a lot, watch T.V." He reported having fun with the test (HSDS). "Thinking about the future. . . . I hadn't done that for awhile. I never gave it much thought and since I've been sick no one seems to care much about (my future) anymore." When asked about his understanding of his medical problems, he reported "At first I was scared to death. . . . I guess I could die, you know. . . . I forgot the rest. . . . Now I just don't think about it. I don't think about much really."

Treatment

Treatment centers around conflicts in self-esteem, loss of control and independence, separation, and death and dying. These conflicts may be addressed directly and/or indirectly. Often activity serves as a vehicle. A major component of treatment is the therapeutic use of self. Counseling is done in conjunction with activity involvement or can be the primary mode of treatment. Appropriate treatment activities can act as precursors to the discussion of role changes, body image, personal worth, and self-management. Applied activities must be meaningful, pleasurable, and appropriate to the patient's physical and emotional tolerance.

A Shift in Role

As a member of a psychiatric consultation-liaison service, the occupational therapist must feel comfortable in a role that requires a high degree of autonomy with little of the customary "team approach." Strong clinical and interpersonal skills are necessary for the therapist. Many times the therapist is the only psychiatric professional working with a particular patient. Thus the therapist must be able to articulate psychological and rehabilitative concepts fluently at a variety of levels. Ideas and recommendations prescribed to unit staff may be new and/or unpopular and may not be readily welcomed.

Working with acute medically ill patients requires a period of adjustment to the signs, symptoms, and physical treatment of illness, such as the Hickman catheters, ileostomies, suctioning, and dialysis. Having an active interest in medical conditions is essential to developing a working hypothesis about symptomatology. For example, how incapacitating is the patient's pain, nausea, or fever in relation to his or her current medical status, and are these symptoms symbolic of a deteriorating psychological condition?

In this capacity the occupational therapist feels the primary nature of each relationship and the subsequent responsibility. Helping a patient to deal with issues regarding the quality of life and death and dying is often painful and complex (Purtilo, 1983). In each relationship, the emotional availability of the therapist is important for listening and deeply understanding the meaning of each person's experience. Supporting the patient to clarify and progress with these issues is another important aspect of this work. The occupational therapist must have basic skills in assessing the family's coping methods in relation to the illness of the patient. Interventions with patients and their families may tangibly reduce symptoms or complaints (Shapiro, 1986). Helping someone to live a more satisfactory, if brief, life is its own reward.

References

Blumenfield, M. (1983). Patients' fantasies about physical illness. *Psychotherapy & Psychosomatics, 39*, 171-179.

Bustamente, J. P., & Ford, C. V. (1981). Characteristics of general hospital patients referred for psychiatric consultation. *Journal of Clinical Psychiatry, 42*(9), 338-341.

Cavanaugh, S. (1984). The diagnosis and treatment of depression in the medically ill. In F. G. Guggenheim, & M. F. Weiner (Eds.), *Manual of psychiatric consultation and emergency care* (pp. 211-222). New York: Jason Aronson, Inc.

Cavanaugh, S. (1986). Depression in the hospitalized inpatient with various medical illnesses. *Psychotherapy & Psychosomatics, 45*, 97-104.

Cavanaugh, S., Clark, D. C., & Gibbons, R. D. (1983). Diagnosing depression in the hospitalized medically ill. *Psychosomatics, 24*(9), 809-815.

Cohen-Cole, S. A., & Friedman, C. P. (1983). The language problem: Integration of psychosocial variables in medical care. *Psychosomatics, 24*(1), 54-60.

Groves, J. E. (1978). Taking care of the hateful patient. *The New England Journal of Medicine, 298*(16), 883-887.

Hengeveld, M. W., Rooymans, H. G., & Hermans, J. (1987). Assessment of patient-staff and intrastaff problems in psychiatric consultations. *General Hospital Psychiatry, 9,* 25-30.

Kahana, R. J., & Bibring, G. L. (1964). Personality types in medical management. In N. E. Zinberg (Ed.), *Psychiatry and medical practice in a general hospital* (pp. 108-123). New York: International University Press.

Kielhofner, G., Shepherd, J., Stabenow, C. A., Bledsoe, N., Furst, G., Green, J., Harlin, B. H., McLellan, C. L., & Owens, J. (1985). Physical disabilities. In G. Kielhofner (Ed.), *A model of human occupation: Theory and application* (pp. 170-247). Baltimore: Williams & Wilkins.

Mailick, M. D. (1985). The short-term treatment of depression of physically ill hospital patients. *Social Work in Health Care, 9*(3), 51-61.

Millon, T. (1981). *Disorders of personality DSM-III: Axis II.* New York: Wiley-Interscience.

Pasnau, R. (1982). *Consultation-liaison psychiatry.* Kalamazoo, MI: Upjohn.

Perl, M., & Shelp, E. E. (1982). Psychiatric consultation masking moral dilemmas in medicine. *The New England Journal of Medicine, 307*, 618-621.

Purtilo, R. B. (1983). Ethical issues in cancer. *Journal of Psychosocial Oncology, 1*(1), 3-15.

Robinson, L. (1984). *Psychological aspects of the care of hospitalized patients.* Philadelphia: F. A. Davis.

Saltz, C. C., & Magruder-Habib, K. (1985). Recognizing depression in patients receiving medical care. *Health and Social Work, 10,* 15-22.

Shapiro, J. (1986). Assessment of family coping with illness. *Psychosomatics, 27*(4), 262-271.

Silverberg, R. A. (1985). Men confronting death: Management versus self-determination. *Clinical Social Work Journal, 13*(2), 157-169.

Strain, J. J. (1978). *Psychological interventions in medical practice.* New York: Appleton-Century-Crofts.

Strain, J. J., & Grossman, S. (1975). *Psychological care of the medically ill: A primer in liaison psychiatry.* New York: Appleton.

Watson, L. J. (1986). Psychiatric consultation-liaison services in the acute physical disabilities setting. *American Journal of Occupational Therapy, 40*(5), 338-342.

Chapter 66

The Remediation of Role Disorders Through Focused Group Work

Hilda P. Versluys, MeD, OTR

D espite advances in medicine and rehabilitation, a high percentage of patients are discharged from the hospital unprepared to meet the demands of daily living and are not motivated to reach and maintain projected functional levels of performance. Their return to the community may be followed by social withdrawal, depression, regression, and multiple readmissions.

Harber and Smith define disability as the inability to perform the usual role activities as a result of a physical or mental impairment of long-term duration (1). The idea central to this paper is that loss of or change in valued personal roles can result in role disorders. Role disorders may produce social, psychological, and behavioral problems more profound than the disabling condition (2, 3) and signal the need for occupational therapy intervention.

Role Theory

The therapist committed to restoring a patient's physical function should also consider the patient's need to continue to meet role responsibilities. An understanding of the developmental aspects of role acquisition and the tasks and social skills that support adult roles is indispensable both in the evaluation of role loss and disorder and in the design of treatment programming (4, 5).

Berger states that Man directs considerable energy and commitment to the development of a variety of role functions resulting in the formation of personal identity and a unique life style (6). This process is a continual life task and might be thought of as part of Man's career.

Reilly and Moorehead [sic] have described the hierarchical development of a role through play, chores, and activities. This development is conceived of as a fluid process continuing through the life span and requiring continual adaptations and acquisitions of new skills and habits (7, 8).

Sociologists agree that the genesis of the adult role occurs in childhood through play, exploration, and relationships developed within the family and community. The child tests out or practices the role tasks and social interactional skills that allow adult roles to be successfully performed. These early maturational experiences of the child may be viewed as a learning laboratory or clinic where role models can be observed and role possibilities experienced, thus providing an indispensable process leading to adult role taking (6).

The resulting adult roles—such as sexual, occupational, family, avocational, and social—allow an individual to participate in his or her culture and to satisfy human needs. The mature, well adjusted person integrates all his or her roles into a balanced life style (7, 9).

Role Disorders

Physical illness and disability may adversely affect personal role functions on a continuum from minor changes to complete obliteration of all major roles. A hospitalized and disabled patient struggling to maintain role responsibilities may experience a reduction or fragmentation in functional role skills that undermines confidence and may lead to depression, formation of a poor self-image, and lack of motivation for the rehabilitation task. Functional role skills include maintenance tasks such as shopping and cooking, and work/occupational tasks such as driving, using the telephone, and caring for children. Patients may also temporarily have to shelve role tasks such as meeting financial obligations, maintaining personal standards, and meeting social commitments (10,11).

Role disorders are often compounded by the patients' fears that their customary life styles will change irrevocably. Patients may deal with these anxieties by resorting to maladaptive behaviors such as dependence, denial, and regression (12, 13). For example, a cardiac event may precipitate fear, anxiety, and depression, which may result in unnecessary retirement, the termination of many adult roles, and entrenchment in a sick role (14).

The residual effects of disability may prevent the performance of those "physical" skills that make the execution of major roles possible and thereby result in the exacerbation of role disorders (3). For example, the loss of the physical skills that allow driving cancels the patient's ability to drive a car. Driving can be a vocational necessity and also influence participation in recreation and social activities. The loss of these physical skills severely limits the patient's ability to meet his or her human needs and prevents a balanced and rewarding life style.

Avocational experiences fill needs for creativity and physical action. The loss of physical functions required to dance or ski may not only lead to the termination of pleasurable recreation, but also affect the release of tension through activity. The inability to perform these physical skills means that the role or role tasks must be changed and human and occupational needs must be met in a different manner (15).

Patients vary in their ability to deal with role loss and to accept role substitutes. The loss of a valued role may present a barrier to role substitution for those patients who had invested time and effort in roles that increased status and self-esteem.

The time required for medical treatment, the stress of rehabilitation, the lack of mobility, and concern with changing personal appearance may precipitate a number of crises for the patient. The patient's response to this stressful or traumatic situation may be the development of avoidance behaviors that protect him or her from fear of rejection and contribute to social isolation. A family role such as father and provider carries certain expectations and responsibilities. Discontinuation of these roles, even for a short time, may result in crisis for both the patient and the family (10, 13).

Although dedicated to rehabilitation, the hospital system has its own overt and covert rules for patients' conduct and behaviors that may contribute to role dysfunction. Patients are no longer in charge of their own destiny and may find that they are unable to exert control over the use of their own time (i.e., when to eat, when to go to bed, and when to leave the hospital to visit their family). The patient is expected to adhere to decisions made by others, often without his [or her] knowledge or input. The patient's special skills prized in the community or at work are not useful in the hospital nor are they recognized by the hospital staff as significant. Personal initiative and problem solving are discouraged (10).

Goals of rehabilitation should include the preservation and maintenance of adult roles or the development of strategies to compensate for the loss of social, task, and performance skills that make major role performances possible.

Factors Influencing Role Transformation

Occupational therapy intervention into role disorders is first aimed at assisting the patient to adjust to and understand the hospital system, and thus be in a better psychological position to benefit from rehabilitation. The second strategy is to assist the patient in maintaining role responsibilities during the period of treatment. However, if the prognosis indicates permanent dysfunction, including the patient's inability to fill previous life roles, the goals of treatment are to rehabilitate by the transformation and reassignment of roles.

Based upon the premise that adult roles with their resulting identities are socially bestowed and sustained, it follows that role transformation or the reassignment of roles is a social, interactive process. Perhaps the most important influence in role maintenance and transformation is the contribution of the family. The attitudes the family maintains toward the patient's roles, their willingness to reestablish or contribute to role maintenance, and their identification and assignment of roles useful to the family and within the patient's capabilities are essential in reaching rehabilitation goals (5, 10, 16).

Human roles influenced by cultural definition may be limited in the options for role change and reassignment (6). Patients and their families may assume that there is only one way to be a successful man or woman, a worker, or to fill family membership roles. The considerations of alternative life styles and concomitant adult roles may be difficult for the patient and resisted by the family.

The patient may accept the need to try new work options, devise a new life style, and work to experience and develop different leisure time interests. However, these choices must also be supported by family and reflect the reality of the patient's background experiences, interests, and real skills, both physical and intellectual. Failure to achieve in new endeavors may discourage the patient's progress in rehabilitation and his or her wish to become a viable part of the community upon discharge.

Role loss and lack of role acquisition should be assessed developmentally and chronologically before a problem list for treatment programming is identified. The occupational therapist should be aware that the patient's major life roles vary in priority at different times in the life cycle. Treatment goals should consider the patient's present and future role needs. After the degree of physical and role dysfunctions have been determined, treatment emphasis is placed upon guiding the patient in reexperiencing early developmental tasks through role-focused group experiences. Conditions for change within such groups include interpersonal transactions within a human group, opportunities for exploration [and] play, and the choosing and use of activities (6, 7,17). The patient involved in such a treatment program must also identify the need and purpose for maintaining and/or acquiring new skills (18).

Focused Group Work

Occupational therapy believes that change occurs through action and involvement that reinforce the learned tasks or new skills. The patient, after the traumatic event or as a result of long illness and hospitalization, may not have the ego, strength, and energy to handle formal discussions concerning disability, role skills, and psychosocial needs. Didactic or vicarious teaching, independent of an experiential component, is not successful in increasing self-esteem or in helping the patient to explore new role possibilities (10).

Focused Group

A focused group experience provides a training ground where patients test their ability to deal with problems of living, decision making, and risk taking involved in the change process.

Patients are encouraged to continue responsibility for role tasks in the hospital, family, and community. The patient can be assisted in identifying and maintaining major role responsibilities through a problem-solving process. Graded social roles can be designed for and assigned to the patient for practice in the hospital and the community (10, 19).

Cohesive Group

A cohesive group sustains patients while they experiment and master the skills necessary for physical and psychological survival in the community (16, 21). These necessary role skills are called "Weapons of Life," by Kutner (5). To maintain viable adult roles and personal independence, patients need an arsenal of social and interpersonal skills, the ability to deal with everyday problems of living, and to take social responsibility.

Yalom states that, in the intrinsic act of giving, patients receive a boost to their self-esteem and find that they can be altruistic and important to others (20). The physically disabled patient who encourages, responds, and becomes actively involved in supporting and sharing with other group members, including family, feels immediately more confident and useful, more in control, and [more] positive about his/her ability to handle change.

Role-Focused Group

A role-focused group assists in the ventilation of feelings concerning the permanence of disability, allows the patient to see that others have struggled and succeeded, amplifies the motivation for change, [and] encourages the patient to feel more socially acceptable and to plan more realistically toward transition into the community.

Through group interaction patients are exposed to a variety of social roles. Through activities and involvement in encouraging, planning, organizing, helping, and sharing, patients discover they are capable of being productive within their physical and medical limitations (17, 21, 22).

Also important in treatment for the atrophy or loss of adult roles and underlying role skills is the kind of stress inherent in society. The removal of all stress in therapy groups will impoverish role expectations and thus limit the available number and complexity of roles the patient can play (23). It becomes the responsibility of the therapist to estimate when the patient can handle stress and to program experiences to meet individual learning needs.

The design of role-focused groups includes the following six factors: a group of patients that have the potential to become cohesive; role-building experiences that allow the patients to explore and test new behaviors (5); the freedom to seek out and use activities to please the self and others and to feel competent (17); a clear communication system of supportive and realistic feedback that encourages adaptation and reinforces learning (24); social recognition of group members and their role functions; and opportunities for role experiences that are compatible with the patients' values, culture, and preferred life styles (5, 7).

Role Disorders

Certain responsibilities are specifically the therapist's task. The first is evaluation of role disorders. Guidelines include: 1) a diagnostic projection to identify the degree of permanent functional limitation; 2) patient and family interviews to identify the importance to the patient of each adult role and those role areas central to preservation of the patient's self-esteem and identity; 3) an analysis of the elements of each role most prized by the patient to determine whether these needs can be met through substitute role activities, or compensated for by adaptive equipment or acquisition of new task skills; 4) evaluation of the family commitment level and the skills available in the family to achieve role continuity; 5) recognition of cultural and religious influences; and 6) determination of the patient's interests, values, background, experience, and preferred life style.

In addition to evaluating the patient, the occupational therapist should also: 1) facilitate insight concerning coming changes in adult roles and role skills; 2) design strategies to circumvent those role tasks the patient can no longer perform; 3) develop and encourage realistic treatment goals with the patient; 4) counsel and investigate alternative ways of filling role requirements; 5) prevent role saturation by insisting that role acquisition proceed cautiously and progressively so that new role tasks and behaviors become well-integrated within one major role; 6) stimulate development of follow-up programming within the community to strengthen and internalize new roles.

The patient's performance must be facilitated and monitored skillfully. Tasks need to be assigned, and dialogue and feedback that reinforce the direction and pace of new learning must be provided (5, 24).

Rehabilitation staff may feel that role disorders will remedy themselves when patients return to the community, or that the social and emotional needs of patients are not part of the total rehabilitation goals. Such concepts must be rejected since role disorders cannot be treated quickly, at the last minute, or post-discharge. The timing of treatment is important and should occur concurrently with physical rehabilitation, beginning at the time a patient is admitted to the hospital. The

inclusion of experienced handicapped role models as group leaders or group members provides evidence to patients that others have been successful in building satisfying lives.

Role-Focused Group Models

Homemakers' Group

In this group, members consider alternative ways of home management with emphasis on such specialty areas as child care, cooking, architectural and interior design, and social entertaining. They also deal with feelings about change in living style and the loss incurred in relinquishing familiar ways of meeting personal and family needs at home. Techniques the therapist might use include education, problem solving for individual situations, role playing, direct experience at home, and handicapped role models as teachers and consultants. Families are invited to participate (15).

Role Maintenance Group

This group would assist the patient in maintaining role responsibilities while hospitalized. Emphasis is on identification and realistic appraisal of those role tasks that can be maintained during rehabilitation and separation from work and family. The occupational therapist and group members are responsible for facilitation of negotiations with community and family in problem solving as well as in continual feedback and monitoring of the maintenance process. For example, the salesman who can handle some of his accounts at the hospital through meetings with clients who visit him requires cooperation of the hospital administration and the employer. The group helps him negotiate with these authorities. Also, a mother is encouraged to give input to child care, children's activities, and home management via the telephone and family visits. Meeting the family at the hospital to establish role responsibilities may be helpful. A patient's social obligations and committee tasks can be handled via the telephone. Community, work, and family responsibilities can be redesigned to allow patients continued participation. Family, friends, and business associates are encouraged to attend some of these group sessions.

Social Skill Development

In this group, the emphasis is on maintaining social and communication skills by providing structured learning experiences within a patient group. Mature social skills may have atrophied because of isolation and lack of opportunity to practice, or may be developmentally delayed. Treatment is focused on the development of age-appropriate social and communication skills through interactive exercises, social club activities, and expressive media—for example, poetry and literature. The end goals of community participation are stressed. For example, to illustrate this role-focused group, a patient may learn new social games within his or her physical capacities and then join a community group—for example, chess, bowling, musical club.

Sensitivity Training

This group is designed to assist patients in coping with feelings about community re-entry, being visible in the community, and dealing with rejection. Techniques include sequenced social experiences, planned tasks within the community such as shopping, luncheon, or parties, and dialogue with handicapped role models (17, 19). There is an emphasis on group design of experiential community assignments. The patients assigned to community tasks report back to the group on their personal experiences and feelings. The group provides feedback and support, and assists in solving problems encountered in mobility, access to public buildings, and poise in public or social situations.

Family Task-Oriented Groups

These are interhospital groups formed to strengthen and maintain family relationships and encourage the maintenance of the patient's roles within the family constellation. Patients and family are involved in dialogue concerning the adjustments to disability, the treatment process, [and] planning for discharge, and in social and recreational activities. Emphasis is on programming that provides opportunities for families to interact with the handicapped member (16, 25). Participation in task-oriented activity groups helps to reduce the tension a family feels toward relating to the patient who is physically ill or disabled. Activities include dinners prepared by patients and families, trips, game nights, parties, and expressive media experiences. Handicapped role models allow the family to observe the potential for good functioning after rehabilitation. Activities involving the patient and family allow the family to observe how the staff relates to the patient and what independent behavior is possible; for example, the patient's ability to eat independently, [to] organize activities, or to research and present information used for group planning.

Transitional Group

This group offers transitional or bridging activities designed to provide linkage between the hospital and the community. The patients consider ways to participate in family activities and work/social relationships. They prepare to meet their future social and emotional needs by participation in community groups while still hospitalized, and practice the social role skills necessary upon discharge. Group techniques include dialogue and activities with family, friends, community volunteers, and anticipatory guidance by handicapped consultants. Group design of transitional or bridging activities includes both interhospital and community activities, such as patient organization. For example, patients make and carry out plans to go to church, arrange job interviews or preliminary visits to the old work area, participate in volunteer experiences to teach skills to hospital staff or community groups, and find ways to maintain old friendships and to make new ones (5, 21, 22).

Summary

Patients with a physical illness or a disability may find that their usual adult roles must be modified or permanently changed. Role disorders occur when patients are no longer able to meet their usual role responsibilities. The resulting social and psychological disturbances may be a permanent response to the physical trauma and more profound than the residual limitation warrants.

Treatment goals for such patients should include not only the mastery of physical and compensatory skills required for activities of daily living and mobility, but also parallel programming to treat the psychological and social effects of role disorders, hospitalization, and isolation from the family and community.

Remediation of role disorders can occur through an involvement in experience-based activity groups focused on maintaining and/or transforming major adult role functions. Group goals include re-mastery of social and communication skills, role building, the development of new and satisfying role experiences, and the enhancement of family cohesiveness.

Within the transitional programming between the hospital and community, the patient learns that intergroup roles are also relevant to family, work, and the social community.

Role-focused groups are specialized, flexible, and designed to meet the individual and changing needs of a patient population with role disorders secondary to physical disability.

Acknowledgment

This paper is based on a program developed in the occupational therapy department at Highland View Hospital, Cleveland, Ohio, and on a presentation at the AOTA Annual Conference, Detroit, April 26, 1979. The author also appreciates the assistance of Phillip Shannon and Willem Versluys in editing and organization.

References

1. Kutner B: The social psychology of disability. In *Rehabilitation Psychology*, W Neff, Editor. Washington, DC: American Psychological Association, 1971

2. Wright BA: *Physical Disability—A Psychological Approach*, New York: Harper and Row, 1960

3. Kutner B, Rosenberg PP, Berger R, Abramson AS: *A Therapeutic Community in Rehabilitation Medicine*, New York: Albert Einstein College of Medicine of Yeshiva University, 1970

4. Thomas EJ: Problems of disability from the perspective of role theory. *J Health Hum Behav* 7: 2-14, 1966

5. Kutner B: Milieu therapy. *J Rehabil* 34: 14-17, 1968

6. Berger PL: *Invitation to Sociology*, New York: WW Norton Co., 1963

7. Kielhofner G: The evolution of knowledge in occupational therapy—understanding adaptation of the chronically disabled. Unpublished master's thesis, University of Southern California, Los Angeles, 1973

8. Moorhead L: The occupational history, *Am J Occup Ther* 23: 329-334, 1969

9. Duncombe L, Versluys H: *Occupational Therapy Theory in Psychiatry*, Unpublished Course Manual, Occupational Therapy Department, Sargent College of Allied Health Professions, Boston University, 1979 (2nd Edition)

10. Kutner B: Role disorders in extended hospitalization. *Hosp Admin* 12: 52-59, 1967

11. Carmechail HT, Gruber HW, Sletten CO: *Meeting the Social Needs of Long-Term Patients*. Chicago: American Hospital Association, 1963

12. Ouigley JL: Understanding depression—helping with grief. *Rehabil Gazette* 19: 2-6, 1976

13. Siller J: Psychological situation of the disabled with spinal cord injury. *Rehabil Lit* 30: 290-296, 1969

14. Naughton J: Coronary heart disease. In *Rehabilitation Practices with the Physically Disabled*, JF Garrett, ES Levine, Editors. New York: Columbia University Press, 1973

15. Safilios-Rothschild C: *The Sociology and Social Psychology of Disability and Rehabilitation*, New York: Random House, 1970

16. Versluys HP: Psychological adjustment to physical disability. In *Occupational Therapy for Physical Dysfunction*, CA Trombly, AD Scott. Baltimore: The Williams and Wilkins Co., 1977

17. Geis J: The problem of personal worth in the physically disabled patient. *Rahabil Lit* 33: 19-37, 1972

18. Taylor DP: Treatment goals for quadriplegic and paraplegic patients. *Am J Occup Ther* 28: 22-29, 1974

19. Cogswell BE: Self socialization: Readjustment of paraplegics in the community. *J Rehabil* 34: 11-35, 1968

20. Yalom ID: *The Theory and Practice of Group Psychotherapy*, New York: Basic Books, 1970

21. Romano MD: Social skills training with the newly handicapped. *Arch Phys Med Rehabil* 57: 302-303, 1976

22. Gordon EW: Race, ethnicity, social disadvantagement and rehabilitation. In *Rehabilitation Psychology*, W Neff, Editor. Washington, DC: American Psychological Association, 1971

23. Bennett DH: Rethinking rehabilitation: No bedlam in Bethlehem. *Innovations* 2: 13-14, 1975

24. McDaniel JW: *Physical Disability and Human Behavior*, New York: Pergamon Press, 1976. 2nd Edition

25. D'Afflitti JG, Weitz, GW: Rehabilitating the stroke patient through patient and family groups. In *Coping with Physical Illness*, RH Moss, Editor. New York: Plenum Medical Book Co., 1977

Chapter 67

Sexuality and Disability— Treating the Whole Person

Maureen Freda, OTR

This chapter was previously published in *Physical Disabilities Special Interest Section Newsletter* (1985, June), pp. 2-3. Copyright © 1985, The American Occupational Therapy Association, Inc.

Sexuality, our own and others, is at the very core of our personalities. It plays a big part in how we see ourselves and how others see us. It affects our self-image and often our self-esteem. It is expressed in many ways throughout a typical day—through the subtle glances we share across a room, the gentle touch of a hand, the warm embrace of a friend, the tentative handshake of a new acquaintance, and the twinkle in our eyes as we share an idea. Human beings need to touch each other and physically demonstrate their caring to reinforce their positive attitude to life and their feelings of self-worth; they are not, by nature, isolated beings.

There is a great probability that the very people rehabilitation professionals work with on a daily basis will become isolated. This isolation can be caused by many factors. The disabled can become isolated from people in general because our world is basically inaccessible to them, and they can become isolated from human touch because others don't know how to deal with a wheelchair, a walker, or braces. Also disabled persons may isolate themselves because their self-esteem is low or simply because they lack information.

As health professionals, we have a responsibility to break this cycle. As occupational therapists and holistic caregivers, we must begin to address the sexual concerns of our patients. We cannot say we treat the "whole" person if we consistently delete the entire realm of sexuality from our patient programs. By refusing to include this information, we are telling our patients that sexuality is a nonissue. Then we send them out into a society where sexuality plays an integral part in people's lives.

First, we need to analyze our own views on sexuality and the disabled. For instance, when we see a person in a wheelchair, do we recognize in that individual his or her sexuality? Or is that perception blocked by the ever-present wheelchair? When we see a young couple holding hands in the park and one of the two is disabled, do we conjure up the image of romance and love? When we hear that one of our colleagues is dating a disabled person, are we happy for them? Or are we interested in the whys, the hows, and the mechanics?

As professionals we need to expand our horizons and begin to understand and attend to what is possible for the disabled. We must recognize that sexuality is not a privilege reserved for the able-bodied. We can start this process by identifying our feelings and discussing them openly with other professionals. The more we talk and listen, the easier it will be to discard our prejudices. Workshops and seminars are available throughout the country for health professionals who are willing to come out of the Dark Ages. Before we can play a role in addressing these issues with our patients, we must understand our own feelings.

Once we have come to grips with our own beliefs, we can take the second step. We can help to create an environment where it is easy for our patients to ask questions and discuss problems. The patient must feel safe, safe from being judged and ridiculed. We have to be ready to communicate with our patients at whatever level they are comfortable. Most importantly, we must have correct information, anatomical, medical, and sexual. We can do great harm if we give out misinformation or if we try and "fake" it. Of course, we also have to be available; the patient must be made aware that we have the information and will share it whenever he or she is ready. Above all, we must remember the therapeutic purpose of the interaction. We must not give the patient more information than he or she is comfortable receiving; on the other hand, we must not hold back information because it doesn't conform to "our" norm. As nonjudgmental information givers, we must be ready to give what the patient needs for his or her life style.

Occupational therapists are uniquely qualified to be one of the team members involved in the discussion of the patient's sexuality. The occupational therapist has developed a therapeutic relationship with the patient. In addition, he or she is already dealing with the patient's daily functional living skills, and that acts as an easy bridge to the issues of sexuality. After all, isn't sexuality a daily part of life? Once the basic trust has been established and preliminary information has been shared, we, as occupational therapists, can do what we do best—assist in increasing functional ability. The key word here is functional. I do not suggest that all occupational therapists become sex counselors; however, it is entirely appropriate that the occupational therapist attend to the functional aspects of sexuality and the limitations caused by particular disabilities. We can use our medical and clinical knowledge to help the patient face the how-to issues. We can teach what we are famous for, adaptability; we can suggest alternatives and new ideas to those patients who want this kind of information. Finally, when we have accomplished all this, we can say that we do indeed treat the whole person.

Chapter 68

The PLISSIT Model of Sexuality Counseling and Education

Wilma Asrael, OTR, MHDL

The PLISSIT model of sexual counseling, developed by Annon (1), is an approach that rehabilitation and health professionals can easily adapt to the disabled person's needs. Starting at a level requiring only basic therapeutic skills and some specific sexual knowledge, the model goes through three additional levels, the last of which usually requires referral for long-term intervention.

Every occupational therapist who is willing to regard the patient as a total human being has the skills and knowledge necessary to achieve the goals of the first two levels, designated P for Permission and LI for Limited Information. During the first level of counseling, Permission, patients are reassured that regarding themselves as being sexual is OK. Questions in the minds of most traumatically disabled persons might include the following: Can I function as a male or female? Will I be acceptable as a partner? What pleasure can I give and receive? Am I normal to even have these thoughts and feelings? Many patients do not have the courage to pose these questions directly; for sexuality, in spite of the so-called sexual revolution, is still an embarrassing, highly sensitive subject to most people. The key therapeutic intervention at the permission level is to give the patient an opportunity to talk to a nonjudgmental, knowledgeable, relaxed individual who is a good listener and who is willing to reassure the patient that his or her fears and concerns are normal. It is evident that many occupational therapists who have not had specific training may not be nonjudgmental, knowledgeable, and relaxed when dealing with the subject of sexuality. However, when a patient indicates to a specific therapist that he or she needs to discuss sexual concerns, one may assume that the patient feels a strong, positive rapport with that therapist. If questions are ignored, as they often are, the patient is likely to feel rejected and unworthy. Even when the occupational therapist feels uncomfortable with the implied or direct question, she or he must be able to respond at least by saying, "I understand what you are asking. I'm afraid I'm not comfortable with this subject, but it is a very important one. Would you mind if I introduced you to somebody who can give you the information you need." By reacting in this positive manner, the occupational therapist provides the patient with the necessary permission and reassurance.

The second level of the PLISSIT model, Limited Information, provides information to dispel myths and misconceptions about the sexual functioning of disabled men and women. Here are some of the most common myths and misconceptions: disabled people are not sexual; disabled people are oversexed; disabled people use perverted techniques in sexual activity; no one would want to marry a disabled person; disabled persons are a burden to their partners; disabled women should not get married or have children, can only give birth by C-section, and cannot adequately take care of children; disabled men are not fertile, cannot have orgasms if there is no genital sensation, and are inadequate as husbands and fathers. The list is endless. These misconceptions in the minds of the disabled persons, their friends and families, the public in general, and yes, also in the minds of many health professionals, must be dispelled by offering factual information on a one-to-one basis or, as is now the case in many rehabilitation hospitals, in regularly scheduled classes or therapeutic group sessions. Special literature, adapted for the patient's needs, may also be helpful to reinforce the facts. Children who have developmental disabilities need the same factual information as their able-bodied counterparts (many believe they need even more information). Young people need to be informed to enhance their self-esteem and body image and to protect themselves from sexual abuse. The unfortunate fact is that disabled children and adults are abused at a higher rate than able-bodied persons. In addition to providing information on sexuality, it might be necessary to train the disabled in self-protection techniques.

Even further training is needed at the third level of the PLISSIT model, designated SS for Specific Suggestions. Often, although not always, the partner or "significant other" of the disabled person needs to be involved at this level. The counselor helps the couple by discussing their sexual activity before the onset of the disability, discussing the changes that have occurred, setting realistic goals for future activity, and helping plan strategies for achieving such goals. Most occupational therapists would probably not want to be involved at this level, but all could be informed about the proper referrals in their setting and could aid the patient in deciding to seek out such help. Also, occupational therapy intervention at this level would include input on positioning and adapting equipment to meet the patient's needs.

The fourth level of counseling, designated IT for Intensive Therapy, implies long-term treatment for relationship problems and sexual problems that have been in existence for long periods of time and usually since before the onset of the disability. Most rehabilitation settings do not employ the personnel to handle in-depth problems, and the patient would, in many cases, be referred to community resources.

Most patients with physical disabilities can be greatly helped by intervention at the first three levels of the PLISSIT model. The occupational therapist's role can be determined on a personal and professional basis with the needs of the total patient in mind. The input of the occupational therapist who sees all patients first as men or women and only second as disabled can be of great value in a team approach to the sexuality of the disabled.

Related Reading

Sex Disability Problems: Who Cares? A handbook on sex education and counseling services for disabled people. Washington DC: George Washington University, 1979

Reference

1. Annon JS. The behavioral treatment of sexual problems. In *Brief Therapy* (Vol 1) Honolulu: Kapiolani Health Services, 1974

Chapter 69

Psychosocial Occupational Therapy Intervention With AIDS Patients

Victoria J. Schindler, MA, OTR

This chapter was previously published in the *American Journal of Occupational Therapy*, 42, 507-512. Copyright © 1988, The American Occupational Therapy Association, Inc.

The World Health Organization, in November 1983, acknowledged acquired immune deficiency syndrome (AIDS) as a worldwide problem. Accurate reporting has been carried out in the United States since 1981, and as of March 1, 1988, 54,233 cases have been reported to the Centers for Disease Control in Atlanta (Gable, Barnard, Norko, & O'Connell, 1986; Centers for Disease Control, Atlanta, personal communication, March 1988).

AIDS is a complex disease process characterized by a collapse of the body's natural immune system. A virus, now labeled human immunodeficiency virus (HIV), has recently been discovered by investigators as being linked with AIDS (New York State Department of Health, 1987).

Most AIDS cases are found in metropolitan areas; yet cases have been reported in all 50 states (and in all ethnic groups). AIDS occurs most frequently among male homosexuals and bisexuals and intravenous drug users. However, it is also seen in the female sexual partners of men with AIDS or at risk for AIDS, children who acquired AIDS at birth from infected mothers, and persons with hemophilia who received transfusions of infected blood or blood products. Most persons with AIDS are in their early twenties to mid-forties—an age group that does not expect to develop a terminal illness (Christ & Wiener, 1985; New York State Department of Health, 1987).

AIDS is not an easily transmissible disease. Evidence to date indicates that the virus is spread only through blood-to-blood and semen-to-blood contact. Although it was originally feared that the virus could be contracted through casual methods, evidence indicates that the disease cannot be transmitted through casual contact such as sneezing, coughing, or sharing household items with a person with AIDS (New York State Department of Health, 1987; Ungvarski, 1985).

Presently, there is no definitive test to diagnose AIDS; nor is there a vaccine or a cure. However, a blood test has been developed that detects antibodies to the HIV. Some people infected with the virus have no symptoms at all, whereas others may develop mild or temporary symptoms that disappear a few days or weeks after exposure. About 20% of those infected with the virus have developed the severe and fatal form of the disease.

The incubation period for AIDS ranges from a few weeks to many years (New York State Department of Health, 1987).

Because AIDS is a severe immune defect, persons with AIDS are open to a number of opportunistic diseases. About 85% have one or both of two rare diseases: pneumocystis carinii pneumonia, an infection of the lungs, and Kaposi's sarcoma, a rare type of cancer occurring on the skin or in the mouth. A variety of antiviral drugs are showing some promise of killing or inhibiting the HIV, but most treatment is presently aimed at specific opportunistic infections or cancers (New York State Department of Health, 1987).

Another syndrome associated with the HIV is AIDS-related complex (ARC). The symptoms categorized as ARC are associated with the HIV but are not components of the Centers for Disease Control's definition for AIDS. Some of the symptoms seen with ARC are continued fever, swollen lymph glands, bouts of diarrhea, and thrush. Persons with ARC may die of their infections without ever developing full-blown AIDS (New York State Department of Health, 1987).

Effect of AIDS on Life Roles and Tasks

Patients with AIDS require a massive adjustment upon diagnosis of the syndrome. They are suddenly faced with the issue of contagion and must worry about transmitting the disease to others, and dealing with the responses and fears of lovers, parents and other family members, co-workers, and the public. They must also be concerned about protecting themselves from opportunistic diseases. During the first 100 days after the diagnosis the AIDS patient is vulnerable to reactive psychiatric symptoms, such as depression, anxiety, and preoccupation with the illness. This vulnerability to AIDS-related distress is at least as serious and widespread among ARC patients as it is among AIDS patients. In a comparative study of gay men with AIDS (n = 89), gay men with ARC (n = 39), and gay men with no physical symptoms (n = 149), ARC patients scored at least as high as, if not higher than, AIDS patients on multiple parameters of both general and AIDS-specific distress. This is believed to be secondary to the persistent uncertainty about developing AIDS (Holland & Tross, 1985).

Other issues may require adjustment: The patients may not have resolved issues regarding their homosexuality or drug abuse. Additionally, because the public is ambivalent about the illness and the major high-risk populations who contract it, AIDS patients tend to be denied some of the psychological benefits of the sick role that other terminally ill patients receive. For example, because of the fear of contagion, AIDS patients are often isolated and have difficulty obtaining benefits,

employment, and care. Moreover, public fear and anxiety about homosexuality and drug addiction can contribute to a social rejection of the patient (Christ & Wiener, 1985).

AIDS patients also need to cope with declining function in physical, psychosocial, and cognitive functioning. General physical problems include weight loss, progressive weakness, and decreased endurance. Denton (1987) cited evidence that 40% of AIDS patients manifest neurological impairment such as paraparesis, sensory perception changes, peripheral neuropathies, and dysphagia. Additionally, recent studies indicate that the HIV directly affects the central nervous system and may cause psychiatric symptoms such as dysphoric mood, apathy, impaired concentration and memory, and anxiety, before other signs of immune deficiency, cognitive impairment, or neurological abnormalities emerge. For example, patients with AIDS who had been relatively well adjusted and had no psychiatric history developed depression, major affective disorder, and psychosis before acquiring other medical AIDS/ARC-associated conditions (Perry & Jacobsen, 1986).

Because this disease usually strikes persons in their early to middle adulthood, it has a huge impact on the developmental tasks of this period. Overall, the young adult (25-45 years old) is expected to enter new roles at work, home, and in society and develop the values, attitudes, and interests attributed to these roles (Christ & Wiener, 1985; Murray & Zentner, 1979).

In family relationships, the young adult is expected to be independent of the parents' direct care although he or she may receive some indirect assistance. Work becomes a major focus and the young adult is expected to choose an occupation that will provide a livelihood for him- or herself and possibly for dependents. Much time and energy is focused on this process, and work becomes a central part of the adult self-concept. Leisure is now viewed as a time of earned recreation and relaxation from work and often takes the form of exercise, sports, and hobbies (Murray & Zentner, 1979).

During young adulthood, a person has reached his or her optimum mental and motor functioning. Thinking and learning are objective, realistic, and problem-centered, and the person can cognitively combine or integrate steps in addition to considering alternatives and synthesizing information. Emotionally, the young adult is in Erikson's (as discussed by Murray & Zentner, 1979) developmental crisis of intimacy versus self-isolation in which he or she will form an intense commitment to another person, cause, or institution or become withdrawn, lonely, or self-centered. Sexuality is powerful, and there is a need to find adequate and satisfying sexual experiences (Murray & Zentner, 1979).

Patients diagnosed with AIDS or ARC are suddenly thrown to a much later developmental period without adequate opportunity to master the life tasks for young adulthood. At a time when the young adult is expected to be independent from his or her parents and establish an occupation, he or she is now facing less financial independence with increased dependence on others. Additionally, patients often do not have the energy or physical or mental capabilities to maintain their performance at work. Leisure, a time which had been reserved for refreshment from work, now becomes the major focus of the person's schedule; yet participation in some of the usual recreational activities may no longer be possible because of the patient's decreased physical status. All of these changes can cause a negative effect on a person's self-concept.

Physiologically, the patient with AIDS is often very weak and ill at a time when he or she should be functioning at peak efficiency. Cognitively, the thought processes can be severely disabled if there is any neurological manifestation of the illness. Emotionally, the patient may not have the energy or opportunity to seek and form intimate relationships and may feel isolated and lonely and withdrawn. Although sexuality is usually powerful at this stage, the person with AIDS may have a very weakened sexual drive or may experience guilt or conflictual feelings about practicing sexual intercourse since it is a major method for transmitting the disease.

All of these changes interrupt every facet of life for the young adult with AIDS/ARC. The young adult is forced into a developmental period usually experienced by persons who are 20-40 years older; he or she has to face retirement from work, separation and/or the loss of intimate relationships, and decreased physiological and mental functioning.

Despite the alarming facts regarding the disease, studies have shown that patients with AIDS are surviving for significant periods of time after diagnosis. A study of 178 patients conducted in Britain between 1982 and 1985 showed that three quarters of the patients died up to 28 months after diagnosis. With the development of the new drug AZT these time periods are increasing (Guiles & Allen, 1987). Patients will therefore often survive for a considerable length of time after diagnosis and will often be well enough to live outside of the hospital with varying amounts of assistance (Guiles & Allen, 1987).

Because the syndrome has such a debilitating effect on the patient's ability to perform the physical and psychosocial aspects of work, leisure, social interaction, and self-care and because the patient needs to cope with these changes for 2 or more years, occupational therapy intervention is of great benefit.

Occupational Therapy Intervention

My review of the occupational therapy literature revealed that only three articles on AIDS have been published (Caestle, 1986; Denton, 1987; Guiles & Allen, 1987). I incorporated the information from these articles with literature from other allied health professions on AIDS. During the review I also found that the occupational behavior model, which had previously been incorporated with terminally ill patients, can be used in the treatment of patients with AIDS.

Principles of Occupational Behavior

Kielhofner defines occupation as "the purposeful use of time by humans to fulfill their own internal urges toward exploring and mastering their environment that at the same time fulfills the requirements of the social group to which they belong and personal needs for self-maintenance" (Kielhofner, 1980, p. 659). Through the course of normal development people explore their environment and make choices. However, terminal illness disrupts this process. The ability to control and master life situations ceases and life goals may be abandoned. Temporal adjustment to a shortened life span and to the present, with its problems, may be difficult. Physical, psychosocial, and cognitive disabilities can limit a person's ability to explore and master his or her environment. This is especially a problem for patients with AIDS since most are in the early to middle adult period of their life, and have chosen or are beginning to choose an occupation and have formed or are beginning to form enduring relationships. The younger ones among them are still solidifying their identity. Additionally, not only may they be partially or completely unable to fulfill the requirements of their social group, they may be shunned by members of society, not only for their serious illness, but also because their illness labels them as people having a different sexual orientation or having an addiction.

For example, A., a 35-year-old homosexual man, 2 years after he had received a diagnosis of AIDS, was severely emaciated, had peripheral neuropathy, and was confined to a wheelchair. He was enrolled in a weekly outpatient support group for persons with AIDS, which was co-led by a psychiatric resident and an occupational therapist. Because of generalized muscle weakness, he did not have the strength and endurance to care for any of his needs and required a 24-hour home health aide. This man, who had been a stand-up comedian until 4 years earlier, now stayed home all day, limiting his activities to watching television, and he had become very depressed. He was shunned by the members of his family, who were hurt and angry after learning about his homosexuality at the time of diagnosis. Many of his friends had died of complications from AIDS. This man was no longer able to explore and master his environment and he was shunned by or lost contact with his small social group.

Evaluation and Treatment—Occupational Behavior Model

Evaluation. In the evaluation phase the occupational therapist formally assesses role performance and addresses treatment to those areas in which the patient prefers to remain in control. The patient's present skills and deficits (both physical and psychosocial) are evaluated in the areas of work, leisure, and activities of daily living with an emphasis on the areas the patient wants to maintain or improve. If there is severe weakness, the patient may want to build up his or her strength and endurance in order to carry out specific activities. If the patient is depressed, he or she may want to work toward improving his or her psychosocial functioning to return to the highest level of functioning possible.

Evaluation should also address the three subsystems (volitional, habituation, and performance) outlined in the occupational behavior model. Because of the disabilities that result from the physical, neurological, and psychological opportunistic diseases, the components of the three subsystems may undergo extreme changes (Kielhofner & Burke, 1980).

In the volitional subsystem, the therapist would evaluate the patient's personal causation (image of him- or herself as a competent or incompetent person), valued goals, and interests. With the disruption in accomplishing or maintaining specific developmental milestones, such as financial independence, the patient may experience a negative change in his or her sense of competence and goals and interests. In the habitual subsystem, the therapist would assess the patient's habits and internalized roles. Habits and roles that have been incorporated into daily life may now be difficult to accomplish. For example, independent self-care habits could be limited by a physical disability that resulted from an opportunistic illness, or a patient may no longer be able to fulfill selected life roles, such as a worker role. Finally, in the performance subsystem, the therapist would assess the patient's present skills. The motoric, psychosocial, cognitive, and sensory aspects of the skills could be dysfunctional. For instance, limited motor ability could affect a person's ability to complete a self-care task. After a thorough evaluation, the next aspect would be to assist the patient in setting concrete, measurable goals that reflect the time constraints imposed by a terminal illness (Pizzi, 1984).

Treatment. Despite the severe life changes imposed by a terminal illness, occupation, as the tool of the occupational therapist, can enhance the quality of life for AIDS patients by assisting them to develop skills, set priorities, maximize occupational roles, and gain a sense of mastery and competence over the present environment, the self, and the disease process (Pizzi, 1984). For example, A., because his cognitive functioning and speech were still intact, was encouraged to tell his comedy routines into a tape recorder. A. enlisted the help of a friend to write down the jokes, hoping to get them printed for fellow comedians or possibly published. In this way, he was able to enhance skills that had been abandoned, maximize his role as a comedian, and gain a sense of mastery over his goals, his environment, and the disease.

More specifically, the occupational behavior frame of reference (Kielhofner, 1980; Kielhofner & Burke, 1980) can be incorporated into the treatment of the AIDS population, as it would be with any other population, through assisting the patient to move through a process that begins with exploration and leads to competency and achievement in physical, cognitive, and psychosocial tasks (Kielhofner, 1980). This method allows for trial and error, which is essential for developing problem-solving and decision-making skills (Tigges & Sherman, 1983). This process also addresses the three subsystems through assisting the patient in acquiring skills, forming roles and habits, and developing interests, goals, and a positive sense of personal causation. I have incorporated Kielhofner's (1980) framework with the case study described below.

Another patient, G., a 28-year-old, single, white, heterosexual woman with no prior psychiatric history, was admitted to an inpatient psychiatric unit for adults with acute problems with a 1-week history of labile and elated affect, grandiose delusions, auditory hallucinations, agitation, hyperactivity, sexual preoccupation, and numerous spending sprees. Prior to admission the patient had been living with her boyfriend in an apartment and had been working as a pharmacist in a major metropolitan hospital. The patient's condition was initially diagnosed as bipolar affective disorder—manic phase, and she was treated with a variety of medications, including lithium, none of which had positive effects. As the patient continued in treatment, she began to develop fevers and weight loss in addition to psychosis and disorientation. Although initial medical tests were nonconclusive, later tests showed pneumocystis carinii pneumonia. At this time the patient's boyfriend acknowledged he was bisexual and had probably transmitted the HIV to her.

After her mania subsided, G. began to regress physically, cognitively, and psychosocially. She had been very attractive, but now she began to lose weight and was unable to consistently tend to her grooming and hygiene needs. Although her periods of regression were increasing, she did have lucid periods in which she would become quite depressed about her situation. One look in the mirror would intensify her depression. Her clothes had become much too large for her, her hair had lost its style, and she no longer continued her routine of applying makeup and manicuring her nails. Since she stated a desire to become more feminine again, a goal was set to increase her independence in self-care and grooming.

It had been quite a few months since she had tended to these needs, and in the interim she had lost some of the cognitive skills (judgment and sequencing) necessary to carry out these tasks. Therefore the process began with exploration and experimentation with different kinds of makeup, nail products, and hair styles. Although she required relearning and assistance initially, G. was able to become more competent with practice. A visit to the hospital thrift shop was arranged where G. purchased appropriate clothing. Eventually G. was able to carry out these tasks independently and continued to do so as long as her cognitive ability permitted. Although her health continued to slowly decline, she was able to master a goal that was important to her.

Issues for Therapists Working with AIDS Patients

Working with persons with AIDS can raise many fears and concerns in the occupational therapist. The fear of contagion, although unwarranted, presently appears to be the most widespread and persistent issue for several reasons.

First, there has been an unrealistic desire for absolute proof of absence of risk. Secondly, it remains difficult to believe that a virus capable of causing a cruel and fatal disease is not easily transmitted. Thirdly, because the HIV has been isolated from other bodily fluids, such as saliva, tears, and urine, there is concern that contact with these fluids can lead to infection. However, the evidence to date is that only blood and semen are involved in the transmission of the virus. Finally, there has been an overemphasis on isolated and unusual cases of HIV transmission in health care workers. On further inspection of these cases, it has been documented that blood-to-blood contact was involved ("AIDS: Health Prevention," 1987; Friedland & Klein, 1987).

In reality there are no data to suggest AIDS can be transmitted via an airborne route. Also, not a single case of occupational transmission, outside of the health care environment, has been reported (Gerberling & Sande, 1987). A study of 101 household contacts of 39 AIDS patients with oral candidiasis, all of whom lived in the household with the person with AIDS for at least 3 months and shared household items and facilities, re-

vealed that only 1 of the contacts had become infected with the virus. This contact was a 5-year-old who contracted the HIV perinatally. The study concluded that household contacts who are not sex partners of, or born to, persons with AIDS are at minimal or no risk of infection from the HIV (Friedland et al., 1986).

The inoculation with infected blood during accidental needle stick injury has been linked to the transmission of AIDS in 4 of 2,400 health care workers (Gerberling & Sande, 1987). These isolated cases underscore the need for infection control, but they do not imply a high risk of transmission ("AIDS: Health Prevention," 1987; Friedland & Klein, 1987). Infection control procedures for the therapist include hand washing after all contacts with the patient and the use of sterile equipment and materials during contact with blood or bodily fluids. Infection control for equipment consists of cleaning the equipment with a 9:1 solution of water and household bleach (Denton, 1987).

Several other fears and issues, in addition to the fear of contagion, can influence the therapist's relationship with the patient with AIDS. One is fear of the unknown. To counteract the tendency to treat the person with AIDS as "the other" (Dunkel & Hatfield, 1986), the patient must be recognized as an individual and not as a member of a stereotyped group (Denton, 1987). Another issue is fear of dying. Working with a young person with a terminal illness evokes unresolved feelings regarding one's own mortality. Working with AIDS patients can also raise issues regarding a fear of homosexuality (homophobia). Prior to being diagnosed with AIDS, a person's sexual preference may not have been known or not have been an issue. The AIDS label associates a person with having a same-sex preference or as being an IV drug user, and this raises questions regarding one's own beliefs and values. Therapists can also overidentify with the patient and have difficulty maintaining an objective point of view or may take on a magical belief of omnipotence. The therapist could also experience anger because of feelings of helplessness, fear, and guilt in treating a terminally ill patient. This can result in blaming the patient for having a disease that defies traditional treatment (Dunkel & Hatfield, 1986). Education regarding AIDS, peer support groups, and ongoing supervision can facilitate a therapist's ability to recognize these issues and deal with them in an appropriate, productive manner. These forums can also enable the therapist to ventilate other fears and concerns associated with this challenging population.

Summary

AIDS has been identified as a worldwide problem and a highly debilitating and fatal disease. The epidemiology and clinical picture of AIDS has been described. The disease usually strikes persons in their early twenties to middle forties and greatly influences and interrupts the regular developmental tasks of this period. With occupational therapy's focus on promoting independence in developmental tasks, the role of our profession is emerging as a vital one.

Occupational therapy evaluation and intervention, using the occupational behavior frame of reference (Kielhofner, 1980; Kielhofner & Burke, 1980), can be applied to the AIDS population. In evaluation, the therapist formally assesses role performance via the three subsystems with an emphasis on those areas in which the patient wants to remain in control. Once realistic goals are established, the therapist addresses intervention by assisting the patient to move through a process of exploration to competency to achievement in physical, cognitive, and psychosocial tasks. This process was highlighted in this article with case examples that focused on psychosocial intervention. Working with persons with AIDS also raises many issues and concerns for the therapist. These issues were addressed, and realistic methods to explore these issues were provided.

With all of the physical, psychosocial, and cognitive aspects of the AIDS illness, working with the AIDS population can be a vital role for occupational therapy. However, before successfully assuming this role, occupational therapists need to become knowledgeable about the medical and psychological aspects of the illness, explore the application of occupational therapy theories and treatment with this population, and address the many fears and concerns in working with patients with AIDS. Through application of their knowledge occupational therapists can demonstrate the value of their services for this very challenging population.

References

AIDS: Health prevention for health care workers. (1987, August) *1199 News*, pp. 6, 11.

Caestle, S. (1986, November 5). The emerging role of occupational therapy with AIDS. *Occupational Therapy Forum*, pp. 9-10.

Christ, G. H., & Wiener, L. (1985). Psychosocial issues in AIDS. In V. Devita, Jr., S. Hellman, & S. Rosenberg (Eds.), *AIDS: Etiology, diagnosis, treatment and prevention* (pp. 277-297). Philadelphia, PA: Lippincott.

Denton, R. (1987). AIDS: Guidelines for OT intervention. *American Journal of Occupational Therapy, 41,* 427-432.

Dunkel, J., & Hatfield S. (1986). Countertransference issues in working with persons with AIDS. *Social Work* (March-April), 114-117.

Friedland, G., Saltzman, B., Rogers, M., Kahl, P., Lesser, M., Mayers, M., & Klein, R. (1986). Lack of transmission of HTLV-III/LAV infection to household contacts of patients with AIDS or ARC with oral candidiasis. *New England Journal of Medicine, 314*(6), 344-349.

Friedland G., & Klein R. (1987). Real and perceived risks of AIDS in the family and household. *AIDS: Information on AIDS for the practicing physician* (Vol. 3, pp. 16-22). Chicago: American Medical Association.

Gable R., Barnard, N., Norko, M., & O'Connell, R. (1986). AIDS presenting as mania. *Comprehensive Psychiatry, 26,* 251-254.

Gerberling, J., & Sande, M. (1987). Real and perceived risks of AIDS in the health care and work environment. *AIDS: Information on AIDS for the Practicing Physician.* (Vol. 3, pp. 11-15). Chicago: American Medical Association.

Guiles, G., & Allen, M. E. (1987). AIDS, ARC, and the occupational therapist. *British Journal of Occupational Therapy, 50*(4), 120-122.

Holland, J. C., & Tross, S. (1985). The psychosocial and neuropsychiatric sequelae of the acquired immune deficiency syndrome and related disorders. *Annals of Internal Medicine, 103*(3), 760-4.

Kielhofner, G. (1980). A model of human occupation, part 2. Ontogenesis from the perspective of temporal adaptation. *American Journal of Occupational Therapy, 34,* 657-663.

Kielhofner, G., & Burke, J. (1980). A model of human occupation, part 1. Conceptual framework and content. *American Journal of Occupational Therapy, 34,* 572-581.

Murray, R., & Zentner, J. (1979). *Nursing assessment and health promotion through the life span* (2nd ed.). Englewood Cliffs, NJ: Prentice-Hall.

New York State Department of Health. (1987, May). *AIDS—100 Questions and Answers.* Author.

Perry, S., & Jacobsen, P. (1986). Neuropsychiatric manifestation of AIDS-spectrum. *Hospital and Community Psychiatry, 37*(2), 135-141.

Pizzi, M. (1984). Occupational therapy in hospice care. *American Journal of Occupational Therapy, 37,* 235-238.

Tigges, K. N., & Sherman, L. M. (1983). The treatment of the hospice patient: From occupational history to occupational role. *American Journal of Occupational Therapy, 37,* 235-238.

Ungvarski, P. (1985). Learning to live with AIDS. *Nursing Mirror, 160,* 21-23.

Chapter 70

A Day Treatment Program for Persons With AIDS

Linda Gutterman, OTR

The Village Nursing Home in New York, New York, developed a project to focus on the needs of persons with AIDS. As a result, a three-part plan of action was created to meet these needs. Part 1 entailed the establishment of the AIDS day treatment program, which has been operating since August 1988 under a mental health license and has been serving persons who have both AIDS and a psychiatric disorder. Part 2 entailed the development of a home care program to serve persons with AIDS. Part 3 entailed the opening of a nursing home for persons with AIDS.

The AIDS day treatment program was conceived to provide direct services and a caring environment for persons with AIDS who cannot return to work, require supervision, or need a social support network. Additionally, the program provides the clients' caregivers (spouses or significant others, friends, families) with respite. Adult day care has existed for the elderly and for persons with psychiatric disorders, but it is relatively new for persons with AIDS. Persons with AIDS and elderly persons both experience loss of physical independence, pain, impaired memory and judgment, anxiety and depression, loss of and changes in roles, loss of self-esteem, loss of loved ones, and loss of community. These problems are further compounded for AIDS patients because they must confront these complications of aging without the accompanying chronology. Studies of adult daycare programs have shown significant results regarding the ability of these programs to enhance clients' quality of life by reducing isolation, maintaining and improving activities of daily living skills, improving health status and feelings of well-being, and decreasing the rate of institutionalization (Harder, Gornick, & Burt, 1986).

The holistic approach of the Village Nursing Home's AIDS day treatment program addresses the emotional, psychological, social, physical, spiritual, and environmental needs of the individual and group to establish the highest functioning community possible within the program and to support the highest functioning of the individual.

This chapter was previously published in the *American Journal of Occupational Therapy, 44*, 234-237. Copyright © 1990, The American Occupational Therapy Association, Inc.

Program Overview

Many of the clients in the AIDS day treatment program have housing and homelessness problems or have lived in unsupportive environments. Their conditions have included the following psychiatric diagnoses: (a) history of bipolar illness, personality disorder, or schizophrenia; (b) depression or anxiety in response to a diagnosis of AIDS; and (c) AIDS dementia complex, often resulting from opportunistic infections in the central nervous system. The program's population is approximately 10 men to each woman, with the total number of clients ranging between 100 and 125.

The cause of HIV transmission in this population is due mainly to sexual contact (55%-65%), with the remaining cause being a history of intravenous drug use. Most clients have varying degrees of cachexia, skin and gastrointestinal symptoms, respiratory impairment, neurological involvement, and impaired ambulation and endurance. The clients are referred to the day treatment program by hospitals, clinics, private physicians, other health care professionals, or other clients, and some have walked in off the street. Before admission to the program, the client must have a medical diagnosis from a primary care physician that states the presence of AIDS or AIDS-related complex and a psychiatric disorder. The program is staffed by an occupational therapist, a program director, a medical director (psychiatrist), an infectious disease physician, two nurses, an art therapist, a music therapist, a social worker, a coordinator of volunteers, an operations manager, a dietitian, a substance abuse counselor, an office manager, and an assistant. Volunteer clergy provide pastoral counseling. A psychotherapist from outside the facility leads a staff support group twice per month. Role overlap among disciplines is constant. In this setting, the total multidisciplinary effort is greater than the sum of its parts. Were the staff to remain within their traditional professional roles, there would be large gaps in programming and many unmet needs.

Program Philosophy

The philosophy of the day treatment program and the occupational therapy program is that AIDS is a chronic disease that requires medical and psychiatric attention, rehabilitation (including expressive arts therapies and holistic modalities), psychotherapeutic intervention (including substance abuse counseling), nutritional counseling, and pastoral care. The clients who attend the day program benefit from a milieu that supports their empowerment and facilitates their self-care abilities beyond the usual activities of daily living (e.g., washing, dressing, grooming) to also include self-healing. The incorporation of self-healing into the domain of self-care acknowledges that the spiritual and attitudinal facets of the individual are major forces in the healing process, while noting that healing may not always mean survival. Empowerment and self-healing result from the clients' ability to self-actualize and to discover and respond to their own inner truths. In intense moments of self-revelation, for example, the individual commonly experiences a reduction in or a new perception of pain and a sense of relief in experiencing a self-truth (Ferguson, 1980). For some clients at the day treatment program, empowerment may be a new experience. Although many clients have learned to be "good" patients by becoming passive, the day treatment program encourages them to reclaim their power to direct their own lives. For example, clients can

- Make informed decisions regarding medications and dosages with awareness of drug interactions and adverse reactions.
- Choose to enroll in substance abuse detoxification programs.
- Work with a lawyer to establish a living will or last will and testament, thereby addressing unfinished business and easing the transition for self, family, and friends.
- Use meditation and visualization techniques to control pain, reduce stress, increase coping mechanisms, and facilitate physical and attitudinal healing.

The Occupational Therapist's Role

Health Promotion Groups

While providing traditional occupational therapy services to treat the loss of physical and cognitive function, the occupational therapist at the day treatment program also acts as an agent of change, as depicted in the literature as an educator, an indirect service provider, and a program planner (Grossman, 1977; Laukaran, 1977). The occupational therapist fulfills this role by helping to create a fertile internal and external environment for change. At the day treatment program, the therapist's primary focus is to provide health education and health promotion activities that (a) support clients physically, emotionally, and spiritually; (b) facilitate adaptive behavior; and (c) act as a catalyst for change where there is receptivity and motivation.

Occupational therapy is interested in wellness. Activities with this objective include educational classes that are taught by the therapist or by guest teachers. For example, 20 clients complaining of severe, constant itching; reddened, dry skin; and sores that became infected and were difficult to heal attended a skin care class. This class focused on the use of nontoxic natural and herbal remedies, including salves and baths. A general instruction section followed, as well as a question-and-answer session and an experiential component in which clients gave one another cleansing facials. This was followed at a later date by a workshop in which the clients made salves for themselves.

Another health promotion class addressed nutrition and emphasized the use of unprocessed foods and foods free of preservatives and chemicals, the use of herbal teas to decrease caffeine intake, and the reduction of sugar in the diet. This class was given by a clinical nutritionist who volunteered her time. All clients and staff members received copies of dietary information. A nutritionist was hired recently to oversee the clients' general nutrition. Although caloric intake is crucial to persons with AIDS, calories must be worthwhile and not devoid of nutrients. For example, although sugar is high in calories, it offers little in the way of nutrients and causes the loss of chromium and other minerals from the body. Chromium is necessary for correcting the amino acid balance in the body (Badgley, 1986). Food served in the day treatment program tries to incorporate this information while acknowledging that dietary habits are difficult to change, even for those who are motivated. Whenever possible, the occupational therapist has provided the clients with information about holistic alternatives for maintaining health, because the clients are already overstressed by high doses of medications, such as zidovudine (AZT), which has multiple adverse reactions. The program's medical staff has been interested in this information and supportive of its use.

Spirituality and Holistic Modalities

Occupational therapists examine motivation and attitudes and their direct effect on quality of life. *Motivation* can be defined as that which moves or prompts a person to act in a certain way. Spirit, the force behind motivation, is a crucial aspect of the person and an important one to reach in the healing process. Spirituality and occupational therapy interconnect when we define spirit as the life force within us that tells us who we really are. Occupational therapists can stimulate, or inspire, the client toward self-actualization and insight by teaching or providing opportunities for learning self-healing techniques. Within this framework, the inner spirit is the source. Motivation, or a lack of it, may be indicative of the client's desire to live. In the day treatment program, the occupational therapist teaches the clients the use of visualization and guided imagery to evoke their self-knowledge to help with pain or

anxiety reduction, problem solving, or overall relaxation. Additionally, the occupational therapist, who is also trained in holistic healing, provides supervision as needed to volunteers licensed in massage; certified in yoga instruction; and trained in movement and exercise, therapeutic touch, and other modalities that deal with the electromagnetic field. The occupational therapist and the volunteer coordinator determine the level of competence and professionalism of these volunteers. Licensed volunteers can document their treatment sessions with a client in the client's chart. To receive a particular treatment, a client may request the service or a staff member can make a referral.

One client, C.R., showed severe weight loss, decreased appetite, decreased endurance, and a sunken posture. He had a grayish complexion, and he isolated himself on days when he felt particularly fatigued. The occupational therapist recommended an appointment with the massage therapist who, with C.R., decided on a full body massage lasting 1½ hours. After two massages on different occasions and a myofascial release session with the occupational therapist, C.R. returned to the program with more color in his complexion, a more upright posture, and a greater sense of vitality and well-being. He also actively participated in programming and in helping to set up the tables and chairs for lunch. He commented that although he did not know how the massage and myofascial work helped him physically, he did feel very positive about the prolonged attention and touching (Montague, 1986; Older, 1982).

Occupational Therapy Assessment and Intervention

An initial occupational therapy assessment of the client, in the form of an interview, covers the following:

1. Activities of daily living, including food shopping, meal preparation, and diet.
2. Overall feelings and facts regarding past and present health status.
3. Social environment (e.g., Is there a support network? Are there any involved caregivers, or is the client isolated?).
4. Pain or other problems or concerns that keep the client from performing desired activities.
5. Assessment of strength, coordination, sensation, ambulation, and cognition, as indicated.
6. Time management, including activities engaged in for enjoyment.
7. Substance abuse issues and, if applicable, how they are handled.
8. Work history and how the worker role has changed since the onset of AIDS.

The following are examples of interventions used as a result of this assessment:

- J.M., who has progressive multifocal leukoencephalopathy and who appears much like a person with advanced multiple sclerosis, was given adapted eating utensils that enabled him to feed himself, after months of being fed at home.
- A.G., who lives alone, is ambulatory with decreased endurance, was previously suicidal, is isolated, and was unable to shop or prepare meals. He consumed milkshakes, cakes, and soft drinks when he was at home. The occupational therapist referred him for a home attendant to decrease his isolation and increase the availability of adequate nutrition.
- M.W. complained of severe headaches. He received medications from his psychiatrist and was referred to occupational therapy for pain management. The client learned a basic relaxation and visualization method to physically reduce tension. He began working with this technique on his own, with positive results.
- W.R. had chronic sinus swelling. He learned to apply pressure to specific areas on his face, head, and neck, which improved his nasal breathing.
- A support group led by the occupational therapist addresses time management issues with an emphasis on what people do during their day that makes them feel good. Most clients reveal that when they are not at the day treatment program, they are often in a clinic or hospital waiting room, in line at a welfare agency, or at home watching television. The quality of activity is often not as rewarding as it could be. This group discussion is geared toward a stimulation of the clients' interests and a discovery of ways in which they can pursue these interests.
- Several clients concerned about what they could do to remain well were referred by the occupational therapist to acupuncture clinics that accept third-party payment. One client in particular experienced significant relief in lower extremity pain due to peripheral neuropathy.
- E.D., who was frail, underweight, and wheelchair-bound due to wasting syndrome, was evaluated for mobility by the occupational therapist. After 2 weeks, he was able to use a walker independently at the day treatment program and at home.

Additional Observations

Several additional observations have come from this program. First, since the beginning of this program, the staff has felt a sense of urgency, based in part on the desire to meet clients' needs and to provide the missing link (e.g., change in medication or diet, provision of a walker) that will improve the client's quality of life immediately and in some cases increase life expectancy. This urgency was unexpected before the opening of the day treatment program, but evolved as it became clear that the basic survival needs of persons entering the program were not being met.

Second, several clients have stated that AIDS is not the worst thing that has ever happened to them, and that, in fact, having AIDS has afforded them adequate housing, food, clothing, and medical care for the first time in a long while. Third, it has become evident that clients vary in their outlooks. Whereas some clients may feel hopeless or angry when confronted with options to maintain or improve their strength or health, others are interested in making changes in order to live. Often a person will fluctuate between these two attitudes. A critical role of the day treatment program, therefore, has been to gently guide each person in the direction of self-love and healing.

References

Badgley, L. (1986). *Healing AIDS naturally*. San Bruno, CA: Human Energy Press.

Ferguson, M. (1980). *The Aquarian conspiracy*. Los Angeles: J. B. Tareher.

Grossman, J. (1977). Nationally Speaking—Preventive health care and community programming. *American Journal of Occupational Therapy, 31*, 351-354.

Harder, P. W., Gornick, J. C., & Burt, M. R. (1986). Adult day care: Substitute or supplement? *Milbank Quarterly, 64*(3), 414-441.

Laukaran, V. H. (1977). Nationally Speaking—Toward a model of occupational therapy for community health. *American Journal of Occupational Therapy, 31*, 71-74.

Montague, A. (1986). *Touching: The human significance of the skin* (3rd ed.). New York Harper & Row.

Older, J. (1982). *Touching is healing*. Briarcliff Manor, NY: Stein & Day.

Related Readings

Farber, S. D. (1989). 1989 Eleanor Clarke Slagle Lecture—Neuroscience and occupational therapy: Vital connections. *American Journal of Occupational Therapy 43*, 637-646.

Grunfeld, C. (1989, September/October). Metabolic mechanisms for wasting in AIDS. *Physicians Association for AIDS Care, 5*.

Johnson, J. A. (1986). Wellness and occupational therapy. *American Journal of Occupational Therapy, 40*, 753-758.

Levine, S. (1982). *Who dies?* New York: Anchor Press/Doubleday.

Serinus, J. (Ed.). (1986). *Psychoimmunity and the healing process: A holistic approach to immunity and AIDS.* Berkeley, CA: Celestial Arts.

Siegel, B. (1986). *Love, medicine and miracles.* New York: Harper & Row.

Chapter 71

Adult Day Care: A Model for Changing Times

Laurie Ellen Neustadt, COTA

Day health care for older adults is an exciting and innovative alternative to institutionalization. As will be illustrated below, it is extremely well suited to the skills and interests of many health professionals who assist individuals to attain their maximum levels of independence. This [chapter] discusses the need for adult day care, describes one center's program and offers some ideas for health professionals who are establishing their own programs.

History of Adult Day Care

Adult day care was first developed in Europe in the early 1940's. In 1947 the Menninger Clinic became the first United States adult day care center, followed by the Yale Psychiatric Clinic in 1949. Both were established for psychogeriatric care (Rathbone-McCuan and Elliot, 1976-77). By 1969, there were still only twelve adult day care programs, whereas an estimated 800 centers existed by 1984.

Historically, families provided care for their own relatives. Aging was accepted as a part of the life cycle and not as a sickness. Family units were closer and more interdependent, with one or more family members at home to care for those who needed them. With the societal changes occurring over the past 25 years, the caregiver function of the family has changed.

Society responded to this change in family-provided care by increasing the availability of institutional care. Nursing homes became the alternative to care given at home by the family. Institutionalizing the elderly increased the general perception that aging is an illness, and unfortunately, promoted premature institutionalization for those lacking the family or community support needed to remain independent (Burris, 1981).

While nursing home placement became more widespread, it only provided services for a small segment of the elderly population. The majority were still living in the community and having a great many needs unmet (Kiernat, 1976). With the increased expense of institutionalization, and subsequent burden on families in particular and society as a whole, alternative options for geriatric care have become essential.

The traditional senior center recreational and nutritional programs met some of the community support needs of more self-sufficient older people. However, these programs were not geared to meet the needs of infirm, confused, or disabled adults, lacking the facilities or staff to provide nursing care or therapy.

Adult day centers were developed to provide a supervised, protective environment for participants. Services include nursing, social services, occupational and physical therapy, speech/language pathology, activity programming, transportation, and nutritional meals. Three models of these day care centers evolved—the medical model, the health maintenance model, and the social model—although some overlap exists among the three.

The medical model stresses nursing services, therapy, and rehabilitation while still providing recreational programming. The social model emphasizes socialization and recreation, but can also provide some nursing care and therapy. The health maintenance model is a blend of the two, but does not stress rehabilitation. Most day care centers enable elderly participants to receive coordinated health care at one site. Participants can utilize the program for ongoing health maintenance to avoid institutionalization, or as a temporary setting for rehabilitation after surgery, accident, or illness. The centers provide group involvement and promote wellness and independence which in turn increases the individual's quality of life, contentment, mental functioning, and activity level.

The adult day center also provides needed respite for family members engaged in the caregiver role, and increases the options for those who choose not to place a family member in a nursing home. This assistance often allows the family to continue providing direct care and often improves family relationships by alleviating the stress so common to family caregiver situations.

The following objectives, as established by the Levindale Adult Treatment Center in 1968 (Rathbone-McCuan and Elliot, 1976-77), summarize the overall role of adult day care: "(a) to provide socialization experience to physically and emotionally disabled older people; (b) to help maintain disabled older people in their own homes and communities; (c) to provide an integrated professional service to disabled people living in the community; (d) to preclude the institutionalization of disabled people by providing services through a day care center; and (e) to provide support and relieve the burden of families who care for their older disabled relative" (Rathbone-McCuan and Elliot, 1976-77, p. 159).

The adult day center creates a link in the continuity of care for the elderly between nursing home placement and home care, thus providing a choice for individuals and their families. Maintaining independence in the community, promoting wellness, and offering the option of continued family care, the day center becomes a welcome alternative to institutionalization.

St. Marys Day Health Center for Older Adults

St. Marys Hospital Medical Center in Madison, Wisconsin, hired the Gerontological Planning Associates of Santa Monica, California, in February 1981 as consultants to help clarify the need for services to the elderly in its community. A committee made up of area professionals in aging explored a wide range of possible services, and determined there was a need for a medical model adult day care program in the Madison area. The committee found one-third of the total St. Marys Hospital Medical Center population was 65 years old and over, and discovered that among those elderly patients, the ones suffering from multiple chronic diseases or impairments needed a larger recovery time.

It was determined that the Day Health Center would allow elderly patients to be discharged sooner from the hospital. They would be able to obtain the coordinated therapies, health care, nutritional, and social needs they require, and still benefit from their home environment during recovery. As noted in the Certificate of Need Application, the Day Health Center would alleviate the problem of patients being admitted to nursing homes only because all family members held jobs, and the elderly person could not be left alone for eight hours.

St. Marys Day Health Center for Older Adults opened its doors on July 19, 1982. The Center is open Monday through Friday from 8:00 a.m. to 5:30 p.m., and accommodates up to 20 clients per day.

Program and Staff

St. Marys Day Health Center is a medical model day center established with the following objectives:

1. To promote or maintain independence.
2. To rehabilitate the participant to the maximum extent possible.
3. To maintain the participant in the community as long as it is medically, socially, and economically feasible.
4. To prevent inappropriate or premature institutionalization.
5. To provide daytime respite and educational support for families.

The general philosophy of the Center is to increase the independence of the clients physically, psychologically, and socially, and to assist them in maintaining the highest level of independence possible. Clients are encouraged to involve themselves not only in individual activities but in the life of the Center itself. This approach has developed a sense of community and caring among the clients and the staff.

For each participant, a multidisciplinary team develops an individualized plan of care. Nursing services, social services, occupational and physical therapies, speech/language pathology, activity programming, pastoral care and religious services, transportation services, and a nutritional meal are provided at the Center. The staff includes one full-time Registered Nurse [R.N.] who is the coordinator of the program; one full-time Licensed Practical Nurse [L.P.N.]; one full-time Certified Occupational Therapy Assistant [C.O.T.A.], who is the volunteer and activity coordinator of the program; one part-time Social Worker; one part-time aide; two part-time van drivers; and one part-time secretary.

Occupational and physical therapy and speech/language pathology are contracted through St. Marys Hospital Medical Center on an out-patient basis. Clients who are referred to therapy by their physicians are seen by a hospital therapist at the Day Health Center. A parallel bar, full-view mirror, overhead pulley and weights, treatment tables, hydroculator, exercise bike, and a variety of occupational therapy equipment are on hand for use by the clients.

Nursing services. Nursing services are a vital part of this medical model day center. The R.N. and L.P.N. administer medication and supervise and perform health assessment, counseling, and health education. They monitor specific illnesses such as congestive heart failure, diabetes, pulmonary diseases and hypertension. They provide specific treatments such as dressing changes, catheter care, and monitoring vital signs and weights. Nursing staff also assist with activities of daily living including feeding, toileting, ambulating, bathing, hair care, nail care, teeth or denture care, and shaving. Because of the long-term participation of clients of the Center and low staff turnover, the care given is consistent and personal. All Center participants must have a referral form filled out by their personal physician upon entering the program. The Nurse Coordinator then maintains close communication with the physician to assure the continuity of care given.

Pastoral care. Pastoral care is available, as requested by clients or family, through the Pastoral Care Department of the hospital. Catholic Mass is celebrated on Friday mornings, and most Christian and Jewish holidays are celebrated with the clients.

Social services. Social services at the Center are multidimensional and provide the necessary link between the day center program and the community. The social worker screens prospective clients and conducts initial intake interviews. Once a client has been accepted to the program, the social worker briefs staff members, makes sure the client has a physician, [and] sets up transportation, bathing and medication schedules. The social worker also provides informational services to clients and community agencies. She acts as a liaison between community services, clients, and their families to assure continuity of goals

between services. Individual counseling to clients and families is provided, especially crisis counseling as problems arise. Group counseling is provided regularly on an informal basis through weekly membership meetings between clients and the social worker. An educational program for family caregivers is offered twice a year.

Support staff. The part-time Center aide assists with the activities, shops for supplies, assists clients with activities of daily living, and helps with routine housekeeping at the Center. The secretary acts as receptionist and unit clerk, handles all billing and accounting, keeps Center statistics, and does all the secretarial duties required.

Transportation can be provided for those who need this service by the Center's wheelchair-accessible van. The van accommodates seven individuals and makes two morning and two afternoon runs. The two part-time drivers have developed a particular rapport with the clients and their families and provide essential information on the home environment to the rest of the staff. Other clients are brought to the Center by community transportation services or by their families.

A nutritious noon meal is served daily at the Center, catered by a local business, and served by the staff and volunteers. Specific meals are ordered for those on special diets including diabetic, low salt, vegetarian, and kosher restrictions (Neustadt, 1982). Two snacks are served, one in the morning and one in the afternoon, planned and prepared by the licensed practical nurse.

Basic lab work such as urinalysis and blood work are available. Samples are drawn by the nurse coordinator and processed by the lab at Shared Laboratory Services of Madison.

Volunteers are an essential element of the Day Health Center. They act as an extension of the staff, allowing for a higher level of quality care and diminishing staff burnout. Volunteers assist with activities, visit with clients on an individual basis, help serve and clean up meals and snacks, [and] assist clients to and from activities and [to and from] the Center van. The certified occupational therapy assistant recruits volunteers from the community, universities, and churches, and supervises their activities.

The Center's entire staff meets once a month. The R.N., L.P.N., C.O.T.A., and social worker meet once a week to be briefed on new clients [and to] discuss plans of care and treatment approaches. The Center uses medical model documentation procedures and S.O.A.P. note charting techniques.

The Activities Program

The activities program is central to the success of the Day Health Center program. Through an organized activities program, clients can develop their self-esteem and self-worth, establish support systems, engage in socialization, and become involved with purposeful activity. Activities programming is a medium for creating community among the clients and a means of replacing the occupational and social involvements no longer existent in the clients' lives.

The St. Marys Activity Program is run by a certified occupational therapy assistant. In Adult Day Care Activities one must work with and meet the needs of an extremely varied population with problems ranging from multiple physical handicaps to acute psychological disorders. The C.O.T.A. is trained to work with varying degrees of minimal to multiple handicaps and in acute to chronic stages of disorder, both physical and psychological, and is competent in adapting activities for the problems encountered. The educational training program for C.O.T.A.s—a strong focus on a variety of activities, the skill of needs assessment, and activities adaptation—make the C.O.T.A. a logical candidate for Adult Day Care Activity Programmer.

The occupational behavior frame of reference, with performance components and occupational performance areas, is woven into the fiber of the activity program. Within the performance component areas, the *Physical Component* is addressed in the daily group exercise program, the "Willing Walkers Club," and a daily informal exercise group. Clients presently receiving treatment from the registered occupational therapist [O.T.R.] do supportive exercises during this informal group with the C.O.T.A. *Sensory Integration* is directly addressed through the exercise program. Sensory stimulating props compensate for perceptual and cognitive deficits and assist clients unable to follow verbal cues. All the senses—taste, touch, smell, hearing, and visual stimuli—are incorporated in many of the planned activities. Perceptual deficits are also addressed in the informal exercise group with the C.O.T.A., using input from the O.T.R. Cards and table games, brain teasers, reminiscing groups, discussion groups, story reading, educational programs, and guest lecturers involve the *Cognitive Component*. *Psychological* and *Social Components* are touched upon in weekly membership group meetings. Specific issues that have come up with individuals or the group are discussed. These components are also addressed in other group discussions, programs, and in the daily interpersonal relationships that are an ongoing part of the Center.

The activities also include the occupational performance areas of self-care, work, homemaking, and play/leisure. Most of the clients' self-care needs are addressed by the nursing and occupational therapy staff on an individual basis. Clients are involved in homemaking activities through cooking, sewing, and gardening groups.

Some clients also assist in the homemaking chores of the Center such as watering plants, clearing the table, and helping with dishes. Clients have expressed a need to remain involved in work-oriented projects. Volunteer projects such as preparing mailings, sewing projects, and sorting stamps are brought in from community agencies like the American Red Cross and Retired Senior Volunteer Program. The clients also planned and ran their own Christmas craft bazaar. The group voted to purchase a video recorder with the money it raised. Some clients also needed counseling and assistance in structuring their leisure time both at the Center and at home.

Often, activity programs remain structured and unchanged for many months, if not years. It is important to blend planned, stable events with spontaneity. A structured calendar of activities should exist, but it must allow for daily changes according to the mood, energy level, needs, and interests of the clients present that day. Spontaneity allows for those subtle changes which present themselves day to day, and also allows for those creative moments that cannot be planned. A large store of resources—cognitive games, craft ideas and samples and supplies, group projects, party ideas, and work tasks—make spontaneous activities possible. Offering a wide variety of activities will assist in reaching the varied interests of the participants. There are five group activities a day at the Center with approximately 15 different types of activities per week. (See Table I for a sample activity program.)

Philosophy, Approaches, and Ideas of an Activity Program

Developing an activity program which truly meets the needs of the clientele is always a challenge. Frequently the program represents what staff assume are the needs of the clients, or what might be "good for them." It is a constant challenge to balance the staff's knowledge, skills, and talents with programs based on the actual needs and interests of clients.

"The challenge of activities programming in extended care and long-term care facilities is to provide opportunities for truly meaningful activity. 'Meaningful' is a word that must be individually defined by the (clients) themselves, not by a staff which seeks to involve (clients) in activities which the staff perceives as meaningful. Later maturity is one of several developmental stages in the life continuum and has associated with it specific developmental tasks and human needs. Consequently, activities which are defined as 'meaningful' by a thirty-year old staff member may not be similarly defined by an eighty-year old (client). Careful assessment of (client) problems and needs by perceptive and empathetic professionals who have a thorough knowledge of the developmental tasks of later maturity is essential to gain an understanding of how elderly individuals define 'meaningful activity'" (Curley, 1980).

Clients are approached individually about their specific activity interests. They are encouraged to follow through on individual activities and participate in group activities as they choose. There is a fine line between encouraging clients to attend group activities to in-

client. Verbal and physical affection help establish closer, more rewarding relationships for clients and staff.

Intergenerational programming creates a sense of normalcy which precludes the age separatism so prevalent in institutions. St. Marys Day Health Center is located in a school building that also houses four preschools, two music schools, a gymnastics program, and

Table I. Sample Weekly Activity Calendar

	Monday	Tuesday	Wednesday	Thursday	Friday
8 9	Individual Activity time with snacks, coffee, and juice served. Clients work on individual craft projects [and] occupational therapy exercises, read the newspaper, and participate in the Willing Walkers Club.				
10	Membership Group with the Social Worker	Poetry Group or Health Group	Reminiscing Group	Reading Group or Pet Visit	Current Events
11	Exercise Group to Music	Exercise Group to Music	Exercise Group to Music	Exercise Group to Music	Exercise Group with Children
12	Lunch	Lunch	Lunch	Lunch	Lunch Church Service
	Willing Walkers Club ———————————————————————→				
1	Cooking Group with L.P.N.	Feature Film Presentation of the Week	Volunteer Work Group	Cooking Group with L.P.N.	Brain Teasers
2	Bingo or Bowling	↓	Storyteller from the Community	Drama Group	Stained Glass Workshop
3	Reading Group	Cards and Table Games	Brain Teasers	Crafts	Reading Group
4	Individual Activity time including reading, watching television or listening to music, individual exercise routines and craft projects, individual visiting time with staff and volunteers.				

crease socialization and diminish isolation and depression, and allowing them the freedom to be and do what they want. Staff members need to be aware of the strong need for elderly individuals to reminisce and to be listened to. One of the most important activities for some clients may be talking, and one of the most important activities for the staff may be listening.

Establishing trust is a critical element when working with people in any capacity, and becomes particularly important when working with confused elderly. Consistent approach assures a greater comfort level for the

a grade school. The preschool children join the Center's exercise group once a week and occasionally perform musical programs. The grade school children have conducted taped oral history interviews with clients, practiced storytelling, and performed class plays for the Center. A neighborhood Brownie troop adopted the Center and held their monthly meetings together with the clients. Parties, crafts, and service projects led up to the Brownies flying up ceremony at the Center, with clients escorting the girls across the symbolic bridge to Girl Scouts. The Girl Scouts voted to continue visiting the

Center the following year, with some of the girls establishing one-to-one relationships with special clients. Young children seem to bring out expressions of love and affection from even the most confused and withdrawn of the clients. Between the visiting school children, volunteers, staff, and clients, five generations are integrated into the Center's community.

Most Adult Day Centers are located in churches and school buildings, making it easier to involve resources from the community at large. Helping to keep individuals involved and aware of happenings within their own communities is important when working with the elderly. It is easy to become isolated and uninformed when involvements from the past—jobs, church affiliations, and clubs—are discontinued. The Day Center and its staff become an important link back into the community. Inviting speakers, entertainers and artists to come to the Center is one approach toward reestablishing that link.

The local Humane Society "Love a Pet" program brings Red Cross Volunteers with puppies and kittens to visit twice a month. Community artists have become the Center's resident artists, leading sculpture and stained glass workshops. Often, artists and musicians with City Arts Grants develop programs with this specific purpose in mind. Storytellers, musicians, dancers and choirs have all visited the Center. Speakers from the local Police Department, Save Our Security Organization, Brain Injury Association, [and the] State Historical Society, and area health professionals, have presented their expertise. This outside involvement increases program quality and the level of interaction between the clients and the community.

Developing an internal sense of community is equally important to all the participants in the Day Center program. Clients spend the whole day together and are able to get to know each other and develop a sense of caring and interdependence. By involving clients in the planning and decision-making process, they feel a sense of ownership in the Center. Most staff members lead at least one formal activity, and all are involved in direct care. The continual interaction throughout the day among clients and staff adds considerable depth and vitality to the sense of internal community.

Description of the Population

St. Marys Day Health Center can accommodate 20 clients a day. The Center accepts adults who need continuous individualized medical treatment and rehabilitation. Persons with walkers or wheelchairs, those who require supervision and help with medications, and those who are incontinent are accepted into the program. Clients are referred to the Center by hospitals, clinics, private physicians, health and social service agencies, their families, or by self-referral. Eighty-four

total clients have been served at the Center since its opening. (See Table II.)

In order to be eligible for admission into the Center, potential participants should meet one or more of the following: (1) have a primary physical diagnosis which includes a disability or chronic illness; (2) require continuing medical evaluation, treatment, and follow-up care as well as skilled nursing supervision and care, but

---

Table II. Statistics Collected From July 1982 to January 1984

Total Clients Served: 84

Total Male: 35   Total Female: 49

Age Range of Clients Served: 29 y/o—97 y/o

Age	Number of Clients
20-29	I
30-39	I
40-49	II
50-59	ЖЛ IIII
60-69	ЖЛ ЖЛ I
70-79	ЖЛ ЖЛ ЖЛ IIII
80-89	ЖЛ ЖЛ ЖЛ ЖЛ ЖЛ II
90-99	ЖЛ ЖЛ IIII

---

not to the extent that institutionalization is required; (3) require rehabilitative services to improve or maintain level of independence; (4) require specific training in the taking of prescribed drugs, special diets, special diet preparation, catheter management, and care of the feet because of peripheral vascular disease; (5) the family of the disabled or chronically ill elderly person requires the education and respite support that a day health center offers in order to continue caring for the person at home.

Eligible participants must: (1) be older adults (exceptions are made for younger clients if they need daycare and are at least 18 years of age); (2) not be bedridden, totally disoriented, harmful, or disruptive; (3) be able to tolerate four to eight hours in a day care situation and transportation to and from the Center; (4) have a physician referral; (5) live within metropolitan Madison or provide their own transportation.

Diagnoses submitted by client physicians include: (1) heart and vascular diseases; (2) brain disorders such as tumors, CVA's, Organic Brain Syndrome, and Alzheimer's Disease; (3) bone diseases and fractures; (4) cancer; (5) kidney and bladder disease; (6) vision and hearing impairments; (7) lung disease; (8) depression; and (9) alcohol abuse.

The majority of the Center's clients live either with

their spouse or one of their children. A few clients live with a hired live-in aide or live by themselves. The majority of the clients attend the Center for two or four days a week, with some attending one day a week and some five days a week. Clients arrive between 8:00 and 10:30 in the morning and leave between 3:00 and 5:30 in the evening.

The following case studies illustrate client types served by St. Marys Day Health Center.

Case study Mrs. "R." Mrs. R came to the Center after suffering a right-sided CVA with left hemiplegia. She attends the Center five days a week and receives both physical and occupational therapy. She has shown great improvement with her perceptual exercises and is now walking with assistance. Mrs. R actively participates in most of the Center's activities and has developed many friendships with clients, staff, and volunteers at the Center. The improvement Mrs. R has made while attending the Center has made it feasible for her family to care for her at home.

Case study Mr. "K." This client is a 71 year old male with congestive heart failure who attends the Center Monday, Wednesday, and Friday. Mr. K needs his lungs checked, and his weight, blood pressure and diet monitored by the nursing staff to maintain his delicate physical condition. His wife works during the day and he drives himself from home to the program. He is very alert and social and has many friends both among the clients and staff of the Day Center and among the many children attending preschool in the same building. This client had been physically unstable and frequently required hospitalization before attending the Day Health Center. During his 18 month involvement in the Center, constant monitoring and treatment have prevented further hospitalization.

Case study Mrs. "C." This client is a 77 year old female with severe dementia. She attends the Center Monday through Friday. This client has difficulty communicating her needs and desires and attending to a task. She tends to wander and often requires individual attention for her own safety. Mrs. C participates in some Center activities, especially those involving small children, pets, and music. A number of the clients look out for her well-being and visit with her. Mrs. C lives with her daughter who works full time. Due to the level of care she requires and the expense of in-home care, the Day Health Center provides the only alternative to institutionalization.

Future Program Goals

Future goals of the Day Center staff include: (1) spending more individual time with clients; (2) having more time for staff meetings and in-services; (3) developing regular family conferences and involving families more in the treatment process; (4) developing a formal evaluation for clients and their families to give feedback to the Center; (5) refining and utilizing the assessment tool the staff is now working on to classify levels of client care; (6) developing a system of in-take according to levels of care, percentages of clients in each level of care, and ability of the staff to care for the client accordingly; and (7) developing a work skills program.

St. Marys Day Health Center for Older Adults is a successful medical model day center because of the consistent quality care given by its staff and the enthusiasm of the Madison community. It is a rewarding experience to be involved in an innovative program that may prolong people's independence while helping to relieve the stress experienced in family care-giving situations.

References

Burris, K. Recommending adult day care center. *Nursing and Health Care.* October 1981, 437-441.

Curley, J. *Methodist Health Center Activities Department Statement of Philosophy,* July 1980, unpublished.

Kiernat, J. M. Geriatric day hospitals: A golden opportunity for therapists. *The American Journal of Occupational Therapy,* 1976, *30,* 285-289.

Levy, M. *Certificate of need application.* St. Marys Hospital Medical Center, 1981-82, unpublished.

Neustadt, L. Developing a program for Jewish residents in non-Jewish nursing homes. *Occupational & Physical Therapy in Geriatrics,* 1982, *2,* 13-23.

Rathbone-McCuan, E., & Elliot, M . Geriatric day care in theory and practice. *Social Work in Health Care,* 1976-77, *2,* 13-23.

Robins, E. Keynote Presentation. *Adult day programs for the elderly proceedings,* Publications and Advertising Office, Utica College of Syracuse University, 5-11.

Section IX

Professional Career Development: The Attainment and Maintenance of Excellence

Introduction

Professional career development is a continual lifelong process; It does not end when one receives an academic degree or professional certification (Crist, 1986; Mosey, 1986; Sabari, 1985; Welles, 1988). Rather, a professional career requires an ongoing commitment to the attainment and maintenance of excellence. Competent occupational therapists value this pursuit of excellence and are personally responsible for their professional development (Welles, 1988). Our professional organization, the American Occupational Therapy Association (AOTA), recognizes this need for ongoing career development and has set the ethical standard that "the occupational therapist shall actively maintain and improve one's professional competence. . . . occupational therapists recognize the need for continuing education and where relevant, they obtain training, experience, self-study, or counsel to ensure competent occupational therapy services" (AOTA, 1984, p. 800).

The benefits of a lifelong commitment to one's professional development are numerous. Increased personal pride and satisfaction in one's work; improved health care services for consumers and their families; enhanced professional image among reimbursers, administrators, and the multidisciplinary team; and the prevention of burnout and professional stagnation are all viable outcomes of the continual pursuit of professional excellence (Apter & Kolonder, 1987; Crist, 1986; Davis, 1989; DePoy, 1990; Johnson, 1981; Jones & Kirkland, 1984; Sabari, 1985).

While it is evident that today's health care system offers unique challenges to the health care professional, occupational therapists can respond proactively to these challenges and continue to achieve professional mastery (Bonder, 1987). Rather than bemoan the complexities of today's health care system, readers are challenged to emulate many of this text's authors, who met these challenges head-on throughout their professional careers.

The ongoing development of a professional career requires the individual to utilize numerous resources (Johnson, 1978). Clinical supervision, peer support, professional networks, mentorships, self-study, in-services, workshops, conferences, and post-professional education can all be employed to attain and maintain professional excellence (Baum, 1991; Crist, 1986; DePoy, 1990; Jones and Kirkland, 1984; Mosey, 1986; Welles, 1988). The chapters in this final section explore professional development issues and offer a number of effective strategies for ensuring professional mastery.

In chapter 72, Slater and Cohn present a developmental model for professional growth, which can be utilized for staff development. Developmental concepts are discussed, and relevant clinical examples highlight pertinent points. Practical strategies and recommendations for the implementation of staff development programs are provided. The personal and professional benefits of these programs are emphasized.

A continuum for professional development is also presented in chapter 73, by Rogers, who explores the role of professional sponsorship in selecting and developing leaders for occupational therapy. Rogers explains the diversity of potential sponsorship relationships and defines the qualities, roles, tasks, and benefits of these supportive affiliations. Strategies and examples for implementing sponsorship relationships are provided. The value and efficacy of sponsorship for attaining and maintaining professional excellence is presented.

The personal responsibility of the individual to continue to pursue professional mastery is the focus of chapter 74, by Peloquin. The philosophical and ethical principles underlying the need for a commitment to continued professional learning are discussed. Opportunities available for professional learning are identified; however, the emphasis remains on the individual's responsibility and accountability for professional career development.

A viable outcome of the pursuit of excellence in one's professional career is often the acquisition of a nontraditional professional role. Competent occupational therapists can move confidently into leadership positions and be at the forefront of new and innovative health care programming (Burke, 1984; Moeller, 1991). A number of excellent examples of occupational therapists fulfilling nontraditional roles have been presented in this text (e.g., Wilberding, director of a quarterway house; Moeller, director of a case management program; Watanabe, supervisor of a psychiatric consultation-liaison program; Goldenberg, executive director of a private, non-profit, health care agency; Dasler, Lang, and Kaplan, professional consultants). These model occupational therapists who have assumed leadership roles in today's health care system are just a few of the exemplary occupational therapy practitioners who have utilized their professional expertise to respond proactively to current professional challenges.

The assumption of a nontraditional role in today's health care system requires occupational therapists to generalize and transfer their unique professional skills to a diversity of roles and settings. In chapter 75, Royeen explores the marketable skills occupational therapists possess that enable them to pursue professional roles beyond "the clinic walls." While occupational therapists clearly have the knowledge and skills to acquire nontraditional roles, the assumption of these roles may be deterred by a number of factors. In chapter 76, Adams explores these potential deterrents to nontraditional practice. He provides constructive suggestions to turn these deterrents into opportunities for professional growth.

Another frequent outcome of professional growth is an increased interest in the application of research to clinical practice. Expert practitioners committed to the pursuit of excellence are often curious. They question their theoretical base and seek to improve the efficacy of their interventions. As a result of their research, these practitioners enhance their professional status and refine their clinical practice (Ottenbacher, 1987). However, many therapists are frequently hesitant to participate in clinical research. This hesitancy often limits their professional career development and is frequently based on unfounded misconceptions or fears about the research process. Therefore, the final three chapters in this text

are provided to assist readers in confronting potential resistance to research and to provide a number of effective strategies for implementing clinical research.

Oakley begins this discussion on clinical research by comparing the research process to the process of providing clinical care. She argues that research is a natural extension of an occupational therapist's clinical skills and offers realistic suggestions for incorporating research into clinical practice. Bailey continues this positive discussion of clinical research and adds to Oakley's suggestions by providing practical hints for conducting research in a clinical setting. Her informative advice is supplemented by constructive guidelines for the publication of research studies.

Chapter 79, the last in this section, expands on the use of collaboration as an effective strategy for conducting research in a clinical setting. In their presentation, DePoy and Gallagher describe a seven-step model for faculty-clinician collaboration in clinical research. Realistic guidelines and practical suggestions for implementation of this model are provided. A clinical research example is used to illustrate each step and to highlight the broad potential applications of this model to qualitative and quantitative clinical research designs.

The value of research to the professional growth and career development of occupational therapists is emphasized in all three of these research chapters. As these authors demonstrate, the combination of personal commitment and professional collaboration can greatly enhance one's professional mastery. Readers are challenged to integrate the information and ideas presented in this section as they assume personal responsibility for seeking collaborative relationships and utilizing organizational resources to attain and maintain professional excellence, throughout their occupational therapy careers. References and resources for professional career development are provided at the end of this text. Reflective self-assessment and active utilization of these resources will enable readers to become master clinicians and leaders in today's health care system.

Questions to Consider

1. What is your current level of professional competence? Where are you along the continuum of professional career development?
2. What are your personal and professional values and beliefs? How do these influence your professional growth? Are you actively pursuing excellence in your professional career? If not, what is deterring you?
3. How can you enhance your professional growth and career development? What resources are

available to you to facilitate your attainment and maintenance of professional excellence? How can potential deterrents to growth be changed into professional opportunities?

4. What competencies and strengths do you have to offer others to enhance their professional development? What supportive and collaborative relationships can you establish with others for your mutual professional benefit?

5. How does the attainment and maintenance of professional excellence benefit the individual occupational therapy practitioner? What are the benefits of professional mastery for the occupational therapy profession and for consumers of health care?

6. What clinical skills do occupational therapists possess to enable them to pursue nontraditional professional roles? What are challenges to nontraditional practice facing occupational therapists? How can occupational therapists respond proactively to these challenges to assume leadership roles within today's health care system?

7. How does clinical research relate to one's professional career development? What are research questions you may be interested in exploring? What are practical, realistic strategies you can utilize to implement research within a clinical setting?

8. What are the resources and supports available from AOTA, the American Occupational Therapy Foundation (AOTF), state and local occupational therapy associations, and other professional organizations that can assist occupational therapists in their career development? How can occupational therapists utilize these resources in their ongoing pursuit of excellence?

Burke, J. P. (1984). Occupational therapy in health care: A perspective for our future. In F. S. Cromwell (Ed.), *The changing roles of occupational therapists in the 1980s* (pp. 7-15). New York: Haworth Press.

Crist, P. A. (1986). *Contemporary issues in clinical education.* Thorofare, NJ: Slack.

Davis, C. M. (1989). *Patient practitioner interaction: An experiential manual for developing the art of health care.* Thorofare, NJ: Slack.

DePoy, E. (1990). Mastery in clinical occupational therapy. *American Journal of Occupational Therapy, 44,* 415-422.

Johnson, J. (1978). Nationally speaking: Sixty years of progress: Questions for the future. *American Journal of Occupational Therapy, 32,* 209-213.

Johnson, J. (1981). Old values—new directions: Competence, adaptation, integration. *American Journal of Occupational Therapy, 35,* 589-598.

Jones, J. L., & Kirkland, M. (1984). Nationally speaking: From continuing education to continuing professional education: The shift to lifelong learning in occupational therapy. *American Journal of Occupational Therapy, 38,* 503-504.

Moeller, P. (1991, June). The occupational therapist as case manager in community mental health. *Mental Health Special Interest Section Newsletter,* pp. 4-5.

Mosey, A. C. (1986). *Psychosocial components of occupational therapy.* New York: Raven Press.

Ottenbacher, K. J. (1987). Research: Its importance to clinical practice in occupational therapy. *American Journal of Occupational Therapy, 41,* 213-215.

Sabari, J. S. (1985). Professional socialization: Implications for occupational therapy education. *American Journal of Occupational Therapy, 39,* 96-102.

Welles, C. (1988). Ethics and related professional liability. In S. C. Robertson (Ed.), *Mental health focus: Skills for assessment and treatment* (pp. 3-90—3-106). Rockville, MD: American Occupational Therapy Association.

References

American Occupational Therapy Association (1984). Principles of occupational therapy ethics. *American Journal of Occupational Therapy, 38,* 799-802.

Apter, L. C., & Kolonder, E. L. (1987, September 16). Professional burnout: Are you a candidate? *Occupational Therapy Forum,* pp. 1, 3-4.

Baum, C. (1991). Identification and use of environmental resources. In C. Christiansen & C. Baum (Eds.), *Occupational therapy: Overcoming human performance deficits* (pp. 789-802). Thorofare, NJ: Slack.

Bonder, B. (1987). Occupational therapy in mental health: Crisis or opportunity? *American Journal of Occupational Therapy, 41,* 495-499.

Chapter 72

Staff Development Through Analysis of Practice

Deborah Yarett Slater, MS, OTR/L
Ellen S. Cohn, EdM, OTR/L

This chapter was previously published in the *American Journal of Occupational Therapy, 45*, 1038-1044. Copyright © 1991, The American Occupational Therapy Association, Inc.

In an era in which our profession faces a personnel shortage, the retention of experienced occupational therapists is a timely and critical issue. Bailey's (1990) study of the reasons why occupational therapists have left the field documented that attrition is a serious problem for the profession and for the facilities and persons it serves. Bailey noted that "the largest group of survey respondents who have left the profession [35%] did so after 5 to 10 years in practice" (p. 37). With therapists leaving the profession so early in their careers, we are confronted with a shortage of experienced therapists to serve as role models, supervisors, and mentors for newer staff members. One way that we can increase the retention of experienced therapists is by creating incentives. Innovative staff development programs may serve as a viable, practical, and economical strategy to address attrition and retention.

Like many other health care professions, occupational therapy offers little career mobility. Many staff members believe that if they are competent, they will receive recognition and benefits by promotion into managerial positions. Such promotions, however, take them away from clinical practice. Thirty-one percent of the respondents in Bailey's (1990) study identified poor opportunities for career advancement as a major reason for leaving the profession. The biggest complaint was that our profession is two-tiered, that is, it consists only of clinical staff and department director positions. Despite the existence of career ladders in some facilities, differentiation by salary, title, and responsibilities is limited.

Through their years of practice, seasoned therapists have integrated knowledge and expertise but have received little recognition for their repertoire of clinical skills. The lack of experienced clinicians is particularly problematic when coupled with the complexity of to-day's health care environment. Cost-containment, greater pressure for productivity, shortened lengths of stay, and patients with complicated medical and social needs require the skills of experienced therapists (Brollier, 1985). In this increasingly complex environment, occupational therapists must develop the ability to critically analyze practice situations.

This need for critical thinkers has been a recurrent theme in our profession (American Occupational Therapy Association [AOTA], 1987, 1989 [sic], 1990; Cohn, 1989; Parham, 1987; Rogers, 1983; West, 1990). This need is reinforced by the fact that the best role models for new professionals are committed occupational therapists who use an integrated approach to practice (Christie, Joyce, & Moeller, 1985). Support for the development of clinicians who can analyze their practice and who are committed to providing quality care presents a challenge to supervisors and administrators alike. Such support can be partially provided through programs that focus on meeting the developmental needs of staff. Accordingly, the purpose of the present paper is to describe an approach to staff development in which reflection on and evaluation of ideas are encouraged, rewarded, and expected as a part of everyday performance. The various developmental needs of staff members as they move from novice to expert are described, as are methods that encourage continual reflection on and evaluation of practice.

Staff Development Concepts

Components for successful staff development programs are identified in the management literature. Traditional staff development programs generally consist of formal courses, workshops, conferences, or a series of in-service training events that teach isolated skills and procedures (Pecora & Austin, 1987). These programs focus on immediate gains and productivity as goals rather than on the long-range needs of participants (Kaufman, 1974). Even when supported by the organization, these approaches may not prove to be effective.

Lieberman and Miller (1979) claimed that an effective staff development program should be integrated with the organization's goals and, equally important, integrated with the professionals' goals. They suggested that we focus on the interface between the staff's needs and values and the organization's goals. One way to accomplish this is to use the work itself to stimulate and reinforce professional growth and development. Thus, if the conditions and content of staff development programs are realistic, supervisors will have a better chance of changing behaviors and attitudes. Variation of on-the-job activities to present challenges can create opportunities for self-assessment that provide a basis for ongoing learning. The department director and immediate supervisors play an important role in creating a climate that encourages such self-reflection (Kaufman, 1974).

Another component to be considered in the design of staff development programs is the use of role models, or mentors. This is one of the most powerful strategies available to us for shaping, teaching, coaching, and assisting future therapists (Cohn & Czycholl, 1991; Rogers, 1982; Sabari, 1985; Schön, 1983, 1987). Gitterman and Netter (1968) advocated coupling this notion of role modeling with peer learning to design staff development programs. They suggested setting up situations where staff with varying degrees of experience brainstorm to share their perspectives and ideas.

Conferences, workshops, or other forms of continuing education help clinicians broaden their knowledge base and develop advanced skills. Problems may arise, however, when clinicians have more than adequate knowledge and information about professional issues, strategies, techniques, and skills but simply cannot operationalize such knowledge. One objective of staff development programs, therefore, may be to turn knowledge into action. Analysis of practice can help clinicians break away from procedures and practice concepts that are viewed as fixed formulations and help restore abstractions to their original state. Supervisors can help other clinicians conceptualize patterns of practice, so that learning is not bound to the specific situation in which the learning took place.

To be effective for staff development, supervisors need a thorough understanding of both adult learning and career development. Adult learners are generally "independent, self-motivated learners whose experience orients them to practical issues" (Pecora & Austin, 1987, p. 135). They prefer to apply new knowledge immediately. Thus, effective staff development should focus on skills relevant to the job environment with frequent feedback on the effect of the staff member's actions while the action is taking place (Knowles, 1980). Smith and Elbert (1986) supported this premise by stating that "learning must be integrated with action if training is to produce progress" (p. 129).

The Process Used for Analyzing Practice

The process for analysis of practice developed for the AOTA/American Occupational Therapy Foundation (AOTF) Clinical Reasoning Study, although not conceived as a staff development program, provided an opportunity for the application of some current staff development concepts, such as role modeling, peer learning, the provision of immediate feedback, and the creation of a climate in which the evaluation of ideas was rewarded. The study took place in the occupational therapy department at University Hospital in Boston, Massachusetts, and continued for 2 years. Initially, seven therapists, each with more than 5 years of experience and diverse backgrounds in occupational therapy specialty areas, began analyzing their practice and the reasoning that directed their choice of actions. The principal investigator, an anthropologist, was assisted by occupational therapy graduate students in a process that involved videotaping patient-therapist therapy sessions. Before and after the therapy sessions, interviews with each therapist were videotaped. In the pretherapy interviews, therapists described their work with the patient and imagined or hypothesized how the session would unfold. During the posttherapy interview, the therapists described what happened in the session and identified key points at which specific reasoning resulted in specific actions. Segments of these videotapes were then analyzed and discussed by the therapists themselves, researchers, and other area clinicians in formal study groups. During the second year of the study, an additional group of seven therapists, each with approximately 1 year of experience, joined the study. Because the researchers conducted separate groups for the novice and experienced therapists, we were able to explicate the differences between the reasoning processes of novice and expert clinicians.

Novice to Expert

Integration of the findings from the Clinical Reasoning Study with Dreyfus and Dreyfus's (1986) Model of Skill Acquisition provides an organizing framework for a staff development program. Dreyfus and Dreyfus identified a developmental continuum for growth that involves five career stages: novice, advanced beginner, competent, proficient, and expert. The stages represent increasingly complex ways of responding to practice. Data from the Clinical Reasoning Study demonstrate how these stages apply to the development of occupational therapists.

Stage 1: Novice

The novice recognizes various facts and features relevant to the acquisition of new skills and learns rules for determining actions based on those facts and features. Elements of the patient's disability to be addressed in occupational therapy are so clearly and objectively defined for the novice that they are recognized without reference to the overall situation in which they occur (Dreyfus & Dreyfus, 1986). These elements are called *context-free*, and rules are applied regardless of what else is happening, that is, they are applied in isolation. For example, novice occupational therapists are taught how to assess joint range of motion, muscle tone, or balance and are given rules for how to conduct these procedures. They learn to identify what is normal and what is not, but generally do not consider other aspects of a disability—for example, the effects of joint range limitations on function. Because novices have limited experience with the situation they face, they must be given rules to guide their performance. Consequently, they judge their performance by how well they followed the rules.

In the AOTA/AOTF Clinical Reasoning Study, the novice clinicians focused primarily on objective findings, observable signs, and rules by which to make decisions (Cohn & Czycholl, 1991). Their reports about patients typically included information recalled from course work. They recalled characteristics of the clinical conditions studied and matched them to their patients. For example, a therapist unfamiliar with the diagnosis of Parkinson's disease might read a reference to learn about the symptoms of this illness, yet fail to recognize that the symptoms, such as bradykinesia, will affect the patient's ability to perform routine tasks.

While reflecting on her own development, a relatively new clinician recalled her interactions with patients. She reported that she saw the medical conditions first because she believed that was what she was hired to do—treat the medical condition. She stated, "Once I get my skills down, I can then focus on the interaction." After she became comfortable with the medical focus, she felt free to focus on the patient as a person. Thus, we see that novice occupational therapists focus on context-free elements, that is, the disease processes, free from the context of the patients who have these diseases.

Stage 2: Advanced Beginner

Once novices gain more experience with patients, they learn to consider additional cues, which enable them to consider elements that relate to the patient as an individual. Dreyfus and Dreyfus (1986) called this new element *situational*, in which rules for skill acquisition include both situational and context-free components. For example, occupational therapists at this stage are beginning to consider patients' occupational performance in the context of their patients' expected discharge environments. Advanced beginners recognize the presence and absence of behavior but are not yet able to attach meaning to it, because they are still searching for familiar patterns to assist in problem identification. At this stage, they are still unable to determine priorities. To further clarify this point, try to visualize a patient with spatial perceptual problems performing self-care. The advanced beginner may recognize spatial perceptual impairment in a patient performing self-care but fail to realize that the patient's inability to learn compensation techniques for self-care may be due to a poor attention span as well as decreased motivation. The advanced beginner does not yet see the entire picture.

A relatively young therapist involved in one of the Clinical Reasoning Study groups explained that she structured her treatments according to a framework she learned in school, that is, she had developed a structure to organize her observations for herself. She had a limited ability to sort out significant data, however. The therapist was so focused on the patient's weak right arm that she decided "not to do anything with the other arm because it was okay." However, the patient's potential to function was based on compensatory training of the unimpaired arm. This example illustrates that the therapist was still unable to see the patient's priorities.

Stage 3: Competent

A competent practitioner, according to Dreyfus and Dreyfus (1986), still "sees the situation as a set of facts" (p. 24). Not only do competent practitioners see more facts, but they are also able to identify which facts or observations are relevant. This recognition of crucial facts allows the competent practitioner to determine which aspects of a patient's conditions are most important at a given time. Although competent therapists are able to individualize therapy based on their broader understanding of a patient's problem and are able to handle multiple patient care demands with a feeling of mastery, they lack the flexibility and creativity that characterizes more experienced therapists' work.

Elstein (1978) found that the identification of cues and the generation of multiple hypotheses were two traits demonstrated by successful clinical decision makers. He also found that persons who could gather multiple cues were also able to construct several hypotheses and hold them in abeyance in order to gather additional cues to evaluate the various hypotheses. In the Clinical Reasoning Study, the experienced therapists were able to attend to more patient cues than were novices. They also constructed many hypotheses and seemed to anticipate the need to formulate these hypotheses on a temporary basis. They understood that their initial image of their patients would change as they collected more data. As their images changed, they in turn revised their initial therapy plans.

Stage 4: Proficient

Proficient therapists perceive a situation as a whole rather than as isolated parts. They have a sense of direction and a vision of where the patient should go, and they are able to take steps toward that goal. Proficient therapists are able to recognize and deal with unfamiliar situations and consider options, because they have the experience-based ability to recognize the nuances of a clinical problem. For example, a proficient therapist was able to adapt her handling of a baby addicted to cocaine when she realized that the baby was reactive to tactile input. Consequently, her treatment approach changed dramatically. Proficient therapists are able to see the whole condition. Experience helps proficient therapists identify what typical events to expect in a given situation and how plans need to be modified in response to these events. Proficient therapists can also recognize when the expected picture does not materialize.

By simply learning the diagnosis, such as cerebellar malfunction, the proficient therapist forms a specific mental image of the patient who has this problem and selects evaluation procedures accordingly. The therapist will also hypothesize about the patient's response to therapy before meeting the patient. Once the evaluation is completed, the proficient therapist will modify the initial hypotheses based on unexpected findings.

For the proficient therapist, certain features of a situation stand out as salient and others recede into the background. Once the important elements are identified, the proficient therapist then thinks analytically by combining rules and guidelines to make decisions. As therapy progresses, the salient features, treatment plans, and expectations are modified. No deliberation occurs—It appears just to happen as the therapist draws from similar experiences that trigger plans that have worked in the past and may be reapplied to new situations. Experienced therapists have a mental library full of experiences, whereas novices or students do not (Benner, 1984; Dreyfus & Dreyfus, 1986 [Note. Benner's study of nurses was based on Dreyfus and Dreyfus's original work. Benner's study was published in 1984, whereas Dreyfus and Dreyfus did not formally publish their work until 1986.]).

In the Clinical Reasoning Study, we observed that novice therapists felt less comfortable revising their plans than did experienced therapists. Newer therapists worked hard to develop a treatment plan and were less likely to alter it when they confronted obstacles, whereas proficient therapists seemed to revise their plans automatically.

Stage 5: Expert

Expert therapists use rules and guidelines in a manner completely different from the novice therapists. The rules shift to the background. Experienced therapists appear to have an "intuitive grasp of each situation and zero in on the accurate region of the problem" (Benner,

1984, p. 32). In this context, intuition refers to a thorough understanding of a situation based on reflections of experiences. Intuition is not irrational, unconscious, or guesswork, but rather, the product of situational involvement and recognition of similarity. The rules, then, are unhitched to the sequence in which they were learned and are applied and adapted to a new situation more easily.

In the Clinical Reasoning Study, experienced therapists intuitively knew when to push a patient toward a higher level of function and when to let go to avoid failure (Mattingly, 1988). For example, an expert therapist intuitively knew when to set limits to increase tolerance for structured therapy. This intuitive judgment is based on correct identification of relevant cues at a particular time in the patient's therapy, and a variety of medical, physical, and psychosocial factors are considered. Expert therapists recognized rules but moved beyond the rigid application of these guidelines based on an inner sense of knowing what to do next. "When things are proceeding normally, experts don't solve problems and make decisions; they do what normally works" (Dreyfus & Dreyfus, 1986, p. 31) . However, when confronted with obstacles or new situations, expert therapists demonstrated the analytic abilities described above.

Summary

This continuum of a professional's career can be used as a basis for the design of an effective staff program that influences professional growth from novice to expert. Regardless of their experience, all clinicians may benefit from reflecting on their practice. Experienced staff can instruct those with less experience by example. Because experienced staff may have limited opportunities for advancement in occupational therapy, which is a two-tiered field, sharing their expertise with others in a public forum offers them some recognition. Novice staff members can benefit from observing the broad repertoire of strategies that the proficient and expert clinicians use to engage patients and to reach their collective goals. Other benefits include heightened awareness and interpretation of cues that influence clinicians' actions, identification of successful therapy strategies, and alternatives for meeting treatment goals, all of which lead to a broad approach to practice.

Staff Development Using Case Stories

The basic elements of the process used to analyze practice in the Clinical Reasoning Study were integrated into departmental staff meetings at University Hospital in Boston. Case stories were created around the process of therapy. Some of these stories involved reports of the constant revision of therapy over time or how the patient and the therapy changed. Textbook descriptions of patients' clinical conditions and a listing of short-term and long-term goals were avoided to make the case stories more meaningful. Clinicians selected a therapy session to videotape, then chose a brief segment of that session and identified a number of leading questions to structure the group discussion. These questions included (a) identification of treatment strategies that were or were not successful, (b) identification of points in the therapy session in which the therapist confronted obstacles, (c) naming of the story of the session, (d) identification of choice points where changes in the therapy were made, and (e) "Who is this patient and what does he or she care about?" (i.e., what brings meaning to this patient's life?).

Staff with all levels of experience as well as any students present in the department met so that differing viewpoints, comments, or alternatives could be shared freely among them. As might be expected, staff responses to the process-oriented case story format generated concerns that generally correlated with their stage of professional development. Novice therapists focused on concrete skill acquisition. For example, they enjoyed seeing someone else in action; hearing others in the group discuss alternative approaches, challenges, and techniques that were used when the clinician got stuck; or seeing other specialty treatment areas. Experts, on the other hand, seemed more interested in observing how clinicians engaged their patients. Additionally, the experts were interested in how clinicians create a future with and for their patients, whether there were conflicts in the stories, and how the illness experience affects the patient. These clinicians focused on the more phenomenological aspects of occupational therapy. Although the clinicians viewed and integrated video segments on different levels, they all gained knowledge and benefited from open professional discussions, which often went beyond the specific cases to broader issues affecting the practice of occupational therapy.

Clinicians who had been videotaped articulated tangible ways in which they thought videotaping and analyzing practice in reflective study groups changed their thinking and their approach to practice. Changes noted among clinicians included increased personal insight into their response to patients, increased ability to take a reflective stance toward their practice, different approaches to analyzing and labeling observation, and improved ability to hypothesize about therapy outcomes. These enhanced skills were also observed in supervision. Clinicians became more adept at articulating their own reasoning process. In supervision sessions, the clinicians began to solve problems based on a broader perspective about what might have been happening in therapy.

Additionally, the process of analyzing videotapes

vividly illuminated the complexity of practice and helped clinicians understand why fieldwork students struggle to put it all together. Supervisors were able to differentiate students' problems and restructure the learning experience to facilitate specific skills such as observation, identification of cues, generation of hypotheses, formulation of the patient's future, or engagement of the patient in a collaborative process. Acknowledging the complexity of practice helped clinicians appreciate what they were doing, stimulated their interest, and validated their professional identity. Many participants articulated that the very process of analyzing their practice renewed their interest in, enthusiasm for, and pride in the profession of occupational therapy. It was notable that during the 2 years in which the Clinical Reasoning Study took place, there was no staff turnover. A sense of departmental morale and group cohesiveness were additional outcomes of such study groups (Slater, 1989).

Recommendations for Implementing Staff Development Programs to Facilitate Reflection on Practice

Although this staff development program evolved from a research project, other departments could easily replicate its essential components. Implementation of analysis of practice may be started with staff members who are interested in reflecting on and exploring their own practice. Participation on a voluntary basis would allow therapists to take the initiative and responsibility for planning their own professional development. Persons who volunteer could form two-member teams to interview, observe, and videotape each other. The teams could then meet in larger study groups. The study group leadership might rotate as each clinician showed his or her own videotape and structured the discussion and questions to his or her own developmental needs. Each leader might identify an interesting, difficult, exciting, challenging, or unusual therapy session to videotape and discuss. Another option would be to use an outside facilitator, such as a local occupational therapy faculty member, as a group leader. This facilitator could address potentially threatening situations that may arise as colleagues begin to share their philosophical and personal differences.

Some therapists might find this process threatening. To minimize this possibility, we recommend that supervisors serve as role models by showing that they are willing to risk making their own reasoning process explicit. That is, they must model the process and demonstrate that examination of one's practice can be a rich learning experience. We believe that newer therapists will develop an understanding of their own reasoning processes by observing experienced therapists who question their own practice and by having permission to question others in a nonthreatening manner.

Before the videotaping sessions, the clinician is interviewed. He or she is asked to describe the patient from a narrative perspective, that is, to tell his or her story of the patient (Mattingly, 1990). The clinician is then encouraged to imagine what he or she expects to happen during the therapy session, what accomplishments might occur, or what difficulties might be encountered. Such open-ended questions facilitate a broad perspective and shift the focus away from a description of techniques and a listing of long-term and short-term goals. The clinician may construct a hypothetical story as he or she imagines the session will unfold.

After the videotaping, a posttherapy interview is conducted. The interview format might include a narrative description of what actually happened in the therapy session. The team may view the video together and generate specific questions. Topics of discussion might include specific techniques, patient-clinician interaction, key decision points in the session, frames of reference that inform the clinician's thinking, challenges, surprises, and frustrations. The posttherapy interview serves to enhance clinicians' awareness of what thoughts and actions guide their practice. The teams might then present their case stories to the study group or entire department for a larger discussion.

Given the pressure for productivity and tight schedules common to most occupational therapy departments, successful implementation of this program must be sensitive to time constraints. The process could be integrated into an existing scheduled meeting time during the day. Additional time for this process would be minimal if regular treatment sessions were videotaped and existing supervisory and staff meetings were used for study groups. Ideally, management staff with reduced productivity requirements, personnel from the hospital education department, or student volunteers could be used to videotape the therapy sessions.

Conclusion

We propose that ongoing reflection on practice in the work environment can help experienced clinicians serve as role models and mentors for novice therapists and remain enthusiastic and proud of their profession. This approach may also have a positive effect on staff turnover as therapists develop a renewed investment in their practice. Our experience with the staff at University Hospital has demonstrated the benefits of a process-oriented approach to staff development. By videotaping therapy as well as pretherapy and posttherapy interviews with therapists, followed by group analysis, we encouraged our clinicians to link thought and action in practice. This, in turn, can enhance the quality of care for patients.

Acknowledgment

Parts of this paper appeared in "Facilitating a Foundation for Clinical Reasoning" by E. S. Cohn & C. Czycholl. In E. B. Crepeau & T. LaGarde (Eds.), *Self-Paced Instruction for Clinical Education and Supervision: An Instructional Guide* (pp. 159-182). Rockville, MD: American Occupational Therapy Association. Copyright © 1991 by The American Occupational Therapy Association, Inc.

References

American Occupational Therapy Association. (1987). *Occupational therapy: Directions for the future. Occupational therapy education and practice proposals for action*. Rockville, MD: Author.

American Occupational Therapy Association. (1990). *Directions for the Future Symposium Proceedings*. Rockville, MD: Author.

Bailey, D. M. (1990). Reasons for attrition from occupational therapy. *American Journal of Occupational Therapy, 44*, 23-29.

Benner, P. (1984). *From novice to expert*. Reading, MA: Addison-Wesley.

Brollier, C. (1985). Occupational therapy management and job performance of staff. *American Journal of Occupational Therapy, 39*, 649-654.

Christie, B. A., Joyce, P. C., & Moeller, P. L. (1985). Fieldwork experience, Part 1: Impact on practice preference. *American Journal of Occupational Therapy, 10*, 671-674.

Cohn, E. S. (1989). Fieldwork education: Shaping a foundation for clinical reasoning. *American Journal of Occupational Therapy, 43*, 240-244.

Cohn, E. S., & Czycholl, C. M. (1991). Facilitating a foundation for clinical reasoning. In E. B. Crepeau & T. LaGarde (Eds.), *Self-paced instruction for clinical education and supervision: An instructional guide* (pp. 159-182). Rockville, MD: American Occupational Therapy Association.

Dreyfus, H. L., & Dreyfus, S. E. (1986). *Mind over machine*. New York: Free Press.

Elstein, A. L. (1978). *Medical problem solving: An analysis of clinical reasoning*. Cambridge, MA: Harvard University Press.

Gitterman, A., & Netter, I. (1968). Supervisors as educators. In F. W. Kaslow & Associates (Eds.), *Supervision, consultation and staff training in the helping professions* (pp. 100-114). San Francisco: Jossey-Bass.

Kaufman, H. G. (1974). *Obsolescence and professional career development*. New York: Amacom.

Knowles, M. (1980). *The modern practice of adult education*. New York: Association Press.

Lieberman, A., & Miller, L. (1979). *Staff development: New demands, new realities, new perspectives*. New York: Columbia University Press.

Mattingly, C. (1988). *Educational materials: A new approach for reflecting on clinical practice*. Unpublished report of the AOTA/AOTF Clinical Reasoning Study.

Mattingly, C. (1990). The narrative nature of clinical reasoning in occupational therapy. In M. H. Fleming (Ed.), *Proceedings of the institute on clinical reasoning for occupational therapy educators* (pp. 22-24). Medford, MA: Tufts University, Clinical Reasoning Institute.

Parham, D. (1987). Nationally Speaking—Toward professionalism: The reflective therapist. *American Journal of Occupational Therapy, 41*, 555-561.

Pecora, P., & Austin, M. (1987). *Managing human services personnel*. Newbury Park, CA: Sage.

Rogers, J. C. (1982). Sponsorship: Developing leaders for occupational therapy. *American Journal of Occupational Therapy, 36*, 309-313.

Rogers, J. C. (1983). Eleanor Clarke Slagle Lectureship—1983: Clinical reasoning: The ethics, science, and art. *American Journal of Occupational Therapy, 37*, 601-616.

Sabari, J. S. (1985). Professional socialization: Implications for occupational therapy education. *American Journal of Occupational Therapy, 39*, 96-102.

Schön, D. (1983). *The reflective practitioner: How professionals think in action*. New York: Basic.

Schön, D. (1987). *Educating the reflective practitioner*. San Francisco, CA: Jossey-Bass.

Slater, D. (1989). Clinical reasoning as a staff development process. In *Proceedings of the mini-course in clinical reasoning*. Baltimore: American Occupational Therapy Foundation.

Smith, H. L., & Elbert, N. F. (1986). *The health care supervisor's guide to staff development*. Rockville, MD: Aspen Systems.

West, W. L. (1990). Nationally Speaking—Perspectives on the past and future, Part 2. *American Journal of Occupational Therapy, 44*, 9-10.

Chapter 73

Sponsorship: Developing Leaders for Occupational Therapy

Joan C. Rogers, PhD, OTR

Stogdell defined leadership as "the process (act) of influencing the activities of an organized group in its efforts toward goal setting and goal achievement" (1, p 10). Leaders are needed within occupational therapy to formulate and implement the goals of our professional organization, The American Occupational Therapy Association (AOTA), and to promote the missions of occupational therapy in the health care delivery system. Effective leadership is a learned process. Socialization for leadership may occur in a planned or haphazard fashion. This [chapter] discusses one method of selecting and developing leaders for occupational therapy—professional sponsorship.

Sponsorship

Definition

A sponsor is one who assumes responsibility for another. Hence, a professional sponsor is an individual who takes responsibility for the professional enhancement of another individual. Shapero, Haseltine, and Rowe (2) described the professional sponsorship system as a continuum of advisory and support persons who may be differentiated in terms of levels of influence and impact. Mentors, symbolizing an intense and hierarchical relationship, are at one end of the continuum, and "peer pals," reflecting a less influential and more egalitarian relationship, are at the other (2). The sponsorship system, which is also called *patronage* (2) and *networking* (3-5), is focused on *the politics of career advancement*. The emphasis is on the cultivation of relationships to get ahead professionally. For example, an occupational therapist may seek and develop contacts with those professionals, administrators, and legislators who have power and authority relevant to their career plans.

Mentors

In Greek mythology, Mentor was Odysseus' counselor. In the same spirit, the word *mentor* is used in reference to a trusted advisor or guide. Historically, mentorship represented a formal or informal relationship between a prestigious, established older person and a younger person (6). The type of support given was often financial. Rowe captured the meaning of mentor, as intended in this [chapter], when she remarked, "A mentor is a person who comments on your work, criticizing errors and praising excellence. This person sets high standards and teaches you to set and meet high standards" (7, p 41).

Mentor Roles

The mentor serves as a supporter, educator, and advocate for the protégé. Moral support is necessary for professional as well as for personal growth. A chief function of the mentor is to *believe* in the protégé's abilities. The mentor sets up performance objectives for the protégé and conveys the expectation or message that the protégé can accomplish these. This affirmation assists the protégé in acquiring an image of competence. A self-image of competence, or of the ability to master tasks, facilitates a sense of security, which gives the protégé "growing space" and supports purposeful risk taking (8).

Conformity or imitation is not expected of protégés. Mentors respect the integrity and autonomy of their protégés and help them to discover and explore their own potentials. They do this by directing a career clarification process that includes commenting on ambitions and difficulties, assisting in integrating new ideas and experiences, and aiding in the formulation and ordering of career objectives. Through this dialogue, protégés become more aware of their abilities and shortcomings. This enables more realistic career planning and implementation (8). Epstein (9) viewed mentors as "creators of competence" (p 13). They take pleasure in the achievements of those they have nurtured and are not intimidated by their promotion and success (8).

In the capacity of educator, the mentor provides multiple opportunities for informal or incidental learning. For example, the protégé may be invited to observe the mentor negotiating a contract for a needs assessment for occupational therapy services in a long-term care facility. Observation and discussion of a particular negotiation generally fosters a better understanding and appreciation of the negotiating process than is possible through lecture and reading. The mentor elucidates the interaction by making explicit to the protégé how he or she thought about the negotiation at each step. In a similar manner, the protégé has access to many learning situations that would be unavailable without the mentor.

Another important educational function of the mentor is that of providing insight on professional issues. Written records and reports tend to convey little of the dynamics of decision making. The AOTA Bylaws (10), for instance, document the advent of the Specialty Sections, but the rationale for their emergence is difficult to retrieve. A mentor who served on the Bylaws Committee at the time the Specialty Sections were established would have detailed knowledge about their historical and philosophical significance and could share this with others. The expertise and positions of mentors frequently places them at the center of such decision making and makes them valuable sources of oral history.

Strategies for surviving in bureaucratic environments constitute an important facet of professional behavior. As Rowe stated, one needs to "learn the organizational chart and how the place really works" (7, p 41). The place may be a work setting, such as a hospital or school, or an organization, such as the AOTA. The major concern here revolves around power and politics. The mentor assists the protégé in sensing and understanding the political climate. Knowledge of things such as who owes whom a favor, where the informal power lies, what the unwritten rules are, and how to approach an authoritarian administrator provides an "inside" perspective on group and organizational dynamics. Such assistance is invaluable in managing a bureaucracy efficiently and successfully.

The *prompt* acquisition of information may be as important to survival as the mere receipt of information. Daniels (3) noted that the expeditious relay of information on issues that require fast action allows maximum preparation time and, hence, may make the difference between success and failure. As an established professional, the mentor's position generally provides access to information that is not readily available to the neophyte. This may include notice of job vacancies before public posting, the specific orientation desired in grant applications, and the types of information a particular job interviewer wants to hear. Even where speed is not critical, the mentor can provide assistance that allows tasks to be completed with greater ease. Referral to key references and resource persons reduces the time expended to locate relevant information. Clarification of guidelines for report and proposal writing lessens the anxiety associated with interpreting ambiguous regulations. Such directives constitute labor-saving devices that contribute to work efficiency and productivity.

In addition to being a supporter and educator, the mentor is also an advocate. In this capacity, the mentor introduces the protégé to those in positions of influence and power, recommends the protégé for tasks and responsibilities, and is appropriately assertive when the protégé is criticized. Through such mechanisms the protégé gains visibility and is assisted in establishing a professional communication system. Daniels (3) described the sense of mastery and self-worth that is derived from an understanding of an acceptance into informal networks.

From this discussion, it should be clear that a mentor is more than a role model. Role models exert a passive influence on another. The manner in which they enact their professional role, their personal styles, and their specific characteristics may be emulated. Learning occurs principally through observation and imitation. Role models may, but are not required to, nurture, support, or educate (2, 11).

Qualities of the Mentor

To serve as a supporter, educator, and advocate, certain personal qualities are desirable. The ability to relate well on a one-to-one level, together with such attributes as authenticity, openness, sensitivity, responsiveness, and availability is advantageous (8). Another favorable quality is generativity. Erikson (12) defined generativity as concern with establishing and guiding the next generation. The mentor's motivational power emanates from this concern or caring. These humanistic dimensions are supplemented by professional competence that embodies skill, commitment, and accountability (8). Competence constitutes the essential quality needed by a mentor.

Qualities of the Protégé

It is also advantageous for the protégé to possess certain traits. In view of the commitment of time and effort required to transform talents into competencies, those seeking an advisor need to convince prospective mentors that they are worth an investment in time and effort. Hence, it is desirable for them to display a willingness to learn, and [to] exhibit career directness and trust in the mentor (8). The protégé may invite a mentorship by seeking and offering help. Protégés are appreciative of the help received and acknowledge this, when and as appropriate, to the mentor and others (7).

Mentor-Protégé Relationship

The special qualities of the mentor-protégé relationship emerge from the professional competence and senior position of the mentor. The relationship is hierarchical, not democratic. The protégé with talent, and rudimentary skills, is given a chance to learn from the mentor.

Although hierarchical, the relationship is also mutualistic. Both persons give and receive in a mutually beneficial way. The mentor gives knowledge and support in exchange for the protégé's service. Work with the head is traded for work with the hands, so to speak. Pilette (8) remarked about the spiritedness of the interaction. She observed that after talking with one's mentor one may feel intellectually and physically energized. The perception of mutualism resides between the two parties.

Others may well perceive the relationship to be parasitic; however, if either the mentor or the protégé senses that one party is not adequately reciprocating, the positive quality of the relationship is generally destroyed.

The mentor will generally follow the protégé through a sequence of career developments and will facilitate job entry and mobility at many points along the way (8). The intensity and continuity of the relationship account for its restrictive and exclusionary nature. Since it is difficult for a mentor to sponsor more than a few protégés simultaneously, every learner desiring a mentor may not find one. Buber captured the essence of the mentor-protégé relationship when he said:

> Without either being concerned about it, they learned, without noticing they did the mystery of professional survival. They received the spirit of affirmation. (13, p. 89)

Collegial Relationships

Sponsor relationships range from those that are hierarchical to those that are collegial (2). At the opposite end of the sponsorship continuum from mentors are peer mentors (5), "peer pals" (14), and networks (4, 5). Like mentors, these dyads, groups, or organizations are focused on career development and job-related issues and seek to serve the same functions as mentors—psychological support, advising, information giving, and referral. Peer and network relationships may be distinguished from the mentor-protégé relationship in terms of the egalitarian quality of the former. Each participant in the collegial relationship sometimes acts as a leader and sometimes as a follower. Thus, the notion that sponsors must be more powerful and successful than those they sponsor is contradicted by the concept of peers helping each other to succeed in their careers. These collegial relationships also differ from mentorship in that they are available to more persons and less exclusive.

Networks generally have a broader power base than peer mentorships and "peer pal" groups. According to Welch (5), the peer mentor dyad is based on complementary talents. A clinical specialist wanting to learn research skills and a faculty member possessing such skills and seeking to renew clinical skills would constitute a viable partnership. In the *peer pal* model (14), sharing is encouraged among a small group of people. As the term is commonly used, *networking* implies a larger group than *peer pals*. Also, in networks, there is generally less emphasis on the development of specific vocational or professional skills and more emphasis on upward career mobility. Competence in specific occupational skills is assumed. Networks operate on the principle that it is *who* you know, not *what* you know, that gets you ahead. By participating in a network, one comes in contact with people who are in positions potentially useful to one's career and who know other people who are in positions potentially useful to one's career. Conversely, one's own position and contacts can be useful to others in the network. The interpersonal linkages formed in and through networks are used to advance one's career primarily through referrals and recommendations. Although the impact of networks may be less personal than that of a mentor or a *peer-pal* group, the outreach contact capabilities are much greater.

The Value of Sponsorship for Occupational Therapy

Sponsorship provides an effective, appealing, and personalized strategy for developing leaders for occupational therapy. It is built on a concept of intraprofessional and interprofessional support, which has lacked wide acceptance in "female" professions such as occupational therapy. Levinson and associates (15) observed that women establish fewer mentor relationships than men do. At the same time, Sheehy (16) and Estler (17) documented the importance of a mentor in adult life. The dearth of women in mentorships has been attributed to a lack of opportunity as well as to the general failure to socialize women for leadership positions (18). Others (8, 14) have commented that the sense of distrust and competitiveness among women themselves discourages cooperative interaction. Duncan and Partridge (14) put forth the interesting hypothesis that women may not recognize the association between power and support networks. Whatever the reason, it has become apparent that little has been gained by neglecting sponsorship as a vehicle for leadership development. Recognizing this, women across the country have been joining to form support partnerships and networks to service their career aspirations in much the same way as the *good ole boys'* network has done for men.

Sponsorship can be used by occupational therapists in a variety of ways. The intent of the following discussion is to furnish some examples of its application, rather than an exhaustive list of possibilities.

The concept of hierarchy, as embodied in the mentor-protégé relationship, can be extended to many types of dyads—faculty member-student, instructor-professor, novice clinician-experienced clinician, clinician-administrator. The one-to-one situation is particularly conducive to sharing the subjective aspects of professional behavior. For example, personal experience has indicated that, by verbalizing how one thinks about and reacts to a particular client case, students are assisted in developing clinical reasoning skills and in coping with their reactions to the severely disabled. Similarly, peer reviews

of one's articles and conference proposals may be useful in illustrating that scholarly life is usually a combination of successes and productive failures. Professional meetings and conferences afford opportunities for mentors to introduce their protégés to professional leaders through informal gatherings and spontaneous contacts.

Within occupational therapy, the peer group notion is probably best reflected in the local Special Interest Sections. Such groups may serve as a vehicle for addressing both conceptual and career advancement issues. In gerontology, for example, therapists are needed who can conceptualize practice in the aging services network, including protective services, nutritional sites, and senior citizen centers. The Special Interest Sections provide a logical forum for such exploratory thinking. After roles and functions have been projected, strategies for articulating them to persons in power and authority can be developed, tested, and evaluated. When positions for occupational therapists are created in such settings, members of the Special Interest Section can be instrumental in referring qualified therapists for the position and in preparing them for the application and interview process.

Within the AOTA, the Special Interest Sections, as well as all other organized groups, may be construed as issue-oriented networks. Assuming that the interests of gerontological occupational therapy were being neglected in AOTA policies and actions, the Gerontology Special Interest Section could be mobilized to exert pressure on the policy and decision-making bodies. Application of *networking* principles would involve identifying and patronizing those office holders sympathetic to gerontological issues, persuading and converting other elected and appointed officials, promoting the election and selection of candidates supportive of gerontological issues, and courting the assistance of other AOTA units. These activities would be carried out through person-to-person contacts and organized actions, with the keen recognition that by helping the causes of gerontological practice, gerontological therapists would be helping themselves and each other.

The power base of occupational therapists could be substantially increased if therapists joined *organized* support networks such as the Philadelphia Women's Network or the Bay Area Professional Women's Network. Network contacts can assist in maneuvering occupational therapists into the administrative positions in occupational therapy units, health care settings, social programs, and governmental agencies. They may also be critical for eliciting support for such objectives as licensure legislation and reimbursement by health insurance plans. Networks vary in membership characteristics and degree of structure. Some are restricted to men or women, to certain occupational classifications or job levels, or to personnel in a particular facility. Others cover broad geographical regions and are open to all regardless of occupation, position, or sex. Meeting agendas range from informal career-oriented discussions to planned programs dealing with topics such as agenda planning, the negotiation process, and assertiveness. The selection of a network to join emerges from one's career development needs.

Mechanisms for gaining access to power bases, such as the good ole boys' network, also merit attention. Many of these ties are developed through associations made during the college years. In recognition of this, it may be advisable for occupational therapy students to take their courses in administration and supervision in schools of business and public or hospital administration, which have as their expressed purpose the education of administrators and executives. Such an educational strategy might not only foster a sharp appreciation of how the administrator's mind operates, it might also facilitate collegial relationships with those who will come to exert control over the delivery of occupational therapy services.

Finally, attention should be directed toward the psychological benefits of sponsorship, regardless of the particular form it takes. Professional role strain, also known as "burnout," is prevalent among professionals. Many therapists are disillusioned with their careers. They may work alone. They may not feel like part of a team. They may realize little administrative support and may rarely receive recognition. The information-giving, psychological support, and advocacy inherent in sponsorship could help alleviate such role strain and foster the innovative visions that occupational therapists have about occupational therapy. Sponsorship creates a sense of belonging to a social network designed to help people help people succeed.

In conclusion, sponsorship does not require large expenditures of money and time, or large numbers of therapists to initiate. One therapist can affirm another and, from here, various kinds of social support structures can grow. For each therapist there is a double challenge— to select someone to sponsor and to acquire a sponsor.

Acknowledgment

This paper is based on an address given at the Annual Conference of The American Occupational Therapy Association, San Antonio, Texas, 1981.

References

1. Stogdell RJ: *Handbook of Leadership: A Survey of Theory and Research*, New York: The Free Press, 1974

2. Shapero EC, Haseltine FP, Rowe MP: Moving up: role models, mentors, and the "patron system." *Sloan Management Rev* 19: 51-58, 1978

3. Daniels AK: Development of feminist networks in the health sciences. In *Proceedings of the Conference on Women's Leadership and Authority in the Health Professions*, HEW Contract #HRA 230-76-0269, 1977, pp 25-35

4. Kleiman C: *Women's Networks*, New York: Ballantine Books, 1980

5. Welch M: *Networking*, New York: Warner Books, 1980

6. Kelly LY: Power guide—the mentor relationship. *Nurs Outlook* 26: 339, 1978

7. Rowe MP: Go hire yourself a mentor. In *Proceedings of the Conference on Women's Leadership and Authority in the Health Professions*, HEW Contract #HRA 230-76-0269, 1977, pp 41-42

8. Pilette PC: Mentoring: an encounter of the leadership kind. *Nurs Leadership* 3: 22-26, 1980

9. Epstein CF: Bringing women in: Rewards, punishments, and the structure of achievement. In *Woman and Success*, RB Kundsin, Editor. New York: William Morrow and Co. Inc., 1974, pp 13-21

10. Bylaws. *AOTA Member Handbook*, Rockville, MD: The American Occupational Therapy Association, 1978, pp E-1—E-9

11. Haseltine FP: Why be a role model when you can be a mentor? In *Proceedings of the Conference on Women's Leadership and Authority in the Health Professions*, HEW Contract #HRA 230-76-0269, 1977, pp, 37-39

12. Erikson EH: *Childhood and Society*, New York: W.W. Norton & Co., 1950

13. Buber M: *Between Man and Man*, New York: Macmillan, 1965

14. Duncan J, Partridge R: Peer pals: Overcoming the obstacles to leadership development. *Nurs Leadership* 3: 18-21, 1980

15. Levinson DJ, Darrow CM, Klein EB, Levinson MH, McKee B: The psychosocial development of men in early adulthood and the mid-life transition. In *Life History Research in Psychopathology*, Vol. 3, DR Ricks, A Thomas, M Roff, Editors. Minneapolis: The University of Minneapolis Press, 1974

16. Sheehy G: *Passages*. New York: E.P. Dutton & Co., Inc., 1976

17. Estler S: Women in decision making. In *Proceedings of the Conference on Women's Leadership and Authority in the Health Professions*, HEW Contract #HRA 230-76-0269, 1977, pp 197-208

18. Diamond H: Patterns of leadership. *Educ Horizons* 57: 59-62, 78-79

Chapter 74

Continued Learning: An Adaptive Response

Suzanne Peloquin, MA, OTR

This chapter was previously published in *Mental Health Special Interest Section Newsletter* (1987, March), pp. 2-3. Copyright © 1987, The American Occupational Therapy Association, Inc.

Current issues surrounding our professional preparation are well articulated in the occupational therapy literature. The range of controversial topics, from entry-level requirements to specialization options, reflects a wide variety of compelling themes. Credibility and competence, for example, are two recurrent themes underlying arguments for specialization and standardization of curricula (King, 1986). This [chapter] focuses on the theme of personal responsibility for continued learning as one which merits consideration in any discussion about continued education. Continued learning will be characterized here as an adaptive and accountable response that each of us can formulate.

Continued Learning as an Adaptive Life Response

As mental health practitioners, we scrutinize life experiences. As occupational therapists, we invoke principles and we structure tasks to facilitate healthy responses among our patients. We often speak of achieving a balance and of being adaptive. In advocating a holistic view, we caution our patients and our fellow professionals alike against neglecting significant portions of their lives. We encourage our patients to accept and to assume responsibility for themselves.

In light of our discussion, it seems appropriate to apply these same principles to our life experiences as professionals. If the principles are important, we should benefit from characterizing our professional lives with the principles of balance, adaptive responses, a holistic view, and responsible actions that we recommend to others. In the process of applying these principles to our professional lives, we will be highlighting the theme of personal responsibility for continued learning.

Balance is a principle important to us as therapists. Richard Bolles (1981) describes a balance phenomenon that he calls the "three boxes of life." He refers to a tendency adults have in our culture to sequentially inhabit three distinct life spaces: the world of education, the world of work, and the world of leisure. We proceed through these phases chronologically, and, within each distinct phase, there is the threat of being "boxed in." Young adults (18-22) can spend a disproportionate amount of time in the education box, sometimes to the exclusion of meaningful work or play. Mature adults inhabit the work box, often removed from education, and put off significant play until retirement. Older citizens can become trapped in a leisure box, playing until death. To get out of the boxes, Bolles recommends what he calls life/work planning. What he proposes is endorsed by occupational therapists everywhere: a balance of functions within each life phase.

The portion of Bolles' (1981) thinking that is especially relevant here is adding lifelong education as a component to be balanced within each period of life. As occupational therapists, we speak most often of a work/play balance; Bolles insists that learning must be added to all life phases. He describes lifelong learning as inseparable from work and play because the combination of all three gives life its zest, aim, and mission.

Do occupational therapists perceive education as a lifelong enterprise? Once degree and certification are in hand, do we tend to heave a sigh of relief and end our student role? Do we tend to get "boxed in" by our world of work, depriving ourselves of a vital balance?

Although there is a real probability of getting boxed into a state of imbalance, we need to recognize that we are capable of a different response. We can achieve a balance, and we can commit to learning beyond the box of education.

A second principle that occupational therapists endorse is responding in an adaptive manner. It seems incongruous for therapists who advocate change and adaptation to the environment to be unresponsive professionally to changes around them. Continued learning in our day-to-day practice is an imperative survival strategy. We need to stay current in theories and techniques. It is the rare homemaker who is unaware of the existence of the microwave. Hopefully, it is the rare occupational therapist who is unfamiliar with the contents of DSM-III [-R] or the relevance of DRGs. Continued openness to those issues relating to our practice can be seen as an adaptive professional response.

A third concept therapists value is a holistic view of man. Although we sometimes struggle with our generalist training, we acknowledge its merit in providing us with a more comprehensive understanding of our patients. How could holistic professionals ever justify in practice or in principle any disregard for growth in professional endeavors while developing other aspects of their lives?

A last therapeutic concept we might relate to our professional lives is assuming personal responsibility. Most therapists carry professional liability insurance, a concrete reminder of the responsibility we exercise each day. In the final analysis we are responsible for our professional behaviors. Only continued learning about clinical issues can secure our ability to make responsible clinical decisions in a rapidly changing world.

If we reflect about ourselves as professionals, and if we apply to our professional situation those principles we value, one conclusion is plausible. It is congruent to assume individual responsibility for learning throughout the life span and to find experiences that can facilitate professional development.

Continued Learning as a Form of Accountability

Beyond what we owe ourselves, there are others to whom we are accountable for continued learning. We have a responsibility both to our patients and to our profession. In a service profession, our patients are the reason we exist (Brunyate, 1985). We owe each of our patients the best techniques and alternatives within our means. Our code of ethics commits us to the education of the consumer of health services on matters of health that are within the scope of occupational therapy. Our consumers deserve and increasingly demand our best and most current knowledge. Only through continued learning can we remain accountable to this new breed of informed patient.

We represent a profession. We sit in rounds, report at patient conferences, and serve on committees, representing far more than ourselves. Once certified, we claim the right to be called occupational therapists or occupational therapy assistants. One consequence of this right is the responsibility to represent our titles well. To represent well includes being cognizant of the situation at hand. It requires continued learning. We mastered what was taught when we were in school, but our theoretical mastery cannot stop there.

Our profession conducts the business of occupational therapy. Some of us balk at this notion as if business were the antithesis of service. The fact is that, in our diverse settings, we engage in business endeavors. Prominent business representatives featured in the book *In Search of Excellence* (Peters & Waterman, 1984) report successful business strategies. One strategy is the fostering of creativity, innovation, and continued learning. Success in business requires a commitment to making the business matter and making the business "work." As participants in the business of occupational therapy, we have a vested interest in learning more about how to make it grow and prosper.

When we respond to our patients and our profession with continued learning, we are responding accountably. Given our responsibility to be current and authentically professional, if we do not take the initiative for continued learning and demonstrate that initiative each day, others may step in to structure, legislate, or otherwise ensure our accountability.

Cultivating Opportunities for Continued Learning

If continued learning is vital on many fronts, then commitment to the process must be developed early and rekindled at regular intervals. Throughout this article, use of the phrase *continued learning* in lieu of *continued education* has been deliberate. The two phrases are not necessarily synonymous. While education is a stimulus, it does not always produce a learning response. We may teach facts and skills, but we do not always teach our students to learn.

John Gardner (1963) in *Self-Renewal* reminds us that "the ultimate goal of the educational system is to return to the individual the burden of getting his own education" (p. 12). Our Slagle lecturers have spoken over the years about fostering the drive to learn. Yerxa in 1967 (1985) spoke of the *authentic* professional as that individual who recognizes his or her responsibility to be a lifelong student. Fidler in 1966 described learning as a growth process. She encouraged us to set in operation a learning process that will endure. She cited a passage from a student log illustrating the process being set in motion: "I wonder sometimes if this course is not to teach us so much as it is to make us learn—it would seem that what I am learning is how to learn and teach myself—this conviction grows stronger each week" (1985, p. 149). Once set in motion, the learning process must continue in response to practitioners' needs. And here we face a challenge.

Mental health therapists across the country have markedly different practices and needs, as reported in a survey done by the American Occupational Therapy Association (1982) [sic]. Opportunities for continued education may vary considerably, but opportunities for continued learning always exist. Given the drive to learn, and the mind-set of a lifelong student, therapists can find opportunities everywhere. We have professional colleagues, journals, publications, bibliographies, special interest sections, and other opportunities available to us. If we have the desire to learn, we will find many suitable vehicles. What we may periodically need is the kind of inspiration that we once received from the best of our teachers and mentors.

Our enthusiasm for continued learning may, as it would for any other task, run in spurts. The energy required must be generated. While we must rely primarily on ourselves to maintain the initiative, isn't it good to know that the effort makes a difference to someone? Certainly it helps to remember that the energy expenditure significantly benefits us, our patients, and our profession. But isn't it a revitalizing moment when a co-worker, a colleague, a supervisor, or a former teacher notices the effort? We can help one another to want to continue learning; we can, with the smallest of gestures, make a great difference.

Conclusion

Several controversial premises underlie current discussions about our preparation for practice. The theme of personal responsibility is pertinent to those discussions. As our profession seeks to establish guidelines for educating its members, it is crucial to remember that in the absence of individual commitment to continued learning, structured programs may be meaningless. Therapists must want to learn. They must perceive continued learning as an adaptive and accountable response that benefits them, their patients, and their profession. The drive for and belief in continued learning needs to be carefully cultivated and nurtured as a prerequisite to our ability to grow, serve, and prosper.

References

American Occupational Therapy Association, Division of Continuing Education, (1984). *AOTA competency based curriculum in mental health.* Rockville, MD: AOTA.

Bolles, R. N., (1981). *The three boxes of life.* California: Ten Speed Press.

Brunyate, R. W., (1985). Powerful levers in little common things. In *A professional legacy: The Eleanor Clark Slagle Lectures in occupational therapy* (p. 29). Rockville, MD: American Occupational Therapy Association.

Fidler, G. S. (1985). Learning as a growth process: A conceptual framework for professional education. In *A professional legacy: The Eleanor Clark Slagle Lectures in occupational therapy* (pp. 137-155). Rockville, MD: American Occupational Therapy Association.

Gardner, J. (1963) *Self-Renewal.* New York: Harper & Row.

King, L. J. (1986). Competence and credibility: A challenge to professional self discipline. *Occupational Therapy Forum, 1*(6), 13-14.

Peters, T. J., & Waterman, R. H. (1984). *In search of excellence.* New York: Warner Books.

Yerxa, E. J. (1985). Authentic occupational therapy. In *A professional legacy: The Eleanor Clark Slagle Lectures in occupational therapy* (pp. 155-175). Rockville, MD: American Occupational Therapy Association.

Chapter 75

Employment of Occupational Therapists in Nontraditional Settings

Charlotte Brasic Royeen, PhD, OTR, FAOTA

This chapter was previously published in the *American Journal of Occupational Therapy, 44*, 172-173. Copyright © 1990, The American Occupational Therapy Association, Inc.

Nontraditional occupational therapy can be defined as what is done by an occupational therapist beyond the clinic walls of a hospital, rehabilitation center, or school. What the occupational therapist does in such nontraditional employment settings is usually not direct service and may not even be identified as occupational therapy in the formal job description. Rather, the position can be something that uses an occupational therapist's skills, training, and expertise. Such nontraditional settings as local, state, and federal governments; sales and marketing firms; private industries; and professional associations may all employ occupational therapists. An occupational therapist, for example, may help define and execute policy within government; promote sales of equipment or materials in business; develop habilitation programs for industry; or serve as a lobbyist for a professional association.

Much of an experienced occupational therapist's skills and abilities are transferable to other jobs in nontraditional settings. These marketable skills are (a) responsivity, (b) reasoned judgment, (c) recognition of priorities, (d) realism, and (e) rapport.

Responsivity

Occupational therapists have a tendency toward field dependency; that is, we are sensitive and responsive to our environment and the people in it. We know how to read verbal and nonverbal cues, because the execution of any worthy treatment program requires responsivity to clients and their needs.

Much of the work in business, industry, and government is conducted in groups (e.g., task forces, advisory committees, consultant groups). By perceiving what individuals within the group are doing (independent of what they are saying) as well as perceiving what the group itself is doing (independent of the group mission), one can work well in groups. The group skills training that all therapists receive is invaluable, and an experienced occupational therapist brings more developed group skills to the work setting than do most professionals.

Additionally, we as therapists get along well with almost any type of person because we are trained to read verbal and nonverbal cues and to be sensitive to a person's needs. The ability to get along with others and to be affable and socially adept in work settings is a valuable skill. Thus, social skills and strength in interpersonal relationships based on responsivity are skills that many employers would appreciate.

Reasoned Judgment

Occupational therapists make daily decisions requiring reasoned judgment that affect the lives of clients. Therapists are accountable to clients, supervisors, and third-party payers for their decisions regarding treatment of choice, duration of treatment, and home programs. Thus, experienced occupational therapists have considerable skill in making and explaining reasoned judgments. Reasoned judgments consist of professionally based decisions for which no textbook, scientific paper, or expert can give precise answers—the individual must make them based on the synthesis of available information and past experience.

The ability to execute and justify reasoned judgments can be restated as a commonsense approach to problem identification and problem solving. The ability to justify and explain one's opinions and plan of action is valuable in a nontraditional setting, especially to one's supervisors.

Recognition of Priorities

Occupational therapists set priorities for every testing situation, treatment plan, and treatment session. In the process, they come to accept that not everything can be done and prioritize their work. Many people in nontraditional settings feel burned out because they are unable to prioritize their work. By trying to do it all, they miss important deadlines and feel exhausted and frustrated. But the person who can set priorities brings a real strength to any administrative or management position.

Within the framework of priority setting, flexibility is fundamental. Just as all occupational therapists have considerable experience in setting priorities (e.g., in a treatment program), they also have experience in changing their priorities when an unanticipated event occurs (e.g., the sudden divorce of the parents of a pediatric client). The unanticipated event changes and requires an immediate reordering of the priorities. Thus, priority

setting can be a flexible and dynamic process. By working with many different types of clients and problems, occupational therapists have learned to expect the unexpected. The ability to set and reorder priorities as the situation dictates are high-level management skills crucial to task management.

Realism

One cannot set priorities without a realistic understanding of the situation at hand. Occupational therapists must continually and realistically assess a client's status, progress, and potential. Few of us expect perfection from others, because we understand realistic expectations in terms of function and ability. We are experienced in estimating realistic work loads and task performances for others. We cannot work successfully with clients in their homes, at work, and in social settings without having a realistic understanding of these environments. Thus, occupational therapists have experience working in reality (Fields, 1956). They do not ask "What if?" but rather "What can be accomplished realistically?"

Employees who possess an understanding of what they or others can realistically accomplish, given the available resources, time, and ability, are valued, because this allows for successful plans of action. Thus, possessing realistic viewpoints, or realism, is a valuable skill that occupational therapists can offer employers in nontraditional settings.

Rapport

The hallmark of a successful client-therapist relationship is the establishment of rapport. Occupational therapists are trained in the importance of developing rapport with clients. This ability is also important to the success of a manager in any setting. Successful professionals are usually those who can easily establish rapport with all of the office employees, including janitors, secretaries, and professional staff, because they are best able to motivate others to produce results.

Summary

From my personal experience as a therapist employed in a nontraditional setting, I have identified the skills and abilities of experienced occupational therapists that are germane to work in nontraditional settings or beyond the clinic walls. Our profession can benefit from therapists working in nontraditional settings by gaining recognition and influencing decision makers in ways that will benefit the clientele that occupational therapists serve.

Acknowledgments

This paper is based on presentations made at the Annual Conference of the American Occupational Therapy Association in Phoenix, Arizona, April 1988, and at the Annual Conference of the District of Columbia Occupational Therapy Association, Washington, DC, March 1987.

Reference

Fields, B. (1956). What is realism in occupational therapy? *American Journal of Occupational Therapy 10*, 9-10, 34.

Chapter 76

The Pros and Cons of Nontraditional Practice

Ralph Adams, MS, OTR/L

This chapter was previously published in *Mental Health Special Interest Section Newsletter* (1991, June), pp. 5-6. Copyright © 1991, The American Occupational Therapy Association, Inc.

Numerous deterrents have been identified to explain the comparatively low representation of occupational therapists in nontraditional, particularly community-based, settings. Salaries are generally not competitive. The dearth of occupational therapists to serve as role models and provide peer support is frequently cited as a deterrent. Many therapists are unfamiliar with the structure and dynamic operation of non-hospital-based agencies and facilities. Furthermore, a clearly defined generic role delineation for occupational therapists in such settings is not available. Though none of these deterrents is insurmountable in itself, the whole complex of inhibiting factors can be quite intimidating.

The dog and pony show is a marketing institution, as is the slogan that affirms that "everything is negotiable." Admittedly, many nontraditional settings, particularly those designated as not-for-profit, offer lower and frequently noncompetitive salaries. Administrators, however, are increasingly coming to realize that even not-for-profit organizations operate in a competitive market—a market in which "you get what you pay for" and "the benefit outweighs the cost." The adventurous occupational therapist is able to market personal competence and experience and the direct relevance of occupational therapy with an awareness that salary is negotiable. At the very least, one can suggest a term-fixed renegotiation based on demonstration of productivity and measurable service outcomes.

Though therapists in nontraditional settings frequently do not have other therapists physically present on-site, this does not mean that they are necessarily deprived of role models and peer support. Other professional team members may provide support and guidance in nonclinical areas. Networking with therapists involved in similar endeavors provides opportunity for mutual support and development. If one grants that the process of mentoring is somewhat analogous to professional parenting, then the importance of "quality time," rather than the physical presence of role models, deserves emphasis. Given efficient communication, mentoring can occur across state lines as readily as across the hall.

Though a particular setting may be unfamiliar, the client population generally is not. Granting the uniqueness of each individual, the basic human need for optimum self-actualization remains constant. Occupational therapists are uniquely equipped to address that need. An entrepreneurial therapist can clearly and assertively enunciate the role of occupational therapy as an essential component of rehabilitation. The ability to identify measurable and quantifiable objectives and outcomes and to provide a substantive rationale for specific interventions is second nature to occupational therapists. The vocabulary and thought processes that occupational therapists take for granted are generally not characteristic of the culture of many nontraditional programs. Yet funding sources and granting agencies have consistently begun to require their recipients to demonstrate in their initial proposals and subsequent documentation the type of clinical accountability that characterizes occupational therapy practice. The therapist who speaks the same language as the funding source and is comfortable in that role can readily be recognized as a valuable asset by an astute administrator.

The lack of a clearly defined role for occupational therapists in nontraditional settings might be viewed as an opportunity rather than a deterrent. Therapists in these settings have the opportunity to integrate skills and develop a broad array of competencies. These include program development, management, marketing, development of referral sources, training and supervision of staff, funding skills (e.g., grant writing), and business skills (e.g., budgeting, billing, and reimbursement policy awareness). In addition, therapists are able to personalize their professional roles in a challenging and rewarding way. Experienced therapists may feel that traditional settings do not always provide sufficient challenges, allow for innovation in treatment approaches, or encourage therapists to refine or diversify clinical and nonclinical competencies. Some nontraditional settings may appeal to assertive, experienced therapists because of the greater flexibility of those structures and the greater potential for defining one's personal professional role and identity in a way that is consistent with one's level of professional growth.

For the competent but less experienced therapist, accepting a lower paying job in a nontraditional setting might be considered a career investment. It can be argued that the broader range of experience obtained in many nontraditional settings ultimately places one in a more competitive position in the employment market. A broad array of skills can be developed and honed in nontraditional settings in a comparatively short period of time. Therapists might need to educate themselves in certain areas, use consultants, and make lots of phone calls—but once the skills are developed, the therapists have become more marketable.

Chapter 77

Research and Professional Growth in a Clinical Setting

Frances Oakley, MS, OTR

The occupational therapy mental health program in any clinical setting provides a natural environment for conducting research. In most occupational therapy programs, however, research is not a primary or even secondary activity. One reason for this may be the therapist's misconception about the nature of the research process. Therapists may fear research and consequently mislabel it as some "scary monster" involving numbers and statistics. They may view research as overwhelming, especially in light of patient care responsibilities. They may feel that they lack the time, the skill, the support, the knowledge, or the understanding of its value. This [chapter] compares the research process with the process of providing clinical care to reveal that research is not a scary monster to be feared, rather it is a natural extension of the orderly process occupational therapists follow to provide clinical care. The value of research to our professional growth is discussed as well, followed by suggestions on integrating research into clinical activities.

Stages of Clinical Care

A common goal in all occupational therapy mental health settings is to provide the best possible clinical care. To meet this goal, occupational therapists progress through several stages, including (a) an assessment, (b) the identification of the treatment options and the implementation of treatment, and (c) the evaluation of the treatment outcome (Rogers, 1983). These stages should be guided by a theoretical model that defines the nature of our practice, identifies its guiding principles and tenets, and serves as a framework to organize our thinking throughout the stages of clinical care.

The assessment stage is characterized by a data-gathering process through which we search for facts and information to answer questions about the patient's occupational functioning. Information is obtained, for example, from accurate records of the patient's performance in occupational therapy, interviews with the patient and significant others, and the results of assessment instruments we administer. The assessment instruments and procedures should not only be reliable and valid but also congruent with the theoretical model. The information gleaned from the data-gathering process is then synthesized and analyzed within a theoretical framework to construct an explanation of the patient's occupational functioning. This data set serves as the basis for generating treatment options and establishing goals for occupational therapy intervention.

In the second stage, the treatment options and goals are identified and implemented. After initiating treatment, we evaluate the effectiveness of the plan and determine whether the goals were met. If necessary, the treatment plan is adjusted and its outcome is reevaluated. We gain knowledge about the patient's occupational functioning and draw conclusions about the effectiveness of our clinical care.

Stages of Research

Research is an objective, systematic investigation into a phenomenon to gain an understanding of that phenomenon. The research process, like the process of providing clinical care, should also be guided by a theoretical model.

The first stage in the research process is the identification of a phenomenon or a question for study that is grounded in a theory. A research design, or map, is developed that defines the research procedure. It identifies the instruments that will be used in the study and the manner in which the data will be objectively and systematically collected. The data-collection stage refers to the gathering of information and facts. The instruments used to gather and measure the data must be reliable and valid, because the data collected are no more reliable or valid than the instruments or measures employed. The data are then synthesized and analyzed, and conclusions are drawn that contribute to the knowledge gained about the research question.

Similarities Between Research and Clinical Care

It is a myth that research does not have its place in clinical care; the two go hand-in-hand. Not only does the research process resemble the clinical care process, it also employs similar skills. Both processes are guided by a theoretical framework in which questions are asked and data are collected, synthesized, and analyzed. Conclusions are drawn and knowledge is gained. Research supports the best possible clinical care; at the same time, clinical care is a laboratory for research. A therapist who has integrated theory into clinical practice and is administering reliable and valid assessment instruments has already laid the groundwork for conducting research.

There are, however, few occupational therapy assessments with established reliability and validity. This has important implications for clinical practice and for third-party reimbursement. After all, we are charging people for our service, and our assessments are the basis for our service. The clinical setting is a rich source for establishing the reliability and validity of our instruments, testing our theoretical models, generating new ideas, and identifying areas for future investigation.

The Value of Research

Research must be integrated into our clinical activities. It is relevant and vital to our patients, our profession, and ourselves. Research indicates what works best for the consumers of our services so that we can provide them with the best possible clinical treatment. By examining, validating, supporting, or refuting our clinical practice, we add to the body of knowledge in occupational therapy. It is vital to the future of our profession to provide high-quality, accountable services to secure our place in an increasingly competitive marketplace. Research will also assist us in supporting the fees for our service.

Research supports our professional growth and development by providing a vehicle for seeking, discovering, and answering questions. It presents challenging opportunities in which personal satisfaction, knowledge, and gratification can be derived. Research can also help avoid and counteract professional burnout by creating new challenges for therapists in their practice. For therapists who have mastered their clinical skills and have practiced for several years in the same setting, research can provide a fresh perspective as well as a rewarding opportunity to observe a different kind of outcome from clinical care.

What You Can Do

You do not have to be an expert in all facets (e.g., research design, statistical analysis) of the research process to conduct or participate in research, but you do need to be knowledgeable. It is possible to conduct sound clinical research by using the expertise and guidance of persons who are skilled in each stage of the process. The following are some suggestions for incorporating research into your clinical activities:

- Adopt a theoretical model to guide the clinical care and research processes.
- Generate questions from your own clinical practice that you would like to have answered.
- Become familiar with the research process by reading about it. Read publications by researchers in mental health.
- Identify resources within your facility, such as program analysts or other researchers who can provide guidance and advice.
- Negotiate within your work setting the designation of a resource person to support and coordinate clinical research studies.
- Negotiate with your supervisor the type and kind of patient load that would support research endeavors.
- Develop local study groups; develop a network of therapists and collaborate with them. Weekly staff meetings may be an accessible forum.
- Contact the state occupational therapy association and the American Occupational Therapy Association (AOTA) special interest section for resources and input.
- Use research advisors within AOTA and the American Occupational Therapy Foundation (AOTF). AOTF has identified therapists throughout the country who are skilled in the research process to serve as consultants to therapists.
- Replicate research studies.
- Develop liaisons and collaborate with others who are more experienced in conducting research. For example:
  - Participate in the research symposiums sponsored by AOTF. These symposiums provide the opportunity to participate in research studies already designed by experts in the field.
  - Collaborate with academicians. Many graduate occupational therapy students are required to conduct research for their master's theses. Offer your facility for data collection.

A word of caution: Be prepared. Research proficiency does not happen overnight. Like any new skill, it takes time and practice to perfect. Pinpointing the research question so that the study is manageable is the most difficult part of the research process. But remember that clinical research is an exciting challenge that is well worth the effort.

Reference

Rogers, J. (1983). Eleanor Clarke Slagle lectureship, 1983: Clinical reasoning—The ethics, science, and art. *American Journal of Occupational Therapy, 37*, 601-616.

Chapter 78

The Challenge of Conducting Research in a Clinic

Diana M. Bailey, EdD, OTR, FAOTA

Research can be fun, exciting, and fascinating. Often the student who is required to write a research thesis starts out appalled by the idea yet ends up enjoying the challenge and feeling proud of the results. There is a great sense of satisfaction to be derived from completing this exacting, often complex, always stimulating process. "But how can I find the time and resources for research?" cry busy clinicians, up to their eyes in patients, meetings, and paperwork. Here are some hints that may prove helpful.

Time and Effort

There is no denying that research does take time, resources, and effort and that it is very hard to fit a research project into an already overcrowded schedule. The clinician who makes the difficult decision to take on a research project must understand that it will take priority and that other tasks must go or take a back seat. There will be extra work that must be done in the evenings or on weekends—that is a fact of research. Once the commitment is made and the project is under way, however, I believe clinicians will find it well worth the effort and extra work.

Therapists often ask, "How long will it take to complete a research project?" or, "How long must I spend at it each day or week?" As a faculty advisor, I have found that graduate students take an average of 6 months to a year to identify an issue to be studied, carry out the project, and write up a thesis. In my experience, research conducted by therapists in a clinic tends to take a little longer—12 to 18 months—with some time being spent on the project each week, on average. Of course, certain phases of the research demand more input than others. For example, when a new treatment approach is being investigated, carrying out the actual treatment in the case requires that the therapists adhere to the stipulated amount of preparation, treatment, and record-keeping, according to the research protocol. Meanwhile, reading the literature or writing up the results may be done on one's own time and on a less precise schedule. There are few clinical situations that allow therapists sufficient freedom during the day to do the amount of extra work required to carry out a research study.

Working With a Colleague

When problems with research begin to seem overwhelming, having a colleague can be an enormous help. My guess is that far more studies are completed that have two or more investigators than those that have just one. When the inevitable problems get one person down, the project can still move forward because there is someone else involved who still has some energy with which to deal with these difficulties.

Finding the Right Question and Getting Started

It has been said that finding a research question that is reasonable, doable, interesting, and useful is the most difficult part of the whole process. Talking with fellow therapists or others who have done research in the past is an excellent idea and heartily recommended. However, this can also eventually become a barrier to getting started because everyone has his or her own pet theory about how the project should be carried out. Listening to and acting on some of these ideas can be most helpful in shaping research, but conflicting opinions must somehow be reconciled as well. There comes a point when each therapist must decide that he or she has had enough input from colleagues, family, and friends. At this point, the project must be designed and begun.

The Literature Review

Completing a literature review is perhaps the hardest part of the whole process for many people, but there are some ways to make it less painful. I find it helpful to have a card in front of me containing my research question and the major topics for which I am searching. When I feel I am straying too far afield or have lost sight of the major issues, glancing at the card will get me back on track. A common problem is arriving at the library, finding just the articles you have been looking for, and not having enough change to make the copies. It is wise to take a roll of dimes or one of the copy machine credit cards that are now available. Also, taking down all the reference data immediately will save a great deal of time and trouble when it is time to actually prepare the list. All too often a researcher finds that he or she has lost an article, returned a needed book, loaned an article to someone who has not returned it, or spilled coffee on a volume number. Having all the reference data on index cards will save trouble.

If, during a computer search, you find little or no literature relevant to your topic, there are several possible explanations:

- Your topic does not make sense. No one has written in this area because it is not logical and there is nothing there to research.
- You are looking in the wrong database (e.g., you are looking in Medicine and should be looking in Vocational Counseling).
- You are in virgin territory—nothing has been done in this area. That is very exciting. Go ahead!

Many people find that actually writing up the literature review is a tiresome task—one that they put off as long as possible. Promptness is definitely the best policy, and possibly the only policy that will ensure the completion of the article. It is also easier to write a review when the material is fresh in one's mind and while inspiration is still present.

Confusion of Terms

It is quite common for a researcher to confuse the problem, purpose, and significance of a study. Remember, the *problem* is the larger issue that others have tried to do something about; the *purpose* is what the researcher hopes to accomplish as a result of a small contribution to the larger problem; and the *significance* is the importance of the researcher's particular study and what it will do to help solve the larger problem. It is the "so what" of the study.

People often make the mistake of including in the Assumptions section those notions they hold about the study that can be proved—those that are referenced in scientific literature. Only beliefs that are difficult to prove in any concrete way (i.e., untested beliefs or untestable hypotheses, basic values, or views about the world) should be included as assumptions. The distinction between the assumptions underlying a research project and the scope of the project is sometimes blurred. Assumptions are individual and often unrelated beliefs about the nature of the topic. The scope, on the other hand, presents an encompassing conceptual framework in which to place the whole study. This frame of reference will color all aspects of the research and will provide a backdrop against which the reader may view the entire study.

It is advisable not to give long lists of limitations for studies. After a while, it may look as though the study should never have been conducted when, in fact, it may have proved quite useful in advancing an area of knowledge. There is a happy medium between listing every conceivable problem in the study to being fair with the reader and presenting those things that could truly bias the results. Knowledgeable readers will pick up obvious limitations but will respect an author who acknowledges problems and considers them in the interpretation of findings.

Statistics

Because most health professionals are far from expert with statistics, I recommend that therapists seek the assistance of a statistician when data calls for the use of inferential statistics. Most occupational therapists can handle the descriptive statistics used in nonexperimental research (percentages, means, ranges, and the like) but need help in deciding when and how to use such inferential tests as t tests or analyses of variance. If you are not sure where to find a compatible statistician, ask colleagues who have participated in research, or faculty at the local college. There is usually someone on the faculty whose job it is to assist with statistics, and he or she is often willing to work with private customers. Whomever you find, compatibility and good communication are important. Too often therapists or students struggle to understand what a statistician is saying and feel that the problem is all theirs. Of course, the problem is not all on one side. Often it is the statistician who does not understand the clinical process and is unable to design data collection and analysis methods that are appropriate. Either way, it is best to leave that situation and find someone else. It may take two or three tries to find the right person.

Researchers must also know clearly in their own minds what it is that they hope to find out from the data analysis. Sometimes therapists get talked into performing complex and elegant statistical manipulations by statisticians who are more interested in proving they can do such manipulations than they are in helping therapists achieve their goals. The analysis may look impressive but often does not make much sense in real life. I also recommend that therapists consult with a statistician before beginning to collect data, to ensure that all the necessary data is collected and that it is collected in a useful format.

Human Subjects Committees

Investigators often underestimate the amount of time needed to gain permission from Human Subjects Committees to carry out a study. This process can take anywhere from 1 to 4 months, depending on how frequently the committee meets and whether or not all the materials have been submitted correctly and completely. If components of the protocol need to be revised, the process may take even longer. Much time and irritation can be avoided by finding out ahead of time the exact requirements of the committee. They all vary.

Publishing

Many studies get bogged down when the author receives the article back from the editor and sees that yet more work is needed to get it into publishable shape. Many first-time authors think that drafting the article the first time is all there is to it. Most learn quickly that this is not the case. What appears to an author to be a flawless piece of work appears to others as a piece that can be improved. Generally, the revisions are not as major as they might first appear. After the first disappointment, an author should go through the recommendations one by one to get a more realistic feeling for items that can be changed quickly and sections that will require more work. The author may be too close to the topic to see alternative ways of presenting ideas; a colleague may help shed a more objective light on things and may have suggestions for the more major revisions. It is generally a good idea to set a deadline for all the changes—perhaps within 2 weeks. In my experience, if this stage is not dealt with quickly, the manuscript will sit in the drawer permanently.

If the researcher can push past whichever of these potential stumbling blocks presents a personal bugaboo, he or she will enjoy the challenge and will even have fun conducting a first piece of research in a clinic. The axiom "the more you do something, the easier it gets" is never as true as when conducting research. Therapists will learn about many pitfalls—and ways around pitfalls—from actually designing and carrying out a study. So get started—the time is now.

Chapter 79

Steps in Collaborative Research Between Clinicians and Faculty

Elizabeth DePoy, PhD, MSW, OTR/L
Charles Gallagher, MA, OTR/L

The implementation of clinical research requires two ingredients: a clinical setting and persons who are committed to and knowledgeable about the research process. These two ingredients, however, are rarely found together. Clinicians have access to the clinical setting and to patients but may be hesitant to involve themselves in research due to the time constraints of their jobs, the focus of their work on treatment, or their perceived lack of experience with research methods.

Educators, on the other hand, who should conduct research to gain promotion, merit, and tenure (Rider, 1987; Wilson, 1979), may possess the expertise and experience in research methods but often lack access to the clinical setting. Collaboration between faculty and clinicians is therefore one vehicle through which clinical research can be accomplished, because each party possesses what the other lacks.

Even with the presence of the two ingredients necessary for clinical research, collaborative clinical investigations may still be marred by (a) each party's lack of understanding of the other party's job constraints and responsibilities and (b) the absence of formal *a priori* negotiation of research functions based on each investigator's interest, time, and expertise.

The Colleague Model of Collaborative Investigation, which is presented in this paper, provides a framework collaborators can use to prevent obstacles from emerging, identify potential barriers, and employ strategies to facilitate the completion of clinical research. This model comprises seven steps that guide clinical researchers through the collaborative process (see Table 1). The Colleague Model of Collaborative Investigation has been used successfully in six projects within the past 2 years.

The use of this model is illustrated through a discussion of a recent pilot study by DePoy, Gallagher, Calhoun, and Archer (1989) that explored the extent to which altruistic activity contributed to self-esteem and internal locus of control in a population of elderly patients who were hospitalized for clinical depression.

Table 1. The Colleague Model of Collaborative Investigation

Step No.	Definition	Aim	Outcome
1	Identifying a common research interest	To find a research partner	The beginning of a collaborative research relationship
2	Role taking	To enhance the collaborative relationship	An understanding of the partner's perspective
3	Planning and design	To plan clinical research to soothe clinical irritations	A carefully developed, systematic research plan
4	Negotiation	To meet individual needs and expectations and to use the skills of each collaborator efficiently	A detailed plan of the duties and payoffs for each collaborator
5	Implementation	To carry out the research plan, collect the data, and modify the plan to meet unforessen obstacles	A completed data set for analysis
6	Completion	To analyze the data and create a format for dissemination	A publishable article, formal presentation of findings, or both
7	Evaluation	To assess the project for strengths and weaknesses and to determine future research	A stronger collaborative research relationship

Step 1: Identifying A Common Research Interest

Occupational therapy practitioners and educators have questions about practice. Yerxa (1979) called this inquisitiveness a "clinical irritation" (p. 26) and indicated that it is the initial step in the research process.

In the first step of clinical research, the investigator's aim is to find a colleague who not only has an analogous clinical irritation, but also a complementary ideology of occupational therapy practice and the desire and resources to soothe the irritation through research. The faculty researcher may easily identify a clinical colleague who has similar interests. Any person specializing in the treatment of the population or area of interest is a potential colleague. In the DePoy et al. (1989) pilot study, the student, Archer, discussed a research idea with the faculty member, DePoy. After DePoy refined the idea into a potential research question, she contacted the clinician, Gallagher, who worked in a clinical setting where the study could be implemented. Additionally, DePoy was aware of Gallagher's research experience, compatible philosophical view of occupational therapy, and desire to conduct research. DePoy, Gallagher, and Archer discussed the project further.

Although the clinician may have more difficulty locating a faculty colleague as a research partner, various methods can be used. One such method is for the clinician to contact the educational institution directly to explore the research interests and skills of the faculty. If no faculty member has the desired expertise, the faculty can probably refer the clinician to someone either inside or outside the educational institution who is currently conducting or planning research in the clinician's field of interest. A second method to search for a research partner is through current publications. A person's publication record not only demonstrates that person's interest area, but also indicates his or her ideology, research skills, and ability to communicate findings in writing. A third method by which a clinician can find a potential research partner is by contacting the person designated as research liaison in the state occupational therapy organization.

To ascertain common interests, the interested parties should discuss areas of clinical interest, ideology, and preferred method of investigation. For example, in the area of human occupation, multiple research methods are useful, depending on the nature of the questions. Because of the nature of clinical research and the early level of theory development in occupational therapy, naturalistic studies are often useful for initial descriptions of phenomena of interest. These research methods should be strongly considered when research questions and previous theory development lend themselves to descriptive strategies.

In the DePoy et al. (1989) pilot study, the collaborators agreed that the methodological approach would integrate qualitative and quantitative designs. They also agreed to fit the methodology with the daily routine at the institution by planning experimental and control conditions within the already scheduled occupational therapy program.

If the potential collaborators perceive their research relationship as productive, they are ready for Step 2.

Step 2: Role Taking

Because of the job norm differences between clinical practice and academia, Step 2 is perhaps most fundamental to the establishment of a solid collaborative research relationship. In this step, the collaborators engage in mature role taking behavior (Selman, cited in Wolman, 1980).

Selman (Wolman, 1980) defined *role taking* as cognitive growth that leads to the individual's ability to understand the perspective, thoughts, and feelings of others. The mature role taker is able not only to articulate his or her understanding of the other person but also to adjust behavior to meet the needs of others in a mutually satisfactory manner. In the collaborative process, this step is crucial, particularly when each of the collaborators approaches the research project with different needs, desires, expectations, and external demands.

Each collaborator must identify the following:
1. His or her purpose for conducting the research.
2. Skills he or she possesses.
3. Skills he or she expects the other party to contribute.
4. Personal time constraints and commitments to the project.
5. Which part of the project he or she is willing to complete.
6. Areas of weakness that may interfere with the completion of the project.
7. Feelings about the research process in general.
8. Expected outcomes, particularly for publication and dissemination.
9. Expected use of the results.

A thorough and honest dialogue clarifies the expectations, areas of potential contribution, and expertise of each collaborator so that Step 3 may begin on sound footing. In addition, with the perspectives of the research team clarified, the need for additional resource persons, such as statisticians, data collectors, and consultants, can be evaluated and met.

The collaborators in the DePoy et al. (1989) pilot study talked extensively about their expectations of each other. Although interested in the topic, Archer indicated that she did not have the time or expertise in research to direct the project. She wished to participate with direction from the faculty member and the clinician. Gallagher indicated that his purpose in conducting research was threefold. He was interested in the question, he wished to improve the scholarly reputation of his department, and he wanted to set an example to enhance acceptance of clinical research as a norm for clinical practice. Although Gallagher was knowledgeable about and experienced in research methodology, his job constraints prevented him from taking the primary responsibility for design and report writing. Gallagher, therefore, participated in discussing the design of the project, directing data collection, interpreting the findings, and editing the manuscript. Gallagher also suggested valuable literature that contributed to the theoretical rationale for the project.

DePoy's purpose was to investigate productivity in adulthood and aging. Her commitment to clinical occupational therapy research could be actualized through this project. DePoy agreed to be primarily responsible for articulating and refining the research design, analyzing the data, and writing the report.

Step 3: Planning and Design

Step 3 involves the design and planning phase of the research project. In this step, the collaborators derive the research question and design from a synthesis of their mutual interests, ideologies, skills, and expectations and from consideration of the constraints of the clinical setting. The methodology must be carefully specified during this step so that Step 4 can be accomplished.

The first task in Step 3 is to state a common theoretical approach to occupational therapy treatment that will underpin the research question and design. Once a philosophical foundation has been agreed upon, the research question is formulated. The initial design of the research project can then be founded on the theoretical framework, the research question, and the literature available to support the study. In the DePoy et al. (1989) pilot study, the collaborators agreed that occupation was the core of occupational therapy practice and that an examination of normative occupations in adulthood and aging could constitute the theoretical framework of the research. The integration of current readings on aging with Erikson's (1950) stages of development gave rise to the themes of altruism and giving as norms of adult productive activity. From this theoretical support, the following research questions were derived:

1. What is the effect of altruistic activity on the self-esteem and locus of control of elderly depressed patients?
2. What, if any, clinical changes were observed when patients engaged in altruistic activity?

A quasi-experimental design, enhanced with qualitative data collection techniques, was then selected. Hence, the outcome of this step was clearly stated research questions and a method by which the question was to be answered.

In addition to focusing on the design of the research project, Step 3 must address practical matters such as the articulation of ideas to institution research committees and human subject review boards. In the DePoy et al. (1989) pilot study, a date was set for Gallagher to present the project to the institutional research committee for feedback and approval.

By the end of Step 3, a formal research plan, including the literature review, the question, the design, and the process, should be completed.

Step 4: Negotiation

Step 4 involves the negotiation phase, in which the collaborators determine each of their parts in the project and each of their personal payoffs. The omission of this stage from collaborative research is often responsible for the breakdown of a project because of each investigator's differing norms and expectations (Parham, 1987; Wilson, 1979).

Although the collaborative research process has no formal leadership, the concept of exchange of privilege for expertise fits well in the negotiation phase of this model. In the DePoy et al. (1989) pilot study, the first authorship was granted to DePoy for her contributions in the area of research design, data analysis, and reporting. Gallagher received second authorship for his effort and participation in conceptualizing the project.

The negotiation process is essentially an interactive one in which skills are identified and assessed and privileges and duties are agreed upon to maximize the assets of the research group. Through negotiation, each function of the research process—the mix among skill, time commitment, and payoff—is clarified, and the assignment of research activities and rewards is clearly defined. In other words, during this phase, each collaborator operationalizes his or her commitment, stake in the project, and expected outcome.

In this phase of the planning, creative solutions to time boundaries can be developed. One advantage of a collaborative relationship between faculty and clinicians is that students may be retained as research assistants who can review literature and collect data as part of their education. Both of the student collaborators in the DePoy et al. (1989) pilot study exchanged data collection and literature search activity for authorship. At the end of Step 4, each of the collaborators in the DePoy et al. pilot study had a clear idea of his or her responsibilities and the time frame in which to conduct them. Authorship was also clarified for each participant.

In summary, the product of Step 4 is a concrete research plan, which should include a time line and a scheduled sequence of research activities. With such a plan in place, the research study can be implemented.

Step 5: Implementation

In Step 5, the project is initiated according to the plans made during Step 4. Implementation, however, does not always proceed according to plan. Regular communication and evaluation must therefore be considered as essential during the implementation phase. Researchers and research assistants should meet on a regular basis to report their progress and to discuss any unexpected issues that arise. Communication with research committees and human subject review boards must also be planned as a regular activity in Step 5.

During the course of the research project, periodic formal evaluation not only ensures that the research is proceeding as planned, but also identifies methodological flaws and operational difficulties. This type of evaluation is particularly necessary in clinical research due to the limited control that the researchers have over the research environment.

Formal evaluation should include (a) critical analysis of the initial research plan, (b) determination of the congruence of the plan with the limitations of the research environment, (c) identification of the strengths and weaknesses of carrying out the plan, and (d) strategies to strengthen the research project.

With the data from the evaluation, the collaborators are prepared to mediate any difficulties that may interfere with the research project. In addition, formal evaluation may influence the design and implementation of future research. In the DePoy et al. (1989) pilot study, the original quasi-experimental design was precluded by the admission and discharge patterns of the institution. The initial research, which was to be conducted by a comparison of concurrent control and experimental groups on measures of self-esteem and locus of control and on qualitative observations of competence in the assigned activity, was changed to a design in which groups were conducted sequentially over 2 weeks. The new design was selected so that the subjects served as their own controls, thus eliminating the obstacle posed by a small sample. The new plan resulted in the collection of a complete data set for analysis.

Step 6: Completion

In this step, the data are analyzed and summarized for presentation or publication. Even if the data analysis and the reporting are the responsibility of only one of the researchers, the interpretation of the results is a collaborative affair and should be discussed and agreed upon by each of the collaborators.

In the DePoy et al. (1989) pilot study, a statistician was consulted. After a final analysis of the data, DePoy and Gallagher discussed the findings and developed conclusions. DePoy then wrote the research report, which was reviewed by all of the collaborators. Their comments were incorporated into the final report, which was subsequently published.

Step 7: Evaluation

In this step, the collaborators review their research findings, their methodology, and their working relationship for the purpose of improving future research. This step also adds to the collective knowledge of occupational therapy through a general refinement and improvement of collaborative research. During Step 7, alternative research methodologies, data collection strategies, and operating procedures can emerge. At this final step of the Colleague Model of Collaborative Investigation, the collaborators decide whether to continue, modify, or dissolve the research partnership. The DePoy et al. (1989) pilot study has been expanded to a larger sample and to more diverse populations as a result of Step 7.

Discussion

A model of collaborative research has implications beyond the facilitation of research. The model encourages occupational therapy researchers to explore all of the investigative methods available to answer complex questions about human occupation and health. Stimulation of more diverse types of clinical research can assist occupational therapy's development of a unique epistemology while still addressing the need for accountability in a competitive health care market.

The conduct of collaborative clinical research furthers the occupational therapy profession by enhancing its place as a professional discipline within the academic arena. As discussed by educators (Ottenbacher, 1987; Parham, 1987; Rider, 1987; Yerxa, 1983) occupational therapy faculty must publish research to conform to the norms of scholarship within the university community.

Finally, collaborative research gives the seasoned clinician a professional role into which he or she may grow. As indicated by Johnson (1973), attrition in the field is in large part a function of the linearity of the field. In other words, as a person grows more competent in treating patients, clinical positions do not offer more challenging expectations. Therefore, excellent clinicians often turn to administration or leave the field entirely. As clinical research becomes more the norm than the exception, however, clinicians may assume more challenging tasks within the context of clinical practice. Consideration of clinical research as a norm of clinical practice rather than as an ancillary professional activity can expand occupational therapy's knowledge and provide challenges for professionals interested in further clinical stimulation.

References

DePoy, E., Gallagher, C., Calhoun, L., & Archer L. (1989). Altruistic activity versus self-focused activity: A pilot study. *Topics in Geriatric Rehabilitation, 4*(4), 23-30.

Erikson, E. (1950). *Childhood and society.* New York: Norton.

Johnson, J. (1973). 1972 Eleanor Clarke Slagle Lecture—Occupational therapy: A model for the future. *American Journal of Occupational Therapy, 27,* 1-17.

Ottenbacher, K. J. (1987). Nationally Speaking—Research: Its importance to clinical practice in occupational therapy. *American Journal of Occupational Therapy, 41,* 213-215.

Parham, D. (1987). Nationally Speaking—Toward professionalism: The reflective therapist. *American Journal of Occupational Therapy, 41,* 555-561.

Rider, B. A. (1987). The Foundation—Faculty research: A reply to Deborah Labovitz. *American Journal of Occupational Therapy, 41,* 55-56.

Wilson, L. (1979). *American academics: Then and now.* New York: Oxford University Press.

Wolman, B. (Ed.). (1980). *The handbook of developmental psychology.* Englewood Cliffs, NJ: Prentice Hall.

Yerxa, E. (1979). The philosophical base of occupational therapy. In *Occupational therapy: 2001 AD* (pp. 26-30). Rockville, MD: American Occupational Therapy Association.

Yerxa, E. (1983). Audacious values: The energy source for occupational therapy practice. In Kielhofner, G. (Ed.). *Health through occupation* (pp. 149-162). Philadelphia: F. A. Davis.

Appendix A

Supplemental Reference Lists

The following reference lists provide the reader with resources for further study in a diversity of topics relevant to the practice of occupational therapy. It is not intended to be an all-inclusive reference guide, as an exhaustive bibliography is in itself a book.

I have carefully selected literature for these lists that I have found to be relevant and applicable to current practice. The reference lists at the end of each chapter also provide a wealth of well-researched resources. While reviewing these references, readers will want to consider the commonalities among different patient populations and treatment settings. Often a reference cited for one population or setting is equally relevant to other populations or settings. For example, individuals with psychiatric diagnoses and individuals with traumatic brain injuries both frequently have cognitive impairments and social skill deficits; therefore, references regarding cognitive rehabilitation and social skills training may be applicable to both populations and are worthy of further review by occupational therapists practicing in either area.

Readers who actively explore these resources with an open mind will expand their view of occupational therapy practice, develop their clinical expertise, and attain the highest level of professional excellence.

Activity Group Process

See Intervention Principles and Techniques

Administration: Management and Supervision

American Occupational Therapy Association (1985). Guide to classification of occupational therapy personnel. *American Journal of Occupational Therapy, 39*, 824-830.

American Occupational Therapy Association Practice Division (1991a). *COTA supervision information packet.* Rockville, MD: Author.

American Occupational Therapy Association (1991b). *Self-paced instruction for clinical education and supervision: An instructional guide* (SPICES). Rockville, MD: Author.

American Occupational Therapy Association (1992). *Effective documentation for occupational therapy.* Rockville, MD: Author.

Bailey, D. (1988). Occupational therapy administrators and clinicians: Differences in demographics and values. *Occupational Therapy Journal of Research, 8*(5), 299-315.

Bailey, D. (1990). Ways to retain or reactivate occupational therapists. *American Journal of Occupational Therapy, 44*, 31-37.

Bair, J., & Gray, M. (Eds.). (1992). *The occupational therapy manager* (2nd ed.). Rockville, MD: American Occupational Therapy Association.

Baum, C. M. (1983). Nationally speaking: Strategic integrated management system: SIMS. *American Journal of Occupational Therapy, 37*, 595-600.

Berman, C. (Ed.). (1989, June). Reimbursement [Special issue]. *Mental Health Special Interest Section Newsletter.*

Bordieri, J. E. (1988). Job satisfaction of occupational therapists: Supervision and managers versus direct service staff. *Occupational Therapy Journal of Research, 8*, 155-163.

Bowman, O. J. (1991, September). Managers to play an important role in implementing the Americans with Disabilities Act. *Administration and Management Special Interest Section Newsletter*, pp. 1-2.

Boyt Schell, B. A. (1989). Nationally speaking: Occupational therapy management: Accepting the challenge. *American Journal of Occupational Therapy, 43*, 215-217.

Broiller, C. (1985a). Managerial leadership and staff OTR job satisfaction. *Occupational Therapy Journal of Research, 5*, 170-184.

Broiller, C. (1985b). Occupational therapy management and job performance of staff. *American Journal of Occupational Therapy, 39*, 649-654.

Broiller, C. (Ed.). (1987). Management [Special issue]. *American Journal of Occupational Therapy, 41*.

Carr-Ruffino, N. (1985). *The promotable woman becoming a successful manager.* Belmont, CA: Wadsworth Publishing.

Chilton, H. (1989, September). Today's occupational therapy managers as managers of change. *Administration and Management Special Interest Section Newsletter*, p. 4.

Committee on Education of American Occupational Therapy Association. (1991). *Guide to fieldwork education* (2nd ed.). Rockville, MD: American Occupational Therapy Association.

Crist, P. A. (1986). *Contemporary issues in clinical education.* Thorofare, NJ: Slack.

Daniel, M. (1989, June). A career ladder for registered occupational therapists and certified occupational therapy assistants. *Administration and Management Special Interest Section Newsletter*, pp. 3-4.

Dolh, C. D., & Gruen, H. (1992, March). Is occupational therapy management a cumulative stress disorder? *Administration and Management Special Interest Section Newsletter*, p. 1.

Donnelly, J. H., Gibson, J. L., & Ivancevick, J. M. (1984). *Fundamentals of management.* Plano, TX: Business Publications.

English, C. B. (1984). *Management techniques for physical and occupational therapists.* Sereno, CA: C. B. English Therapy Services.

Foto, M. (1988a). Nationally speaking: Managing changes in reimbursement patterns, part 1. *American Journal of Occupational Therapy, 43*, 563-565.

Foto, M. (1988b). Nationally speaking: Managing changes in reimbursement patterns, part 2. *American Journal of Occupational Therapy, 42*, 629-631.

Frum, D. C., & Opacich, K. J. (1987). *Supervision: Development of therapeutic competence.* Rockville, MD: American Occupational Therapy Association.

Galbraith, J. K. (1983). *The anatomy of power.* Boston: Houghton Mifflin.

Gibson, D. (1983). A guide to women in management. *Occupational Therapy in Mental Health, 3*(1), 55-65.

Gilfoyle, E. F. (1987). Nationally speaking: Leadership and management. *American Journal of Occupational Therapy, 41*, 281-283.

Glantz, C. H., & Richman, N. (1991). *Occupational therapy: A vital link to O.B.R.A.* Rockville, MD: American Occupational Therapy Association.

Gwin, C. H., & Silvergleit, I. (Eds.). (1992). *Managing productivity in occupational therapy.* Rockville, MD: American Occupational Therapy Association.

Hart, G. M. (1982). *The process of clinical supervision.* Baltimore, MD: University Park Press.

Hays, C. (1992). Retention of occupational therapy staff. *Occupational Therapy Practice, 3*(3), 45-52.

Hennig, M., & Jardin, A. (1977). *The managerial woman.* New York: Anchor Press/Doubleday.

Hightower-Vandamm, M. D. (1980). Nationally speaking: Management, marketing, and the real hard facts. *American Journal of Occupational Therapy, 34*, 833-843.

Jacobs, K., & Logigian, M. (1989). *Functions of a manager in occupational therapy.* Thorofare, NJ: Slack.

Kaslow, F. W., & Associates. (1977). *Supervision, consultation, and staff training in the helping professions.* San Francisco: Jossey-Bass.

King, E. S. (1982). Coping with organizational change. *Topics in Clinical Nursing, 4*, 66-73.

Kolodner, E. L., Wiener, W. J., & Frum, D. C. (1989). *Models for mental health fieldwork.* Rockville, MD: American Occupational Therapy Association.

Liebler, J. G., Levine, R. E., & Dervitz, H. L. (1984). *Management principles for health professionals.* Rockville: MD: Aspen Publishers.

Liebler, J. G., Levine, R. E., & Rothman, J. (1992). *Management principles for health professionals* (2nd ed.). Rockville, MD: Aspen Publishers.

Peters, M. E. (1984). Reimbursement for psychiatric occupational therapy services. *American Journal of Occupational Therapy, 38*, 307-312.

Sanderson, S. N. (1992). Making meetings work. *Occupational Therapy Practice, 3*(3), 63-71.

Schwartz, K. B. (1984). An approach to supervision of students in fieldwork. *American Journal of Occupational Therapy, 38*, 393-397.

Scott, S. J., & Acquaviva, J. D. (1985). *Lobbying for health care.* Rockville, MD: American Occupational Therapy Association.

Scott, S. J., & Dennis, D. C. (1988). *Payment for occupational services.* Rockville, MD: American Occupational Therapy Association.

Shapiro, D., & Broun, D. (1981). The delineation of the role of entry level occupational therapy personnel. *American Journal of Occupational Therapy, 35*, 306-311.

Slater, P. Y. (1990, September). A manager's role in shaping practice: The clinical reasoning process. *Administration and Management Special Interest Section Newsletter*, p. 4.

AIDS

Baer, J., Hall, J., Holm, K., & Lewitter Koefield, S. (1987). Challenges in developing an inpatient psychiatric program for patients with AIDS and ARC. *Hospital and Community Psychiatry, 38*, 1299-1303.

Belman, A. L., Diamond, G., Dickson, D., Horoupian, D., Llena, J., & Rubinstein. (1988). Pediatric acquired immunodeficiency syndrome. *American Journal of Developmental Behavior in Pediatrics, 9*, 47-48.

Dekker, A. H. (1988). The impact of AIDS in the pediatric and adolescent populations. *Journal of the American Osteopathic Association, 41*, 427-432.

Denton, R. (1987). AIDS: Guidelines for OT intervention. *American Journal of Occupational Therapy, 41*, 427-432.

Eidson, T. (Ed.). (1988). *The AIDS caregiver's handbook.* New York: St Martin's Press.

Fisher, D. G. (Ed.). (1990). *AIDS and alcohol/drug abuse.* New York: Haworth Press.

Friedman, S. R., & Lipton, D. S. (Eds.). (1991). *Cocaine, AIDS and intravenous drug use.* New York: Haworth Press.

Galantino, M. L. (1992). *Clinical assessment and treatment in HIV.* Thorofare, NJ: Slack.

Goldfinger, S. M. (Ed.). (1990). *Psychiatric aspects of AIDS and HIV infection.* San Francisco: Jossey-Bass.

Gordon, L. (1987, September). An occupational therapy protocol for the AIDS patient. *Physical Disabilities Special Interest Section Newsletter,* pp. 4-5.

Guiles, G., & Allen, M. E. (1987). AIDS, ARC and the occupational therapist. *British Journal of Occupational Therapy, 50*(4), 120-122.

Hansen, R. (1990). The ethics of caring for patients with HIV or AIDS. *American Journal of Occupational Therapy, 44,* 239-242.

Hopp, J., & Rogers, E. (1989). *AIDS and the allied health professions.* Philadelphia: F. A. Davis.

Klug, R. M. (1986). Children with AIDS. *American Journal of Nursing, 10,* 1126-1132.

Kübler-Ross, E. (1978). *To live until we say good-bye.* Englewood Cliffs, NJ: Prentice Hall.

Kübler-Ross, E. (1981). *Living with death and dying.* New York: Macmillan.

Lauer-Listhuass, B., & Walterson, J. (1988). A psychoeducational group for HIV positive patients on a psychiatric service. *Hospital and Community Psychiatry, 39,* 776-777.

Lockhart, L., & Wodarski, J. (1989). Facing the unknown: Children and adolescents with AIDS. *Social Work,* 215-221.

Marcil, W. M., & Tigges, K. N. (1992). *The person with AIDS: A professional and personal perspective.* Thorofare, NJ: Slack.

NYU Regional AIDS Education and Training Center. (1990). *Occupational therapy: The challenge of AIDS—A curriculum guide.* New York: Author.

Peloquin, S. (1990). AIDS: Toward a compassionate response. *American Journal of Occupational Therapy, 44,* 271-278.

Perry, S., & Markowitz, J. (1986). Psychiatric interventions for AIDS—Spectum disorders. *Hospital and Community Psychiatry, 37,* 1001-1005.

Pierme, J., & Bolle, J. (1990). Coping with grief in response to caring for persons with AIDS. *American Journal of Occupational Therapy, 44,* 266-269.

Pizzi, M. (1984). Occupational therapy in hospice care. *American Journal of Occupational Therapy, 37,* 235-238.

Pizzi, M. (1989, November 16). Pediatric AIDS: An OT's overview. *OT Week,* p. 7.

Pizzi, M. (1989, November 23). Pediatric AIDS: OT assessment and treatment. *OT Week,* pp. 7, 10.

Pizzi, M. (1990). The model of human occupation and adults with HIV infection and AIDS. *American Journal of Occupational Therapy, 44,* 257-264.

Pizzi, M., & Johnson, J. (Eds.). (1990). *Productive living strategies for people with AIDS.* New York: Harrington Park Press.

Polan, H. J., Hellerstein, D., & Amchin, J. (1985). Impact of AIDS-related cases on an inpatient therapeutic milieu. *Hospital and Community Psychiatry, 36,* 173-176.

Steich, T. J. (1987). AIDS: Legal, professional and ethical responsibilities. *Occupational Therapy News, 41*(6), 1, 17.

Stuber, M. L. (Ed.). (1991). *Children and AIDS.* Washington, DC: American Psychiatric Association.

Tigges, K. N., & Marcil, W. M. (1988). *Terminal and life-threatening illness: An occupational behavior perspective.* New Jersey: Slack.

Winiarski, M. G. (1991). *AIDS related psychotherapy.* Elmsford, NY: Pergaman Press.

Wofsy, C. B. (1987). Human immunodeficiency virus infection in women. *Journal of the American Medical Association, 257,* 2074-2976.

Assessment/Evaluation Principles and Tools

Allen, C. K. (1985). *Occupational therapy for psychiatric diseases: Measurement and management of cognitive disabilities.* Boston: Little, Brown.

Allen, C. K. (1988). Occupational therapy functional assessment of the severity of mental disorders. *Hospital and Community Psychiatry, 39,* 140-142.

American Psychological Association. (1987). *Diagnostic and statistical manual of mental disorders.* (3rd ed.)(rev.). Washington DC: Author.

Asher, I. E. (1989). *An annotated index of occupational therapy evaluation tools.* Rockville, MD: American Occupational Therapy Association.

Barth, T. (1985). *Barth time construction.* New York: Health Related Consulting Services.

Bendroth, S., & Sothham, M. (1973). Objective evaluation of projective material. *American Journal of Occupational Therapy, 27,* 78-80.

Black, M. M. (1976). Adolescent role assessment. *American Journal of Occupational Therapy, 30,* 73-79.

Brayman, S. S., Kirby, T. F., Misenheimer, A. M., & Short, M. J. (1976). Comprehensive occupational therapy evaluation scale. *American Journal of Occupational Therapy, 30,* 94-100.

Buck, R., & Provancher, M. (1972). Magazine picture collages as an evaluation technique. *American Journal of Occupational Therapy, 26,* 36-39.

Casanova, J. S., & Ferber, J. (1976). Comprehensive evaluation of basic living skills. *American Journal of Occupational Therapy, 30,* 101-105.

Cubie, S. H., & Kaplan, K. (1982). A case analysis method for the model of human occupation. *American Journal of Occupational Therapy, 36,* 645-656.

Cynkin, S., & Robinson, A. M. (1990). *Occupational therapy and activities health: Toward health through activities.* Boston: Little, Brown.

Diasio, K., & Moyer, E. (1980). On psychosocial assessment. *Occupational Therapy in Mental Health, 1*(1), 1-3.

Dowbrowski, L. B. (1990). *Functional needs assessment: Program for chronic psychiatric patients.* Tucson, AZ: Therapy Skill Builders.

Endicott, J., Spitzer, R. L., Fleiss, J. L., & Cohen, J. (1976). The global assessment scale. *Archives of General Psychiatry, 33,* 766-771.

Fillenbaum, G. G. (1988). *Multidimensional functional assessment of older adults: The Duke older Americans resources and services procedures.* Hillsdale, NJ: Lawrence Erlbaum Associates Publishers.

Florey, L. L., & Michelman, S. M. (1982). Occupational role history: The screening tool for psychiatric occupational therapy. *American Journal of Occupational Therapy, 36,* 301-308.

Good-Ellis, M. A., Fine, S. B., Spencer, J. H., & DiVittis, A. (1987). Developing a role activity performance scale. *American Journal of Occupational Therapy, 41,* 232-241.

Hemphill, B. (Ed.). (1981). *The evaluative process in psychiatric occupational therapy.* Philadelphia: Lippincott.

Hemphill, B. (1988). *Mental health assessment in occupational therapy.* New Jersey: Slack.

Hendricks, D. W., Hanlon, M., & Carpenter, W. T. (1984). The quality of life scale: An instrument for rating the schizophrenic deficit syndrome. *Schizophrenia Bulletin, 10,* 388-398.

Houston, D., Williams, S. L., Bloomer, J., & Mann, W. C. (1989). The Bay area performance evaluation: Development and standardization. *American Journal of Occupational Therapy, 43,* 170-183.

Johnson, T. P., Vinnicombe, B. J., & Merrill, G. W. (1980). The Independent Living Skills Evaluation. *Occupational Therapy in Mental Health, 1*(1), 5-18.

Kane, R. A., & Kane, R. L. (1981). *Assessing the elderly.* Lexington, MA: The Rand Corporation.

Kaplan, H. I., & Sadock, B. J. (1985). *Modern synopsis of comprehensive textbook of psychiatry/IV,* (4th ed.). Baltimore, MD: Williams & Wilkins.

Kaplan, K. (1984). Short-term assessment: The need and a response. *Occupational Therapy in Mental Health, 4*(3), 29-45.

Kaplan, K., & Kielhofner, G. (1989). *Occupational case analysis interview and rating scale.* New Jersey: Slack.

Kielhofner, G., Henry, A., & Walens, D. (1989). *A user's guide to the occupational performance history interview.* Rockville, MD: American Occupational Therapy Association.

Lawton, M. P., & Brody, E. M. (1969). Assessment of older people: Self-maintaining and instrumental activities of daily living. *Gerontologist, 9,* 179-186.

Leonardelli, C. (1988). *The Milwaukee evaluation of daily living skills.* Thorofare, NJ: Slack.

Lerner, C. (1979). The magazine picture collage: Its clinical use and validity as an assessment device. *American Journal of Occupational Therapy, 33,* 500-504.

Malm, U., May, P., & Dencker, S. (1981). Evaluation of the quality of life of the schizophrenic outpatient: A checklist. *Schizophrenia Bulletin, 7,* 477-487.

Matsutsuyu, J. S. (1969). The interest checklist. *American Journal of Occupational Therapy, 23,* 368-373.

Moorhead, L. (1969). The occupational history. *American Journal of Occupational Therapy, 23,* 329-334.

Oakely, F., Kielhofner, G., & Barris, R. (1985). An occupational therapy approach to assessing psychiatric patients' adaptive functioning. *American Journal of Occupational Therapy, 39*(3), 147-154.

Peloquin, S. N. (1983). The development of an occupational therapy interview/set procedure. *American Journal of Occupational Therapy, 37,* 457-461.

Robertson, S. C. (Ed.). (1989). *Mental health focus: Skills for assessment and treatment.* Rockville, MD: American Occupational Therapy Association.

Sarno, J. E., Sarno, M. T., & Levito, E. (1973). The functional life scale. *Archives of Physical Medicine and Rehabilitation, 54,* 214-220.

Thibeault, R., & Blackner, E. (1987). Validating a functional performance with psychiatric patients. *American Journal of Occupational Therapy, 41,* 515-521.

Thomson, L. K. (1992). *Kohlman evaluation of daily living skills* (3rd ed.). Rockville, MD: American Occupational Therapy Association.

Van Schroeder, C., Block, M. P., Trottier, E. C., & Stowall, M. S. (1983). *SBC; Schroeder, Block, Campbell: Adult Psychiatric Sensory Integration Evaluation.* Sequin, WA: Schroeder Publishing.

Watts, J. H., Kielhofner, G., Bauer, D. F., Gregory, M. D., & Valentine, D. B. (1986). The assessment of occupational functioning: A screening tool for use in long-term care. *American Journal of Occupational Therapy, 40,* 231-240.

Williams, S. L., & Bloomer, J. (1987). *Bay area functional performance Evaluation* (2nd ed.). Palo Alto, CA: Consulting Psychologists Press.

Case Management

Asley, A. (1988). Case management: The need to define goals. *Hospital and Community Psychiatry, 39,* 499-500.

Bachrach, L. L. (1986). The challenge of service planning for chronic mental patients. *Community Mental Health Journal, 22,* 170-174.

Baker, F., & Weiss, R. (1984). The nature of case manager support. *Hospital and Community Psychiatry, 35,* 925-928.

Bebout, R. R. (1988). The link between inpatient care and case management services. In M. Harris & L. L. Bachrach (Eds.), *Clinical case management* (pp. 53-56). San Francisco: Jossey-Bass.

Berzon, P., & Lowenstein, B. (1984). A flexible model of case management. In B. Pepper & H. Ryglewicz (Eds.), *Advances in treating the young adult chronic patient* (pp. 49-57). San Francisco: Jossey-Bass.

Bond, G. R., Miller, L. D., & Krumwied, R. D, (1988). Assertive case management in three CMHCs: A controlled study. *Hospital and Community Psychiatry, 39,* 411-418.

Borland, A., McRae, J., & Lycan, C. (1989). Outcomes of five years of continuous intensive case management. *Hospital and Community Psychiatry, 40*, 369-376.

Center for Consumer Healthcare Information (1992). *1992 case management resource guide.* Irvine, CA: Author.

Chamberlain, R., & Rapp, C. A. (1991). A decade of case management: A methodological review of outcome research. *Community Mental Health Journal, 27*, 171-188.

Corrigan, P. W., Liberman, R. P., & Engel, J. D. (1990). From noncompliance to collaboration in the treatment of schizophrenia. *Hospital and Community Psychiatry, 41*, 1203-1211.

Deitchman, W. (1980). How many case managers does it take to screw in a light bulb. *Hospital and Community Psychiatry, 31*, 788-789.

Dufresne, G. (1991). Statement: The occupational therapist as case manager. *American Journal of Occupational Therapy, 45*, 1065-1066.

First, R. J., Rife, J. C., & Kraus, S. (1990). Case management with people who are homeless and mentally ill: Preliminary findings from an NIMH demonstration project. *Psychosocial Rehabilitation, 14*, 87-91.

Franklin, J. L., Solovitz, B., Mason, M., Clemons, J. R., & Miller, G. E. (1987). An evaluation of case management. *American Journal of Public Health, 77*, 674-678.

Goering, P., Wasylenki, D., Farkas, M., Lancer, W., & Ballantyne, R. (1988). What difference does case management make? *Hospital and Community Psychiatry, 39*, 272-276.

Harris, M. (1988). New directions in case management. In M. Harris and L. L. Bachrach (Eds.), *Clinical case management* (pp. 87-96). San Francisco: Jossey-Bass.

Harris, M. (1990). Redesigning case-management services for work with character disordered young adult patients. In N. L. Cohen (Ed.), *Psychiatry takes to the streets* (pp. 156-176). New York: Guilford.

Harris, M., & Bachrach, L. L. (1988). A treatment planning grid for clinical case management. In M. Harris & L. L. Bachrach (Eds.), *Clinical case management* (pp. 29-38). San Francisco: Jossey-Bass.

Harris, M., & Bergman, H. C. (1987). Case management with the chronically mentally ill: A clinical perspective. *American Journal of Orthopsychiatry, 57*, 296-302.

Harris, M., & Bergman, H. C. (1988a). Case management and continuity of care for the "revolving-door" patient. In M. Harris & L. L. Bachrach (Eds.), *Clinical case management* (pp. 57-62). San Francisco: Jossey-Bass.

Harris, M., & Bergman, H. C. (1988b). Clinical case management for the chronic mentally ill: A conceptual analysis. In M. Harris & L. Bachrach (Eds.), *Clinical case management* (pp. 5-13). San Francisco: Jossey-Bass.

Harris, M., Bergman, H. C., & Bachrach, L. (1987). Individualized network planning for chronic psychiatric patients. *Psychiatric Quarterly, 58*, 51-56.

Intagliata, J. (1982). Improving the quality of community care for the chronically mentally disabled: The role of case management. *Schizophrenia Bulletin, 8*, 655-673.

Intagliata, J., & Baker, F. (1983). Factors affecting case management services for the chronically mentally ill. *Administration in Mental Health, 11*, 75-91.

Intagliata, J., Willer, B., & Egri, G. (1988). The role of the family in delivering case management services. In M. Harris & L. L. Bachrach (Eds.), *Clinical case management* (pp. 39-50). San Francisco: Jossey-Bass.

Johnson, P., & Rubin, A. (1983). Case management in mental health: A social work domain? *Social Work, 28*, 49-55.

Kanter, J. (1988). Clinical issues in case management. In M. Harris & L. L. Bachrach (Eds.), *Clinical case management* (pp. 15-27). San Francisco: Jossey-Bass.

Kanter, J. (1989). Clinical case management: Definition, principles, components. *Hospital and Community Psychiatry, 40*, 361-368.

Klasson, E. M. (1989). A model of the occupational therapist as case manager: Two case studies of chronic schizophrenic patients living in the community. *Occupational Therapy in Mental Health, 9*(1), 63-90.

Lamb, H. R. (1980). Therapist-case managers: More than brokers of service. *Hospital and Community Psychiatry, 31*, 762-764.

Lehman, A. F., (1988). Financing case management: Making money work. In M. Harris & L. L. Bachrach (Eds.), *Clinical Case Management* (pp. 67-78). San Francisco: Jossey-Bass.

Rapp, C. A., & Chamberlain, R. (1985). Case management services for the chronically mentally ill. *Social Work, 30*, 417-422.

Roberts-DeGennaro, M. (1987). Developing case management as a practice model. *Social Casework: The Journal of Contemporary Social Work, 68*, 466-470.

Sanborn, C. J. (Ed.). (1983). *Case management in mental health services.* New York: Haworth Press.

Schwartz, S., Goldman, H., & Churgin, E. (1982). Case management for the chronic mentally ill: Models and dimensions. *Hospital and Community Psychiatry, 33*, 1006-1009.

Sherman, P. S., & Porter, R. (1991). Mental health consumers as case management aides. *Hospital and Community Psychiatry, 42*, 494-498.

Sullivan, J. (1981). Case management. In J. Talbott. (Ed.), *The chronically mentally ill* (pp. 119-131). New York: Human Sciences Press.

Weil, M., & Karls, J. M. (Eds.). (1985). *Case management in human service practice: A systematic approach to mobilizing resources for clients.* San Francisco: Jossey-Bass.

Willenbring, M., Kidgeley, M. S., Stinchfield, R., & Rose, M. (1991). *Application of case management in alcohol and drug dependence: Matching technique and populations.* Rockville, MD: National Institute in Alcohol Abuse and Alcoholism.

Child and Adolescent Psychiatry

Achenback, T. M. (1979). The child behavior profile: An empirically based system for assessing children's behavioral problems and competencies. *International Journal of Mental Health, 7*, 24-42.

Adelstein, L. A., Barnes, M. A., Murray-Jensen, F., & Baker-Skaggs, C. (1989, March). A broadening frontier: Occupational therapy in mental health programs for children and adolescents. *Mental Health Special Interest Section Newsletter*, pp. 2-4.

American Psychiatric Association (1987). *Diagnostic and statistical manual of mental disorders* (3rd. ed.) (rev.). Washington, DC: Author.

Axline, V. H. (1969). *Play therapy.* New York: Ballantine Books.

Ayres, A. J. (1974). *Sensory integration and learning disabilities.* Los Angeles: Western Psychological Services.

Ayres, A. J. (1981). *Sensory integration and the child.* Los Angeles: Western Psychological Services.

Baker, R., Gaffney, S., & Trocchi, L. (1989, March). Dyadic treatment. *Mental Health Special Interest Section Newsletter*, pp. 4-6.

Baldwin, L. C. (1990). Child abuse as an antecedent to multiple personality disorder. *American Journal of Occupational Therapy, 44*, 978-983.

Baron, K. B. (1987). The model of human occupation: A newspaper treatment group for adolescents with a diagnosis of conduct disorder. *Occupational Therapy in Mental Health, 7*(2), 89-104.

Baron, K. B. (1989, March). Occupational therapy: A program for child psychiatry. *Mental Health Special Interest Section Newsletter*, pp. 6-7.

Baron, K. B. (1991). The use of play in child psychiatry: Reframing the therapeutic environment. *Occupational Therapy in Mental Health, 11*(2/3), 37-56.

Barris, R., & Kielhofner, G. (1985). Adolescence. In G. Kielhofner (Ed.), *A model of human occupation: Theory and application* (pp. 99-111). Baltimore: Williams & Wilkins.

Berman, A. L., & Jobes, D. A. (1991). *Adolescent suicide: Assessment and intervention.* Washington, DC: American Psychological Association.

Blakeney, A. B. (1985). Adolescent development: An application to the model of human occupation. *Occupational Therapy in Health Care, 2*, 19-40.

Brandenburg, N. A., Friedman, R. M., & Silver, S. (1990). The epidemiology of childhood psychiatric disorders: Prevalent findings from recent studies. *Journal of the American Academy of Child and Adolescent Psychiatry, 29*, 76-83.

Briere, J. (Ed.). (1991). *Treating victims of child sexual abuse.* San Francisco, CA: Jossey-Bass.

Clark, P. N., & Allen, A. (Eds.). (1985). *Occupational therapy for children.* St. Louis: Mosby.

Coons, P. M. (1986). Child abuse and multiple personality disorder: Review of the literature and suggestions for treatment. *Child Abuse and Neglect, 10*, 455-462.

Ebb, E. W., Coster, W., & Duncombe, L. (1989). Comparison of normal and psychosocially dysfunctional male adolescents. *Occupational Therapy in Mental Health, 9*(2), 53-74.

Erikson, E. H. (1969). *Identity, youth and crisis.* New York: Norton.

Esman, A. H. (1992). Treatment and services for adolescents: An introduction. *Hospital and Community Psychiatry, 43*, 616.

Fazio, L. S. (1992). Tell me a story: The therapeutic metaphor in the practice of pediatric occupational therapy. *American Journal of Occupational Therapy, 46*, 112-119.

Giles, G. M., & Schell, D. (1988). Occupational therapy in a behavior modification setting. In D. W. Scott & N. Katz (Eds.), *Occupational therapy in mental health: Principles in practice* (pp.105-115). New York: Taylor and Francis.

Goldston, S. E., Heinicke, C. M., Pynoos, R. S., & Yager, J. (Eds.). (1990). *Preventing mental health disturbances in childhood.* Washington, DC: American Psychiatric Press.

Hardison, J., & Llorens, L. A. (1988). Structured craft group activities for adolescent delinquent girls. *Occupational Therapy in Mental Health, 8*(3), 101-117.

Harrington, R. G. (Ed.). (1986). *Testing adolescents: A reference guide for psychological assessments.* Kansas City, MI: Test Corporation of America.

Herman, B. E. (1980). A sensory integration approach to the psychotic child. *Occupational Therapy in Mental Health, 1*(1), 57-68.

Jemerin, J. M., & Philips, I. (1988). Changes in inpatient child psychiatry: Consequences and recommendations. *Journal of the American Academy of Child and Adolescent Psychiatry, 27*, 397-403.

Jones, D., & McQuiston, M. G. (1988). *Interviewing the sexually abused child.* Washington, DC: American Psychiatric Press.

Kaufman, C. H., Daniels, R. D., Laverdure, P., Moyer, R., & Campana, L. (1988). Pediatric occupational therapy within a cognitive-behavioral setting. In D. W. Scott & N. Katz (Eds.), *Occupational therapy in mental health: Principles in practice* (pp. 88-104). New York: Taylor and Francis.

Keith, C. (1984). *The aggressive adolescent.* New York: Basic Books.

Kernberg, P. F. (1983). Update of borderline disorders in children. *Occupational Therapy in Mental Health, 3*(3), 83-91.

Kistenbaum, C. J., & Williams, D. T. (Eds.). (1988). *Handbook of clinical assessment of children and adolescents.* New York: University Press.

Klerman, G. L. (Ed.). (1986). *Suicide and depression among adolescents and young adults.* Washington, DC: American Psychiatric Press.

Kluft, R. P. (Ed.). (1985). *Childhood antecedents of multiple personality disorders.* Washington, DC: American Psychiatric Press.

Lahey, B., & Kazden, A. (Eds.). (1980). *Advances in child clinical psychology.* London: Pergamon.

Lancaster, J., & Mitchell, M. (1991). Occupational therapy treatment goals, objectives and activities for improving low self-esteem in adolescents with behavioral disorders. *Occupational Therapy in Mental Health, 11*(2/3), 3-22.

Llorens, L. A., & Rubin, E. (1967). *Developing ego functions in disturbed children.* Detroit: Lafayette Clinic.

Looney, J. G. (Ed.). (1988). *Chronic mental illness in children and adolescents.* Washington, DC: American Psychiatric Press.

Mayberry, W. (1990). Self-esteem in children: Considerations for measurement and intervention. *American Journal of Occupational Therapy, 44*, 729-734.

McKibbin, E., & King, J. (1983). Activity group counseling for learning-disabled children with behavior problems. *American Journal of Occupational Therapy, 36*, 433-437.

Melia, M. A., & Weikert, K. (1987). Evaluation and treatment of adolescents on a short-term unit. *Occupational Therapy in Mental Health, 7*(2), 51-66.

Nelson, D. L. (1989). *Children with autism and other pervasive disorders of development and behavior: Therapy through activities.* Thorofare, NJ: Slack.

Nelson, D. L. (1980/81). Evaluating autistic clients. *Occupational Therapy in Mental Health, 1*, 1-22.

Nemiroff, M. A., & Annunziata, J. (1990). *A child's first book of play therapy.* Washington, DC: American Psychological Association.

Neville, P., Kielhofner, G., & Royeen, C. B. (1985). Childhood. In G. Kielhofner (Ed.), *A model of human occupation: Theory and application* (pp. 82-98). Baltimore: Williams & Wilkins.

Ollendick, T. H., & Hersen, M. (Eds.). (1983). *The handbook of child psychopathology.* New York: Plenum.

Olson, L., Heaney, C., & Soppas-Hoffman, B. (1989). Parent-child activity group treatment in preventative psychiatry. *Occupational Therapy in Health Care, 6*, 29-43.

Ottenbacher, K. J. (1982). Vestibular processing dysfunction in children with severe emotional and behavioral disorders: A review. *Physical and Occupational Therapy in Pediatrics, 2*, 3-12.

Pennington, V., & Sharrot, G. W. (1985). The developmental tasks of adolescence and the role of occupational therapy. *Occupational Therapy in Health Care, 2*, 7-18.

Peterson, T. W. (1986). Recent studies in autism: A review of the literature. *Occupational Therapy in Mental Health, 6*(4), 63-75.

Pezzuti, L. (1985). Self-concept/self-esteem development: Its relevance to occupational therapy. *Occupational Therapy in Health Care, 2*, 41-48.

Pfeffer, C. R. (Ed.). (1989). *Suicide among youth: Perspectives on risk and prevention.* Washington, DC: American Psychiatric Press.

Popper, C. (Ed.). (1987). *Psychiatric pharmacosciences of children and adolescents.* Washington, DC: American Psychiatric Press.

Rapoport, J. L. (Ed.). (1989). *Obsessive-compulsive disorder in children and adolescents.* Washington, DC: American Psychiatric Press.

Reilly, M. (1974). *Play as exploratory behavior.* Newbury Park, CA: Sage.

Robinson, A. L. (1977). Play, the arena for acquisition of rules for competent behavior. *American Journal of Occupational Therapy, 31*, 248-253.

Robson, K. S. (1986). *Manual of child psychiatry.* Washington, DC: American Psychiatric Press.

Rutter, M., Tom, A. H., & Lann, I. S. (1988). *Assessment and diagnosis in child psychopathology.* New York: Guilford.

Santostefano, S. (1985). *Cognitive control therapy with children and adolescents.* Elmsford, NY: Pergamon Press.

Shafi, M., & Shafi, S. L. (Eds.). (1991). *Clinical guide to depression in children and adolescents.* Washington, DC: American Psychiatric Press.

Shannon, P. D. (1972). The adolescent experience. *American Journal of Occupational Therapy, 26*, 284-287.

Sholle-Martin, S., & Alessi, N. E. (1990). Formulating a role for occupational therapy in child psychiatry: A clinical application. *American Journal of Occupational Therapy, 44*, 871-882.

Sholle-Martin, S. (1987). Application of the model of human occupation: Assessment in child and adolescent psychiatry. *Occupational Therapy in Mental Health, 7*(2) 3-22.

Silver, L. B. (1991). *Attention-deficit hyperactivity disorder: A clinical guide to diagnosis and treatment.* Washington, DC: American Psychiatric Press.

Symntek, L., Barris, R., & Kielhofner, G. (1985). The model of human occupation applied to functional and dysfunctional adolescents. *Occupational Therapy in Mental Health, 5*(1), 21-39.

Trafford, G., & Boyd, S. (1988). Child and family psychiatry. In D. W. Scott & N. Katz (Eds.), *Occupational therapy in mental health: Principles in practice* (pp. 77-87). New York: Taylor and Francis.

Varni, J. W. (1983). *Clinical behavioral pediatrics—An interdisciplinary biobehavioral approach.* Elmsford, NY: Pergamon Press.

Weissenberg, R., & Giladi, N. (1989). Home economics day: A program for disturbed adolescents to promote acquisition of habits and skills. *Occupational Therapy in Mental Health, 9*(2), 89-103.

Wiener, J. M. (Ed.). (1991). *Textbook of child and adolescent psychiatry.* Washington, DC: American Psychiatric Press.

Willis, D. J., Bogwell, W., & Campbell, M. M. (Eds.). (1991a). *Child abuse: Abstracts of the psychological and behavioral literature, volume 1, 1967-1985.* Washington, DC: American Psychological Association.

Willis, D. J., Broyhill, G. C., & Campbell, M. M. (Eds.). (1991b). *Child abuse: Abstracts of the psychological and behavioral literature, volume 2, 1986-1990.* Washington, DC: American Psychological Association.

Documentation, Goal Setting, and Treatment Planning

Allen, C. K., Earhart, C. A., & Blue, T. (1992). *Occupational therapy treatment goals for the physically and cognitively disabled.* Rockville, MD: American Occupational Therapy Association.

American Occupational Therapy Association (1989). Uniform terminology for occupational therapy (2nd ed.). *American Journal of Occupational Therapy, 43*, 808-815.

American Occupational Therapy Association (1992). *Effective documentation for occupational therapy.* Rockville, MD: Author.

Denton, P. L. (1987). *Psychiatric occupational therapy: A workbook of practical skills.* Boston: Little, Brown.

Dunn, W., & McGourty, L. (1989). Application of uniform terminology to practice. *American Journal of Occupational Therapy, 43*, 817-831.

Hansen, S. (1983). Documentation simplified in acute psychiatry. *Mental Health Special Interest Section Newsletter, 6*(4), 1, 4.

Hemphill, B. J., Peterson, M. S., & Werner, P. C. (1991). *Rehabilitation in mental health: Goals and objectives for independent living.* New Jersey: Slack.

Kettenbach, G. (1990). *Writing S.O.A.P. notes*. Philadelphia: F. A. Davis.

Pagonis, J. F. (1989). Documentation. In K. Jacobs & M. Logigian (Eds.), *Functions of a manager in occupational therapy* (pp. 111-144). Thorofare, NJ: Slack.

Payton, O. D., Nelson, C. E., & Ozer, M. N. (1990). *Patient participation in program planning: A manual for therapists*. Philadelphia: F. A. Davis.

Pelland, M. J. (1987). A conceptual model for the instruction and supervision of treatment planning. *American Journal of Occupational Therapy, 41*, 351-359.

Peloquin, S. (1986). Uniform terminology as a basis for goal formation. *Occupational Therapy in Mental Health, 6*(4), 49-63.

Scott, A. H., & Haggarty, E. J. (1984). Structuring goals via goal attainment scaling in occupational therapy groups in a partial hospitalization setting. *Occupational Therapy in Mental Health, 4*(2), 39-59.

Eating Disorders

Agras, W. S., & Kraemer, H. C. (1983). The treatment of anorexia nervosa: Do different treatments have different outcomes? *Psychiatric Annals, 13*, 928-935.

Alexander, N. (1986). Characteristics and treatment of families with anorectic offspring. *Occupational Therapy in Mental Health, 6*(1), 117-135.

Anderson, A. E. (1985). *Practical comprehensive treatment of anorexia nervosa and bulimia*. Baltimore: Johns Hopkins University Press.

Bailey, M. K. (1986). Occupational therapy for patients with eating disorders. *Occupational Therapy in Mental Health, 6*(1), 89-116.

Barris, R. (1986). Occupational dysfunction and eating disorders: Theory and approach to treatment. *Occupational Therapy in Mental Health, 6*(1), 27-45.

Birtchnell, S. A., Lacey, J. H., & and Harte, A. (1985). Body image distortion in bulimia nervosa. *British Journal of Psychiatry, 147*, 408-412.

Brotman, A. W., Herzok, D. B., & Hamburg, P. (1988). Long-term course in 14 bulimic patients treated with psychotherapy. *Journal of Clinical Psychiatry, 49*, 157-160.

Bruch, H. (1973). *Eating disorders, obesity, anorexia nervosa and the person within*. New York: Basic Books.

Bruch, H. (1978). *The golden cage: The enigma of anorexia nervosa*. Cambridge, MA: Harvard University Press.

Bruch, H. (1982). Anorexia nervosa: Therapy and theory. *American Journal of Psychiatry, 139*, 1531-1538.

Brumberg, J. J. (1989). *Fasting girls: The history of anorexia nervosa*. New York: New American Library.

Cooper, R. C., Halmi, K. A., Goldberg, S. C., Eckert, E.D., & Davis, J. M. (1979). Disturbance in body image estimation as related to other characteristics and outcome of anorexia nervosa. *British Journal of Psychiatry, 134*, 60-66.

Crisp, A. H., Norton, K. R. S., Jurczak, S., Bowyer, C., & Duncan, S. (1985). A treatment approach to anorexia nervosa—25 years on. *Journal of Psychiatric Research, 19*(2/3), 393-404.

Darby, P. L., Garfinkel, P. E., Garner, D. M., & Coscina, D. V. (Eds.). (1983). *Anorexia nervosa*. New York: Liss.

Fairburn, C. (1981). A cognitive-behavioral approach to bulimia. *Psychological Medicine, 11*, 707-711.

Garfinkel, P. E., & Garner, D. M. (1982). *Anorexia nervosa: A multidimensional perspective*. New York: Brunner/Mazel.

Garfinkel, P. E., Garner, D. M., & Goldbloom, D. S. (1987). Eating disorders: Implications for the 1990s. *Canadian Journal of Psychiatry, 32*, 624-631.

Garner, D. M., & Garfinkel, P. E. (1980). Sociocultural factors in the development of anorexia nervosa. *Psychological Medicine, 10*, 647-656.

Giles, G. M. (1985). Anorexia nervosa and bulimia: An activity oriented approach. *American Journal of Occupational Therapy, 39*, 510-517.

Giles, G. M., & Allen, M. E. (1986). Occupational therapy in the rehabilitation of the patient with anorexia nervosa. *Occupational Therapy in Mental Health, 6*(1), 47-66.

Hall, A. (1987). The place of family therapy in the treatment of anorexia nervosa. *Australian and New Zealand Journal of Psychiatry, 21*, 568-574.

Lucus, A. R. (1981). Toward an understanding of anorexia nervosa as a disease entity. *Mayo Clinic Proceedings, 56*, 254-264.

McColl, M. A., Friedland, J., & Kerr, A. (1986). When doing is not enough: The relationship between activity and effectiveness in anorexia nervosa. *Occupational Therapy in Mental Health, 6*(1), 137-150.

McGee, K. T., & McGee, J. P. (1986). Behavioral treatment of eating disorders. *Occupational Therapy in Mental Health, 6*(1), 15-25.

Meyers, S. K. (1989). Occupational therapy treatment of an adult with an eating disorder: One woman's experience. *Occupational Therapy in Mental Health, 9*(1), 33-47.

Minuchin, S., Rosman, B. L., & Baker, L. (1978). *Psychosomatic families: Anorexia nervosa in context*. Cambridge, MA: Harvard University Press.

Piran, N., & Kaplan, A. S. (1990). *A day hospital group treatment program for anorexia nervosa and bulimia nervosa*. New York: Brunner/Mazel.

Posobiec, K., & Renfrew, J. W. (1988). Successful self management of severe bulimia: A case study. *Journal of Behavior Therapy and Experimental Psychiatry, 19*(1), 63-68.

Roth, D. (1986). Treatment of the hospitalized eating disorder patient. *Occupational Therapy in Mental Health, 6*(1), 67-87.

Russell, G. F. (1985). The changing nature of anorexia nervosa: An introduction to the conference. *Journal of Psychiatric Research, 19*(2/3), 101-109.

Shimp, S. L. (1989, September). Short-term treatment for eating disorder patients with a high-level of functioning. *Mental Health Special Interest Section Newsletter*, pp. 1-3.

Slade, P. (1985). A review of body image studies in anorexia nervosa and bulimia nervosa. *Journal of Psychiatric Research, 19*(2/3), 253-265.

Stanton, E., Mann, W. C., & Klyczek, J. P. (1991). Use of the Bay area functional performance evaluation with eating disordered patients. *Occupational Therapy Journal of Research, 11*, 227-237.

Vandereycken, W. (1985). Inpatient treatment of anorexia nervosa: Some research guides change. *Journal of Psychiatric Research, 19*(2/3), 413-422.

Vigersky, R. A. (Ed.). (1977). *Anorexia nervosa*. New York: Raven Press.

Weinstein, H. M., & Richman, A. (1984). The group treatment of bulimia. *Journal of American College Health, 32*, 208-215.

Wilson, G. I., Rossiter, E., Kleifield, E. I., & Lindholm, L. (1986). Cognitive behavioral treatment of bulimia nervosa: A controlled evaluation. *Behavior Research and Therapy, 24*(3), 277-288.

Yager, J. (1988). The treatment of eating disorders. *Journal of Clinical Psychiatry, 49*, 18-25.

Yates, W. R., & Sreleni, B. (1987). Anorexia and bulimia. *Primary Care: Clinics in Office Practice, 14*, 737-744.

Education

See Vocational Rehabilitation and Education

Family and Social Supports

Abrams, A. J., & Abrams, M. A. (1990). *The first whole rehab catalog: A comprehensive guide to products and services for the physically disadvantaged*. Crozet, VA: Betterway Publications, Inc.

Allen-Burhet, G. (1988). *Time well spent: A manual for visiting older adults*. Madison, WI: Bi-Folkal Productions.

American Association of Homes for the Aging. (1985). *Guide to caring for the mentally impaired elderly*. Washington, DC: Author.

American Association of Retired Persons (1985). *Your home, your choice. A workbook for older people and their families*. Washington, DC: Author.

Anderson, C. M., Hogarty, W., & Reiss, D. J. (1980). Family treatment of adult schizophrenic patients: A psychoeducational approach. *Schizophrenia Bulletin, 6*, 490-505.

Anderson, C. M., Reiss, D. J., & Hogarty, C. E. (1986). *Schizophrenia and the family: A practitioner's guide to psychoeducation and management*. New York: Guilford.

Anderson, J., & Hinojosa, J. (1984). Parents and therapists in a professional partnership. *American Journal of Occupational Therapy, 38*, 452-461.

Anthony-Bergstone, C., Zarit, S. H., & Gatz, M. (1988). Symptoms of psychological distress among caregivers of dementia patients. *Psychology and Aging, 3*, 245-248.

Arieti, S. (1979). *Understanding and helping the schizophrenic: A guide for family and friends*. New York: Simon & Schuster.

Asrael, W. (1982). An approach to motherhood for disabled women. *Rehabilitation Literature, 43*(7-8), 214-218.

Baker, B. L., & Brightman, A. J. (1989). *Steps to independence: A skills training guide for parents and teachers of children with special needs* (2nd ed.). Baltimore: Paul H. Brookes Publishing Company.

Barnes & Crutchfield. (1984). *The patient at home*. Thorofare, NJ: Slack.

Bass, D. M., & Noelker, L. S. (1987). The influence of family caregivers on elder's use of in-home services: An expanded conceptual framework. *Journal of Health and Social Behavior, 28*, 184-196.

Baxter, W. E. (1992). *Stigma*. Washington, DC: Hospital and Community Psychiatry Service.

Beck, A. (1988). *Love is never enough*. New York: Harper & Row.

Begmagin, V., & Hirn, K. (1979). *Aging is a family affair*. New York: Thomas Y. Crowell.

Bernheim, K. F., & Lehman, A. F. (1985). *Working with families of the mentally ill*. New York: Norton.

Biegel, D. E., & Blum, A. (Eds.). (1990). *Aging and caregiving: Theory, research and policy*. Newbury Park, CA: Sage.

Biegel, D. E., & Yamatani, H. (1987). Help-giving in self-help groups. *Hospital and Community Psychiatry, 38*, 1195-1197.

Blandin, M. (1987, December). Concurrent support groups for persons with early-stage Alzheimer's disease and for their caregivers. *Gerontology Special Interest Section Newsletter*, p. 5.

Bowers, B. J. (1987). Intergenerational caregiving: Adult caregivers and their aging parents. *Advanced Nursing Science, 9*, 20-31.

Brinson, M. H. (1989, December). Support groups for families of persons with mental illness. *Mental Health Special Interest Section Newsletter*, pp. 3-5.

Brody, E. M. (1985). Patient care as a normative family stress. *Gerontologist, 25*, 19-29.

Burnfield, A. (1985). *Multiple sclerosis: A personal exploration*. New York: Demos Publications.

Butin, D. (1989, November/December). Helping Alzheimer's patients live at home. *Senior Patient*, 72-76.

Cantor, M. (1983). Strain among caregivers: A study of experience in the United States. *Gerontologist, 23*, 597-603.

Cantor, N. M. (1979). Neighbors and friends: An overlooked resource in the informal support system. *Research on Aging, 1*, 434-463.

Carroll, D. (1989). *When your loved one has Alzheimer's disease*. New York: Harper & Row.

Chenoweth, B., & Spencer, B. (1986). Dementia: The experience of family caregivers. *Gerontologist, 26*, 267-272.

Clark, N. M., & Rakowski, W. (1983). Family caregivers of older adults: Improving helping skills. *Gerontologist, 23*, 637-642.

Cohen, D., & Eisendorfer, C. (1986). *The loss of self: A family resource for the care of Alzheimer's disease and related disorders*. New York: Norton.

Cohler, B., Groves, L., Borden, W., & Lasarus, L. (1989). Caring for family members with Alzheimer's disease. In E. Light & B. Lebowitz (Eds.), *Alzheimer's disease, treatment, and family stress: Directions for research* (pp. 50-105). Washington, DC: U.S. Government Printing Office.

Cole, H. A. (1991). *Helpmates*. Louisville, KY: Westminster/John Knox Press.

Committee on Psychiatry and the Community (1987). *A family affair: Helping families cope with mental illness.* New York: Brunner/Mazel.

Coons, D. H., Metzelaar, L., Robinson, A., & Spencer, B. (Eds.). (1986). *A better life: Helping family members, volunteers, and staff improve the quality of life of nursing home residents suffering from Alzheimer's disease and related disorders.* Columbus, OH: The Source for Nursing Home Literature.

Cotton, D. H. (1990). *Stress Management: An integrated approach to therapy.* New York: Brunner/Mazel.

Covell, M. (1983). *The home alternative to hospitals and nursing homes.* New York: Holt, Rinehart & Winston.

Curley, J. (1987, December). Care for the caregiver: A support group for caregivers of persons with Alzheimer's disease. *Gerontology Special Interest Section Newsletter,* pp. 4-8.

Dayton-Ingersoll, B., Chapman, N., & Neal, M. (1990). A program for caregivers in the workplace. *Gerontologist, 29,* 195-202.

DeBoskey, D. S., Hecht, J. S., & Calub, C. (1991). *A guide for families of the head injured.* Rockville, MD: Aspen Publishers.

Deimling, G., & Bass, D. M. (1986). Symptoms of mental impairments among elderly adults and their effects on family caregivers. *Journal of Gerontology, 41,* 778-784.

Deimling, G., Bass, D. M., Townsend, A., & Noelker, L. (1989). Care-related stress: A comparison of spouse and adult child caregivers in shared and separate households. *Journal of Aging and Health, 1,* 67-82.

Eggert, G., Granger, C., Morris, K., & Pendleton, S. (1977). Caring for the patient with long-term disability. *Geriatrics, 32,* 102.

Evans, R., Held, S., Kleinman, L., & Halar, E. (1985). Family stroke education: Increasing patient and family involvement in rehabilitation. *Occupational Therapy in Health Care, 2*(1), 63-71.

Eyde, D. R., & Rich, J. A. (1983). *Psychological distress in aging: A family management model.* Rockville, MD: Aspen Systems.

Fallon, I. R. H., Boyd, J. L., & McGill, C. W. (1985). *Family care of schizophrenia.* New York: Guilford.

Featherstone, H. (1981). *A difference in the family: Living with a disabled child.* New York: Penguin.

Felder, L. (1991). *When a loved one is ill: How to take better care of your loved one, your family, and yourself.* Levittown, PA: The Phoenix Society.

Fewell, R., & Vadasy, P. (Eds.). (1986). *Families of handicapped children: Needs and supports across the life span.* Austin, TX: Pro-Ed.

Fieve, R. (1975). *Moodswing.* New York: Bantam Books.

Figley, C. (1989). *Treating stress in families.* New York: Brunner/Mazel.

France, R. D., & Krishnan, K. R. (Eds.). (1988). *Chronic pain.* Washington, DC: American Psychiatric Press.

Freeman, D., & Trute, B. (Eds.). (1981). *Treating families with special needs.* Alberta, Canada: Alberta Association of Social Workers.

Gallagher, D., Rose, J., Rivera, P., Lovett, S., & Thompson, L. W. (1989). Prevalence of depression in family caregivers. *Gerontologist, 29,* 449-456.

Gartner, A., Lipsky, D. K., & Turnbell, A. P. (1991). *Supporting families with a child with a disability.* Baltimore: Paul H. Brookes Publishing Company.

Gatz, M., Bengtson, V. L., & Blum, M. J. (1990). Caregiving families. In J. E. Birren & K. W. Schaie (Eds.), *Handbook of the psychology of aging* (3rd ed.) (pp. 405-426). New York: Academic Press.

George, L., & Gwyther, L. (1986). Caregiver well-being: A multidimensional examination of family caregivers of demented adults. *Gerontologist, 26,* 253-259.

Geralis, E. (Ed.). (1991). *Children with cerebral palsy: A parent's guide.* Rockville, MD: Woodbine House Inc.

Gessert, V. G. (1987, December). Living room: A support group for families with aging relatives. *Gerontology Special Interest Section Newsletter,* pp. 1-3.

Giles, J. (1988). *Caregiving: When someone you love grows old.* Wheaton, IL: Harold Shaw Publishers.

Goldfarb, L. A., Brotherson, M. J., Summers, J. A., & Turnbull, A. (1986). *Meeting the challenge of disability or chronic illness: A family guide.* Baltimore: Paul H. Brookes Publishing Company.

Greene, V. L., & Monahan, D. J. (1989). An analysis of the effect of a support and education program on stress and burden among family caregivers to frail elderly. *Gerontologist, 29,* 472-477.

Hasselkus, B. R. (1988). Meaning in family caregiving: Perspectives on caregiver/professional relationships. *Gerontologist, 28,* 686-691.

Hasselkus, B. R. (1989). The meaning of daily activity in family caregiving for the elderly. *American Journal of Occupational Therapy, 43,* 649-656.

Hasselkus, B. R., & Brown, M. (1983). Respite care for the community elderly. *American Journal of Occupational Therapy, 37,* 83-88.

Hatfield, A. B. (1983). *Coping with mental illness in the family.* College Park, MD: University of Maryland Press.

Hatfield, A. B. (1990). *Family education in mental illness.* New York: Guilford.

Hatfield, A. B., & Lefley, H. P. (Eds.). (1987). *Families of the mentally ill: Coping and adaptation.* New York: Guilford.

Hinkley, J., & Hinkley, J. (1985). *Breaking points.* Grand Rapids, MI: Chosen Books.

Hinojosa, J., Anderson, J., & Strauch, C. (1988). Pediatric occupational therapy in the home. *American Journal of Occupational Therapy, 43,* 17-22.

Horne, J. (1985). *Caregiving: Helping an aging loved one.* Washington, DC: AARP Books.

Howell, M. (1973). *Helping ourselves: Families and the human network.* Boston: Beacon Press.

Ipeler, B. (1986). *Parenting your disabled child.* Philadelphia: Westminister.

Jacob, M., Frank, E., Kupfer, D., Cornes, C., & Carpenter, L. (1987). A psychoeducational workshop for depressed patients, family, and friends: Description and evaluation. *Hospital and Community Psychiatry, 38,* 968-972.

Jed, J. (1989). Social support for caregivers and psychiatric rehospitalization. *Hospital and Community Psychiatry, 40,* 1297-1299.

Kaplan, H. B. (Ed.). (1983). *Psychosocial stress: Trends in theory and research.* New York: Academic Press.

Keitner, G. I. (Ed.). (1990). *Depression and families: Impact and treatment.* Washington, DC: American Psychiatric Press.

Kenny, J., & Spicer, S. (1984). *Caring for your aging parents: A practical guide to the challenges, the choices.* Cincinnati, OH: St. Anthony Messenger Press.

Killeffer, E. H., & Bennett, R. (Eds.). (1990). *Successful models of community long-term care services for the elderly.* New York: Haworth Press.

Kinney, J. M., & Stephens, M. A. P. (1989a). Caregiving hassles scale: Assessing the daily hassles of caring for a family member with dementia. *Gerontologist, 29,* 328-332.

Kinney, J. M., & Stephens, M. A. P. (1989b). Hassles and uplifts of giving care to a family member with dementia. *Psychology and Aging, 4,* 402-408.

Korpell, H. (1984). *How you can help: A guide for families of psychiatric patients.* Washington, DC: American Psychiatric Press.

Kyle, S., & Taylor, P. (1983). Developing a group for friends and families of schizophrenics: A hospital model. *Canadian Mental Health, 31*(4), 14, 25.

Lawton, M. P., Brody, E. M., & Saperstein, A. R. (1989). A controlled study of respite services for caregivers of Alzheimer's patients. *Gerontologist, 29,* 8-16.

Lebowitz, B. D. (1985). Family caregiving in old age. *Hospital and Community Psychiatry, 36,* 457-458.

Lefley, H. P. (1992). Expressed emotion: Conceptual, clinical and social policy issues. *Hospital and Community Psychiatry, 43,* 591-598.

Lefley, H. P., & Johnson, D. L. (Eds.). (1990). *Families as allies in treatment of the mentally ill: New directions for mental health professionals.* Washington, DC: American Psychiatric Press.

Lester, A., & Lester, J. (1980). *Understanding aging parents.* Philadelphia: Westminster.

Liberman, R. P., Mueser, K. T., Wallace, C. J., Jacobs, H. E., Eckman, T., & Massell, H. K. (1986). Training skills in the psychiatrically disabled: Learning coping and competence. *Schizophrenia Bulletin, 12,* 631-647.

Liebermann, M. (1979). *Self-help groups for coping with crisis: Origins, members, processes and impact.* San Francisco: Jossey-Bass.

Lieff, J. D. (1984). *Your parent's keeper: A handbook of psychiatric care for the elderly.* Cambridge, MA: Ballinger Publishing.

Lindsay, A. M., & Hughes, E. M. (1981). Social support and alternatives to institutionalization for the at-risk elderly. *Journal of the American Geriatric Society, 24,* 308-314.

Litwak, E. (1985). *Helping the elderly: The complementary roles of informal networks and formal systems.* New York: Guilford.

Lobato, D. J. (1990). *Brothers, sisters and special needs: Information and activities for helping young siblings of children with chronic illnesses and developmental disabilities.* Baltimore: Paul H. Brookes Publishing Company.

Ludwig, F. M. (1987, December). Caregiving and developmental issues during middle age. *Gerontology Special Interest Section Newsletter,* pp. 2-6.

Mace, N., & Rabins, P. (1981). *The 36-hour day: A family guide to caring for persons with Alzheimer's disease, related dementia illnesses and memory loss in later life.* Baltimore: Johns Hopkins University Press.

Maddox, S. (1987). *Spinal network: The total resource for the wheelchair community.* Boulder, CO: Spinal Network.

Matorin, S., & Greenberg, L. (1992). Family therapy in the treatment of adolescents. *Hospital and Community Psychiatry, 43,* 625-629.

McClurg, E. (1986). *Your Down syndrome child: Everything today's parents need to know about raising their special child.* New York: Doubleday.

Middleton, L. (1984). *Alzheimer's family support groups: A manual for group facilities.* Tampa, FL: Sun Coast Gerontology Center.

Miller, T. (1988). Advances in understanding the impact of stressful life events in health. *Hospital and Community Psychiatry, 39,* 615-621.

Montgomery, R. J. V., & Borgatta, E. F. (1989). The effects of alternative support strategies on family caregiving. *Gerontologist, 29,* 457-464.

Montgomery, R. J. V., Gonyea, J. G., & Hooyman, N. R. (1985). Caregiving and the experience of subject and objective burden. *Family Relations, 34,* 19-26.

Morycz, R. K. (1985). Caregiving strain and the desire to institutionalize family members with Alzheimer's disease. *Research on Aging, 7,* 329-361.

Mosher, L., & Keith, S. (1980). Psychosocial treatment: Individual, group, family and community support approaches. In Mosher and Keith (Eds.), *Special report: Schizophrenia, 1980* (pp. 127-158). Washington, DC: National Institute of Mental Health.

Myers, J. E. (1988). The mid/late life generation cap: Adult children with aging parents. *Journal of counseling and development, 66,* 331-335.

Nassif, J. Z. (1985). *The home health care solution: A complete consumer guide.* New York: Harper & Row.

National Council on the Aging. (1982). *Adult day care annotated bibliography.* Washington, DC: Author.

New York City Alzheimer's Resource Center. (1985). *Caring: A family guide to managing the Alzheimer's patient at home.* New York: Author.

Niebuhr, S., & Royse. (1989). *Take care: A guide for caregivers on how to improve their self-care.* St. Paul, MN: The Wilder Foundation.

Noelker, L. S., & Bass, D. M. (1989). Home care for elderly persons: Linkages between formal and informal caregivers. *Journal of Gerontology, 44,* 563-572.

North, C. S. (1987). *Welcome silence: My triumph over schizophrenia.* New York: Simon & Schuster.

Park, C., & Shapiro, L. (1976). *You are not alone: Understanding and dealing with mental illness.* Boston: Little, Brown.

Pearlin, L. I., Mullan, J. T., Semple, S. J., & Skaff, M. M. (1989). *Caregiving and the stress process: An overview of concepts and their measures.* Paper presented at the 42nd annual scientific meeting of the Gerontological Society of America, Minneapolis, MN.

Pearlin, L. I., Turner, H. A., & Semple, S. J. (1989). Coping and the mediation of caregiver stress. In E. Light & B. Lebowitz (Eds.), *Alzheimer's disease treatment and family stress: Directions for research* (pp. 198-217). Washington, DC: National Institute of Mental Health.

Pelletier, K. R. (1983). Stress management: An approach to optimum health and longevity. *Generations, 7*(3), 26-29.

Petrila, J. P., & Sadoff, R. L. (1992). Confidentiality and the family as caregiver. *Hospital and Community Psychiatry, 43*, 136-139.

Pierce, D. (Ed.). (1989, March). Occupational therapy and the family [Special issue]. *Developmental Disabilities Special Interest Section Newsletter.*

Pitzele, S. K. (1985). *We are not alone: Learning to live with chronic illness.* New York: Workman Publishing.

Post, K. (Ed.). (1989, June). Childbearing and parenting by persons with physical disabilities [Special issue]. *Physical Disabilities Special Interest Section Newsletter.*

Poulshock, W., & Deimling, G. (1984). Families caring for elders in residence: Issues in the measurement of burden. *Journal of Gerontology, 39*, 230-239.

Powell, C. S. (1989, December 11). How can we, as therapists, help the families of the critically ill? *Occupational Therapy Forum,* pp. 8-11.

Powell, L. S. (1983). *Alzheimer's disease: A guide for families.* Reading, MA: Addison-Wesley.

Powell, T. J. (1990). *Working with self-help.* Silver Spring, MD: NASW Press.

Powers, P. W. (1985). Family coping behaviors in chronic illness: A rehabilitation perspective. *Rehabilitation Literature, 46*(3-4), 78-83.

Pruchno, R. A., & Resch, N. L. (1989). Aberrant behaviors and Alzheimer's disease: Mental health effects on spouse caregivers. *Journal of Gerontology: Social Sciences, 44*(5), S177-182.

Pueschel, S., Bernier, J., & Weidenmann, L. (1988). *The special child.* Baltimore: Paul H. Brookes Publishing Company.

Radomski, M. V., & Dougherty, P. M. (Eds.). (1990). *The caregiving alliance: Enhancing collaboration between therapist and caregiver.* Rockville, MD: Aspen Publishers.

Register, C. (1988). *Living with chronic illness: Days of patience and passion.* New York: Macmillan.

Reisberg, B. (1983). *A guide to Alzheimer's disease for families, spouses, and friends.* New York: Free Press.

Roach, M. (1985). *Another name for madness.* Boston: Houghton Mifflin.

Robinson, B. (1983). Validation of a caregiver strain index. *Journal of Gerontology, 38*, 344-348.

Rosenfeld, A. H. (1982). Closing the revolving door through family therapy. Optimal community management of schizophrenia. *Hospital and Community Psychiatry, 33*(11), 893-894.

Rossner, L. J. (1987). *Multiple sclerosis: New hope and practical advice for people with MS and their families.* Englewood Cliffs, NJ: Prentice Hall.

Rzetelney, H., & Mellor, J. (1981). *Support groups for caregivers of the aged: A training manual for facilitators.* New York: Community Services Society.

Sachs, P. R. (1991). *Treating families of brain-injury survivors.* New York: Springer.

Scheinberg, L., & Holland, N. (1987). *Multiple sclerosis: A guide for patients and their families* (2nd ed.). New York: Raven Press.

Scheinberg, L., & Schneider, D. (1987). *Voluntary health organizations: A guide to patient services.* New York: Demos Publications.

Schlacter, G., & Weber, R. D. (1990). *Financial aid for the disabled and their families.* San Carlos, CA: Reference Service Press.

Schmidt, G. L., & Keyes, B. (1985). Group psychotherapy with family caregivers of demented patients. *Gerontologist, 25*, 347-350.

Schuman, R., & Schwartz, J. (1988). *Understanding multiple sclerosis: A new handbook for families.* New York: Charles Scribers Sons.

Seeman, M., Littman, S., Thornton, J., Jeffries, J., & Plummer, K. (1982). *Living and working with schizophrenia.* New York: Plume Books.

Seligman, M., & Benjamin, D. (1989). *Ordinary families: Special children: A system approach to childhood disability.* New York: Guilford.

Shanas, E. (1979). The family as a social support system in old age. *Gerontologist, 19*, 169-174.

Silver, L. (1988). *The misunderstood child: A guide for parents of learning disabled children.* New York: McGraw-Hill.

Silverman, I. (1989). Children of psychiatrically-ill parents: A prevention perspective. *Hospital and Community Psychiatry, 40*, 1257-1265.

Silverstone, B., & Hyman, H. (1976). *You and your aging parent: The modern family's guide to emotional, physical, and financial problems.* New York: Pantheon Books.

Springer, D., & Brubaker, T. (1984). *Family caregiving and dependent elderly.* Beverly Hills, CA: Sage.

Stoller, E. P., & Earl, L. L. (1983). Help with activities of everyday life: Sources of support for the non-institutionalized elderly. *Gerontologist, 23*, 64-70.

Stone, R., Cafferata, G. L., & Sangl, J. (1986). *Caregivers of the frail elderly: A national profile.* Rockville, MD: National Center for Health Services Research.

Strachan, A. M. (1986). Family intervention for the rehabilitation of schizophrenia. Toward protection and coping. *Schizophrenia Bulletin, 12*, 678-698.

Strong, M. (1988). *Mainstay: For the well spouse of the chronically ill.* Boston: Little, Brown.

Taylor, R. L., Lam, D. J., Roppel, C. E., & Barter, J. (1984). Friends can be good medicine: An excursion into mental health promotion, mass media and intensive community participation. *Community Mental Health Journal, 20*, 294-303.

Tessler, R. C., Bernstein, A. G., Rosen, B. M., & Goldman, H. H. (1982). The chronically mentally ill community support systems. *Hospital and Community Psychiatry, 33*, 208-211.

Thompson, C. E. (1986). *Raising a handicapped child: A helpful guide for parents of the physically disabled.* New York: William Morrow.

Tingey-Michaelis, C. (1983). *Handicapped infants and children: A handbook for parents and professionals.* Austin, TX: Pro-Ed.

Torrey, E. F. (1983). *Surviving schizophrenia: A manual for families.* New York: Harper & Row.

Toseland, R. W., Rossiter, C. M., & Labrecque, M. S. (1989). The effectiveness of peer-led and professionally-led groups to support family caregivers. *Gerontologist, 29*, 465-471.

Turnbull, A. P., & Turnbull, H. R. (1985). *Parents speak out: Then and now.* Columbus, OH: Merrill Publishing Company.

Turnbull, A. P., & Turnbull, H. R. (1986). *Families, professionals, and exceptionality: A special partnership.* Columbus, OH: Merrill Publishing Company.

Vine, P. (1982). *Families in pain.* New York: Pantheon Books.

Walsh, N. (1985). *Schizophrenia: Straight talk for families and friends.* New York: William Morrow.

Wasow, M. (1982). *Coping with schizophrenia: A survival manual.* Palo Alto, CA: Science and Behavior.

Wolf, J. (1991). *Fall down seven times, get up eight: Living well with multiple sclerosis.* Rutland, VT: Academy Books.

Wolf, J. (Ed.). (1987). *Mastering multiple sclerosis: A handbook for MSers and families.* Rutland, VT: Academy Books.

Wood, J. (1987, August/September). Labors of love: What will you do when it's your turn to take care of a loved one? *Modern Maturity,* pp. 28-34, 90-94.

Zarit, S., Orr, N., & Zarit, J. (1985). *The hidden victims of Alzheimer's disease: Families under stress.* New York: University Press.

Zisserman, L. (1981). The modern family and rehabilitation of the handicapped: A macrosociological view. *American Journal of Occupational Therapy, 35*, 13-20.

Zweben, A. (1979). Family care for the mentally ill: A new perspective. *Social Work in Health Care, 5*(2), 205-217.

Frames of Reference/Practice Models

Allen, C. K. (1985). *Occupational therapy for psychiatric diseases: Measurement and management of cognitive disabilities.* Boston: Little, Brown.

Anthony, W. A. (1980). *The principles of psychiatric rehabilitation.* Baltimore: University Park Press.

Anthony, W., Cohen, M., & Cohen, B. (1983). The philosophy, treatment process and principles of the psychiatric rehabilitation approach. *New Directions in Mental Health, 17*, 67-79.

Barris, R. (1982). Environmental interactions: An extension of the model of human occupation. *American Journal of Occupational Therapy, 36*, 637-644.

Barris, R., Keilhofner, G., & Watts, J. (1983). *Psychosocial occupational therapy: Practice in a pluralistic arena.* Laurel, MD: RAMSCO.

Bruce, M. A., & Borg, B. (1987). *Frames of reference in psychosocial occupational therapy.* Thorofare, NJ: Slack.

Christiansen, C. H., & Baum, C. M. (Eds.). (1991). *Occupational therapy: Overcoming human performance deficits.* Thorofare, NJ: Slack.

Clark, P. N. (1979a). Human development through occupation: A philosophy and conceptual model for practice, part 1. *American Journal of Occupational Therapy, 33*, 505-514.

Clark, P. N. (1979b). Human development through occupation: A philosophy and conceptual model for practice, part 2. *American Journal of Occupational Therapy, 33*, 577-585.

Cynkin, S. (1979). *Occupational therapy toward health through activities.* Boston: Little, Brown.

Cynkin, S., & Robinson, A. M. (1990). *Occupational therapy and activities health: Toward health through activities.* Boston: Little, Brown.

Diasio, K. (1968). Psychiatric occupational therapy: Search for a conceptual framework in light of psychoanalytic ego psychology and learning theory. *American Journal of Occupational Therapy, 22*, 400-414.

Early, M. B. (1987). *Mental health concepts and techniques for the occupational therapy assistant.* New York: Raven Press.

Fidler, G. S., & Fidler, J. W. (1963). *A communication process in psychiatry: Occupational therapy.* New York: Macmillan.

Fidler, G. S., & Fidler, J. W. (1978). Doing and becoming: Purposeful action and self-actualization. *American Journal of Occupational Therapy, 32*, 305-310.

Fine, S. B. (1983). *Occupational therapy: The role of rehabilitation and purposeful activity in mental health practice.* Rockville, MD: American Occupational Therapy Association.

Howe, M. C., & Briggs, A. K. (1982). Ecological systems: Model for occupational therapy. *American Journal of Occupational Therapy, 36*, 322-327.

Katz, N. (1985). Occupational therapy's domain of concern: Reconsidered. *American Journal of Occupational Therapy, 39*, 518-524.

Kielhofner, G. (1978). General systems theory: Implications for theory and action in occupational therapy. *American Journal of Occupational Therapy, 32*, 637-645.

Kielhofner, G. (1982). A heritage of activity: Development of theory. *American Journal of Occupational Therapy, 36*, 723-730.

Kielhofner, G. (Ed.). (1985). *A model of human occupation: Theory and practice.* Baltimore: Williams & Wilkins.

Kielhofner, G. (1992). *Conceptual foundations of occupational therapy.* Philadelphia: F. A. Davis.

King, L. J. (1985). Toward a science of adaptive responses. In AOTA (Ed.), *A professional legacy: The Eleanor Clark Slagle lectures in occupational therapy, 1955-1984* (pp. 311-329). Rockville, MD: Editor.

Liberman, R. P., & Foy, D. W. (1983). Psychiatric rehabilitation for chronic mental patients. *Psychiatric Annals, 13*, 539-545.

Lillie, M. D., & Armstrong, H. E. (1982). Contributions to the development of psychoeducational approaches to mental health service. *American Journal of Occupational Therapy, 36,* 438-443.

Llorens, L. A. (1976). *Application of developmental theory for health and rehabilitation.* Rockville, MD: American Occupational Therapy Association.

Llorens, L. A. (1984). Theoretical conceptualization of occupational therapy: 1960-1982. *Occupational Therapy in Mental Health, 4*(2), 1-14.

Madden, A. (1984). Explaining psychiatric occupational therapy: An art in itself? *British Journal of Occupational Therapy, 47,* 15-17.

Miller, B. R. J., Sieg, K. W., Ludwig, F. M., Shortridge, S. D., & Van Deusen, J. (1988). *Six perspectives on theory for the practice of occupational therapy.* Rockville, MD: Aspen Publishers.

Mosey, A. C. (1974). An alternative: The biopsychosocial model. *American Journal of Occupational Therapy, 28,* 137-140.

Mosey, A. C. (1981). *Occupational therapy—Configuration of a profession.* New York: Raven Press.

Mosey, A. C. (1985). Eleanor Clarke Slagle lecture, 1985—A monistic or a pluralistic approach to professional identity. *American Journal of Occupational Therapy, 39,* 504-509.

Mosey, A. C. (1986). *Psychosocial components of occupational therapy.* New York: Raven Press.

Mosey, A. C. (1992). *Applied scientific inquiry in the health care professions: An epistemological orientation.* Rockville, MD: American Occupational Therapy Association.

Neville, A. (1985, March). The model of human occupation and depression. *Mental Health Special Interest Section Newsletter,* pp. 1, 3-4.

Reed, K. L. (1984). *Models of practice in occupational therapy.* Baltimore: Williams & Wilkins.

Rogers, J. C. (1982). Order and disorder in medicine and occupational therapy. *American Journal of Occupational Therapy, 36,* 199-202.

Serrett, K. D. (Ed.). (1985). Philosophical and historical roots of occupational therapy [Special issue]. *Occupational Therapy in Mental Health, 5*(3).

Sharrott, G. W. (1985/86). An analysis of occupational therapy theoretical approaches for mental health: Are the profession's major treatment approaches truly occupational therapy? *Occupational Therapy in Mental Health, 5*(4), 1-16.

Sharrott, G. W., & Cooper-Traps, C. (1986). Theories of motivation in occupational therapy: An overview. *American Journal of Occupational Therapy, 40,* 249-257.

Stein, S. (1982). A current review of the behavioral frame of reference and its application to occupation therapy. *Occupational Therapy in Mental Health, 2*(4), 35-62.

Williamson, G. G. (1982). A heritage of activity: Development of theory. *American Journal of Occupational Therapy, 36,* 723-730.

Yerxa, E. J. (1979). The philosophical base of occupational therapy. In AOTA, *Occupational therapy—2001 AD* (pp. 26-30). Rockville, MD: American Occupational Therapy Association.

Zenke, R., & Gratz, R. R. (1982). The role of theory: Erikson and occupational therapy. *Occupational Therapy in Mental Health, 2*(3), 45-64.

Homelessness

American Psychiatric Association. (1984). Recommendations of the APA's task force on the homeless mentally ill. *Hospital and Community Psychiatry, 35,* 908-909.

Bachrach, L. L. (1987). Homeless women: A context for health planning. *Milbank Quarterly, 65,* 371-396.

Bassuk, E. L., Rubin, L., & Lauriet, A. (1984). Is homelessness a mental health problem? *American Journal of Psychiatry, 141,* 1546-1550.

Batty, J. (1988, August 4). Homeless offered a new beginning at transitional center. *OT Week,* pp. 16-17.

Belcher, J. R. (1988). Defining the service needs of the homeless mentally ill. *Hospital and Community Psychiatry, 39,* 1203-1205.

Benda, B. B., & Datallo, P. (1988). Homelessness: Consequence of a crisis or a long-term process? *Hospital and Community Psychiatry, 39,* 884-886.

Blanhertz, L., & White, K. K. (1990). Implementation of a rehabilitation program for the dually diagnosed homeless. *Alcoholism Treatment Quarterly, 7*(1), 149-164.

Brack, C. (1988, June 13). Pathways—Community outreach: The road to a new life for the homeless mentally ill. *Occupational Therapy Forum, 1,* 3-6.

Breten, M. (1984). A drop-in program for transient women: Promoting competence through the environment. *Social Work, 29,* 542-546.

Chafetz, L. (1988). Perspective for psychiatric nurses on homelessness. *Issues in Mental Health Nursing, 9,* 325-335.

Cohen, N. L. (Ed.). (1991). *Psychiatric outreach to the mentally ill.* San Francisco: Jossey-Bass.

Cohen, N. L. (1992). What we must learn from the homeless mentally ill. *Hospital and Community Psychiatry, 43,* 101.

Del Vecchio, A. L., & Kearney, P. C. (1990, March). Homeless women's dinner program: Adapting traditional interventions to a nontraditional environment. *Mental Health Special Interest Section Newsletter,* pp. 2-4.

Feitel, B., Margetsen, N., Chamas, J., & Lipman, C. (1992). Psychosocial backgrounds and behavioral and emotional disorders of homeless and runaway youth. *Hospital and Community Psychiatry, 43,* 155-159.

Harris, M., & Bachrach, L. L. (1990). Perspectives on homeless mentally ill women. *Hospital and Community Psychiatry, 41,* 253-254.

Isaac, R. J., & Armat, V. C. (1990). *Madness in the streets.* New York: Free Press.

Lamb, H. R. (Ed.). (1984). *The homeless mentally ill.* Washington, DC: American Psychiatric Association.

Levine, I. S., & Rog, D. J. (1990). Mental health services for homeless mentally ill persons: Federal initiatives and current service trends. *American Psychologist, 45,* 963-968.

Levine, M. (1988, February 1). OT intervention and the homeless. *Occupational Therapy Forum,* pp. 11-12.

Lipton, F. R., Sabatini, A., & Katz, S. E. (1983). Down and out in the city: The homeless mentally ill. *Hospital and Community Psychiatry, 34,* 817-821.

Martin, M. A., & Wayowith, S. A. (1988). Creating community: Groupwork to develop social support networks with homeless mentally ill. *Social Work With Groups, 11*, 78-93.

National Alliance for the Mentally Ill. (1990). *Homeless and missing mentally ill network handbook.* Arlington, VA: Author.

Rosenheck, R. A., Sallup, P., & Leda, C. (1991). Vietnam veterans among the homeless. *American Journal of Public Health, 81*, 643-646.

Rossi, P. (1989). *Down and out in America: The causes of homelessness.* Chicago: University of Chicago Press.

Roth, D., & Bean, G. J. (1986). New perspectives on homelessness: Findings from a state-wide epidemiological study. *Hospital and Community Psychiatry, 37*, 712-719.

Schutt, R. K., & Garret, G. R. (1988). Social background, residential experience and health problems of the homeless. *Psychosocial Rehabilitation Journal, 12*, 67-70.

Solarz, G., & Bogat, S. A. (1990). When social support fails: The homeless. *Journal of Community Psychiatry, 18*, 79-96.

Susser, E., Strueming, E. L., & Canover, S. (1988). Psychiatric problems in homeless man: Lifetime psychosis, substance use, and current distress in new arrivals at New York City shelters. *Archives of General Psychiatry, 46*, 845-850.

Torrey, E. F. (1988). *Nowhere to go: The tragic odyssey of the homeless mentally ill.* New York: Harper & Row.

Watson, S., & Austerbary, H. (1986). *Housing and homelessness: A feminist perspective.* London: Routledge & Kegan Paul.

Intervention Principles and Techniques/ Treatment Programs

Adler, D. A. (Ed.). (1990). *Treating personality disorders.* San Francisco: Jossey-Bass.

Agacinski, K., & Stern, D. (1984). A two track program enhances therapeutic gains for chronically ill in a day hospital population. *Occupational Therapy in Mental Health, 4*, 15-22.

Allen, C. K. (1985). *Occupational therapy for psychiatric diseases: Measurement and management of cognitive disabilities.* Boston: Little, Brown.

Allen, C. K., & Earhart, C. A. (1992). *Occupational therapy treatment goals for the physically and cognitively disabled.* Rockville, MD: American Occupational Therapy Association.

Allen, G., & Peppers, S. (1988, March). Use of a therapeutic choir as an agent of change in patients. *Mental Health Special Interest Section Newsletter*, pp. 2-3.

American Occupational Therapy Association. (1986). *Depression: Assessment and treatment outcome.* Rockville, MD: Author.

American Occupational Therapy Association. (1987). *The chronically mentally ill: Issues in intervention proceedings.* Rockville, MD: Author.

American Psychiatric Association (1982). *The young adult chronic patient.* Washington, DC: Author.

Anthony, W. A. (1980). *The principles of psychiatric rehabilitation.* Baltimore: University Park Press.

Anttinen, E. E., & Ojanen, M. (1985). An integrative, progressive rehabilitation model for long term schizophrenic patients. *World Hospital, 21*(3), 54-58.

Ascher-Svanum, H., & Krause, A. A. (1991). *Psychoeducational groups for patients with schizophrenia: A guide for practitioners.* Rockville, MD: Aspen Publishers.

Bachrach, L. (1980). Overview: Model programs for chronic mental patients. *American Journal of Psychiatry, 137*, 1023-1031.

Bailey, D. S., Cooper, S. O., & Bailey, D. R. (1984). *Therapeutic approaches to the care of the mentally ill* (2nd ed.). Philadelphia: F. A. Davis.

Bair, J. (Ed.). (1987). *Occupational therapy in acute care settings: A manual.* Rockville, MD: American Occupational Therapy Association.

Bakker, C. B., & Armstrong, H. E. (1976). The adult development program: An educational approach to the delivery of mental health services. *Hospital and Community Psychiatry, 27*, 330-334.

Barter, J. T., Qerirolo, J. F., & Ekstrom, S. P. (1984). A psycho-educational approach to educating chronic mental patients about community living. *Hospital and Community Psychiatry, 35*, 793-797.

Bavaro, S. M. (1991). Occupational therapy and obsessive-compulsive disorder. *American Journal of Occupational Therapy, 45*, 456-458.

Beard, J. H. (1976). Psychiatric rehabilitation of Fountain House. In J. Jeislin (Ed.), *Rehabilitation medicine and psychiatry* . Springfield, IL: Charles C. Thomas.

Becker, R. E., & Page, M. S. (1973). Psychotherapeutically oriented rehabilitation in chronic mental illness. *American Journal of Occupational Therapy, 27*, 34-38.

Beidel, D. C., Bellack, A. S., Turner, S. M., Hersen, M., & Luber, R. F. (1981). *Social skills training for chronic psychiatric patients: A treatment manual.* Pittsburgh, PA: Western Psychiatric Institute.

Bennett, S. H. (1991, September). Managing sensory impairments in group settings. *Mental Health Special Interest Section Newsletter*, pp. 3-4.

Berry, B. L., & Lukens, H. C. (1975). Integrating occupational therapy into other activities in a day treatment program. *Hospital and Community Psychiatry, 26*, 569-574.

Biegel, A., Hollenbach, H., Gurgerich, S., Scanlon, J., & Geffen, J. (1977). Practical issues in developing and operating a halfway house program. *Hospital and Community Psychiatry, 28*, 601-607.

Borg, B., & Bruce, M. (1991). *The group system: The therapeutic activity group in occupational therapy.* Thorofare, NJ: Slack.

Brabender, V., & Fallon, A. E. (1992). *Models of inpatient group psychotherapy.* Washington, DC: American Psychological Association.

Brady, J. P. (1984a). Social skills training for psychiatric patients, I: Concepts, methods, and clinical results. *American Journal of Psychiatry, 141*, 333-341.

Brady, J. P. (1984b). Social skills training for psychiatric patients, II: Clinical outcome studies. *American Journal of Psychiatry, 141*, 491-498.

Brammer, L. M. (1985). *The helping relationship: Process and skills* (3rd ed.). Englewood Cliffs, NJ: Prentice Hall.

Brigs, A. K., & Agrin, A. R. (Eds.). (1981). *Crossroads: A reader for psychological occupational therapy.* Rockville, MD: American Occupational Therapy Association.

Brockema, M. C., Danz, K. H., & Schloemer, C. V. (1975). Occupational therapy in a community after care program. *American Journal of Occupational Therapy, 29,* 22-27.

Brown, T., Harwood, K., Heckman, J., & Short, J. (Eds.). (1989). *Mental health protocols.* Baltimore: Chess Publications.

Brucki, H. L. (1986). An overview of incest with suggestions for occupational therapy treatment. *Occupational Therapy in Mental Health, 5*(4), 63-76.

Burton, L. (1984). Introducing the concept of occupational therapy to patients in an acute psychiatric unit. *British Journal of Occupational Therapy, 47*(7), 178-183.

Campbell, M. (1981). The three-quarterway house—A step beyond the halfway house toward independent living. *Hospital and Community Psychiatry, 32,* 330-334.

Campenelli, P., Leiberman, H., & Triyillo, M. (1983). Creating residential alternatives for the chronic mentally ill. *Hospital and Community Psychiatry, 34,* 166-167.

Carberry, H. (1983). Psychological methods for helping the angry, resistant and negative patient. *Cognitive Rehabilitation, 1*(4), 4-5.

Casarino, J., Wilner, M., & Maxey, J. (1982). American association for partial hospitals, standards and guidelines for partial hospitalization. *International Journal of Partial Hospitalization, 1,* 5-22.

Caton, C. (1984). *Management of chronic schizophrenia.* New York: Oxford University Press.

Chacko, R. C. (Ed.). (1985). *The chronic mental patient in a community context.* Washington, DC: American Psychiatric Press.

Christiansen, C. H., & Baum, C. M. (Eds.). (1991). *Occupational therapy: Overcoming human performance deficits.* Thorofare, NJ: Slack.

Cohen, N. L. (Ed.). (1991). *Psychiatric outreach to the mentally ill.* San Francisco: Jossey-Bass.

Corrigan, P. W., Liberman, R. P., & Engel, J. D. (1990). From noncompliance to collaboration in the treatment of schizophrenia. *Hospital and Community Psychiatry, 41,* 1203-1211.

Coviensky, M. (1986, June). Addressing performance components in day treatment: A program description. *Mental Health Special Interest Newsletter,* pp. 3-4.

Cromwell, F. S. (Ed.). (1985). *The roles of occupational therapists in continuity of care.* New York: Haworth Press.

Curran, J. P., & Monti, P. M. (Eds.). (1982). *Social skills training: A practical handbook for the assessment and treatment.* New York: Guilford.

Cynkin, S. (1979). *Occupational therapy: Toward health through activities.* Boston, MA: Little, Brown.

Cynkin, S., & Robinson, A. M. (1990). *Occupational therapy and activities health: Toward health through activities.* Boston: Little, Brown.

Davis, S., & Keene, N. (1983). Making social skills work with outpatients. *British Journal of Occupational Therapy, 46,* 257-259.

DeCarlo, J. J., & Mann, N. C. (1985). The effectiveness of verbal versus activity groups in improving self-perceptions of interpersonal communication skills. *American Journal of Occupational Therapy, 39,* 20-27.

Denton, P. (1987). *Psychiatric occupational therapy: A workbook of practical skills.* Boston: Little, Brown.

Dickey, B., Cannon, N., McGuire, T., & Gudeman, J. (1986). The quarterway house: A two year study of an experiential residential program. *Hospital and Community Psychiatry, 37,* 1136-1143.

Dombrowski, L. B. (1990). *Functional needs assessment program for chronic psychiatric patients.* Tucson, AZ: Therapy Skill Builders.

Donohue, M. (1982). Designing activities to develop a woman's identification group. *Occupational Therapy in Mental Health, 2*(1), 1-19.

Duncombe, L. W., & Howe, M. C. (1985). Group work in occupational therapy: A survey of practice. *American Journal of Occupational Therapy, 39,* 163-169.

Early, M. B. (1987). *Mental health concepts and techniques for the occupational therapy assistant.* New York: Raven Press.

Falk-Kessler, J., Momick, C., & Perel, S. (1991). Therapeutic factors in occupational therapy groups. *American Journal of Occupational Therapy, 45,* 59-66.

Fidler, G. S. (1984). *Design of rehabilitation services in psychiatric hospital settings.* Rockville, MD: American Occupational Therapy Association.

Fine, S. (1983). *Occupational therapy: The role of rehabilitation and purposeful activity in mental health practice.* Rockville, MD: American Occupational Therapy Association.

Frye, B. (1990). Art and multiple personality disorder: An expressive framework for occupational therapy. *American Journal of Occupational Therapy, 44,* 1013-1022.

Gibson, D. (Ed.). (1983). Occupational therapy with borderline patients [Special issue]. *Occupational Therapy in Mental Health, 3*(3).

Gibson, D. (Ed.). (1986). Treatment of the chronic schizophrenic patient [Special issue]. *Occupational Therapy in Mental Health, 6*(2).

Gibson, D. (1987). Caring for the chronically mentally ill in the 1990s. In AOTA (Ed.), *The chronically mentally ill: Issues in intervention proceedings* (pp. 10-26). Rockville, MD: Editor.

Gibson, D. (Ed.). (1988). Group process and structure in psychosocial occupational therapy [Special issue]. *Occupational Therapy in Mental Health, 8*(3).

Gibson, D., & Kaplan, K. (Eds.). (1984). Short-term treatment in occupational therapy [Special issue]. *Occupational Therapy in Mental Health, 4*(3).

Glynn, S., & Muesser, K. (1986). Social learning for chronic mental inpatients. *Schizophrenia Bulletin, 12,* 648-668.

Goldmeier, J., Shore, M., & Mannino, F. (1977). Cooperative apartments: New programs in community mental health. *Health and Social Work, 2*(1), 119-140.

Goldstein, A. P., Gershaw, N. J., & Sprafkin, R. P. (1975). Structured learning therapy: Skill training for schizophrenics. *Schizophrenia Bulletin, 14*, 83-86.

Goodman, G. (1982). The borderline patient and occupational therapy treatment. *Mental Health Special Interest Newsletter, 5*(4), 1-3.

Gorman, P. (1985a). Sensory integration and the treatment of chronic schizophrenia, part 1. *Occupational Therapy Forum, 1*(22), 24-25.

Gorman, P. (1985b). Sensory integration and the treatment of chronic schizophrenia, part 2. *Occupational Therapy Forum, 1*(22), 32-33.

Grogan, G. (1991a). Anger management: A perspective for occupational therapy, part 1. *Occupational Therapy in Mental Health, 11*(2/3), 135-148.

Grogan, G. (1991b). Anger management: Clinical applications for occupational therapy, part 2. *Occupational Therapy in Mental Health, 11*(2/3), 149-171.

Grotjohn, M., Kline, F. M., & Friedmann, C. (Eds.). (1983). *Handbook of group therapy*. New York: Van Nostrand Reinhold.

Group for the Advancement of Psychiatry—Committee on Psychopathology. (1990). *Beyond symptom suppression: Improving long-term outcomes of schizophrenia*. Washington, DC: American Psychiatric Press.

Gutheil. (1985). The therapeutic milieu: Changing times and theories. *Hospital and Community Psychiatry, 36*, 1279-1285.

Harris, B. (1984). Short-term treatment of the acute schizophrenic episode. *Occupational Therapy in Mental Health, 4*(3), 75-87.

Hibbard, T., Campitelli, J., & Lieberman, H. J. (1989). Off-unit activities programming for long-stay psychiatric inpatients: Clinical and administrative effects. *Occupational Therapy in Mental Health, 9*(1), 49-61.

Hickerson-Crist, P. A., Thomas, P. P., & Stone, B. L. (1984). Prevocational and sensorimotor training in chronic schizophrenia. *Occupational Therapy in Mental Health, 4*(2), 23-37.

Heirholzer, R., & Liberman, R. (1986). Successful living: A social skills and problem solving group for the chronic mentally ill. *Hospital and Community Psychiatry, 37*, 913-918.

Higden, J. F. (1990). Expressive therapy in conjunction with psychotherapy in the treatment of persons with multiple personality disorder. *American Journal of Occupational Therapy, 44*, 991-993.

Howe, M., & Schwartzburg, S. (1986). *A functional approach to group work in occupational therapy*. Philadelphia: Lippincott.

Hughes, P. L., & Mullins, L. (1981). *Acute psychiatric care: An occupational therapy guide to exercises in daily living skills*. Thorofare, NJ: Slack.

Hutchins, D. E., & Cole, C. S. (1986). *Helping relationships and strategies*. Pacific Grove, CA: Brooks/Cole.

Johnson, D. W., & Johnson, F. P. (1982). *Joining together: Group theory and group skills*. Englewood Cliffs, NJ: Prentice Hall.

Kane, R. A., & Kane, R. L. (1987). *Long-term care: Principles, programs and policies*. New York: Springer.

Kaplan, K. (1988). *Directive group therapy: Innovative mental health treatment*. Thorofare, NJ: Slack.

Kavanagh, M. (1990, March). Way station: A model community support program for persons with severe mental illness. *Mental Health Special Interest Section Newsletter*, pp. 6-8.

Keller, P., & Murray, R. L. (Eds.). (1982). *Handbook of rural community mental health*. New York: Human Sciences Press.

Kielhofner, G. (Ed.). (1983). *Health through occupation: Theory and practice in occupational therapy*. Philadelphia: F. A. Davis.

Klasson, E. M., & MacRae, A. (1985). A university-based occupational therapy clinic for chronic schizophrenics. *Occupational Therapy in Mental Health, 5*(2), 1-13.

Klimowicz, R. (1987). Sensorimotor activities on a short-term inpatient unit. *Occupational Therapy Forum, 4*(2), 1, 3-6.

Klyczek, J. P., & Mann, W. C. (1986). Therapeutic modality comparisons in day treatment. *American Journal of Occupational Therapy, 40*, 606-611.

Knill, M., & Knill, C. (1987). *Activity programs for body awareness, contact and communication*. Tucson, AZ: Therapy Skill Builders.

Korb, K. L., Azok, S. K., & Leutenberg, E. A. (1989). *Life management skills*. Beechwood, OH: Wellness Reproductions.

Korb, K. L., Azok, S. K., & Leutenberg, E. A. (1991). *Life management skills II*. Beechwood, OH: Wellness Reproductions.

Krauss, J., & Slavinsky, A. (1982). *The chronically ill psychiatric patient and the community*. New Haven, CT: Yale University School of Nursing.

Kresky, M., Maeda, E., & Rothwell, N. (1976). The apartment program: A community living option for halfway house residence. *Hospital and Community Psychiatry, 27*, 153-154, 159.

Krupa, T., Hayashi, C., Murphy, M., & Thornton, J. (1985). Occupational therapy issues in the treatment of the long-term mentally ill. *Canadian Journal of Occupational Therapy, 52*, 107-111.

Kupers, T. A. (Ed.). (1990). *Using psychodynamic principles in public mental health*. San Francisco: Jossey-Bass.

Lamb, H. R. (1976). An educational model for teaching living skills to long-term patients. *Hospital and Community Psychiatry, 27*, 875-877.

Lamb, H. R. (1982). *Treating the long-term mentally ill*. San Francisco: Jossey-Bass.

Lamb, H. R., & Goertzel, V. (1977). The long-term patient in the era of community treatment. *Archives of General Psychiatry, 34*, 679-682.

Leopold, B. (1987). A short-term psychiatric unit: Description and philosophy. *Occupational Therapy in Mental Health, 7*(1), 1-16.

Levy, S. T., & Ninan, P. T. (1990). *Schizophrenia: Treatment of acute psychotic episodes*. Washington, DC: American Psychiatric Press.

Liberman, R. P. (Ed.). (1988). *Psychiatric rehabilitation of chronic mental patients*. Washington, DC: American Psychiatric Press.

Liberman, R. (Ed.). (1991). *Handbook of psychiatric rehabilitation*. New York: Pergamon Press.

Liberman, R. P., DeRisi, W. J., & Mueser, K. T. (1989). *Social skills training for psychiatric patients*. New York: Pergamon Press.

Liberman, R. P., & Foy, D. W. (1983). Psychiatric rehabilitation for chronic mental patients. *Psychiatric Annals, 13*, 539-545.

Liberman, R. P., Massell, H. K., Mosk, M. D., & Wong, S. E. (1985). Social skills training for chronic mental patients. *Hospital and Community Psychiatry, 36*, 396-403.

Liberman, R. P., Mueser, K. T., Wallace, C. J., Jacobs, H. E., Eckman, T., & Massell, H. K. (1986). Training skills in the psychiatrically disabled: Learning coping and competence. *Schizophrenia Bulletin, 12*, 631-647.

Lillie, M., & Armstrong, H. (1982). Contributions to the development of psychoeducational approaches to mental health services. *American Journal of Occupational Therapy, 36*, 438-443.

Lloyd, C. (1987). Sex offender programs: Is there a role for occupational therapy? *Occupational Therapy in Mental Health, 7*(3), 55-66.

Maslen, D. (1982). Rehabilitation training for community living skills: Concepts and techniques. *Occupational Therapy in Mental Health, 2*(1), 33-49.

Matson, J., Ziess, A., Ziess, R., & Bowman, W. (1980). A comparison of social skills training and contingent attention to improve behavioral deficits of chronic psychiatric patients. *British Journal of Social and Clinical Psychology, 19*, 57-64.

Mauras-Corsino, E., Daniewicz, C. V., & Swan, L. C. (1985). The use of community networks for chronic psychiatric patients. *American Journal of Occupational Therapy, 39*, 374-378.

Maves, P. A., & Schulz, J. W. (1985). Inpatient group treatment on short-term acute care units. *Hospital and Community Psychiatry, 36*, 69-73.

May, P. R. A., Tuma, H., & Dixon, W. J. (1981). Schizophrenia: A follow-up study of the result of five forms of treatment. *Archives of General Psychiatry, 38*, 776-784.

McFadden, S. (1987). Private practice and mental health: A point of view. In AOTA (Ed.), *The chronically mentally ill: Issues in intervention proceedings* (pp. 56-68). Rockville, MD: Editor.

McSurp, E., Howard, L., & Schlitt, D. (1990). The planning group: An example of learning through doing. *Occupational Therapy Forum, 5*(1), 1, 3-5.

Mechanic, D., & Aiken, L. H. (1987). Improving the care of patients with chronic mental illness. *The New England Journal of Medicine, 317*, 1634-1638.

Mendel, W. M. (1989). *Treating schizophrenia.* San Francisco: Jossey-Bass.

Meyerson, A. T., & Herman, G. S. (1983). What's new in aftercare? A review of the literature. *Hospital and Community Psychiatry, 34*, 333-341.

Meyerson, A. T., & Soloman, P. (Eds.). (1990). *New developments in psychiatric rehabilitation.* San Francisco: Jossey-Bass.

Michael, P. S. (1991, June). Occupational therapy in prison? You must be kidding! *Mental Health Special Interest Section Newsletter*, pp. 3-4.

Mosey, A. C. (1973). *Activities therapy.* New York: Raven Press.

Mosey, A. C. (1986). *Psychosocial components of occupational therapy.* New York: Raven Press.

Mosher, L., & Keith, S. (1980). Psychosocial treatment: Individual, group, family and community support approaches. In Mosher & Keith (Eds.), *Special report: Schizophrenia, 1980* (pp. 127-158). Washington, DC: National Institute of Mental Health.

Mueser, K. T., Levine, S., Bellack, A. S., Douglas, M. S., & Brady, E. U. (1990). Social skills training for acute psychiatric inpatients. *Hospital and Community Psychiatry, 41*, 1249-1251.

Nachajski, S. B., & Gordon, C. Y. (1987). The use of Trivial Pursuit in teaching community living skills to adults with developmental disabilities. *American Journal of Occupational Therapy, 41*, 10-15.

Napier, R. N., & Gershenfeld, M. K. (1983). *Making groups work: A guide for group leaders.* Boston: Houghton Mifflin.

Paschke, M. J. (1984). Day care within a community mental health center. *Physical and Occupational Therapy in Geriatrics, 3*(4), 67-70.

Pasnau, R. O. (Ed.). (1984). *Diagnosis and treatment of anxiety disorders.* Washington, DC: American Psychiatric Press.

Pato, M. T., & Zohar, J. (Eds.). (1991). *Current treatments of obsessive-compulsive disorder.* Washington, DC: American Psychiatric Press.

Payton, O. D., Nelson, C. E., & Ozer, M. N. (1990). *Patient participation in program planning: A manual for therapists.* Philadelphia: F. A. Davis.

Perry, S., Frances, A., & Clarkin, J. (1990). *A DSM III-R casebook of treatment selection.* New York: Brunner/Mazel.

Peters, C. P. (1990). Critical issues in the evaluation and treatment of the borderline patient. *Occupational Therapy in Mental Health, 10*(4), 79-84.

Poirier, S. (Guest Ed.). (1986, June). Community mental health [Special issue]. *Mental Health Special Interest Section Newsletter.*

Radonsky, V. E., Jackson, H., Barton, S., Fedak, K., & Martin, M. (1986). Step ahead—Occupational therapy in the community. *Occupational Therapy in Mental Health, 6*(2), 79-87.

Raish, H., & Rog, D. (1975). Psychiatric halfway house: How is it measuring up? *Community Mental Health Journal, 11*(12), 310-317.

Ranz, J. M., Horen, B. T., McFarlane, W. R., & Zito, J. M. (1991). Creating a supportive environment using staff psychoeducation in a supervised residence. *Hospital and Community Psychiatry, 42*, 1154-1159.

Remocker, A. J., & Storch, E. (1987). *Action speaks louder: A handbook of structured group techniques.* New York: Churchill Livingstone.

Rider, B. A. (1978). Sensorimotor treatment of chronic schizophrenics. *American Journal of Occupational Therapy, 32*, 451-455.

Richert, G. Z., & Berglard, C. (1992). Treatment choices: Rehabilitation services used by patients with multiple personality disorder. *American Journal of Occupational Therapy, 46*, 634-638.

Robertson, S. C. (Ed.). (1989). *Mental health focus: Skills for assessment and treatment.* Rockville, MD: American Occupational Therapy Association.

Rosie, J. (1987). Partial hospitalization: A review of recent literature. *Hospital and Community Psychiatry, 38*, 1291-1299.

Ross, M. (1987). *Group process: Using therapeutic activities in chronic care.* Throrofare, NJ: Slack.

Ross, M. (1991). *Integrative group therapy: The structured five stage approach.* Thorofare, NJ: Slack.

Sampson, E. E., & Marthas, M. (1981). *Group process for the health professionals* (2nd ed.). New York: John Wiley and Sons.

Schulberg, H. C., & Killilea, M. (Eds.). (1982). *The modern practice of community mental health.* San Francisco: Jossey-Bass.

Schwartzberg, S. L., Howe, M. C., & McDermott, A. (1982). A comparison of three group formats for facilitating social interaction. *Occupational Therapy in Mental Health, 2*(4), 1-16.

Scott, D. W., & Katz, N. (1988). *Occupational therapy in mental health: Principles in practice.* New York: Taylor and Francis.

Shelton, J. L., & Levy, R. L. (1981). *Behavioral assignments and treatment compliance: A handbook of clinical strategies.* Champaign, IL: Research Press.

Shulman, L. (1984). *The skills of helping individuals and groups* (2nd ed.). Itasca, IL: F. E. Peacock.

Skinners, S. T. (1987). Multiple personality disorder: Occupational therapy intervention in acute care psychiatry. *Occupational Therapy in Mental Health, 5*(4), 47-58.

Snyder, S. (1985). Comprehensive inpatient treatment for the young adult patient. *Occupational Therapy in Mental Health, 5*(4), 47-58.

Spivak, G., Siegel, J., Sklaver, D., Deuschle, L., & Garrett, L. (1982). The long-term patient in the community: Life-style patterns and treatment implications. *Hospital and Community Psychiatry, 33*, 291-295.

Stein, F., & Tallant, B. (1988). Applying the group process to psychiatric occupational therapy, part 2: A model for a therapeutic group in psychiatric occupational therapy. *Occupational Therapy in Mental Health, 8*(3), 29-52.

Stein, L., & Test, M. (Eds.). (1978). *Alternatives to mental hospital treatment.* New York: Plenum.

Stein, L., & Test, M. (1980). Alternative to mental hospital treatment, I: Conceptual model, treatment programs and clinical evaluation. *Archives of General Psychiatry, 37*, 392-397.

Stierlin, H., Wynne, L. C., & Wirshing, M. (Eds.). (1983). *Psychosocial intervention in schizophrenia.* Berlin: Springer.

Stratoudakis, J. P. (1986). Rehabilitation of the mentally ill: Psychosocial, vocational, and community support perspectives. *Annual Review of Rehabilitation, 5*, 255-284.

Strauss, J. S., Boker, W., & Brenner, H. D. (Eds.). (1987). *Psychosocial treatment of schizophrenia.* Toronto: Hans Huber.

Stream, H. S. (1990). *Resolving resistance in psychotherapy.* New York: Brunner/Mazel.

Stroul, B. A. (1989). Community support services for persons with long-term mental illness: A conceptual framework. *Psychosocial Rehabilitation Journal, 12*, 9-26.

Talbott, J. (Ed.). (1981). *The chronic mentally ill: Treatment, programs, systems.* New York: Human Services Press.

Talbott, J. (Ed.). (1984). *The chronic mental health patient five years later.* New York: Grune and Stratton.

Taube, C. A., Thompson, J. W., Rosenstein, M. J., Rosen, B. M., & Goldman, H. H. (1983). The "chronic" mental hospital patient. *Hospital and Community Psychiatry, 34*, 611-615.

Tessler, R. C., Bernstein, A. G., Rosen, B. M., & Foldman, H. H. (1982). The chronically mentally ill community support systems. *Hospital and Community Psychiatry, 33*, 208-211.

Test, M. A., & Stein, L. (1976). Practical guidelines for the community treatment of markedly impaired patients. *Community Mental Health Journal, 12*, 72-82.

Vander Roest, L. L., & Clements, S. T. (1983). *Sensory integration: Rationale and treatment activities for groups.* Grand Rapids, MI: South Kent Health Services, Inc.

Van Schroeder, C., & Herbert, A. K. (1981). *Adult psychiatric sensory integration treatment manual.* Sequin, WA: Schroeder Publishing and Consulting.

Vinogradov, S., & Yalom, I. D. (1989). *Concise guide to group psychotherapy.* Washington, DC: American Psychiatric Press.

Webb, L. J. (1973). The therapeutic social club. *American Journal of Occupational Therapy, 27*, 81-83.

Westland, G. (1985). Dipping into community mental health: An aspect of the occupational therapist's role. *British Journal of Occupational Therapy, 48*(9), 260-262.

Wilberding, D. (1987). Rehabilitation through activities for the chronic schizophrenic patient. In AOTA (Ed.), *The chronically mentally ill: Issues in intervention proceedings* (pp. 34-47). Rockville, MD: Editor.

Wilder, J., & Gadlen, W. (1977). A halfway house in a mental health care center. *Community Mental Health Journal, 13*(2), 168-174.

Wilson, M. (1983). *Occupational therapy in long-term psychiatry.* New York: Churchill Livingstone.

Wilson, H. S. (1982). *Deinstitutionalized residential care for the mentally disordered: The Soteria House approach.* New York: Grune and Stratton.

Wodarski, J. S. (1983). *Rural community mental health practice.* Baltimore: University Park Press.

Wolf, M. E., & Mosnaim, A. K. (1990). *Post traumatic stress disorder: Etiology, phenomenology, and treatment.* Washington, DC: American Psychiatric Press.

Woodside, H. (1984). Community care for the chronic mentally ill. *Canadian Journal of Occupational Therapy, 51*(4), 181-187.

Yalom, I. (1975). *The theory and practice of group psychotherapy.* New York: Basic Books.

Yalom, I. D. (1983). *Inpatient group psychotherapy.* New York: Basic Books.

Neuroscience and Psychopharmacology

Abrams, R., & Taylor, M. A. (1983). The genetics of schizophrenia: A reassessment using modern criteria. *American Journal of Psychiatry, 140*, 171-175.

Andreasen, N. C. (1982). Negative symptoms in schizophrenia. *Archives of General Psychiatry, 39*, 784-788.

Andreasen, N. C. (1984). *The broken brain: The biological revolution in psychiatry.* New York: Harper & Row.

Andreasen, N. C. (Ed.). (1989). *Brain imaging: Applications in Psychiatry.* Washington, DC: American Psychiatric Press.

Arnadottir, G. (1990). *The brain and behavior: Assessing cortical dysfunction through activities of daily living.* St. Louis: Mosby.

Barris, R. (1985, September). Review of current research on schizophrenia. *Mental Health Special Interest Section Newsletter,* pp. 1-2.

Baxter, W. E. (1991a). *Psychopharmacology review.* Washington, DC: Hospital and Community Psychiatry Service.

Baxter, W. E. (1991b). *Tardive dyskinesia update.* Washington, DC: Hospital and Community Psychiatry Service.

Beck, M. A., & Callahan, D. K. (1980). Impact of institutionalization on the posture of chronic schizophrenic patients. *American Journal of Occupational Therapy, 34,* 332-335.

Blakeney, A. B., Strickland, L. R., & Wilkinson, J. H. (1983). Exploring sensory integrative dysfunction in process schizophrenia. *American Journal of Occupational Therapy, 37,* 399-406; 850-851.

Boll, T., & Bryant, B. K. (Eds.). (1988). *Clinical neuropsychology and brain function: Research, measurement and practice.* Washington, DC: American Psychological Association.

Carpenter, W. T., & Schooler, N. R. (Eds.). (1983). *New directions in drug treatment for schizophrenia.* Rockville, MD: National Institute of Mental Health.

Ciccone, C. D., & Wolf, S. L. (Eds.). (1990). *Pharmacology in rehabilitation.* Philadelphia: F. A. Davis.

Deutsch, S. I., & Davis, K. L. (1983). Schizophrenia: A review of diagnostic and biological issues. *Hospital and Community Psychiatry, 34,* 423-437.

Easton, K., & Link, I. (1986-87). Do neuroleptics prevent relapse? Clinical observations in a psychosocial rehabilitation program. *Psychiatric Quarterly, 58*(1), 42-50.

Eimon, M. C., Eimon, P. L., & Cermak, S. A. (1983). Performance of schizophrenic patient on a motor-free visual perception test. *American Journal of Occupational Therapy, 37,* 327-332.

Filskov, S. B., & Boll, T. J. (Eds.). (1981). *Handbook of clinical neuropsychology.* New York: John Wiley and Sons.

Gorman, J. (1990). *The essential guide to psychiatric drugs.* New York: St. Martin's Press.

Grabowski, J., & Vanden Bros, G. R. (Eds.). (1992). *Psychopharmacology: Basic mechanisms and applied interventions.* Washington, DC: American Psychological Association.

Greden, J. F., & Tandon, R. (Ed.). (1990). *Negative schizophrenic symptoms: Pathophysiology and clinical implications.* Washington, DC: American Psychiatric Press.

Hyman, S. E., & Nestler, E. (1992). *The molecular foundations of psychiatry.* Washington, DC: American Psychiatric Press.

Kane, J. M. (1992). *Tardive dyskinesia: A task force report of the American Psychiatric Association.* Washington, DC: American Psychiatric Association.

King, L. J. (1983). Occupational therapy and neuropsychiatry. *Occupational Therapy in Mental Health, 3*(1), 1-15.

Lawson, G. W., & Cooperrider, C. C. (1988). *Clinical psychopharmacology: A practical reference for nonmedical psychotherapists.* Rockville, MD: Aspen Publishers.

Lezak, M. D. (1983). *Neuropsychological assessment* (2nd ed.). New York: Oxford University Press.

Lindquist, J. E. (1981). Activity and vestibular function in chronic schizophrenia. *The Occupational Therapy Journal of Research, 1*(1), 56-78.

Linn, M. W., Caffey, E. M., Klett, C. J., Hogarty, G. E., & Lamb, H. R. (1978). Day treatment and psychotropic drugs in the after-care of psychiatric patients. *Archives of General Psychiatry, 36,* 1055-1066. Reprinted in *Occupational Therapy in Mental Health* (1980) *1*(1), 77-105.

Long, J. W. (1992). *The essential guide to prescription drugs, 1992 edition.* New York: Harper & Row.

Moak, G. S., Stein, E. M., and Rubin, J. E. (1989). *The over-50 guide to psychiatric medications.* Washington, DC: American Psychiatric Association.

Popper, C. (Ed.). (1987). *Psychiatric pharmacosciences of children and adolescents.* Washington, DC: American Psychiatric Association.

Rieder, R. O., Mann, L. S., Weinberger, D. R., van Kammen, D. P., & Post, R. M. (1983). Computed tomographic scans in patients with schizophrenia, schizo-affective, and bipolar affective disorder. *Archives of General Psychiatry, 40,* 735-739.

Satz, P., & Fletcher, J. M. (1981). Emergent trends in neuropsychology: An overview. *Journal of Consulting and Clinical Psychology, 49,* 851-865.

Schatzberg, A. F., & Cole, J. O. (1991). *Manual of clinical psychopharmacology.* Washington, DC: American Psychiatric Press.

Shamoian, C. A. (Ed.). (1992). *Psychopharmacological treatment complications in the elderly.* Washington, DC: American Psychiatric Press.

Strauss, D., & Solomon, K. (1983). Psychopharmacologic intervention for depression in the elderly. *Clinical Gerontologist, 2*(1), 3-29.

Sturgess, J., & Clancy, H. (1981). The case for a sensory-integrative approach to schizophrenia: An evaluative review. *British Journal of Occupational Therapy, 44,* 182-186.

Swonger, A. K., & Constantine, L. L. (1983). *Drugs and therapy: A handbook of psychotropic drugs.* Boston: Little, Brown.

Talbott, J. A. (Ed.). (1990). Clozapine [Special issue]. *Hospital and Community Psychiatry, 41.*

Tucker, G. J., Campion, E. M., & Sieberfarb, P. M. (1975). Sensorimotor functions and cognitive disturbance in psychiatric patients. *American Journal of Psychiatry, 132*(1), 17-21.

U. S. Department of Health and Human Services. (1984). *The neuroscience of mental health.* Rockville, MD: National Institute of Mental Health.

Utley, E. R., & Robertson, D. (1981). Activity and vestibular function in chronic schizophrenia. *The Occupational Therapy Journal of Research, 1,* 179-183.

Wahba, M., Donlon, P. T., & Meadow, A. (1981). Cognitive changes in acute schizophrenia with brief neuroleptic treatment. *American Journal of Psychiatry, 138,* 1307-1310.

Yudofsky, S. C., & Hales, R. E. (Eds.). (1992). *American Psychiatric Press textbook of neuropsychiatry* (2nd ed.). Washington, DC: American Psychiatric Press.

Yudofsky, S. C., Hales, R. E., & Ferguson, T. (1991). *What you need to know about psychiatric drugs: A consumer's guide to the full range of psychiatric medications.* Washington, DC: American Psychiatric Press.

Zubin, J., & Spring, B. (1977). Vulnerability: A new view of schizophrenia. *Journal of Abnormal Psychology, 86*, 103-126.

Prevention, Health Promotion, and Wellness

Also see Stress Management

Adam, C. T. (1981). A descriptive definition of primary prevention. *Journal of Primary Prevention, 2*, 67-79.

Ardell, D. (1982). *14 days to a wellness lifestyle.* Mill Valley, CA: Whatever Publishing, Inc.

Barter, J. T., & Talbott, S. W. (Eds.). (1986). *Primary prevention in Psychiatry: State of the art.* Washington, DC: American Psychiatric Press.

Benzing, P., & Strickland, R. (1983). Occupational therapy in a community-based prevention program. *Occupational Therapy in Mental Health, 3*(1), 15-31.

Brandon, J. E. (1985). Health promotion and wellness in rehabilitation services. *Journal of Rehabilitation, 51*(4), 54-58.

Broderick, T., & Glazer, B. (1983). Leisure participation and retirement. *American Journal of Occupational Therapy, 37*, 15-23.

Buckner, J. C., Trickett, E. J., & Corse, S. J. (1985). *Primary prevention in mental health: An annotated bibliography.* Rockville, MD: National Institute of Mental Health.

Cantor, S. G. (1981). Occupational therapists as members of pre-retirement resource teams. *American Journal of Occupational Therapy, 35*, 638-644.

Commission on the Prevention of Mental-Emotional Disabilities (1986). *The prevention of mental-emotional disabilities.* Alexandria, VA: National Mental Health Association.

Ellsworth, P. D., & Rambaugh, J. H. (1980). Community organization and planning consultation: Strategies for community-wide assessment and preventative program design. *Occupational Therapy in Mental Health, 1*(1), 33-56.

Finn, G. L. (1972). The occupational therapist in prevention programs. *American Journal of Occupational Therapy, 26*, 59-66.

George, N. M., Braun, B. A., & Walker, J. M. (1982). A prevention and early intervention program for disadvantaged preschool children. *American Journal of Occupational Therapy, 36*, 99-106.

Gill, A. A., Veigl, V. L., Shuster, J. J., & Notelovitz, M. (1984). A well woman's health maintenance study comparing physical fitness and group support programs. *Occupational Therapy Journal of Research, 4*, 286-308.

Gonski, G., & Miyake, S. (1985). The adolescent life/work planning group: A prevention model. *Occupational Therapy in Health Care, 2*, 139-150.

Grossman, J. (1977). Nationally speaking: Preventive health care and community programming. *American Journal of Occupational Therapy, 31*, 351-354.

Grossman, J. (1991). A prevention model for occupational therapy. *American Journal of Occupational Therapy, 45*, 33-41.

Jaffe, D. T. (1980). *Healing from within.* New York: Alfred A. Knopf.

Jaffe, E. (1982). Role of occupational therapy as a community consultant: Primary prevention mental health programming. *Occupational Therapy in Mental Health, 1*(2), 47-62.

Jaffe, E. (1986). The role of occupational therapy in disease prevention and health promotion. *American Journal of Occupational Therapy, 40*, 749-758.

Johnson, J. (1985). Wellness: Its myths, realities and potential for occupational therapy. *Occupational Therapy in Health Care, 2*(2), 117-138.

Johnson, J. (1986). *Wellness: A context for living.* Thorofare, NJ: Slack.

Kirchman, M. M., Reichenback, V., & Giambalvo, B. (1982). Preventive activities and services for the well elderly. *American Journal of Occupational Therapy, 36*, 236-242.

Laukaran, V. H. (1977). National speaking: Toward a model of occupational therapy for community health. *American Journal of Occupational Therapy, 31*, 71-74.

Lord, J., & Farlow, D. M. (1990, Fall). A study of personal empowerment: Implications for health promotion. *Health Promotion*, pp. 2-8.

Maguire, G. A. (1979). Volunteer program to assist the elderly to remain in home settings. *American Journal of Occupational Therapy, 33*, 98-101.

Mungai, A. (1985). The occupational therapist's role in employee health promotion programs. *Occupational Therapy in Health Care, 2*, 67-77.

Opatz, J. P. (1985). *A primer of health promotion.* Washington, DC: Oryn Publishing, Inc.

Perlmutter, F. D. (Ed.). (1982). *Mental health promotion and primary prevention.* San Francisco: Jossey-Bass.

Rider, B. A., & White, V. K. (1986). Occupational therapy education in health promotion and disease prevention. *American Journal of Occupational Therapy, 40*, 781-783.

Robinson, V. (1977). *Humor and the health professions.* Thorofare, NJ: Slack.

Sachs, S. R. (1990). A brief history of the center for preventive psychiatry. *Journal of Preventive Psychiatry and Allied Disciplines, 4*(1), 97-100.

Simson, S., Wilson, L. B., Hermalin, J., & Hess, R. (Eds.). (1983). *Aging and prevention: New approaches to preventing health and mental health problems in older adults.* New York: Haworth Press.

Szekais, B. (1985). Risk factors for institutionalization in a community elderly population. *Physical and Occupational Therapy in Geriatrics, 4*(1), 33-43.

Travis, J. W., & Ryan, S. R. (1981). *Wellness workbook.* Berkeley, CA: Ten Speed Press.

White, V. K. (Ed.). (1986). Health promotion [Special issue]. *American Journal of Occupational Therapy, 40*.

Wiemer, R. B. (1972). Some concepts of prevention as an aspect of community health. *American Journal of Occupational Therapy, 26*, 1-9.

Zins, J. E., Wagner, D. I., & Maher, C. A. (Eds.). (1985). *Health promotion in the schools.* New York: Haworth Press.

Professional Career Development

American Occupational Therapy Association (1991). *Re-entry/refresher packet*. Rockville, MD: Author.

Bochannon, R. W. (1985) Mentorship: A relationship important to professional development: A special communication. *Physical Therapy, 65*, 920-923.

Boissoneau, R. (1980). *Continuing education in the health professions*. Rockville, MD: Aspen Systems.

Boyt-Schell, B. A. (1992). Setting realistic career goals. *Occupational Therapy Practice, 3*(3), 11-20.

Brienes, E. B. (1988). The issue is: Redefining professionalism for occupational therapy. *American Journal of Occupational Therapy, 42*, 55-57.

Bucher, R., & Stelling, J. G. (1977). *Becoming professional*. Newbury Park, CA: Sage.

Carr, E. M. (1982). Networking: A resource for change. *Nurse Practitioner, 7*, 32-34.

Cook, H. L., Beery, M., Sauter, S. V. H., & DeVellis, R. F. (1987). Continuing education for health professionals. *American Journal of Occupational Therapy, 41*, 652-65.

Cooper, R. K. (1991). *The performance edge: New strategies to maximize your working effectiveness and competitive edge*. Boston: Houghton Mifflin.

Cottrell, R. F. (1990). Perceived competence among occupational therapists in mental health. *American Journal of Occupational Therapy, 44*, 118-123.

Davidson, D. A. (1991). The issue is: Facilitating a balance between career and family: A crucial challenge. *American Journal of Occupational Therapy, 45*, 84-85.

Donohue, M. (1990). The issue is: Progressive career patterns versus mandated entry-level education. *American Journal of Occupational Therapy, 44*, 759-762.

Dunn, W., & Huss, A. J. (1992). Personal perspectives on career development: Interviews with occupational therapy leaders. *Occupational Therapy Practice, 3*(3), 1-6.

Fidler, G. S. (1990). Reflections on choice. *Occupational Therapy in Mental Health, 10*(1), 77-84.

Fine, S. B. (1990). The promise of occupational therapy: Professional challenges, personal rewards. *Occupational Therapy in Mental Health, 10*(1), 63-75.

Grant, H. K. (1992). Job satisfaction: Whose responsibility. *Occupational Therapy Practice, 3*(3), 72-8.

Grossman, J. (1992). Commentary: Professionalism in occupational therapy. *Occupational Therapy Practice, 3*(3), 7-10.

Hein, E., & Nicholson, M. J. (Eds.). (1986). *Contemporary leadership behavior: Selected readings* (2nd ed.). Boston: Little, Brown.

Houle, C. O. (1980). *Continued learning in the professions*. San Francisco: Jossey-Bass.

Jaffe, E. G., & Epstein, C. F. (Eds.). (1992). *Occupational therapy consultation: Theory, principles and practice*. St. Louis: Mosby.

Jones, J. L., & Kirkland, M. (1984). Nationally speaking: From continuing education to continuing professional education: The shift to lifelong learning in occupational therapy. *American Journal of Occupational Therapy, 38*, 503-504.

McCrum Griffin, R. (1992). Controlling stress to attain career goals. *Occupational Therapy Practice, 3*(3), 39-44.

Mitchell, M. M. (1985). Professional development: Clinician to academician. *American Journal of Occupational Therapy, 39*, 368-373.

Morgan, M. K., & Irby, D. M. (Eds.). (1978). *Evaluating clinical competence in the health professions*. St. Louis: Mosby.

Neuhaus, B. E., Rodriguez, L., Zukas, R., Chandler, B., & Morris, A. O. (1991). *Reactivation—Returning to the OT workforce*. Rockville, MD: American Occupational Therapy Association.

Numerof, R. (1983). *Managing stress: A guide for health care professionals*. Rockville, MD: Aspen Systems.

Parnham, D. (1987). The reflective therapist. *American Journal of Occupational Therapy, 41*, 555-561.

Peters, T., & Austin, N. (1986). *A passion for excellence*. New York: Warner Books.

Peters, T. J., & Waterman, R. H. (1982). *In search of excellence*. New York: Warner Books.

Robertson, S. C. (1992). *Find a mentor or be one*. Rockville, MD: American Occupational Therapy Association.

Rogers, J. C. (1986). Mentoring for career achievement and advancement. *American Journal of Occupational Therapy, 40*, 79-82.

Sabari, J. S. (1985). Professional socialization: Implications for occupational therapy. *American Journal of Occupational Therapy, 39*, 96-102.

Schon, D. A. (1983). *The reflective practitioner: How professionals think in action*. New York: Basic Books.

Smith, B. C. (1992). Mentoring: The key to professional growth. *Occupational Therapy Practice, 3*(3), 21-28.

Program Development and Evaluation

Anthony, W., & Farkas, M. (1982). A client outcome planning model for assessing psychiatric rehabilitation interventions. *Schizophrenia Bulletin, 3*, 13-38.

Fidler, G. S. (1991). *Design of rehabilitation services in psychiatric hospital settings*. Rockville, MD: American Occupational Therapy Association.

Fitz-Gibbon, C. T., & Morris, L. L. (1978). *How to design a program evaluation*. Beverly Hills, CA: Sage.

Gelatt, J. P. (1989). *Planning for excellence: How to position and fund rehabilitation and education programs*. Rockville, MD: Aspen Publishers.

Haller, R. A., & Shaw, K. J. (1984). *A manual on program evaluation*. Bethesda, MD: Goodwill Industries of America.

Joe, B. E., Lawlor, M. C., Scott, T., and Thein, M. (1992). *Quality assurance in occupational therapy: A practitioner's guide to setting up a QA system using three models*. Rockville, MD: American Occupational Therapy Association.

Kagan, R. M. (1984, September). Organizational change and quality assurance in a psychiatric setting. *Quality Review Bulletin*, pp. 270-277.

Liberman, D. (Ed.). (1991). *Clinician's guide to program evaluation*. Rockville, MD: Aspen Publications.

Loschen, E. L. (1986). The challenge of providing quality psychiatric services in a rural setting. *Quality Review Bulletin, 12*(11), 376-379.

McColl, M., & Quinn, B. (1985). Quality assurance method for community occupational therapy. *American Journal of Occupational Therapy, 39*, 570-577.

Robertson, S. C. (Ed.). (1986). *Strategies, concepts, and opportunities for program development and evaluation: An occupational therapy curriculum*. Rockville, MD: American Occupational Therapy Association.

Robertson, S. C. (Ed.). (1988). *Mental health focus: Skills for assessment and treatment*. Rockville, MD: American Occupational Therapy Association.

Schulberg, H. C., & Baker, F. (1979). *Program evaluation in the health fields, VII*. New York: Human Science Press.

Skorupka, P. C., & Cooley, S. J. (1983). The development of a partial hospitalization program evaluation tool. *International Journal of Partial Hospitalization, 2*, 57-66.

Psychogeriatrics

Albert, M. S. (1981). Geriatric neuropsychology. *Journal of Consulting and Clinical Psychology, 49*, 835-850.

Arie, T. (Ed.). (1985). *Recent advances in psychogeriatrics*: New York: Churchill Livingstone.

Billig, N. (1987). *To be old and sad: Understanding depression in the elderly*. Lexington, MA: Lexington Books/Heath.

Breslau, L. D., & Haug, M. R. (Ed.). (1983). *Depression and aging. Causes, care, and consequences*. New York: Springer.

Brink, T. L. (Ed.). (1986). *Clinical gerontology: A guide to assessment and intervention*. New York: Haworth Press.

Burnside, I. M. (Ed.). (1986). *Working with the elderly: Group process and techniques* (2nd ed.). Boston: Jones and Bartlett Publications.

Caplaw-Lindner, E., Harpaz, L., & Samberg, S. (1979). *Therapeutic dance/movement—Expressive activities for older adults*. New York: Human Sciences Press.

Carnes, M. (1984). Diagnosis and management of dementia. *Physical and Occupational Therapy in Geriatrics, 3*, 11-24.

Chaisson-Stewart, G. M. (Ed.). (1985). *Depression in the elderly: An interdisciplinary approach*. New York: John Wiley and Sons.

Christenson, I. (1984). Self-help groups for depressed elderly in the nursing home. *Physical and Occupational Therapy in Geriatrics, 3*(4), 39-47.

Davis, C. M. (Ed.). (1986). Psychosocial considerations in geriatric practice. *Topics in Geriatric Rehabilitation, 1*(2), 1-82.

Davis, L. J., & Kirkland, M. (Eds.). (1986). *Role of occupational therapy with the elderly*. Rockville, MD: American Occupational Therapy Association.

Davis, J. (1983). Mental well being of elders: Seeking positive solutions. *Generations, 7*(3), 30-33, 67.

Edelson, J. S., & Lyons, W. H. (1985). *Institutional care of the mentally impaired elderly*. New York: Van Nostrand Reinhold.

Erikson, E. H., Ericson, J. M., & Kivinick, H. Q. (1986). *Vital involvement in old age*. New York: Norton.

Farrell-Holtan, J. (1990). The occupational therapist's role in interdisciplinary team assessment of the cognitively impaired elderly. *Occupational Therapy in Mental Health, 10*(3), 53-63.

Feil, N. (1982). *Validation—The Feil method: How to help the disoriented old-old*. Cleveland, OH: Feil Productions.

Fry, P. S. (1986). *Depression, stress and adaptations in the elderly: Psychological assessment and intervention*. Rockville, MD: Aspen Publishers.

Gelfand, D. E. (1983). *Mental health concerns of older women*. College Park, MD: National Policy Center on Women and Aging.

Glickstein, J. K. (1988). *Therapeutic interventions in Alzheimer's disease—A program of functional communication skills for activities of daily living*. Rockville, MD: Aspen Publishers.

Haley, W. E. (1983). A family-behavioral approach to the treatment of the cognitively impaired elderly. *Gerontologist, 23*, 18-20.

Hall, B. A. (Ed.). (1984). *Mental health and the elderly*. Orlando, FL: Grune & Stratton.

Hamill, C. M., & Oliver, R. C. (1980). *Therapeutic activities for the handicapped elderly*. Rockville, MD: Aspen Publishers.

Harvey, L. (1984). Advocacy and the aged: A case for the therapist advocate. *Physical and Occupational Therapy in Geriatrics, 3*(2), 5-15.

Harwood, K. J., & Wenzl, D. (1990). Admissions to discharge: A psychogeriatric transitional program. *Occupational Therapy in Mental Health, 10*(3), 79-100.

Hasselkus, B. R. (1992). The meaning of activity: Day care for persons with Alzheimer's disease. *American Journal of Occupational Therapy, 46*, 199-206.

Hasselkus, B. R., & Kiernat, J. M. (1989). Not by age alone: Gerontology as a speciality in occupational therapy. *American Journal of Occupational Therapy, 43*, 78.

Hellen, C. R. (1992). *Alzheimer's disease: Activity-focused care*. Stoneham, MA: Andover Medical Publishers.

Helm, M. (Ed.). (1987). *Occupational therapy with the elderly*. New York: Churchill Livingstone.

Hirano, A., & Miyoshi, K. (1983). *Neuropsychiatric disorders in the elderly*. New York: Igaku-Shoin Medical Publishers.

Holden, U. P., & Woods, R. T. (1982). *Reality orientation: Psychological approaches to the confused elderly*. New York: Churchill Livingstone.

Hughston, G. A., & Merriam, S. B. (1982-83). Reminiscence: A non-formal technique for improving cognitive functioning in the aged. *International Journal of Aging and Human Development, 15*(2), 139-149.

Kermis, M. D. (1986). *Mental health in late life: The adaptive process*. Boston: Jones and Bartlett Publishers.

Kiernat, J. M. (1991). *Occupational therapy and the older adult: A clinical manual.* Rockville, MD: Aspen Publishers.

Kultgen, P., & Habenstein, R. (1984). Processes and goals in aftercare programs for deinstitutionalized elderly mental patients. *Gerontologist, 24,* 167-173.

Levy, L. (1990). Activity, social role retention and the multiply disabled aged: Strategies for intervention. *Occupational Therapy in Mental Health, 10*(3), 1-30.

Levy, L. L. (1987a). Psychosocial intervention and dementia, part 1: State of the art, future directions. *Occupational Therapy in Mental Health, 7*(1), 69-107.

Levy, L. L. (1987b). Psychosocial intervention and dementia, part II: The cognitive disability perspective. *Occupational Therapy in Mental Health, 7*(4), 13-36.

Lewis, S. C. (1979). *The mature years: A geriatric occupational therapy text.* Thorofare, NJ: Slack.

Lewis, S. C. (1989). *Elder care in occupational therapy.* Thorofare, NJ: Slack.

Mace, N. L. (1987). Principles of activities for persons with dementia. *Physical and Occupational Therapy in Geriatrics, 5*(3), 13-27.

Martin, R. M. (1989). Update on dementia of the Alzheimer type. *Hospital and Community Psychiatry, 40,* 593-604.

McEvoy, C. L., & Patterson, R. L. (1986). Behavioral treatment of deficit skills in dementia patients. *Gerontologist, 26,* 475-478.

Norman, A. N., & Crosby, P. M. (1990). Meeting the challenge: Role of occupational therapy in a geriatric day hospital. *Occupational Therapy in Mental Health, 10*(3), 65-78.

Oakley, F. (1987). Clinical application of the model of human occupation in dementia of the Alzheimer's type. *Occupational Therapy in Mental Health, 7*(4), 37-50.

Ostrow, A. C. (1984). *Physical activity and the older adult: Psychological perspectives.* Princeton, NJ: Princeton Book Company.

Paire, J. A., & Karney, R. J. (1984). The effectiveness of sensory stimulation for geropsychiatric inpatients. *American Journal of Occupational Therapy, 38,* 505-509.

Parish, B., & Landsberg, G. (1984). Developing a geriatric mental health outreach unit in a rural community. *Journal of Gerontological Social Work, 7*(3), 75-82.

Paschke, M. J. (1984). Day care within a community mental health center. *Physical and Occupational Therapy in Geriatrics, 3*(4), 67-70.

Rabinowitz, E. (1986). Day care and Alzheimer's disease: A weekend program in New York City. *Physical and Occupational Therapy in Geriatrics, 4*(3), 95-103.

Reisberg, B. (1986). Dementia: A systematic approach to identifying reversible causes. *Geriatrics, 41,* 30-46.

Rogers, J. C. (1986). Occupational therapy services for Alzheimer's disease and related disorders [Position paper]. *American Journal of Occupational Therapy, 40,* 822-824.

Rogers, J. C., Marcus, C. L., & Snow, T. L. (1987). Maude: A case of sensory deprivation. *American Journal of Occupational Therapy, 41,* 673-676.

Ross, M., & Burdick, D. (1981). *Sensory integration: A training manual for therapists and teachers for regressed, psychiatric and geriatric patient groups.* Thorofare, NJ: Slack.

Rubin, E. H., Zorumski, C. F., & Burke, W. J. (1988). Overlapping symptoms of geriatric depression and Alzheimer-type dementia. *Hospital and Community Psychiatry, 39,* 1074-1079.

Sadavoy, J., Lazarus, L. W., & Jarvik, L. F. (Eds.). (1991). *Comprehensive review of geriatric psychiatry.* Washington, DC: American Psychiatric Press.

Saxon, S. V., & Etten, M. J. (1984). *Psychosocial rehabilitative programs for older adults.* Springfield, IL: Charles C. Thomas.

Shamoian, C. A. (Ed.). (1985). *Treatment of affective disorders in the elderly.* Washington, DC: American Psychiatric Press.

Sheridan, C. (1987). *Failure-free activities for the Alzheimer's patient: A guidebook for caregivers.* San Francisco: Cottage Books.

Skolaski-Pellitteri, T. (1983). Environmental adaptations which compensate for dementia. *Physical and Occupational Therapy in Geriatrics, 3,* 25-32.

Skolaski-Pellitteri, T. (1984). Environmental intervention for the demented person. *Physical and Occupational Therapy in Geriatrics, 3,* 55-59.

Stafford, F. (1986). *Caring for the mentally impaired elderly: A family guide.* New York: Henry Holt and Company.

Taira, E. D. (Ed.). (1986). Therapeutic interventions for the person with dementia [Special issue]. *Physical and Occupational Therapy in Geriatrics, 4*(3).

Teitelman, J. L. (1982). Eliminating learned helplessness in older rehabilitation patients. *Physical and Occupational Therapy in Geriatrics, 1*(4), 3-10.

Teri, L., & Lewinsohn, M. (Eds.). (1986). *Geropsychological assessment and treatment: Selected topics.* New York: Springer.

Weiner, M. F. (1991). *The dementias: Diagnosis and management.* Washington, DC: American Psychiatric Press.

Weinstein, W. S., & Prabha, K. (1986). *Depression in the elderly: Conceptual issues and psychotherapeutic intervention.* New York: Philosophical Library.

Whanger, A. D., Myers, A. C., Blazer, D. G., & Matteson, M. A. (1984). *Mental health assessment and therapeutic intervention with older adults.* Rockville, MD: Aspen Publishers.

Williams, J., Drinka, T., Greenberg, J., Farrell-Holtan, J., Euhardy, R., & Schram, M. (1991). Development and testing of the assessment of living skills and resources (ALSAR) in elderly community dwelling veterans. *Gerontologist, 31,* 84-91.

Wilson, D. S., Allen, C. K., McCormick, G., & Burton, G. (1989). Cognitive disability and routine task behaviors in a community-based population with senile dementia. *Occupational Therapy Practice, 1*(1), 58-66.

Woods, R. T., & Britton, P. G. (1985). *Clinical psychology with the elderly.* Rockville, MD: Aspen Publishers.

Zarit, S. H. (1980). *Aging and mental disorders: Psychological approaches to assessment and treatment.* New York: Free Press.

Zogola, J. M. (Ed.). (1987). *Doing things: A guide to programming activities for persons with Alzheimer's disease and related disorders.* Baltimore: Johns Hopkins University Press.

Psychosocial Aspects of Physical Disabilities

Arnetz, B. (1985). Gerontonic occupational therapy—Psychological and social predictors of participation and therapeutic benefits. *American Journal of Occupational Therapy, 39,* 460-465.

Burnfield, A. (1985). *Multiple sclerosis: A personal exploration.* New York: Demos Publications.

Charash, L., Lovelace, R., Wolf., S., Kutscher, A., Roye, D. P., & Leach, C. (Eds.). (1987). *Realities in coping with progressive neuromuscular disorders.* Philadelphia: Charles Press.

Copley, J. (1986). Development of a psychosocial group for the chronic physically disabled adult. *Advance, 2*(4), 1, 2, 7.

Davoud, N. (1985). *Where do I go from here? The autobiography of a remarkable woman.* London: Judy Platkus, Ltd.

De Loach, C., & Greer, B. J. (1981). *Adjustment to severe disability.* New York: McGraw Hill.

Downey, J., Reidel, G., & Kitischer, A. (Eds.). (1981). *Bereavement of physical disability: Recommitment to life, health, and function.* New York: Arno Press.

Falvo, D. R. (1991). *Medical and psychosocial aspects of chronic illness and disability.* Rockville, MD: Aspen Publishers.

Henderson, G., & Bryan, W. V. (1984). *Psychosocial aspects of disability.* Springfield, IL: Charles C. Thomas.

Kaminsky, J. (1988, July 28). Group therapy provides extra push for motivating rehabilitation clients. *OT Week,* pp. 4-5.

Kruger, D. W. (Ed.). (1984). *Emotional rehabilitation of physical trauma and disability.* New York: SP Medical and Scientific Books.

Kübler-Ross, E. (1978). *To live until we say good-bye.* Englewood Cliffs, NJ: Prentice Hall.

Kübler-Ross, E. (1981). *Living with death and dying.* New York: Macmillan.

Marinelli, R. P., & Dell Orto, A. E. (1984). *The psychological and social impact of physical disability* (2nd ed.). New York: Springer.

Miller, J. F. (1983). *Coping with chronic illness, overcoming powerlessness.* Philadelphia: F. A. Davis.

Moos, R. H. (Ed.). (1977). *Coping with physical illness.* New York: Plenum.

Murphy, R. F. (1987). *The body silent.* New York: Henry Holt.

O'Hara, C. C., & Harren, M. (1987). *Rehabilitation with brain injured survivors: An empowerment approach.* Rockville, MD: Aspen Publishers.

Register, C. (1988). *Living with chronic illness: Days of patience and passion.* New York: Macmillan.

Rogers, J. C., & Figone, J. J. (1979). Psychosocial parameters in treating the person with quadriplegia. *American Journal of Occupational Therapy, 33,* 432-439.

Rousso, M., O'Malley, S. G., & Severance, M. (1988). *Disabled, female and proud: Stories of ten women with disabilities.* Boston: Exceptional Parent Press.

Schontz, F. C. (1975). *The psychological aspects of physical illness and disability.* New York: Macmillan.

Sienkiewicz-Mercer, R., & Kaplan, S. (1989). *I raise my eyes to say yes.* New York: Houghton Mifflin.

Tickle, L. S., & Yerxa, E. J. (1981a). Need satisfaction of older persons living in the community and in institutions, part 1: The environment. *American Journal of Occupational Therapy, 35,* 644-649.

Tickle, L. S., & Yerxa, E. J. (1981b). Need satisfaction of older persons living in the community and in institutions, part 2: Role of activity. *American Journal of Occupational Therapy, 35,* 650-655.

Tigges, K. N., & Marcil, W. M. (1986, January/February). Maximizing quality of life for the homebound patient. *The American Journal of Hospice Care,* pp. 21-23.

Tigges, K. N., & Marcil, W. M. (1988). *Terminal and life-threateninq illness: An occupational behavior perspective.* Thorofare, NJ: Slack.

Wright, B. A. (1983). *Physical disability: A psychological approach* (2nd ed.). New York: Harper & Row.

Research Principles and Methods

American Psychological Association (1983). *Publication manual of the American Psychological Association.* Washington, DC: Author.

Barlow, D. H., Hayes, S. C., & Nelson, R. O. (1984). *The Scientist-practitioner: Research and accountability in clinical settings.* New York: Pergamon.

Bundy, A. C., Pendergast, N., Steffan, J. A., & Thorn, D. (1990). *Reviews of selected literature on occupation and health.* Rockville, MD: American Occupational Therapy Association.

Christiansen, C. H. (1983). Research: An economic imperative. *Occupational Therapy Journal of Research, 3,* 195-198.

Gelfand, H., & Walker, C. J. (1990). *Mastering APA style: Student's workbook and training guide.* Washington, DC: American Psychological Association.

Greenstein, L. R. (1980). Teaching research: An introduction to statistical concepts and research terminology. *American Journal of Occupational Therapy, 34,* 320-327.

Hasselkus, B. R. (1991). Qualitative research: Not another orthodoxy. *Occupational Therapy Journal of Research, 11*(1), 3-7.

Herring, K. L. (Ed.). (1987). *APA's guide to research support* (3rd ed.). Washington, DC: American Psychological Association.

Johnson, E. (Ed.). (1990). *Readings in occupational therapy research.* Rockville, MD: American Occupational Therapy Association.

Kazdin, A. E. (Ed.). (1992). *Methodological issues and strategies in clinical research.* Washington, DC: American Psychological Association.

Mann, W. C. (1985). Survey methods. *American Journal of Occupational Therapy, 39,* 640-648.

Marks, R. G. (1980). Choosing the appropriate design and analysis of a research project. *Occupational Therapy in Mental Health, 1*(1), 69-76.

Marks, R. G. (1987). Statistical design considerations to incorporate into published research articles. *Occupational Therapy in Mental Health, 7*(3), 37-53.

Mitcham, M. D. (1985). *Integrating research into occupational therapy.* Rockville, MD: American Occupational Therapy Foundation.

Ostrow, P. C., & Kaplan, K. L. (Eds.). (1987). *Occupational therapy in mental health: A guide to outcomes research.* Rockville, MD: American Occupational Therapy Association.

Royeen, C. B. (1988). *Philosophy and methodologies of research tradition in occupational therapy: Process, philosophy and status.* Thorofare, NJ: Slack.

Royeen, C. B. (1989). *Clinical research handbook: An analysis for the service professions.* Thorofare, NJ: Slack.

Stein, F. (1989). *Anatomy of clinical research: An introduction to scientific inquiry in medicine, rehabilitation and related health professions.* Thorofare, NJ: Slack.

Sexuality

Andamo, E. (1980). Treatment model: Occupational therapy for sexual dysfunction. *Sexuality and Disability, 3*, 26-38.

Anderson, T., & Cole, T. (1975). Sexual counseling of the physically disabled. *Postgraduate Medicine, 58*, 117-123.

Ayrault, E. (1981). *Sex, love, and the physically handicapped.* New York: Continuum Publishing.

Barrett, M. *Sexuality and multiple sclerosis.* New York: New York City Multiple Sclerosis Society.

Bidgood, F. E. (1974). Sexuality and the handicapped. *SIECUS Report, 2*(3).

Bullard, D., & Knight, S. (Eds.). (1981). *Sexuality and physical disability: Personal perspectives.* St. Louis: Mosby.

Chipouras, S., Cornelius, D., Daniels, S., & Makas, E. (1982). *Who cares? A handbook on sex education and counseling services for disabled people* (3rd ed.). Baltimore: University Park Press.

Clements, M. (1989, November 13). Sexual rehabilitation with spinal cord injured individuals. *Occupational Therapy Forum,* pp. 10-14.

Cole, T., & Cole, S. (1982). How physical disabilities affect sexual health. *Medical Aspects of Human Sexuality, 16*, 136-151.

Comfort, A. (Ed.). (1978). *Sexual consequences of disability.* Philadelphia, PA: George Strickley.

Conine, T., Christie, G., Hammond, G., & Smith, M. (1979). An assessment of occupational therapists' roles and attitudes toward sexual rehabilitation of the disabled. *American Journal of Occupational Therapy, 33*, 515-519.

Conine, T., & Evans, J. (1981). Sexual adjustment in chronic obstructive pulmonary disease. *Respiratory Care, 26*, 871-874.

Conine, T., & Evans, J. (1982). Sexual reactivation of chronically ill and disabled adults. *Journal of Allied Health, 11*, 251-269.

Craft, A., & Craft M. (Eds.). (1983). *Sex education and counseling for mentally handicapped people.* Austin, TX: University Park Press.

Dawe, N., & Shephard, H. (1985, June). Occupational therapy in the sexuality program of a rehabilitation hospital. *Physical Disabilities Special Interest Section Newsletter,* pp. 1-2.

Enby, H. (1975). *Let there be love—Sex and the handicapped.* New York: Taplinger Publishing.

Evans, J. (1985). Performance and attitudes regarding sexual habilitation of pediatric patients. *American Journal of Occupational Therapy, 39*, 664-670.

Evans, J., & Conine, T. (1982). Development of sexuality in children with chronic obstructive pulmonary disease. *Journal of Allied Health, 14*, 79-87.

Finger, A. (1990). *Past due: A story of disability pregnancy and birth.* Seattle, WA: Seal Press.

Frames, R. (1989, Fall). Sexual dysfunction: Dare we discuss it? *Inside Multiple Sclerosis,* pp. 24-31.

Klein, E., & Kroll, K. (1992). *Enabling romance: A guide to love, sex and relationships for the disabled (and the people who care about them).* Southbridge, MA: Harmony Books.

Lefebvre, K. A. (1990). Sexual assessment planning. *Journal of Head Trauma and Rehabilitation, 5*(2), 25-30.

Miller, W. T. (1984). An occupational therapist as a sexual health clinician in the management of spinal cord injuries. *Canadian Journal of Occupational Therapy, 51*, 172-175.

Neustadt, M. (1988, May 12). Sexuality: Part of quality life for the head injured. *OT Week,* pp. 6, 30.

Neustadt, M., & Freda, M. (1987). *Choices: A guide to sex counseling with physically disabled adults.* Melbourne, FL: Robert E. Krieger Publishing Company.

Novak, P., & Mitchell, M. (1988). Professional involvement in sexual counseling for patients with spinal cord injuries. *American Journal of Occupational Therapy, 42*, 105-112.

Robmault, J. P. (1978). *Sex, society and the disabled.* New York: Harper & Row.

Rudolph, M. (1988, March 21). Arthritis and sexuality. *Occupational Therapy Forum,* pp. 7-9.

Saydah, A. (Ed.). (1992). Sexuality and neurologic damage [Special issue]. *Headlines, 3*(1).

Schover, L., & Jensen, S. (1988). *Sexuality and chronic illness: A comprehensive approach.* New York: Guilford.

Sidman, J. M. (1977). Sexual functioning and the physically disabled adult. *American Journal of Occupational Therapy, 31*, 81-85.

Walbroehl, G. S. (1987). Sexuality in the handicapped. *American Family Physician, 36*(1), 129-133.

Zasler, N. D. (1990). Rehabilitative management of sexual dysfunction. *Journal of Head Trauma Rehabilitation, 5*(2) 14-24.

Social Skills Training

See Intervention Principles and Techniques

Stress Management

Also see Prevention, Health Promotion, and Wellness

Blumenthal, J. A. (1985). Relaxation therapy, biofeedback and behavioral medicine. *Psychotherapy, 22*, 516-530.

Brown, B. (1977). *Stress and the art of biofeedback*. New York: Bantam Books.

Charlesworth, E. A., & Nathan, R. G. (1984). *Stress management: A comprehensive guide to wellness*. New York: Antheneum.

Cotton, D. H. (1990). *Stress management: An integrated approach to therapy*. New York: Brunner/Mazel.

Davis, M., McKay, M., & Eskelman, R. (1982). *The relaxation and stress reduction workbook* (2nd ed.). Oakland, CA: New Harbinger.

Fine, S. B. (1991). Resilience and human adaptability: Who rises above adversity. 1990 Eleanor Clark Slagle lecture. *American Journal of Occupational Therapy, 45*, 493-503.

Folkman, S. (1984). Personal control and stress and coping processes: A theoretical analysis. *Journal of Personality and Social Psychology, 46*, 839-852.

Gage, M. (1992). The appraisal model of coping: An assessment and intervention model for occupational therapy. *American Journal of Occupational Therapy, 46*, 353-362.

Gal, R., & Lazarus, R. S. (1975). The role of activity in anticipating and confronting stressful situations. *Journal of Human Stress, 1*, 4-20.

Greenberg, J. S. (1983). *Comprehensive stress management*. Dubuque, IA: William C. Brown Company.

Hamberger, L. K., & Lohr, J. M. (1984). *Stress and stress management: Research and applications*. New York: Springer.

Hansen, M., Ritter, G., Gutmann, M., & Christiansen, B. (1990). *Understanding stress: Strategies for a healthier mind and body*. Rockville, MD: American Occupational Therapy Association.

Hiebert, B., Cardinal, J., Dumka, L., & Marx, R. W. (1983). Self-instructed relaxation: A therapeutic alternative. *Biofeedback and Self-Regulation, 8*, 601-617.

Hoover, R. M., & Parnell, P. K. (1984). An inpatient educational group on stress and coping. *Journal of Psychosocial Nursing and Mental Health Services, 22*(6), 16-22.

Kaplan, H. B. (1983). *Psychosocial stress: Trends in theory and research*. New York: Academic Press.

Lazarus, R. S., & Folkman, S. (1984). *Stress appraisal and coping*. New York: Springer.

McLean, A. (1974). *Occupational stress*. Springfield, IL: Charles C. Thomas.

Miller, T. W. (1988). Advances in understanding the impact of stressful life events on health. *Hospital and Community Psychiatry, 39*, 615-622.

Monat, A., & Lazarus, R. S. (Eds.). (1985). *Stress and coping: An anthology* (2nd ed.). New York: Columbia University Press.

Safranek, R., & Schill, T. (1982). Coping with stress: Does humor help? *Psychological Reports, 51*(1), 222.

Schafer, W. E. (1987). *Stress management for wellness*. New York: Holt, Rinehart & Winston.

Selye, H. (1956). *The stress of life*. New York: Bantam Books.

Selye, H. (1974). *Stress without distress*. New York: New American Library.

Selye, H. (1977). *The stress of my life*. Toronto: McClellan and Stewart.

Steinmetz, J. I., Kaplan, R. M., & Miller, G. L. (1982). Stress management: An assessment questionnaire for evaluating interventions and comparing groups. *Journal of Occupational Medicine, 24*, 923-931.

Tubesing, N., & Tubesing, D. (1983). *Structured exercises in stress management*. Duluth, MN: Whole Person Press.

Woolfolk, R. L., & Lehrer, P. M. (Eds.). (1984). *Principles and practice of stress management*. New York: Guilford.

Substance Abuse

Ackerman, R. (1983). *Children of alcoholics: A guide for parents educators, and therapists*. New York: Simon & Schuster.

Alterman, A. I. (Ed.). (1985). *Substance abuse and psychology*. New York: Plenum.

American Psychiatric Association. (1987). *Diagnostic and statistical manual of mental disorders—Revised* (3rd ed.). Washington, DC: Author.

Atkinson, R. M. (1985). Persuading alcoholic patients to seek treatment. *Comprehensive Therapy, 11*, 16-24.

Baumrind, D., & Moselle, K. (1985). *Alcohol and substance abuse in adolescence*. New York: Haworth Press.

Bergman, H. C., & Harris, M. (1985). Substance use among young adult chronic patients. *Psychosocial Rehabilitation Journal, 9*, 49-54.

Bjodstrup, B. (1986). Treating the chemically dependent adolescent. *Occupational Therapy Forum, 1*(5), 1, 3-6.

Brown, L., & Ostrow, F. (1980). The development of an assertiveness program on an alcoholism unit. *International Journal of the Addictions, 15*, 323-328.

Caton, C. L. M., Gralnick, A., Bender, S., & Simon, R. (1989). Young chronic patients and substance abuse. *Hospital and Community Psychiatry, 40*, 1037-1040.

Carruth, B., & Mendenhall, W. (Eds.). (1988). *Co-dependency: Issues in treatment and recovery*. New York: Haworth Press.

Cassidy, C. L. (1988). Occupational therapy intervention in the treatment of alcoholics. *Occupational Therapy in Mental Health, 8*(2), 17-26.

Cermack, T. (1986). *Diagnosing and treating co-dependence*. Minneapolis, MN: Johnson Institute.

Ciranlo, D. A., & Shader, R. I. (1991). *Clinical manual of chemical dependence*. Washington, DC: American Psychiatric Press.

Cox, W. M. (Ed.). (1986). *Treatment and prevention of alcohol problems: A resource manual*. New York: Academic Press.

Drake, R. E., & Wallach, M. A. (1989). Substance abuse among the chronic mentally ill. *Hospital and Community Psychiatry, 40*, 1041-1045.

Edwards, J. T. (1990). *Treating chemically dependent families: A practical systems approach for professionals*. Minneapolis, MN: Johnson Institute.

Emrick, C. D. (1987). Alcoholics anonymous: Affiliation processes and effectiveness as treatment. *Alcoholism: Clinical and Experimental Research, 2*(5), 416-423.

Evans, K., & Sullivan, J. M. (1990). *Dual diagnosis: Counseling the mentally ill substance abuser.* New York: Guilford.

Fox, S. (1990). Fetal alcohol syndrome: The hidden handicapped. *Advance for Occupational Therapists, 6*(17), 1-2.

Frances, R. J., & Franklin, J. E. (1989). *Concise guide to treatment of alcoholism and addictions.* Washington, DC: American Psychiatric Press.

Gangle, M. L. (1987). The effectiveness of an occupational therapy program for chemically dependent adolescents. *Occupational Therapy in Mental Health, 7*(2), 67-88.

Glantz, M., & Pickens, R. (Eds.). (1991). *Vulnerability to drug abuse.* Washington, DC: American Psychological Association.

Hossack, J. R. (1952). Clinical trial of occupational therapy in the treatment of alcohol addiction. *American Journal of Occupational Therapy, 6,* 265-266, 282.

Jaffe, S. L. (1990). *The step workbook for adolescent chemical dependency recovery: A guide to the first five steps.* Washington, DC: American Psychiatric Press.

Kaminer, Y., & Frances, R. J. (1992). Inpatient treatment of adolescents with psychiatric and substance abuse disorders. *Hospital and Community Psychiatry, 42,* 894-896.

Minkoff, K. (1989). An integrated treatment model for dual diagnosis of psychosis and addiction. *Hospital and Community Psychiatry, 40,* 1031-1036.

Mitiguy, J. (1991, Summer). Alcohol and head trauma: Cycles of abuse. *Headlines,* pp. 3-4, 6-9.

Monti, P. M., Abrams, D. B., Dadden, R. M., & Cooney, N. L. (1989). *Treating alcohol dependence: A coping skills training guide.* New York: Guilford.

Moyers, P. A. (1988). An organizational framework for occupational therapy in the treatment of alcoholism. *Occupational Therapy in Mental Health, 8*(2), 27-46.

Moyers, P. A. (1991). Occupational therapy and treatment of the alcoholic's family. *Occupational Therapy in Mental Health, 11*(1), 45-64.

Moyers, P. A. (1992). Occupational therapy intervention with the alcoholic's family. *American Journal of Occupational Therapy, 46,* 105-111.

Moyers, P. A., & Barrett, C. E. (1990, September). Treating the alcoholic's family. *Mental Health Special Interest Section Newsletter,* pp. 2-4.

Neville-Jan, A., Bradley, M., Bunn, C., & Gehri, B. (1991). The model of human occupation and individuals with co-dependency problems. *Occupational Therapy in Mental Health, 11*(2/3), 73-97.

New York State Commission on Quality of Care for the Mentally Disabled. (1986). *The multiple dilemmas of the multiply disabled: An approach to improving services for the mentally ill chemical abuser.* Albany, NY: Author.

O'Rourke, G. C., Blaisdell, M., & Carter-Fenton, E. (1990, September). Substance abuse fieldwork: An alternative recruitment strategy. *Mental Health Special Interest Section Newsletter,* pp. 5-6.

Osher, F. C., & Kofoed, L. L. (1989). Treatment of patients with psychiatric and psychoactive substance abuse disorders. *Hospital and Community Psychiatry, 40,* 1025-1030.

Raymond, M. (1990, September). Life skills and substance abuse. *Mental Health Special Interest Section Newsletter,* pp. 1-2.

Rice-Licare, J., & Delany-McLoughlin, K. (1990). *Cocaine solutions: Help for cocaine abusers and their families.* New York: Haworth Press.

Ridgeley, M. S., Osher, F. C., & Talbott, J. A. (1987). *Chronically mentally ill young adults with substance abuse problems: Treatment and training issues.* Baltimore: University of Maryland School of Medicine.

Rivinus, T. (1988). *Alcoholism/chemical dependency and the college student.* New York: Haworth Press.

Scarth, P. P. (1990, September). Services for chemically dependent adolescents. *Mental Health Special Interest Section Newsletter,* pp. 7-8.

Schroff, J. T. (1992, March 20). The role of an OTR consultant in a medical detoxification unit. *Occupational Therapy Forum,* pp. 4-6, 11.

Schuckit, M. A. (1984). *Drug and alcohol abuse: A clinical guide to diagnosis and treatment.* New York: Plenum.

Shore, J. H., & Kofoed, L. (1984). Community intervention in the treatment of alcoholism. *Alcoholism: Clinical and Experimental Research, 2,* 151-159.

Slobetz, F. W. (1970). The role of occupational therapy in heroin detoxification. *American Journal of Occupational Therapy, 24,* 340-342.

Smith, T. M., & Glickstein, C. S. (1981). Art as a therapeutic modality for individuals with alcohol-related problems in a milieu setting. *Occupational Therapy in Mental Health, 1,* 33-44.

Solomon, J. (Ed.). *Alcoholism and clinical psychiatry.* New York: Plenum.

Stamner, M. E. (1991). *Women and alcohol: The journey back.* New York: Gardner Press.

Stensrud, M. K., & Lushbough, R. S. (1988). The implementation of an occupational therapy program in an alcohol and drug dependency treatment center. *Occupational Therapy in Mental Health, 8*(2), 1-15.

Strachan, J. G. (1982). *Alcoholism: Treatable illness.* Center City, MN: Hazelden.

Van Deusen, J. (1989). Alcohol abuse and the occupational therapist's role. *American Journal of Occupational Therapy, 43,* 384-390.

Viik, M. K., Watts, J. H., Madigan, M. J., & Bauer, D. (1990). Preliminary validation of the assessment of occupational functioning with an alcoholic population. *Occupational Therapy in Mental Health, 10*(2), 19-33.

Wegscheider, D., & Wegscheider, S. (1975). *Family illness: Chemical dependency.* Minneapolis, MN: Johnson Institute.

Welsh, J. (1959). Occupational therapy contributions in the treatment of alcoholism. *American Journal of Occupational Therapy, 13,* 157-161, 176.

Willenbring, M., Ridgely, M. S., Stinchfield, R., & Rose, M. (1991). *Application of case management in alcohol and drug dependence: Matching techniques and populations.* Rockville, MD: National Institute on Alcohol Abuse and Alcoholism.

Treatment Programs
See Intervention Principles and Techniques

Trends and Issues in Mental Health Practice

American Occupational Therapy Association. (1985). *Occupational therapy manpower: A plan for progress.* Rockville, MD: Author.

Anthony, W. A., & Liberman, R. P. (1986). The practice of psychiatric rehabilitation: Historical, conceptual and research base. *Schizophrenia Bulletin, 12,* 542-559.

Bachrach, L. L. (Ed.). (1983). *New directions for mental health services series: Deinstitutionalization.* San Francisco: Jossey-Bass.

Baum, C. (1991). Professional issues in a changing environment. In C. Christiansen & C. Baum (Eds.), *Occupational therapy: Overcoming human performance deficits* (pp. 807-817). Thorofare, NJ: Slack.

Bonder, B. R. (1987). Occupational therapy in mental health: Crisis or opportunity? *American Journal of Occupational Therapy, 41,* 495-499.

Bonder, B. R. (1988, December). Occupational therapy: Issues in mental health. *Mental Health Special Interest Section Newsletter,* pp. 1-3.

Bowman, O. J. (1992). Nationally speaking: Americans have a shared vision: Occupational therapists can help create the future reality. *American Journal of Occupational Therapy, 46,* 391-396.

Bruhn, J. G. (1991). Nationally speaking: Occupational therapy in the 21st century: An outsider's view. *American Journal of Occupational Therapy, 45,* 775-780.

Cottrell, R. F. (1990). Perceived competence among occupational therapists in mental health. *American Journal of Occupational Therapy, 44,* 118-123.

Ethridge, D. A. (1984). Issues and trends in mental health practice. *Occupational Therapy in Health Care, 1*(1), 75-87.

Ethridge, D. A. (1986, September). Issues and trends in mental health practice: An update. *Mental Health Special Interest Section Newsletter,* pp. 1-2.

Fine, S. B. (1987). Looking ahead: Opportunities for occupational therapy in the next decade. *Occupational Therapy in Mental Health, 7*(4), 3-12.

Fine, S. B. (1988). Nationally speaking: Working the system: A perspective for managing change. *American Journal of Occupational Therapy, 42,* 417-426.

Gralnick, A. (1985). Build a better hospital: Deinstitutionalization has failed. *Hospital and Community Psychiatry, 36,* 738-741.

Grossman, J. (1986, December). Deinstitutionalization and the chronic mental patient: The community mental health movement. *Mental Health Special Interest Section Newsletter,* pp. 1-4.

Gutheil, (1985). The therapeutic milieu: Changing times and theories. *Hospital and Community Psychiatry, 36,* 1279-1285.

Haiman, S. (1990). Education and enticement: A recruitment strategy. *Occupational Therapy in Mental Health, 10*(1), IX-XVI. New York: Haworth Press.

Johnson, J. (1983). The changing medical marketplace as a context for the practice of occupational therapy. In G. Kielhofner (Ed.), *Health through occupation* (pp. 163-177). Philadelphia: F. A. Davis.

Kleinman, B. L. (1992). The issue is: The challenge of providing occupational therapy in mental health. *American Journal of Occupational Therapy, 46,* 555-557.

Koyanagi, C., & Goldman, H. H. (1991). The quiet success of the national plan for the chronically mentally ill. *Hospital and Community Psychiatry, 42,* 899-905.

Lamb, H. R. (1981). What did we really expect from deinstitutionalization? *Hospital and Community Psychiatry, 32,* 105-109.

Lamb, H. R., & Peele, R. (1984). The need for continuing asylum and sanctuary. *Hospital and Community Psychiatry, 35,* 798-801.

Okin, R. (1985). Expand the community care system: Deinstitutionalization can work. *Hospital and Community Psychiatry, 36,* 742-745.

Page, M. (Ed.). (1990, December). Special issue on recruitment and retention. *Mental Health Special Interest Section Newsletter,* pp. 1-8.

Scott, A. H. (1990). A review, reflections and recommendations: Speciality preference of mental health in occupational therapy. *Occupational Therapy in Mental Health, 10*(1), 1-28.

Struthers, M. S., & Schell, B. B. (1991). Public policy and its influence on performance. In C. Christiansen & C. Baum (Eds.), *Occupational therapy: Overcoming human performance deficits* (pp. 179-196). Thorofare, NJ: Slack.

Walens, D. (1992, March). Occupational therapists who specialize in mental health: An endangered or evolving species? *Mental Health Special Interest Section Newsletter,* pp. 1-4.

West W. L. (1968). The 1967 Eleanor Clark Slagle Lecture: Professional responsibility in times of change. *American Journal of Occupational Therapy, 22,* 9-15.

Vocational Rehabilitation and Education

American Occupational Therapy Association. (1985). *PIVOT: Planning and implementing vocational readiness in OT.* Rockville, MD: Author.

Anderson, A. P. (1985). Work potential evaluation in mental health. *American Journal of Occupational Therapy, 39,* 659-663.

Anthony, W. A., & Blanch, A. (1987). Supported employment for persons who are psychiatrically disabled: An historical and conceptual perspective. *Psychosocial Rehabilitation, 11*(2), 5-23.

Anthony, W., & Jansen, M. (1984). Predicting the vocational capacity of the chronically mentally ill: Research and policy implications. *American Psychologist, 39,* 537-544.

Baker, B. L., & Bughtman, A. J. (1989). *Steps to independence: A skills training guide for parents and teachers of children with special needs* (2nd ed.). Baltimore: Paul H. Brookes Publishing Company.

Bigge, J. L. (1982). *Teaching individuals with physical and multiple disabilities* (2nd ed.). Columbus, OH: Charles E. Merrill Publishing Company.

Bolton, B. (1982). *Vocational adjustment of disabled persons*. Baltimore: University Park Press.

Brolin, D. E. (1979). *Career education for handicapped children and youth*. Columbus, OH: Charles E. Merrill Publishing Company.

Brolin, D. E. (Ed.). (1982). *Vocational preparation of persons with handicaps* (2nd ed.). Columbus, OH: Charles E. Merrill Publishing Company.

Creighton, C. (1985). Three frames of reference in work-related occupational therapy. *American Journal of Occupational Therapy, 39*, 331-334.

Crist, P., & Stoffel, V. (1992). The Americans with Disabilities Act of 1990 and employees with mental impairments: Personal efficacy and the environment. *American Journal of Occupational Therapy, 46*, 434-443.

Crist, P. A. H., Thomas, P. P., & Stone, B. L. (1984). Prevocational and sensorimotor training in chronic schizophrenia. *Occupational Therapy in Mental Health, 4*(2), 23-37.

Cromwell, F. S. (Ed.). (1985). *Work-related programs in occupational therapy*. New York: Haworth Press.

Demers, L. M. (1992). *Work hardening: A practical guide*. Stoneham, MA: Andover Medical Publishers.

Denniston, Lust, & Hutcheson. (1980). *It isn't easy being special. Let's help special needs learners: A resource guide for vocational educators*. Columbus, OH: National Center for Research in Vocational Education.

Distefano, M. K., Jr., & Pryer, M. W. (1970). Vocational evaluation and successful placement of psychiatric clients in a vocational rehabilitation program. *American Journal of Occupational Therapy, 24*, 205.

Dooley, S. (1985, December). Program description: Prevocational assessment center. *Mental Health Special Interest Section Newsletter*, p. 3.

Fortune, J. R., & Eldredge, G. M. (1982). Predictive validation of the McCarron-Dial evaluation system for psychiatrically disabled sheltered workshop workers. *International Journal of Rehabilitation Research, 5*, 540-541.

Harrington, T. F. (1982). *Handbook of career planning for special needs students*. Rockville, MD: Aspen Systems.

Harvey, K. L. (1985). The concept of work in OT: A historical review. *American Journal of Occupational Therapy, 39*, 301-307.

Hayden, M. J. (1992). Disability awareness workshop: Helping businesses comply with the Americans with Disabilities Act of 1990. *American Journal of Occupational Therapy, 46*, 461-465.

Heard, C. (1977). Occupational role acquisition: A perspective on the chronically disabled. *American Journal of Occupational Therapy, 31*, 243-247.

Helmes, E., & Fekken, G. C. (1986). Effects of psychotropic drugs and psychiatric illness on vocational attitude and interest assessment. *Journal of Clinical Psychology, 42*, 569-576.

Howe, M. C., Weaver, C. T., & Dulay, J. (1981). The development of a work-oriented day center program. *American Journal of Occupational Therapy, 35*, 711-718.

Jacobs, K. (1985). *Occupational therapy: Work-related programs and assessments*. Boston: Little, Brown.

Kanellos, M. (1985). Enhancing vocational outcomes of spinal cord-injured persons: The occupational therapist's role. *American Journal of Occupational Therapy, 39*, 726-733.

Kemp, B., & Kleinplatz, F. (1985). Vocational rehabilitation of the older worker. *American Journal of Occupational Therapy, 39*, 322-326.

Kirk, S., & Gallagher, J. (1989). *Educating exceptional children* (6th ed.). Burlington, MA: Houghton Mifflin.

Kramer, L. W. (1984). Score: Solving community obstacles and restoring employment [Special issue]. *Occupational Therapy in Mental Health, 4*(1).

Lewin, J. V., & Lewin, R. A. (1987). On treatment integration: Psychotherapy and work therapy. *Occupational Therapy in Mental Health, 7*(3), 21-36.

Litterest, T. A. (1987, March). Work: A central element in acute-term psychiatric programming. *Work Programs Special Interest Section Newsletter*, pp. 1, 5.

Lynch, K. P., Kiernan, W. E., & Stark, J. A. (Eds.). (1982). *Prevocational and vocational education for special needs youth: A blueprint for the 1980s*. Baltimore: Paul H. Brookes Publishing Company.

Mancuso, L. L. (1990). Reasonable accommodation for workers with psychiatric disabilities. *Psychosocial Rehabilitation Journal, 14*, 3-19.

Matheson, L. (1984). *Work capacity evaluation: Interdisciplinary approach to industrial rehabilitation*. Trabuco Canyon, CA: Eric.

Matheson, L., & Ogden, L. D. (1983). *Work tolerance screening*. Trabuco Canyon, CA: Rehabilitation Institute of Southern California.

Matheson, L., Ogden, L., Violette, K., & Schultz, K. (1985). Work hardening: Occupational therapy in industrial rehabilitation. *American Journal of Occupational Therapy, 39*, 314-321.

McKinney, Vreeberg, & West. (1985). *Extending horizons: A resource for assisting handicapped youth in their transition from vocational education to employment*. Columbus, OH: National Center for Research in Vocational Education.

Mcloughlin, C. S., Garner, J. B., & Callahan, M. (Eds.). (1987). *Getting employed, staying employed: Job development and training for persons with severe handicaps*. Baltimore: Paul H. Brookes Publishing Company.

Meers. (Ed.). (1980). *Handbook of special vocational needs education*. Rockville, MD: Aspen Publishers.

Mellen, V., & Danley, K. (Eds.). (1987). Supported employment for persons with severe mental illness [Special issue]. *Psychosocial Rehabilitation Journal, 11*(2).

Palmer, F., & Barrows, C. (1985, December). Vocational activities for adolescents: A program description. *Mental Health Special Interest Section Newsletter*, pp. 1-2.

Radonsky, V. E., Haffenbreidel, J., Harper, C., Kligman, K., & Timms, C. (1987). Occupational therapy in vocational readiness. *Occupational Therapy in Mental Health, 7*(3), 83-92.

Reynolds-Lynch, K. (1987, March). Work programs in mental health: An evaluation checklist. *Work Programs Special Interest Section Newsletter*, p. 4.

Reichle, J., York, J., & Sigafoos, J. (1991). *Implementing augmentative and alternative communication: Strategies for learners with severe disabilities*. Baltimore, MD: Paul H. Brookes Publishing Company.

Richert, G. Z., & Merryman, M. B. (1987). The vocational continuum: A model for providing vocational services in a partial hospitalization program. *Occupational Therapy in Mental Health, 7*(3), 1-20.

Rubin, S. E., & Roessler, R. T. (Eds.). (1983). *Foundations of the vocational rehabilitation process* (2nd ed.). Baltimore: University Park Press.

Salz, C. (1983). A theoretical approach to the treatment of work difficulties in borderline personalities. *Occupational Therapy in Mental Health, 3*(3), 33-46.

Sarkees and Scott. (1985). *Vocational special needs*. Alsip, IL: American Technical Publishers, Inc.

Scheiber, B., & Talpers, J. (1987). *Unlocking potential: College and other choices for learning disabled people, a step-by-step guide*. Bethesda, MD: Adler & Adler.

Sheer, S. J. (1990). *Multidisciplinary perspectives in vocational assessment of impaired workers*. Rockville, MD: Aspen Publishers.

Shore, K. (1986). *The special education handbook: A comprehensive guide for parents and educators*. New York: Teachers College Press.

Smith, Hopkins, & Creasy. (1982). *Career planner: A guide for students with disabilities* (2nd ed.). Alta Loma, CA: Educational Resource Center.

Stockdell, S. M., & Crawford, M. S. (1992). An industrial model for assisting employers to comply with the Americans with Disabilities Act of 1990. *American Journal of Occupational Therapy, 46*, 427-433.

Straugh, C., & Colby, M. S. (1987). *Lovejoy's college guide for the learning disabled* (2nd ed.). New York: Simon & Schuster.

Tindall, L. (1980). *Puzzled about educating special needs students?* Madison, WI: University of Wisconsin-Madison.

Tindall, L. (1985). (Ed.). *Partnership in business and education: Helping handicapped students become a part of the job training partnership act*. Madison, WI: University of Wisconsin-Madison.

Tweed. (1989). *Colleges that enable: A guide to support services to physically disabled students on 40 U. S. campuses*. Oil City, PA: Park Avenue Press.

U.S. Department of Education. *The pocket guide to federal help for the disabled person*. Publication #20202. Washington, DC: U.S. Government Printing Office.

Wehman, P., & Moon, M. S. (1988). *Vocational rehabilitation and supported employment*. Baltimore: Paul H. Brookes Publishing Company.

Wehman, P., Wood, W., Everson, J. M., Goodwyn, R., & Conley, S. (1988). *Vocational education for multihandicapped youth with cerebral palsy*. Baltimore: Paul H. Brookes Publishing Company.

Wegg, L. (1957). The role of the occupational therapist in vocational rehabilitation. *American Journal of Occupational Therapy, 11*, 252-254.

Weisgerber, Dahl, & Applby. (1980). *Training the handicapped for productive employment*. Rockville, MD: Aspen Publishers.

Wircenski, J. (1982). *Employability skills for the special needs learner*. Rockville, MD: Aspen Publishers.

Appendix B

Supplemental Resource Lists

These resource lists provide information about organizations and companies that strive to facilitate the development of functional living skills and to enhance the quality of life of persons with disabilities, and their families. Most of the resources listed offer comprehensive educational literature and maintain active mailings to distribute up-to-date information. These mailings are often invaluable to a busy occupational therapist who cannot independently conduct frequent literature and product reviews in all areas of interest. The resources also assist the therapist by providing an excellent referral base for patients and their families. While therapists cannot personally address all areas of concern for all patients, they can easily supply patients with the names and addresses of relevant resources.

Resources listed include professional service organizations and publishers; consumer and family support groups; vocational, educational, and recreational programs; and therapeutic activities and suppliers. These annotated lists include resources relevant to psychosocial and physical disabilities practice. Physical disabilities resources are included, for rarely does a treatment situation only encompass psychosocial issues. The mother who is depressed due to the recent diagnosis of her child with muscular dystrophy, the adult son whose mania is exacerbated by his caregiving responsibilities for his father who has Parkinson's disease, the teenager who is angry and "acting out" his frustration due to his learning disabilities; all of these individuals and families may be seen in a mental health clinical setting, and all can benefit from information and referrals about their nonpsychiatric diagnostic concerns.

Readers will note that most of the resources are nationally based, as a state-by-state, community-by-community listing would be copious. Readers are encouraged to contact national organizations to identify local resources and to join those organizations related to their clinical practice and areas of professional interest. Readers are also urged to contact their state divisions of mental health and offices for persons with disabilities, as these state agencies can provide vital information on resources, services, and policies unique to each state.

Readers who actively utilize national, regional, and local resources will enhance their professional career development, improve the relevance of their occupational therapy programs, and empower clients and their families with vital information and appropriate referrals to enhance the quality of their lives.

Leisure and Recreation

Also see Professional Organizations, Family and Social Supports; and Publishers and Information Centers, as many of these professional and consumer resources provide a diversity of information and services relevant to leisure pursuits and recreational activities (e.g., books, videos, games, exercise groups, swimming programs, field trips, discount tickets, and transportation).

American Canoe Association

Kayaking/Disabled Paddlers Committee
8580 Cinderbed Road
P.O. Box 1190
Newington, VA 22122
703-550-7495
An organization promoting recreational and compet-

itive canoeing and kayaking for the disabled. These sports primarily require upper extremity strength, so athletes with lower-level disabilities can compete equally with non-disabled competitors.

American Waterski Association

Disabled Ski Committee
681 Bailey Woods Road
Dacula, GA 30211
404-995-8528

An organization providing entry-level programs and instructor workshops to promote waterskiing for the disabled. Adaptive equipment is available.

American Wheelchair Bowling Association (AWBA)

N54 W15858 Larkspur Lane
Menomonee Falls, WI 53051
414-781-6976

A national organization to promote wheelchair bowling. Local league play and tournaments are provided. "Mixed" bowling between disabled and non-disabled persons is encouraged. Adaptive equipment is available.

Childswork/Childsplay Center for Applied Psychology, Inc.

P.O. Box 1586
King of Prussia, PA 19406
800-962-1141

A distributor of therapeutic games, self-help books, and reference materials that focus on addressing the mental health needs of children and their families. Many of its self-awareness and esteem building products are suitable for all ages.

Choice Magazine Listening

85 Channel Drive
Port Washington, NY 11050
516-883-8280

A free bimonthly recorded service for persons unable to use regular print because of visual or physical disabilities. Choice Magazine Listening provides, on 4-track cassette tapes, 8 hours of unabridged articles, fiction, and poetry from such publications as *Smithsonian*; *The New Yorker*; *Foreign Affairs*; *The New York Times Magazine*; *The Atlantic*; *Esquire*; *Sports Illustrated*; *Audubon*; and *The Wall Street Journal*. Talking book 4-track cassette tape players are available free from the Library of Congress, National Library Service for the Blind and Physically Handicapped, Washington, DC.

Coalition for Disabled Musicians

P.O. Box 1002M
Bay Shore, NY 11706
516-586-0366

A self-help, non-profit organization that gives persons with disabilities the opportunity to pursue their musical dreams. Accessible rehearsal and studio space, music workshops, seminars, and lessons are provided. Amateurs and professionals can join a diversity of studio and stage bands.

Freedom's Wings International

1832 Lake Avenue
Scotch Plains, NJ 07076
908-232-6354

A membership organization providing flight training with FAA-certified instructors, hand-control equipped aircraft, and support equipment for persons with disabilities who wish to become pilots.

Handicap Introductions (HI)

P.O. Box 1215
152 Brigantine Road
Manahawkin, NJ 08050
609-660-0606

A network for persons with disabilities and non-disabled people who do not view disabilities as barriers to an active social life. HI operates as an international dating service with most "matches" occurring across the United States via phone calls and mailed correspondence. Successful "matches" have resulted in strong friendships, social dates, interstate visits, and more than 100 marriages.

Handicapped Scuba Association

116 W. El Portal, Suite 104
San Clemente, CA 92672
714-498-6128

An organization providing diving classes for the disabled. A dive club, refresher courses, diving excursions, videos, and lecture presentations are available.

Itinerary Magazine

P.O. Box 1084
Bayonne, NJ 07002-1084
201-858-3400

A bimonthly travel magazine for persons with disabilities. Travel guides, access reports, and new products are featured to make travel easier for persons with disabilities.

The Lighthouse, Inc.

Low Vision Products
36-02 Northern Boulevard
Long Island City, NY 11101
800-453-4923

A non-profit vision rehabilitation agency providing a diversity of consumer services. Its product catalog offers a number of assistive devices, games, and hobbies for the visually impaired. Many items are also appropriate for persons with physical and/or cognitive disabilities.

Mobility International USA (MIUSA)

P.O. Box 3551
Eugene, OR 97403
503-343-1284

A national non-profit organization that helps integrate people with disabilities into travel programs. It offers educational exchange programs, international workcamps, and travel information and referral services for individual or group travel. A quarterly newsletter, resource texts, travel guides, and videotapes are available.

Modern Talking Picture Service
Theatrical Captioned Films/Videos Program
for the Deaf

5000 Park Street North
St. Petersburg, FL 33709
813-541-7571 (Voice/TTY)
800-237-6213 (Voice/TTY)

A free loan service of educational and theatrical captioned films/videos to assist deaf/hearing impaired persons in their educational and recreational pursuits. Classic features, the latest Hollywood releases, short subjects, continuing educational titles, and after-school specials are available.

National Amputee Golf Association

11 Walnut Hill Road
P.O. Box 1228
Amherst, NH 03031
800-633-6242

A membership organization open to anyone who has an upper or lower extremity amputation and who enjoys golfing. Learn-to-golf clinics for the physically disabled, and modified golf equipment are available.

National Association for the Visually Handicapped (NAVH)

22 West 21 Street
New York, NY 10010
212-889-3141

NAVH serves as an information and referral agency for the partially sighted. An extensive, free, large print library is available to the visually impaired and/or physically disabled. Books on a diversity of topics for all ages can be borrowed from the library via a convenient free mail order service.

National Foundation of Wheelchair Tennis (NFWT)

940 Calle Amanecer, Suite B
San Clemente, CA 92672
714-361-6811

An organization promoting recreational and competitive wheelchair tennis through instructional clinics, camp programs, and competitive tournaments. Publications and videos are available.

National Handicapped Sports (NHS)

National Headquarters
451 Hungerford Drive, Suite 100
Rockville, MD 20850
301-217-0960

NHS's nationwide network of nearly 70 community-based chapters and affiliates offers a wide variety of activities, including camping, hiking, biking, horseback riding, l0K runs, water skiing, white water rafting, rope courses, mountain climbing, sailing, yachting, canoeing, kayaking, aerobic fitness, and snow skiing. Special youth programs are also available.

National Library Service for the Blind and Physically Handicapped

The Library of Congress
1291 Taylor Street, N.W.
Washington, DC 20542
202-707-5100

A free national library for individuals who cannot use standard printed materials due to visual or physical limitations (e.g., low vision, paralysis, weakness, incoordination). Talking books, and large print and braille books, magazines, and musical scores are available. Special cassette players, phonographs, amplifiers, and remote controls are also loaned for free. A diversity of topics ranging from adventures, mysteries, classics, cookbooks, drama, fine arts, history, humor, music, science and nature, science fiction, westerns, travel, and best sellers are offered for all age ranges.

National Ocean Access Project

410 Severn Avenue, Suite 107
Annapolis, MD 21403
301-280-0464

An organization providing learn-to-sail programs for persons with disabilities. "Tall Ship" sailing opportunities, adaptive equipment, and information on all water sports are available.

The National Theatre Workshop of the Handicapped (NTWH)

106 West 56th Street
New York, NY 10019
212-757-8549

NTWH is a training, production, and advocacy organization serving physically disabled adults who are talented in the performing arts. Live theatre experience and skills training for actors, playwrights, and directors are provided. NTWH maintains a professional repertory theatre company that showcases the talents of its students in every form of theatre.

National Wheelchair Basketball Association (NWBA)

110 Seaton Building
University of Kentucky
Lexington, KY 40506
606-257-1623

A national organization to promote wheelchair basketball. NWBA has 175 teams competing in 25 conferences annually. A wheelchair basketball training camp is also provided.

National Wheelchair Softball Association (NWSA)

1616 Todd Court
Hastings, MN 55033
612-437-1792

NWSA is the national governing body for wheelchair softball in the United States. Local league play and tournaments are available.

North American Riding Association for the Handicapped Association

P.O. Box 33150
Denver, CO 80233
303-452-1212

A national organization with specially trained teachers and horses available for use by riders with disabilities. Adaptive saddles are available.

Sports and Spokes

5201 N. 19th Avenue
Suite 111
Phoenix, AZ 85015
602-224-0500

A bimonthly journal on competitive sports and recreation for persons with disabilities. Junior, adult, and wheelchair sports are featured.

Theatre Access Project (TAP)

Theatre Development Fund
1501 Broadway
New York, NY 10036
212-221-0885

TAP's aim is to increase the access of New York's theatre to the physically disabled. Services include sign-interpreted performances, preferential seating, ticket ordering by mail, and discounted tickets to plays, musicals, concerts, and dance recitals. While TAP only serves the New York theatre, many major cities provide similar accessibility services. For information contact each city's office for the disabled.

Traveling Nurses' Network

P.O. Box 129
Vancouver, WA 98666-0129
206-694-2462

The Traveling Nurses' Network provides registered nurses to accompany persons with disabilities when they travel. The network consists of registered nurses with expertise in all medical areas including: diabetes, dialysis, cardiology, respiratory disease, spinal cord injury, vision-impairment, hearing-impairment, developmental disability, and psychiatry. Costs vary depending on individual need. Arrangements for special equipment that will be needed by the traveler (e.g., oxygen equipment, wheelchair accessible vans) can also be made through this network.

U.S. Wheelchair Weightlifting Federation

3595 E. Fountain Blvd.
Suite L-10
Colorado Springs, CO 80910
719-574-1150

An organization to promote recreational wheelchair weightlifting and competition for men and women throughout the United States. Each year a weightlifting team is organized for international competition.

Very Special Arts (VSA)

The John F. Kennedy Center for the Performing Arts
Washington, DC 20566
800-933-VSA1

A non-profit organization dedicated to enriching the lives of individuals with physical and/or mental disabilities through participation in the arts. VSA coordinates programs in music, dance, creative dramatics, and the visual arts. Publications, videos, technical assistance, demonstrations, conferences, seminars, workshops, and arts festivals are offered throughout the country for all age groups.

Voyageur Outward Bound School

10900 Cedar Road
Minnetonka, MN 55343
800-328-2943

Voyageur Outward Bound's mission is to conduct adventure-based educational courses structured to inspire self-esteem, self-reliance, concern for others, and care for the environment. A "Mixed Ability" course designed for both physically challenged and able-bodied participants is offered to enable persons with physical disabilities to participate in the Outward Bound experience.

Wheelchair Archery Sports Section

3595 E. Fountain Blvd., Suite L-10
Colorado Springs, CO 80910
719-574-1150

An organization promoting recreational and competitive archery for persons with disabilities. Adaptive equipment is available to enable persons with upper extremity weakness to participate in archery events.

Wheelchair Athletics of the USA/NWAA

3595 E. Fountain Blvd., Suite L-10
Colorado Springs, CO 80910
719-574-1150

An organization that promotes a number of recreational and competitive wheelchair sports, including track, field, and road racing.

Wilderness on Wheels Foundation

7125 W. Jefferson Avenue
No. 155
Lakewood, CO 80235
303-988-2212

This foundation has constructed a mile-long accessible boardwalk through the Rockies. People with disabilities can hike, fish, cook out, and camp along the trail.

World At Large

Dept. M
P.O. Box 19033
Brooklyn, NY 11219
800-285-2743
800-AT-LARGE

A weekly, tabloid-size, large-type subscription news magazine that presents stories selected from and published simultaneously by U.S. *News and World Report*, *Time*, and other magazines. World and national news, educa-

tion, health, the arts, sports, and crossword puzzles are among its featured articles.

Professional Organizations, Family and Social Supports

Alexander Graham Bell Association for the Deaf

3417 Volta Place, N.W.
Washington, DC 20007
202-337-5220

A non-profit organization providing advocacy services and financial assistance to children and adults with hearing impairments. Financial aid for newborns and school-aged children, and college scholarships for young adults and adults are provided. General information and a catalog of educational publications are available.

Alzheimer's Disease and Related Disorders Association (ADRDA)

919 North Michigan Avenue
Suite 1000
Chicago, IL 60611
800-621-0379

A national, non-profit organization serving individuals with Alzheimer's disease or related dementias, and their families. Diagnostic and treatment referrals, information packets and fact sheets, local support groups and respite care, legal and financial assistance, an autopsy assistance network, educational seminars and research abstracts, and a print and video library are available to members.

American Association of Retired Persons (AARP)

1909 K Street
Washington, DC 20049
202-434-2277

A membership organization for persons over 50 providing a diversity of educational and service programs. Health care referrals and consumer advocacy, pre-retirement planning, a Volunteer Talent bank, tax assistance and financial counseling, criminal justice assistance, widow-persons services, audio-visual and print publications, and the bimonthly journal *Modern Maturity*, are provided to members. AARP is a member of the Long-term Care Campaign and has special initiatives focusing on minority affairs, women, and worker equity.

American Cancer Society

1599 Clifton Road, N.E.
Atlanta, GA 30329
800-ACS-2345
404-320-3333

A national, non-profit organization dedicated to serving the needs of individuals with cancer, and their families. Public education, consumer information, treatment referrals, advocacy, and research are national priorities. State and local chapters provide a diversity of direct services, including patient and family support groups, peer counseling, rehabilitation programs, home care equipment and supplies, and transportation to and from treatment appointments. Audiovisuals, publications, newsletters, research briefs, workshops, and a national conference are available.

American Council of the Blind

1155 15th Street, N.W.
Washington, DC 20005
202-467-5081
800-424-8666

A national membership organization concerned with improving the quality of life for blind and visually impaired people. Services include toll-free information and referrals, scholarship assistance to post-secondary students, public education and awareness training, legal assistance, and consumer advocacy. *The Braille Forum*, a free bimonthly magazine, and an annual national convention are available to members.

American Diabetes Association

National Service Center
P.O. Box 25757
1660 Duke Street
Alexandria, VA 22314
703-549-1500
800-ADA-DISC

A private, non-profit, membership organization concerned with the diagnosis, treatment, and research for a cure of diabetes. Public, patient, family, and professional educational services and literature are available. A monthly periodical and an annual conference are provided to members.

American Foundation for the Blind (AFB)

1615 M Street, N.W.
Suite 250
Washington, DC 20036
202-457-1487
800-232-5463

AFB is a non-profit organization whose mission is to enable people who are blind or visually impaired to achieve equality of access and opportunity to ensure freedom of choice in their lives. AFB operates the National Technology Center, which serves as a resource for research and development, evaluations, and information services on technology for blind and visually impaired people and their families, professionals in blindness and low vision fields, employers, educators, researchers, and private industry. AFB also operates an Americans with Disabilities Act (ADA) Consulting Group, the Careers and Technology Information Bank, and a Talking Book program. Regional support centers are available nationwide. Publications, adaptive equipment, health care information, and leisure activities are available from AFB's product catalog.

American Heart Association

7320 Greenville Avenue
Dallas, TX 75231
800-242-8721
214-373-6300

A national, non-profit organization serving individuals with heart disease, and their families. Educational information, treatment referrals, prevention programs, patient and family support groups, and research funding are provided.

American Paralysis Association

500 Morris Avenue
Springfield, NJ 07081
201-379-2690
800-526-3456

A non-profit organization providing a toll-free spinal cord injury (SCI) Hotline. The hotline provides information and referrals to individuals who have sustained an SCI, and their families. Referrals include resources for peer support, rehabilitation facilities, professional experts, and local SCI organizations.

American Parkinson's Disease Association (APDA)

Suite 401
60 Bay Street
Staten Island, NY 10301
718-981-8001
800-223-2732

A non-profit organization dedicated to finding a cure and easing the burden of Parkinson's disease. APDA funds research to increase knowledge and improve the treatment of Parkinson's disease. Local support groups for patients and their families, and educational publications are available.

Amyotrophic Lateral Sclerosis (ALS) Association

15300 Ventura Boulevard
Sherman Oaks, CA 91403
818-990-2151

A non-profit organization devoted to research on ALS

and to the provision of information and supportive services to persons with ALS, and their families.

Andrus Gerontology Center

University of Southern California
University Park MC-0191
Los Angeles, CA 90089-0191
213-740-6060

The Andrus Gerontology Center has a phone network program for caregivers who are unable to leave their homes to attend caregiver support groups. The center has developed a series of audiotapes entitled "Care-line" that can be used by phone network members to develop social support, increase coping skills, provide information on practical concerns, and develop strategies to manage their caregiving tasks and responsibilities. The Care-line audiotapes (with a program guide) are available for purchase from the Andrus Gerontology Center.

Arthritis Foundation

1314 Spring Street, N.W.
Atlanta, GA 30309
404-872-7100
800-283-7800

A non-profit organization serving the needs of individuals with rheumatoid arthritis, osteoarthritis, ankylosing spondylitis, scleroderma, systemic lupus erythematosus, juvenile arthritis, or fibrositis. Educational packets, treatment information, research findings, and support groups are available for consumers, their families, and the professionals who work with them. The Arthritis Health Professions Association (AHPA), a section of the Arthritis Foundation, serves as a professional membership organization, publishes professional literature, and conducts continuing education programs annually.

Association for Children and Adults with Learning Disabilities

4156 Library Road
Pittsburgh, PA 15234
412-881-2253

A private, non-profit, membership organization devoted to learning disabilities. A national center, regional offices, and local chapters provide educational information, diagnostic testing, treatment referrals, remedial centers' newsletters, and publications to consumers, their families, and health care professionals.

The Association for Persons with Severe Handicaps (TASH)

11201 Greenwood Avenue North
Seattle, WA 98133
206-361-8870

TASH is an international non-profit membership organization dedicated to improving the quality of life and providing education and advocacy for persons with severe cognitive disabilities. A monthly newsletter, the quarterly *Journal for Persons with Severe Handicaps*, numerous print and audiovisual publications, and an annual conference are provided to members.

Association for Retarded Citizens (ARC)

National Headquarters
500 East Border Street
Suite 300
P.O. Box 300649
Arlington, TX 76010
817-261-6003

ARC is a non-profit national association devoted to improving the welfare of all children and adults with mental retardation, and their families. ARC provides services to parents and other individuals, organizations, and communities for jointly meeting the needs of people with mental retardation. Fact sheets, informational booklets, a bimonthly newsletter, and an electronic mail and information service are available.

Autism Society of America

8601 Georgia Avenue
Suite 503
Silver Spring, MD 20910
301-565-0433

A national agency dedicated to the education and welfare of people with autism. Priorities are research and education. An information and referral service, publications, reading lists, and a quarterly newsletter are provided.

Canine Companions for Independence

P.O. Box 446
1221 Sebastapol Road
Santa Rosa, CA 95402
707-528-0830

A non-profit organization that trains dogs to help persons with disabilities perform activities of daily living and maintain their independence. A promotional and educational video, "What a difference a dog makes," is available.

Children of Aging Parents (CAP)

1609 Woodbourne Road
Woodbourne Office Campus
Suite 302-A
Levittown, PA 19067
215-945-6900

A national organization providing education, information, and referrals on elder care. Peer counseling and support groups are available to assist family caregivers.

Children's Hospice International

901 North Washington Street
Alexandria, VA 22314
703-684-0330

A non-profit organization that provides medical and technical assistance, treatment referrals, education, and research on hospice care for children.

Council for Exceptional Children (CEC)

1920 Association Drive
Reston, VA 22091-1589
703-620-3660

CEC is a private, non-profit, membership organization for persons interested in special education for children who are gifted or who have disabilities. Information packets, two journals, an annual conference, and 17 special interest divisions are available to members. CEC also operates the ERIC Clearinghouse on Handicapped and Gifted Children.

Epilepsy Foundation of America (EFA)

4351 Garden City Drive
Landover, MD 20785
301-459-3700
800-332-1000

EFA is a national, non-profit organization for persons with epilepsy, their families, and the professionals who work with them. Public education, consumer advocacy, treatment referrals, phone counseling, and support groups are provided. Educational publications, information packets, and newsletters are available.

Family Survival Project

425 Bush Street
Suite 500
San Francisco, CA 94108
415-434-3388
800-445-8106

A resource center for families, friends, and professionals who are caregivers for adults with brain injuries. Fact sheets and consultations on legal, financial, and respite care concerns are available.

Gay Men's Health Crisis, Inc. (GMHC)

129 West 20th Street
New York, NY 10011
212-807-6655

GMHC is a comprehensive, non-profit, educational and health care organization serving persons with AIDS

of all ages, regardless of sexual orientation. GMHC develops and distributes materials that address the various aspects of AIDS (general information, risk reduction, medical and psychological issues, testing, health insurance, legal concerns, etc.) to fulfill the needs of different audiences. It conducts public forums, seminars for health care professionals, workshops for people at risk, and educational research programs. GMHC also provides support services for all people with AIDS, which includes crisis intervention counseling; a "buddy" program (helping with daily living tasks); recreational programs; pediatrics programs; support and therapy groups (for people with AIDS and their care partners); and legal, financial, and health care advocacy.

Handykappers, Inc.

P.O. Box 4294
Naperville, IL 60567-42
708-350-5263

A consumer-owned company specializing in educational seminars and videotapes designed to help persons utilizing wheelchairs adjust to their physical challenges.

Helen Keller National Center for Deaf/Blind Youth and Adults

111 Middle Neck Road
Sands Point, NY 11050
516-944-8900

A national facility that offers diagnostic evaluation, comprehensive rehabilitation training, and job preparation for deaf/blind persons from every state and territory in the United States. It also operates a national network of field services through its regional offices and affiliated programs. Training seminars for professionals and parents are conducted at the headquarters in Sands Point and across the nation. The Center maintains a national register of deaf/blind persons, conducts research to develop and/or modify aids and devices for the deaf/blind population, provides community education, publishes a national magazine, and provides publications on curriculum and services.

Help for Incontinent People, Inc. (HIP)

P.O. Box 544
Union, SC 29739
803-579-7900
800-BLADDER

A not-for-profit organization dedicated to improving the quality of life for people with incontinence. HIP functions as a clearinghouse of information and services on incontinence for consumers, their families, and health care professionals. It provides education, advocacy, and support about the causes, prevention, diagnosis, treatment, and management alternatives for incontinence. The *Resource Guide of Incontinent Products and Services*, a newsletter, audio/visual programs, and educational leaflets are available.

Helping Hands: Simian Aides for the Disabled, Inc.

1505 Commonwealth Avenue
Boston, MA 02135
617-787-4419

A non-profit organization that trains capuchin monkeys to provide skilled assistance to quadriplegics, enabling them to perform numerous activities of daily living independently.

Huntington's Disease Society of America

Dept. P
140 W. 22nd Street
New York, NY 10011
800-345-4372

A non-profit organization devoted to research education and the provision of services to persons with Huntington disease, and their families.

International Hearing Dog, Inc.

5901 East 89th Avenue
Henderson, CO 80640
303-287-3277

A non-profit organization that trains dogs to respond to sounds in the home. The "hearing ear" dogs are placed free with individuals who are deaf or hearing impaired, increasing their safety and independence.

Learning Disabilities Association (LDA)

4156 Library Road
Pittsburgh, PA 15234
412-341-1515

LDA is a private, non-profit organization devoted to providing support and advocacy services for children and adults with learning disabilities. Informational and referral services are provided to consumers, families, and professionals. State and local chapters, a national legislative committee, bimonthly newsbriefs, and an annual conference are available.

Let's Face It

P.O. Box 711
Concord, MA 01742
508-371-3186

An international mutual self-help organization dedicated to helping people with facial difference, their families, and the professionals who work with them to understand and solve the problems of living with facial disfigurement.

Life Services for the Handicapped, Inc.

352 Park Avenue South
Suite 703
New York, NY 10010-1709
212-532-6740

A non-profit organization that has set up a discretionary trust fund and life service program to enable families to leave resources to their children with disabilities without their children losing public entitlements. Assistance to help families plan for the long-term, life-care needs of their family members with disabilities is available. A quarterly newsletter, *Life Lines*, provides current information on long-term care issues, trends, benefits, and programs.

Lighthouse National Programs

Lighthouse National Center for Vision and Aging
Lighthouse National Center for Vision and Child Development
800 Second Avenue
New York, NY 10017
212-808-0077
212-808-5544 (TDD)
800-334-5497

A non-profit rehabilitation organization that provides information and resources for care across the United States for persons with visual impairments. Patient clinics, technical assistance, consultation, professional training, and professional and public education through print and audiovisual publications are provided.

The Long-Term Care Campaign

P.O. Box 27394
Washington, DC 20038
202-393-2092

The Long-Term Care Campaign is a coalition of 140 national organizations, including AOTA, dedicated to enacting comprehensive legislation to protect American families against the devastating costs of long-term care. Professional and consumer information, and print and audiovisual publications are available.

Lupus Foundation of America

1717 Massachusetts Avenue, N.W.
Washington, DC 20036
800-558-0121

A non-profit organization providing funds for research, education, and patient and family information.

Support groups are available for persons with systemic lupus erythematsus and related disorders.

Muscular Dystropy Association (MDA)

3300 East Sunrise Drive
Tucson, AZ 85718
602-529-2000

A non-profit organization funding research to find potential cures and effective treatments for 40 neuro-muscular disorders. Local chapters provide a diversity of services to patients and their families. Services include diagnostic clinics; occupational, physical, and speech therapy; genetic counseling; equipment supplies and repairs; support groups for patients and their families; and summer camp programs for persons aged 6 to 21. Information packets on many neuromuscular disorders, MDA research, and services are available.

National Alliance for Research on Schizophrenia and Depression (NARSAD)

60 Cutter Mill Road
Great Neck, NY 11021
516-829-0091

NARSAD raises and distributes funds for scientific research into the causes, cures, treatments, and prevention of severe mental illnesses, primarily the schizophrenias and the depressions.

National Alliance for the Mentally Ill

2101 Wilson Boulevard
Suite 302
Arlington, VA 22201
800-950-NAMI

NAMI is a self-help, support, and advocacy organization for persons with mental illnesses, their families and friends, and concerned professionals. NAMI provides educational publications, informational packets, audiovisuals, and research support on a multitude of topics. Its goals are to enable members to share concerns, learn about mental illnesses, and receive practical advice on treatment and community resources. Special interest networks offer additional support regarding children and adolescents, consumers (patients), culture and language concerns, curriculum and training (for professionals), forensic issues, guardianships and trusts, the homeless and missing, religious outreach, siblings and adult children, and veterans. NAMI is a strong advocate for improved services for persons with severe mental illnesses and for increased research funding into the causes and treatments of mental illnesses.

National Aphasia Association

Murray Hill Station
P.O. Box 1807
New York, NY 10156-0611
800-922-4622

A non-profit organization devoted to increasing the public's awareness of aphasia and providing information and service referrals to persons with aphasia, and their families. Information packets, reading lists, communication hints, newsletters, and local support groups are available.

National Association for the Dually Diagnosed (NADD)

110 Prince Street
Kingston, NY 12401
800-331-5362

A multidisciplinary membership association devoted to serving those who have both mental illness and mental retardation. Newsletters, regional and local workshops, a national conference, and information dissemination are provided.

National Association for Parents of the Visually Impaired

P.O. Box 317
Watertown, MA 02272-0317
800-562-6265

A self-help organization that addresses the needs of parents and families of visually impaired children and promotes public understanding of the needs and rights of the child with a visual impairment. Six regional support networks are available.

National Association for Visually Handicapped (NAVH)

22 West 21st Street
New York, NY 10010
212-889-3141

NAVH is a non-profit organization that serves as a national information and referral agency for all partially sighted (not totally blind) persons. It offers large-print textbooks, testing materials, visual aids, leisure reading, large-print periodic newsletters for adults and children, and informational literature for the partially sighted and their families, and the professionals and paraprofessionals working with them.

National Ataxia Foundation (NAF)

750 Twelve Oaks Center
15500 Wayzata Boulevard
Wayzata, MN 55391
612-473-7666

A non-profit organization serving individuals with hereditary ataxia, and their families. NAF provides educational publications and referral services to patients, families, and health care professionals. Genetic counseling and research are strongly supported, as there is no screening test, cure, or effective treatment for the hereditary ataxias.

National Center for Learning Disabilities (NCLD)

999 Park Avenue
New York, NY 10016
212-687-7211

A private, non-profit organization dedicated to improving the lives of children and adults with learning disabilities. NCLD's computerized database serves as a nationwide information and referral service. Public education, legislative advocacy, client services, innovative treatment programs, seminars, workshops, and publications are provided. General informational packets, newsletter updates, and a five-part video series, "We Can Learn," are available.

The National Council on the Aging, Inc. (NCOA)

409 Third Street, S.W.
Washington, DC 20024
202-479-1200

A private, non-profit, membership organization committed to improving the lives of older persons. NCOA serves as a national source of information, training, technical assistance, advocacy, and research on virtually every aspect of aging. Specialized units focus on the areas of adult day care, community-based long-term care, seniors centers, senior housing, health promotion, rural aging, older worker employment, spirituality and aging, and financial services for elders. A bimonthly magazine, *Perspective on Aging*, the quarterly *Abstracts in Social Gerontology: Current Literature on Aging*, the bimonthly NCOA *Networks*, and numerous publications, workshops, and conferences are available to members.

National Depressive and Manic-Depressive Association (NDMDA)

730 North Franklin
Suite 501
Chicago, IL 60610
312-642-0049

A non-profit organization dedicated to improving the availability and quality of health care, eliminating discrimination and stigma, and developing and maintaining support groups for persons with depressive and/or manic-depressive illnesses. Research and partnerships with professionals are also emphasized. Informational literature, a newsletter, audiovisuals, service referrals, research support, a national clearinghouse, and an annual conference are available.

National Diabetes Information Clearinghouse

P.O. Box NDIC
9000 Rockville Pike
Bethesda, MD 20892
301-468-2162

A national informational and referral service on diabetes and its complications for consumers, their families, professionals, and the general public. Topical bibliographies, educational publications, conference proceedings, and monographs are available.

National Down Syndrome Congress

1800 Dempster Street
Park Ridge, IL 60068-1146
800-232-NDSC

A private, non-profit, national organization serving individuals of all ages who have Down syndrome, and their families. Educational information and a referral service are available.

National Easter Seal Society

70 East Lake Street
Chicago, IL 60601
312-726-6200
800-221-6827

A national, non-profit organization dedicated to helping people with disabilities achieve maximum independence. Prevention programs, rehabilitation services, technological assistance, public education, and advocacy services are provided through a nationwide network of affiliates and chapters. An extensive library, including print and audiovisual publications on diagnostic and clinical topics, caregiving, and the Americans with Disabilities Act (ADA) may be accessed.

National Head Injury Foundation

1140 Connecticut Avenue, N.W.
Suite 812
Washington, DC 20036
202-296-6443
800-444-6443

A national, non-profit organization devoted to issues affecting persons with brain injuries, and their families. The dissemination of information, educational resources, publications, and referrals are provided.

National Information Center for Children and Youth with Disabilities (NICHCY)

[Acronym refers to previous name]
P.O. Box 1492
Washington, DC 20013
800-999-5599
703-893-6061

NICHCY provides free information to assist parents, educators, care-givers, advocates, and others in helping children and youth with disabilities become participating members of the community. As a national information clearinghouse, NICHCY maintains databases with current information on disability topics; provides information on local, state, and/or national disability groups for parents and professionals; distributes information packets on a multitude of disabilities; and provides technical assistance to parent and professional groups. NICHCY publishes *News Digest*, an issue paper that compiles articles on current research and relevant program information, and *Transition Summary*, which reports on current effective practices that assist persons with disabilities in the transition from school to work, other postsecondary programs, and to independent living in the community.

National Information Center on Deafness

Gallaudet University
800 Florida Avenue, N.E.
Washington, DC 20002
202-651-5051

A private information and referral service for persons who are deaf or hearing impaired. Resource listings and fact sheets are available.

National Multiple Sclerosis Society

733 3rd Avenue
New York, NY 10017
800-624-8236
212-986-3240

A non-profit organization dedicated to serving persons with Multiple Sclerosis (MS) and their families, while supporting research to find the cure for and cause of MS. National, regional, and local chapters provide a wide range of direct services to clients and their families, including medical clinics, support groups, individual counseling, career development services, water therapy, occupational therapy, home health aide assistance, recreational programs, transportation assistance, equipment loan programs, a mail-order prescription plan, and advocacy services. Print and video publications, professional education and training programs, a newsletter, and a journal are available to members.

National Organization for Rare Disorders (NORD)

P.O. Box 8923
New Fairfield, CT 06812-1783
203-746-6518

NORD is a private, non-profit, health-care service that serves as an information clearinghouse on rare disorders. (Rare disorders are defined as those affecting 200,000 people or fewer). Individualized information packets on symptoms, treatment, research, support groups, and self-help organizations are provided for a multitude of rare disorders. NORD will research consumer requests and help members and/or their families network with persons who are affected with the same or similar rare disorder.

National Organization on Disability (NOD)

910 16th Street, N.W.
Suite 600
Washington, DC 20006
202-293-5960
800-248-ABLE

A private, non-profit organization that aims to increase acceptance of all men, women, and children with physical or mental disabilities and to increase their participation in every aspect of life. Educational publications, training manuals, technical assistance, and a computerized database are available. Special emphasis is placed on local community integration for persons with disabilities through a national network of Community Partnership Programs.

National Osteogenesis Imperfecta Foundation, Inc. (OIF)

P.O. Box 14807
Clearwater, FL 34629-4087
813-855-7077

A national voluntary organization dedicated to serving the needs of individuals with Osteogenesis Imperfecta (OI) or Brittle Bone Disorder. Services include a quarterly newsletter, extensive literature, educational videos, a nationwide parent contact network, and national conferences.

National Rehabilitation Association (NRA)

1910 Association Drive
Suite 205
Reston, VA 22091-1502
703-715-9090

A national membership organization of consumers, family members, and professionals interested in the advocacy of programs and services for people with disabilities. Special divisions include the National Association for Independent Living, the Job Placement Division, the National Association of Rehabilitation Instructors, the National Association of Service Providers in Private Rehabilitation, and the Vocational Evaluation and Work Adjustment Association. State, regional, and national conferences; educational seminars; and numerous publications, including the *Journal of Rehabilitation*, *Rehab USA*, and NRA *Newsletter*, are available to members.

National Self-Help Clearinghouse

25 West 43rd Street
New York, NY 10036
212-642-2944

A national clearinghouse providing information and referrals on self-help groups and organizations. Publications and resource lists are available.

National Stroke Association

300 East Hampden Avenue
Englewood, CO 80110-2622
303-762-9922

A non-profit organization whose aim is to reduce the incidence and severity of stroke through prevention, treatment, rehabilitation, and research. Professional and consumer education, print and audiovisual publications, family and self-help groups, and a quarterly newsletter are provided.

Orton Dyslexia Society

Chester Building
Suite 382
8600 La Salle Road
Baltimore, MD 21284
410-296-0232

A membership organization that provides information on dyslexia to the general public, consumers, families, and professionals. Regional and national conferences, a quarterly newsletter, and an annual scholarly journal are available to members.

Paralyzed Veterans of America

801 18th Street, N.W.
Washington, DC 20006
202-USA-1300
800-424-8200

A national organization dedicated to ensuring that veterans with paralysis receive all the benefits and services they are entitled to. Patient education, medical research, consumer advocacy, accessibility, legal assistance, and sports programs are emphasized. The monthly jour-

nal *Paraplegia News*, the bimonthly *Sports and Spokes*, and many educational publications are available to members.

Recovery, Inc.

802 North Dearborn Street
Chicago, IL 60610
312-337-5661

An international self-help organization for former patients and other persons with mental health problems. Recovery stresses cooperation and education with professionals. Its purpose is to prevent relapses and to forestall chronicity in former and current patients. Literature, weekly meetings, and panel demonstrations are available.

Self-Help for Hard-of-Hearing People

7800 Wisconsin Avenue
Bethesda, MD 20814
301-657-2248
301-657-2249 (TDD)

A non-profit, consumer organization dedicated to serving the needs of people with hearing loss, their families, and their friends. Public education, advocacy, treatment referrals, support groups, and research funding into the causes and potential cures for hearing loss are provided.

Shared Housing Resource Center, Inc.

431 Pine Street
Burlington, VT 05401
802-862-2727

A national clearinghouse for more than 400 shared housing programs throughout the country. This center promotes shared housing, answers consumer inquiries, and assists professionals in the development and implementation of shared housing programs.

The Sibling Information Network

The A. J. Pappanikou Center
991 Main Street
East Hartford, CT 06108
203-282-7050

The Network serves as a clearinghouse of information, ideas, projects, literature, and research regarding siblings and other issues related to the needs of families with members who have disabilities. A newsletter containing program descriptions, requests for assistance, conference announcements, reviews of research, literature summaries, discussion articles, and research reports is published quarterly. A newsletter insert specifically for children ages 5 through 15, called "SIBPAGE," is also available.

Siblings for Significant Change

105 East 22nd Street
New York, NY 10010
212-420-0776

Siblings for Significant Change is a non-profit organization designed to unite siblings of individuals with disabilities, to advocate for services, and to improve conditions for their families. The dissemination of information, a speaker's bureau, conferences, and workshops are provided to promote greater public awareness of the needs of the disabled and their families.

Support Dogs for the Handicapped, Inc.

301 Sovereign
Suite 113
St. Louis, MO 63011
314-394-6163

An organization that trains dogs to help persons with disabilities perform activities of daily living and maintain functional independence.

Support Source

420 Rutgers Avenue
Swarthmore, PA 19081
215-544-3605

Publisher of caregiver education manuals and caregiver seminar workbooks.

United Cerebral Palsy, Inc. (UCP)

1522 K Street, N.W.
Suite 1112
Washington, DC 20005
202-371-0622

A private, non-profit, national organization serving adults and children with cerebral palsy, their families, and the professionals who work with them. Educational information, treatment referrals, and advocacy services are available. Services provided by local chapters include early intervention programs, summer camps, assisted living programs, family support groups, and peer counseling. Emphasis is placed on community integration, competitive employment opportunities, and the utilization of environmental control units and assistive technologies to maximize the independence and quality of life for persons with cerebral palsy.

Well Spouse Foundation (WSF)

P.O. Box 28876
San Diego, CA 92198-0876
619-673-9043

WSF is a non-profit, national organization with more than 50 regional support groups, devoted to meeting the needs of the 7 to 9 million individuals who care for spouses with chronic illness or disability. Support groups, networking contacts, monthly bulletins, and a quarterly newsletter are available to give emotional support, and to raise consciousness about and advocate for the spouses and children of the chronically ill.

Publishers and Information Centers

Also see resources for Professional Organizations, Family and Social Supports, as these agencies frequently publish and distribute highly relevant newsletters, pamphlets, journals, and books.

ABLEDATA

Newington Children's Hospital
181 East Cedar Street
Newington, CT 06111
800-344-5405
203-667-5405

ABLEDATA is the largest information source in the nation on disability-related products. ABLEDATA is a continually updated product database with more than 15,000 commercially available products from upwards of 1,900 manufacturers. Detailed information is included on products for use in all aspects of independent living, including personal care, transportation, communication, and recreation. Single copies of product fact sheets are free. Extensive product searches incur a nominal charge.

Accent on Living

P.O. Box 700
Bloomington, IL 61701
309-378-2961

A quarterly magazine focusing on the needs and concerns of persons with disabilities. Articles cover organizations, products, and ideas for daily living, recreation, and humor. A *Buyer's Guide*, a sourcebook on products and services, is also available.

American Psychiatric Press, Inc.

1400 K Street, N.W.
Suite 1101
Washington, DC 20005
800-368-5777

The official publisher of the American Psychiatric Association. Textbooks and journals on neuropsychiatry, psychogeriatrics, pediatrics, community mental health, and substance abuse are available. The subscription journal *Hospital and Community Psychiatry* (H&CP) is particularly relevant to occupational therapists, as occupational therapists serve on H&CP's editorial board, and occupational therapy is frequently featured in the "Interdisciplinary Update" section.

American Psychological Association

P.O. Box 2710
Washington, DC 20784-0710
800-374-2721

A membership organization and publisher. Texts and journals on psychopharmacology, substance abuse, psychotherapy, psychological testing, and research are available.

Andover Medical Publishers, Inc.

80 Montvale Avenue
Stoneham, MA 02180
800-366-2665

A publication company offering a number of journals and books for health care professionals. Subscription publications include *Work: A Journal of Prevention Assessment and Rehabilitation; Journal of Vocational Rehabilitation; Technology and Disability;* and *Neurorehabilitation: An Interdisciplinary Journal.*

Aspen Publishers, Inc.

200 Orchard Ridge Drive
Gaithersburg, MD 20878
301-417-7500

Publisher of the subscription journal *Occupational Therapy Practice,* and many health care, special education, allied health, medical, legal, and occupational therapy textbooks.

Center for Consumer Healthcare Information

4000 Birch Street
Suite 112
Newport Beach, CA 92660
800-627-2244

Publisher of the *Case Management Resource Guide,* an annually updated reference book that covers more than 50 categories of health care resources, including home care, rehabilitation, psychiatric and addiction treatment, and long-term care services. Entries contain detailed information on services, credentials, staffing, admission restrictions, special programs, contact names, phone numbers, and addresses.

Childswork/Childsplay

Center for Applied Psychology
P.O. Box 1586
King of Prussia, PA 19406
800-862-1441

A distributor of self-help books, therapeutic games, and reference materials that focus on addressing the mental health needs of children and their families. Many of the self-awareness and esteem-building products are suitable for all ages.

Churchill Livingstone, Inc.

650 Avenue of the Americas
New York, NY 10011
212-206-5000

A publisher of health care professional books, including many occupational therapy texts.

Computer Solutions for Clinicians

P.O. Box 6587
Danville, VA 24543
804-793-1375

Distributor of clinical computer software, including the "Mental Health Assessment Program System," a menu-driven software product that completes assessment and progress notes.

Consumer Information Center

P.O. Box 100
Pueblo, CO 81002
719-948-3334

A publisher and distributor of consumer education information sheets and booklets. Topics include health, education, federal benefit programs, the Americans with Disabilities Act (ADA), mental illness, AIDS, cancer, and Alzheimer's disease. Most publications are free. Others have a nominal charge. Many are excellent for use as consumer education tools in psychoeducational groups.

The Disability Rag

P.O. Box 145
Louisville, KY 40201
502-459-5343

A bimonthly periodical focusing on civil rights issues, discrimination, and "disability pride" among persons with physical disabilities.

Exceptional Parent: Parenting Your Child with a Disability

1170 Commonwealth Avenue
Boston, MA 02134
617-730-5800

A subscription magazine devoted to providing practical advice and resources to parents of children with physical, mental, and/or developmental disabilities.

F. A. Davis Company

1915 Arch Street
Philadelphia, PA 19103
215-568-2270
800-523-4049

A publisher of occupational therapy, allied health, nursing, and medical textbooks.

Haworth Press, Inc.

10 Alice Street
Binghamton, NY 13904-1580
800-3-HAWORTH

A publication company specializing in books and journals for health care professionals. Subscription journals available include *Occupational Therapy in Mental Health*; *Physical and Occupational Therapy in Geriatrics*; *Occupational Therapy in Health Care*; *Physical and Occupational Therapy in Pediatrics*; *Activities, Adaptation and Aging*; *Home Health Care Quarterly*; *Women and Health*; and many others. Individual monographs are also available for purchase.

Headlines

14 Central Avenue
Lynn, MA 01901-9925
617-598-9230
800-676-6000

A free, multidisciplinary, subscription journal focusing on advancing health care professionals' knowledge of neurologic injuries and conditions. Research, evaluation and intervention principles and techniques, case studies, and suggested readings are included in each bimonthly issue.

Jossey-Bass, Inc. Publishers

433 California Street
San Francisco, CA 94101
415-433-1767

A publisher specializing in books and journals on higher education, independent living, and health care issues and trends. The subscription quarterly, *New Directions in Mental Health Services*, and many monographs and texts on health care and increasing access for persons with disabilities are relevant to occupational therapy.

Kaleidoscope

A. J. Pappanikau Center
991 Main Street
East Hartford, CT 06108
203-282-7050

A quarterly newsletter aimed towards families who have a member with a disability. Each issue contains information about current literature, films, research, treatment programs, and health care trends.

Menniger Video Productions

Dept. B58
The Menniger Clinic
P.O. Box 829
Topeka, KS 66601-0829
800-345-6036

Producer and distributor of audiovisuals on numerous mental health issues. Many are suitable for staff training and patient education programs.

Moving Forward

P.O. Box 3553
Torrance, CA 90510-3553
310-320-8793

A national newspaper for people with disabilities. Regular features include national and international news relevant to persons with disabilities, legal and ADA information, research reports, sports, travel, and opinion columns.

National Rehabilitation Information Center (NARIC)

8455 Colesville Rd.
Suite 935
Silver Spring, MD 20910-3319
800-346-2742
301-588-9284

A library and information center on disability and rehabilitation. NARIC produces and distributes free guidebooks, texts, and journals on many topics and disabilities. ADA information is also available.

Raven Press

1140 Avenue of the Americas
New York, NY 10036
212-930-9500

Publisher of occupational therapy, medical, and allied health books and journals including *Psychosocial Components of Occupational Therapy* and *Alzheimer's Disease and Associated Disorders—An International Journal*.

Rehab Management

4676 Admiralty Way
Suite 202
Marina del Rey, CA 90292
310-306-2206

A free, bimonthly, interdisciplinary subscription journal. Current issues and trends, facility profiles, case studies, practice and department management, rehab engineering, and professional resources are featured in each issue.

Slack, Inc.

6900 Grove Road
Thorofare, NJ 08086
609-848-1000

A major publisher of occupational therapy, allied health, and medical textbooks. Publications include *Mental Health Assessment in Occupational Therapy*; *Elder Care*; *The Group System*; *Acute Psychiatric Care*; *Frames of Reference in Psychosocial Occupational Therapy*; *Directive Group Therapy*; *Neurological Assessment in Occupational Therapy*; and many other relevant texts.

RESNA

1101 Connecticut Avenue, N.W.
Suite 700
Washington, DC 20036-4303
202-857-1199

An interdisciplinary association for the advancement of rehabilitation and assistive technologies. RESNA publishes a quarterly journal, *Assistive Technology*, a bimonthly newsletter, *RESNA News*, and numerous sourcebooks, workbooks, and directories. RESNA also conducts regional and national conferences to disseminate information on the development and delivery of state-of-the-art technologies.

Team Rehab Report

P.O. Box 3640
Culver City, CA 90231-9895
310-337-9717
800-543-4116

A free, multidisciplinary, subscription magazine. Advances in rehabilitation and assistive technology for persons with disabilities are the journal's main focus.

Therapy Skill Builders

3830 E. Bellevue
P.O. Box 42050-H92
Tucson, AZ 85733
602-323-7500

A publisher and distributor of texts, videos, patient education manuals, games, and equipment suitable for a variety of patient populations. *Cognitive Rehabilitation: Group Games and Activities* is particularly relevant to many practice settings.

TRACE Research and Development Center

S-151 Waisman Center
1500 Highland Avenue
Madison, WI 53705
608-262-6966

A multidisciplinary information and training center on technology for persons with disabilities. Products, textbooks, and videotapes on assistive technology, augmentative communication, and adaptive equipment are available.

Twin Peaks Press

P.O. Box 129
Vancouver, WA 98666-0129
206-694-2462
800-637-2256

A publisher and distributor of directories and books for persons with disabilities. Its free Disability Bookshop Catalog lists more than 400 books of interest for persons with disabilities, which are available for mail-order purchase.

U.S. Government Printing Office

Washington, DC 20402-9325
202-512-1356

The official source for government publications, including documents from the National Institute of Health, the National Institute of Mental Health, and many Presidential Commissions. Topics include all major illnesses, treatment protocols, research findings, and trends within the health care system. Subject bibliographies are available upon request.

University of Illinois Film Center

1325 S. Oak Street
Champaign, IL 61820
800-FOR-FILM

A distributor of thousands of educational and health-related videos. Videos are available for sale or short-term and long-term rentals. Many are relevant to patient education and/or staff training programs.

Wellness Reproductions, Inc.

23945 Mercantile Road
Beachwood, OH 44122-5924
800-669-9208
216-831-1355

An OT-owned publishing company specializing in life management skills and coping with mental illness. Posters, videos, texts, and a self-esteem game are available to develop functional life skills.

West Virginia University Research and Training Center

One Dunbar Plaza
Suite E
Dunbar, WV 25064
304-766-7138
304-348-6340

A distributor of videos, audiocassettes, and textbooks focusing on the Americans with Disabilities Act (ADA).

Whole Persons Associates

1702 E. Jefferson
Duluth, MN 55812
800-247-6789

A distributor of print and audiovisual publications that address the areas of stress management and wellness promotion. Complete course packages are available.

Therapeutic Activities

Also see Leisure and Recreation resources.

Attainment Company

504 Commerce Parkway
Verona, WI 53593
800-327-4269

Distributor of Life Skill Programs for people with developmental or acquired disabilities. Products include step-by-step illustrated materials for shopping, cooking, community activities, grooming, and housekeeping.

BiFolkal Productions, Inc.

809 Williamson Street
Madison, WI 53703
608-251-2818

A non-profit corporation producing materials for use in activities with older adults. Multi-sensory kits are designed to encourage reminiscence and the inter-generational sharing of memories. A comprehensive catalog and a free quarterly newsletter of program ideas are available.

Childswork/Childsplay

Center for Applied Psychology, Inc.
P.O. Box 1586
King of Prussia, PA 19406
800-962-1141

A distributor of therapeutic games, self-help books, and reference materials that focus on addressing the mental health needs of children and their families.

Craft Resources

P.O. Box 828
Fairfield, CT 06430
800-243-2874

A distributor of needlecraft, arts and crafts kits, and supplies.

Creative Crafts International

16 Plains Road
P.O. Box 819
Essex, CT 06426
800-666-0767
203-767-2101

A distributor of arts and crafts equipment and supplies.

Cross Creek Recreational Products

P.O. Box 409A
Amenia, NY 12501
212-685-3672

A distributor of therapeutic activities developed for people with Alzheimer's disease and related dementia diseases, multi-infarct stroke patients, the developmentally disabled, mentally retarded adults, and the psychiatrically impaired.

Dick Blick Company

P.O. Box 1267
Galesburg, IL 61401
309-343-6181 x235
800-933-2542

A distributor of arts and crafts materials, including kits and open stock materials.

Fred Sammons, Inc.

P.O. Box 3697, Dept. A90
Grand Rapids, MI 49501-3697
800-323-5547

A distributor of evaluation, treatment, and rehabilitation supplies and equipment.

Geriatric Resources Inc.

5450 Barton Drive
Orlando, FL 32807
407-282-8711
800-359-0390

Producers and distributors of products to help improve the quality of life and manage potentially problematic behaviors for persons with dementia. Products are grouped functionally according to cognitive abilities and level of cognitive decline. Products include memory aids, reminiscent games, puzzles, sensory stimulation products, audio cassettes, and educational texts.

Glanz-Richman Rehabilitation Associates, Ltd.

1560 Indian Trail
Riverwoods, IL 60015
708-945-1917

Publisher and distributor of evaluation, treatment, and activity manuals for the psychogeriatric patient population. Publication emphasis is on meeting the needs of clients residing in nursing homes, and complying with OBRA regulations.

Knight's Woodcraft For Therapeutic Activities

P.O. Box 900888
San Diego, CA 92190-9988
619-265-1668
A distributor of woodcraft kits, tools, and supplies.

The Leather Factory

P.O. Box 50429
Ft. Worth, TX 76105
817-496-4414
A distributor of leather, leathercraft tools, and supplies.

Nasco

901 Janesville Avenue
Fort Atkinson, WI 53538-0901
800-558-9595
A distributor of arts and crafts, teaching aids, supplies, and equipment.

Play With Success

13005 8th Avenue N.W.
Seattle, WA 98177
800-779-5291
206-363-8104
Manufacturer and distributor of toys that can be used for therapy for the very young to the very old. Each toy lists age ranges and specific purposes for which it can be used.

The Rom Institute

3601 Memorial Drive
Madison, WI 53704
608-249-6670
Producer of the ROM Dance Instructional Media kit, which is a tool for teaching range of motion exercise, relaxation, and pain management to elderly, arthritic, or Parkinson's disease patients.

S&S Arts And Crafts

Department 2082
Colchester, CT 06415
800-243-9232, Dept. 2082
A distributor of arts and crafts supplies and equipment. Many products are assigned cognitive level rat-

ings by Claudia Allen, according to her Cognitive Disabilities frame of reference.

Tandy Leather Company

P.O. Box 2934
Ft. Worth, TX 76113
817-551-9778
A distributor of leather craft projects, kits, tools, and books.

Therapro, Inc.

225 Arlington Street
Framingham, MA 01701
508-872-9494
Producer and distributor of therapeutic activities to stimulate sensation, perception, and cognition. Adaptive equipment, developmental learning materials, books, and assessments are also sold.

Therapy Skill Builders

3830 E. Bellevue
Tucson, AZ 85716
602-323-7500
A distributor of textbooks, videos, and activity materials for pediatric through adult clients.

Vanguard Crafts

1081 East 48th Street
Brooklyn, NY 11234
718-377-5188
An arts and crafts supplier and distributor. Project packs and individual materials are available.

Veteran Leather Company, Inc.

204 25th Street
Brooklyn, NY 11232
718-768-0300
A manufacturer and distributor of leather, tools, kits, and other leathercraft supplies.

Wellness Reproductions, Inc.

23945 Mercantile Road
Beachwood, OH 44122-5924
216-831-9209
800-669-9208
Producers and distributors of therapeutic products and psychoeducational materials. Its publications, *Life Management Skills* I and *Life Management Skills* II, each contain 50 reproducible activity handouts covering a wealth of functional skills (e.g., stress management, assertiveness, goal setting, discharge planning, leisure, and community integration). Posters, games, and videos

are also available. All products can be easily graded and utilized with a diversity of patient populations.

World Wide Games

Department 2082
Colchester, CT 06415
800-243-9232, Dept. 2082

A distributor of games to generate social interaction and to improve coordination and concentration. Many are suitable for one hand, wheelchair use, or for the vision-impaired.

Vocational Rehabilitation and Education

ABLEDATA

8455 Colesville Road
Suite 935
Silver Spring, MD 20910-3319
800-346-2742
301-588-9284

A national computerized data bank giving information about commercially available rehabilitation aids and equipment. It also provides the names of local distributors, repair and service centers, and resources for custom design.

Alliance for Technology Access (ATA)

1307 Solano Avenue
Albany, CA 94706-1888
415-528-0747

ATA provides information on micro-computer technology to aid children and adults with disabilities.

American Printing House for the Blind (APH)

1839 Frankfort Avenue
P.O. Box 6085
Louisville, KY 40206-0085
502-895-2405

APH is the official source of educational texts for visually handicapped students (primary through secondary level) throughout the United States and its possessions. It maintains the *Central Catalog*, which is a listing of textbooks available in large type, braille, and recorded format that are produced by APH, volunteers, and commercial companies. It also engages in research, manufactures and sells assistive devices, and produces recreational and religious literature in special format.

Association for Education and Rehabilitation of the Blind and Visually Impaired

206 North Washington Street
Suite 320
Alexandria, VA 22314
703-548-1884

This organization promotes the advancement of education, guidance, and vocational rehabilitation of blind and visually impaired children and adults. It maintains job exchange services and a speakers' bureau, offers continuing education seminars, and publishes several journals and newsletters.

Association on Handicapped Student Service Programs in Postsecondary Education (AHSSPPE)

P.O. Box 21192
Columbus, OH 43221-0192
614-488-4972

AHSSPPE is a membership organization for individuals involved in the provision of quality support services to disabled students in higher education. A quarterly publication, *Journal of Postsecondary Education and Disability*; a newsletter, the *Alert*; and numerous informational publications are provided to members. It also has several special interest groups, training workshops, and conferences.

Breaking New Ground

Resource Center
Arrgricultural Engineering Department
Purdue University
West Lafayette, IN 47907
317-494-5022

The Breaking New Ground Resource Center assists farmers and ranchers who are physically disabled. Publications include newletters, technical articles, resource manuals, and video tapes/slide sets. Major areas of focus include technical devices, prosthetics, worksite modifications, and hand controls to enable farmers and ranchers to continue their work.

CAREERS and the disABLED

Equal Opportunity Publications, Inc.
44 Broadway
Greenlawn, NY 11740
516-273-0066

A career magazine for people with disabilities, published three times per year. A nominal subscription fee is charged.

Center On Education And Training For Employment (CETE)

The Ohio State University
1900 Kenny Road
Columbus, OH 43210
614-292-4353
800-848-4815

CETE is a non-profit organization that provides access to current research, curricular resources, and other products pertaining to vocational education and training.

Closing The Gap (CTG)

P.O. Box 68
Henderson, MN 56044
612-248-3294

CTG disseminates information on up-to-date computer technologies that enable persons with disabilities to utilize computers for education, work, and independent living. A bimonthly newspaper, workshops, and an annual conference are provided.

Council For Exceptional Children (CEC)

1920 Association Drive
Reston, VA 22091-1589
703-620-3660

CEC is a non-profit organization dedicated to quality education for all exceptional children: preschool, gifted, culturally and linguistically diverse, physically disabled, learning disabled, and youth in transition from school to work. CEC has more than 1,000 chapters in the U.S. and Canada and publishes the journals *Teaching Exceptional Children* and *Exceptional Children*. CEC's Center for Special Education Technology distributes information on assistive technology, funding, and training.

Crestwood Company

6625 N. Sidney Place
Milwaukee, WI 53209-3259
414-352-5678

Distributor of communication aids for children and adults and adapted toys for children with special needs.

Disability Rights Center

1346 Connecticut Avenue, N.W.
Suite 1124
Washington, DC 20036
202-223-3304

A public interest organization working to strengthen the rights of persons with physical and/or mental disabilities. The center focuses primarily on employment rights of the disabled. It publishes reports and testimony on implementation of federal affirmative action, and disseminates materials to persons with disabilities.

Disabled Journalists of America

484 Hammond Drive
Griffin, GA 30223
404-228-6491

A member organization for journalists who are disabled. The promotion of employment opportunities for qualified, disabled journalists and the sharing of ideas and information about the industry is its primary focus.

The Dole Foundation

1819 H Street, N.W.
Suite 850
Washington, DC 20006
202-457-0318

A non-profit organization dedicated to expanding employment opportunities for persons with disabilities. It disseminates information, provides grants, and distributes numerous publications to assist employers in making accomodations for workers with disabilities.

Heath Resource Center

(Higher Education and the Handicapped)
One Dupont Circle, N.W.
Suite 800
Washington, DC 20036
202-939-9320
800-544-3284

Heath is the national clearinghouse on post-secondary education for persons with disabilities in the United States. It publishes a news bulletin three times a year and develops and disseminates fact sheets and packets of materials of concern to disabled students, post-secondary administrators, campus support service providers, and advisors of students with disabilities. Heath responds to individual questions by mail or telephone. All its publications are free.

Electronic Industries Foundation (EIF)

The Rehabilitation Engineering Center (REC)
1901 Pennsylvania Avenue, N.W.
Suite 700
Washington, DC 20006
202-955-5810

EIF operates the Rehabilitation Engineering Center, which provides general information on assistive devices and their applications, as well as alternative financing mechanisms for the acquisition of assistive devices for persons with disabilities.

Job Accommodation Network (JAN)

1331 F Street, N.W.
Washington, DC 20004-1107
202-376-6200
800-526-7234
800-ADA-WORK

JAN is an information and consulting service providing individualized accommodation solutions to enable persons with disabilities to work. It is a free service provided by the President's Committee on Employment of People with Disabilities.

Job Opportunities for the Blind (JOB)

1800 Johnson Street
Baltimore, MD 21230
800-638-7518
301-659-9314

A nationwide employment listing and referrel service for persons who are blind.

Lift, Inc.

P.O. Box 1072
Mountainside, NJ 07092
908-789-2443
800-552-5438

Lift is a non-profit organization that recruits, trains, and hires severely disabled individuals as computer professionals for corporate clients throughout the country. A comprehensive 6-month at-home training program, and advanced technological aids, are provided. Job placements at corporate sites and/or at home using telecommunications are available.

Mainstream, Inc.

1200 15th Street, N.W.
Washington, DC 20005
202-833-1136

A non-profit organization that seeks to create greater employment opportunities for persons with disabilities. It uses a newsletter, special publications on topics such as insurance and medical standards, and a speaker's bureau to provide information on the issues involved in employing disabled persons. Its Project LINK matches qualified applicants who have physical and/or mental disabilities with competive employment opportunities. Services are free to employers and applicants.

Mobility International USA (MIUSA)

P.O. Box 3551
Eugene, OR 97403
503-343-1284

A non-profit organization whose aim is to integrate persons with disabilities into international educational exchange programs and travel. MIUSA publishes A *Guide to International Educational Exchange, Community Service, and Travel for Persons with Disabilities* and A *Manual for Integrating Persons with Disabilities into International Educational Exchange Programs.*

Modern Talking Picture Service Educational Captioned Films/Videos Program for the Deaf

5000 Park Street North
St. Petersburg, FL 33709
813-541-7571 (Voice/TTY)
800-237-6213 (Voice/TTY)

A free loan service of captioned educational films/videos to assist deaf/hearing impaired persons in their educational pursuits. Titles in clearly defined school subject areas and student interest levels from preschool through postsecondary are available.

National Employment and Training Program Association for Retarded Citizens

National Headquarters
2501 Avenue J
Arlington, TX 76006
817-640-0204

A nationwide network of job placement personnel to help workers with mental retardation get jobs in the competitive workforce.

President's Committee on Employment of People with Disabilities

1331 F Street, N.W.
Washington, DC 20004-1107
202-376-6200

The President's Committee on Employment of People with Disabilities publishes and distributes free pamphlets, publications, and posters covering such topics as education, employment, accessibility, and adapting the work site. *Worklife,* a quarterly journal, and *Tips and Trends,* a monthly newsletter, are available free upon request. Collaboration with employers is emphasized, and all disabilities (physical, psychological, and/or learning) are considered.

Recording for the Blind (RFB)

20 Roszel Road
Princeton, NJ 08540
609-452-0606

RFB is a non-profit service organization that provides recorded educational books and related library services to people with print disabilities (i.e., blindness, low vision, learning disabilities, or other physical impairments that affect reading). RFB has an extensive lending library of books already recorded, including educational texts, fiction, drama, and poetry. The recordings come in a number of languages. There is also a recording service for additional titles.

RESNA

1101 Connecticut Avenue, N.W.
Suite 700
Washington, DC 20036-4303
202-857-1199

A membership organization that addresses research, development, dissemination, and utilization of knowledge in rehabilitative and assistive technology. A journal (*Assistive Technology*), a newsletter, numerous publications, and an annual conference are provided.

Stout Vocational Rehabilitation Institute (SVRI)

School of Education and Human Services
University of Wisconsin—Stout
Menomonie, WI 54751
715-232-2475

SVRI provides vocational rehabilitation services, conducts research, provides training, and produces and disseminates information to further the potential of persons with disabilities. SVRI is comprised of six centers to meet the needs of persons with disabilities and their service providers effectively. These centers are the Center for Independent Living, Projects with Industry Center, Materials Development Center, Center for Rehabilitation Technology, Research and Training Center, and Vocational Development Center.

The Association for Persons with Severe Handicaps (TASH)

11201 Greenwood Avenue North
Seattle, WA 98133
206-361-8870

TASH is a membership organization involved in a range of issues concerning the living, working, and educational environments of persons with disabilities. Referral services, consumer advocacy, annual conferences, teaching guidebooks, bibliographies, a monthly newsletter, and a quarterly journal are available to members. TASH is primarily concerned with research and trends in services to persons with severe disabilities from birth to adulthood.

Trace Research and Development Center for Communications, Control, and Computer Access for Handicapped Individuals (TRACE)

Waisman Center
1500 Highland Avenue
Madison, WI 53705
608-262-6966

A center for the development and evaluation of technological aids, computers, and adaptive devices. It provides free information related to non-vocal communication, computer access, and technology for persons with disabilities. Trace also maintains an international software registry of programs and modifications created or adapted for individuals with disabilities.

Vocational Studies Center

University of Wisconsin—Madison
964 Educational Sciences Building
1025 West Johnson Street
Madison, WI 53706
608-263-2929

The Vocational Studies Center is a research, development, and service center that provides technical assistance and products to vocational educators and rehabilitation therapists. Resources available include curriculum development aids, audiovisual materials, and textbooks. Many products are specific to persons with disabilities and are suitable for diverse educational levels and age ranges.

Index

E

Index compiled by Susan Lohmeyer, Chesapeake Indexing Associates